Nutritional Epidemiology

MONOGRAPHS IN EPIDEMIOLOGY AND BIOSTATISTICS

Edited by Jennifer L. Kelsey, Michael G. Marmot,
Paul D. Stolley, Martin P. Vessey

Monographs in Epidemiology and Biostatistics
Volume 30

NUTRITIONAL EPIDEMIOLOGY
SECOND EDITION

WALTER WILLETT, M.D.

Professor of Epidemiology and Nutrition
Harvard School of Public Health
Profesor of Medicine
Harvard Medical School

New York   Oxford
OXFORD UNIVERSITY PRESS
1998

Oxford University Press

Oxford   New York
Athens   Auckland   Bangkok   Bogota   Bombay
Buenos Aires   Calcutta   Cape Town   Dar es Salaam
Delhi   Florence   Hong Kong   Istanbul   Karachi
Kuala Lumpur   Madras   Madrid   Melbourne
Mexico City   Nairobi   Paris   Singapore
Taipei   Tokyo   Toronto   Warsaw

and associated companies in
Berlin   Ibadan

Library of Congress Cataloging-in-Publication Data
Willett, Walter.
Nutritional epidemiology / Walter Willett.—2nd ed.
p. cm.—(Monographs in epidemiology and biostatistics ; 29)
Includes bibliographical references and index.
ISBN 0-19-512297-6
1. Nutritionally induced diseases—Epidemiology.
2. Diet in disease—Research—Methodology.
3. Nutrition Surveys—Methodology.
4. Nutrition—Research—Methodology.
I. Title. II. Series.
[DNLM: 1. Nutrition. 2. Diet—adverse effects. 3. Epidemiologic Methods.
W1 MO567LT v.29 1998 / QU 145 W713n 1998] RA645.N87W54 1998
614.5'939—dc21   DNLM/DLC   for Library of Congress   97-37809

5 7 9 8 6 4

Printed in the United States of America
on acid-free paper

To Gail

Preface

This book is written for individuals seeking to understand the relation between diet and long-term health and disease. A basic premise is that our understanding of biologic mechanisms remains far too incomplete to predict confidently the ultimate consequences of eating a particular food or nutrient. Thus, epidemiologic studies directly relating intake of dietary components to risk of death or disease among humans play a critical complementary role to laboratory investigations. A great expansion of the literature in nutritional epidemiology and the development of a firmer quantitative basis for this science occurred in the 1980's. Most important: the substantial variation in diet among individuals was quantified in numerous populations; standardized dietary questionnaires were developed for use in large epidemiologic studies, and the ability of these questionnaires to measure diet was documented. Although many of the major questions about diet and disease remain unresolved, the foundations for obtaining this information are now firmly in place. The first edition of *Nutritional Epidemiology*, published in 1990, represented an attempt to consolidate this substantial new body of methodologic information.

In the short time since the first edition, the literature of nutritional epidemiology has grown enormously. Although the basic principles and approaches have remained intact, the new work has extended the scope of investigation to different populations, examined new aspects of diet, and addressed many methodologic topics in greater detail. Also, large studies started in the 1980's have begun to provide substantial data on diet and disease relationships, raising important issues about the analysis, presentation, and interpretation of complex nutritional data. Thus, three entirely new chapters have been added to this edition: the first addresses the analysis and presentation of data; the second describes applications to nutritional surveillance; and the third provides an additional example using the relation between folic acid and neural tube defects. Considerable new information has been added to all of the previous chapters. Importantly, additional colleagues, Drs. Buzzard, Lenart, Alberg, Stampfer, Byers, and Colditz, have joined with Drs. Hunter, Samet, and me to produce this edition.

This book is designed specifically for researchers actively engaged in studies of diet and disease and for persons seriously attempting to read and interpret published epidemiologic information relating to nutrition. As a field develops, the methodologic cutting edge inevitably becomes more distant from the level of knowledge needed by someone entering the area. Thus, creating a book that provides an introduction to the field and also serves as a resource for investigators becomes increasingly challenging. This edition still attempts to meet both needs. For this reason, though, some parts of the later methodologic chapters could be skipped by the newcomer to nutritional epidemiology without sacrificing the essential concepts. The book is not intended for the casual reader seeking to learn what is currently known about the effects of diet and nutrition on human disease; such a work would rapidly be out of date. Also, this book does not address issues related to child growth and studies of nutritional deficiency in developing countries; both are important topics, but outside the scope of this text. However, I am confident that those involved in nutritional studies in developing countries can benefit from the material presented, as many of the principles are relevant.

Though I have not attempted to define or explain basic epidemiologic terms, most of the chapters can be read by someone with elementary statistical knowledge but with no epidemiologic background. Readers without exposure to epidemiology would profit by referring to an introductory text such as MacMahon and Trichopoulos' *Principles of Epidemiology*, Ahlbom and Norell's *Introduction to Modern Epidemiology*, Friedman's *Primer of Epidemiology*, Kahn and Sempos' *Statistical Methods in Epidemiology*, Hennekens and Buring's *Epidemiology in Medicine*, or Rothman and Greenland's *Modern Epidemiology*—the last being the most advanced. Similarly, epidemiologists without formal exposure to nutrition can benefit by reading Guthrie's *Introductory Nutrition* or Ziegler's *Present Knowledge in Nutrition* and referring to standard texts such as Davidson and Passmore's *Human Nutrition and Dietetics* or Goodhart and Shils' *Modern Nutrition in Health and Disease*.

The first edition was almost exhaustive in covering the published literature in nutritional epidemiology. However, due to the great expansion of the literature since 1990, it was no longer possible to discuss all relevant papers and still provide a readable text for those entering this field. This forced me to be selective about citations in some areas, and I apologize to colleagues if in some cases their contributions seem to have been overlooked. Despite this, this book is almost twice as long as the previous edition; I hope that the insight and knowledge gained by reading it will increase proportionally.

As the content of the different chapters varies considerably in depth, many readers will want to reserve some sections for future reference rather than read the whole book from cover to cover. Chapter 1 provides an overview of nutritional epidemiology for those unfamiliar with the field; experienced epidemiologists may want to skim this material. Chapter 2, written together with Marilyn Buzzard, addresses the various perspectives from which diet can be viewed and discusses the calculation of nutrient intakes from data on food consumption.

Chapter 3 provides a conceptual background regarding sources of variation in diet for the novice to this field and also assembles data on dietary variation that may be of use to the serious investigator. Chapter 4, written by Marilyn Buzzard, reviews the strengths, limitations, and appropriate applications of short-term recalls and dietary records as methods for measuring intake. Because of the central role of food frequency questionnaires in nutritional epidemiology, the design and evaluation of these questionnaires are examined in detail in Chapters 5 and 6. Recall of diet from the remote past is of potential importance for diseases with a long latency; the small but growing literature on this topic is reviewed in Chapter 7. The use of spouse surrogates for reporting of diet is common in case-control studies; this topic is covered in Chapter 8 by Anthony Alberg and Jon Samet, who has made important contributions in this area.

Chapter 9, written by my former graduate student and present colleague, David Hunter, is divided into two parts. The first deals with conceptual and general issues in the use of biochemical indicators for assessing intake of specific dietary factors. The second part provides detailed information on the biochemical measurement of specific nutrients; many readers will probably want to use this material for reference. This chapter provides an epidemiologic perspective on the role of biochemical indicators in epidemiologic studies. Dr. Hunter points out that close collaboration between laboratory scientists and epidemiologists is essential when embarking on studies that involve biochemical measurement. Chapter 10 addresses the use of measures of body size and composition, also with a special emphasis on epidemiologic applications.

Chapters 11, 12, and 13, in contrast with others, probe issues in the analysis, interpretation, and presentation of epidemiologic data. Issues relating to total energy intake are considered in detail in Chapter 11. The effect of measurement error in epidemiologic studies and statistical methods to compensate for measurement error are addressed in Chapter 12. This is an active area of development in epidemiology and statistics in general, but much of the stimulus has arisen from studies of diet. Although it is of general epidemiologic interest, I have included a chapter on this topic because of the important implications for nutritional studies. Some of the later sections of Chapters 11 and 12 go beyond the needs of an entrant to this field and could be skipped in a first read.

Chapters 14 to 18 address substantive applications of nutritional epidemiology, and are included to reinforce the principles covered in the earlier chapters. Tim Byers has written a new chapter on nutritional surveillance, drawing on his experience in this field. The other chapters on vitamin A and lung cancer, dietary fat and breast cancer, diet and heart disease, and folic acid and neural tube defects address topics of substantial current interest.

Many chapters on the relation of diet and disease remain to be written. The brief final section of this book attempts to anticipate the direction of future research and to encourage activity in areas that seem most promising.

Boston, Mass.   W. W.
November 1997

Acknowledgments

The concepts in this book owe much to the work and ideas of many predecessors, present colleagues, and former students. In particular, I am grateful for the encouragement, support, and ideas of my colleagues, Frank Speizer, Meir Stampfer, Graham Colditz, Bernard Rosner, Laura Sampson, Frank Sacks, Simonetta Salvini, Mauricio Hernandez, David Hunter, Jelia Witschi, Charles Hennekens, Sue Hankinson, Eric Rimm, Donna Spiegelman, and Ed Giovannucci at the Channing Laboratory and Harvard School of Public Health. Jon Samet provided strong initial encouragement to begin the book and provided further concrete support in the form of a chapter. Brian MacMahon first stimulated to me to think seriously about diet as a possible cause of cancer, which led to much of the research underlying this book. Further development of ideas and approaches to the study of diet and disease have evolved from intellectual exchanges with Jim Marshall, Saxon Graham, John Potter, Dimitrios Trichopoulos, Peter Boyle, Richard Peto, Geoffrey Howe, and Larry Kushi. Fred Stare provided continued support to extend epidemiologic approaches to issues of nutrition.

Much of the material for this book was developed over the last eighteen years, while I was teaching courses on nutritional epidemiology at the Harvard School of Public Health and the New England Epidemiology Institute. My efforts have benefitted immensely from the ideas and comments of many students in these courses and from my doctoral students and post-doctoral fellows at Harvard School of Public Health.

The developmental work and data described in this book would not have been possible without a career development award and the funding of research grants, particularly the Nurses' Health Study, from the National Institutes of Health. I am thus most grateful for the constructive comments of the many anonymous peer reviewers who have supported this work. Our work and the whole field of nutritional epidemiology also owe much to the encouragement and support of Dr. Joe Patel of the National Cancer Institute.

Susan Newman and Stefanie Parker provided critical support in the production of the first edition of this book and Liz Lenart, Jill Arnold, and Alice Smythe have done the same for the second. Meir Stampfer, Graham Colditz, John Potter, and Matt Longnecker each reviewed the first edition at one stage or another and gave invaluable advice. Mary Fran Sowers, Hugh Joseph, Eric Rimm, Barbara Underwood, Susan Roberts, Donna Speigelman, Ed Giovannucci, Adrianne Bendich, Godfrey Oakley, David Hunter, Wafaie Fawzi, Bernie Rosner, Donald Miller, and Sue Hankinson reviewed specific chapters and provided important comments. Jeffrey House at Oxford University Press gave essential support and counsel during the production of the book. Debbie Flynn kept the rest of my academic life from disintegrating during the process.

Contents

Nutritional Epidemiology

1

Overview of Nutritional Epidemiology

The field of nutritional epidemiology has developed from interest in the concept that aspects of diet may influence the occurrence of human disease. Although it is relatively new as a formal area of research, investigators have used basic epidemiologic methods for more than 200 years to identify numerous essential nutrients. In the mid-eighteenth century, observations that fresh fruits and vegetables could cure scurvy led Lind (1753) to conduct one of the earliest controlled clinical trials; lemons and oranges had the "most sudden and good effects" on the course of this disease, which was ultimately found to be the result of vitamin C deficiency. In an example from the late nineteenth century, the unusual occurrence of beri-beri among sailors subsisting largely on polished rice led Takaki to hypothesize that some factor was lacking in their diet; the addition of milk and vegetables to their rations effectively eliminated this disease (Williams, 1961). Decades later a deficiency of thiamine was found to be primarily responsible for this

syndrome (Davidson et al., 1973). Similarly, Goldberger (1964) used epidemiologic methods to determine that pellagra was a disease of nutritional deficiency, primarily associated with a corn meal subsistence diet in the southern United States. More recently, Chinese investigators determined by epidemiologic means that selenium deficiency is responsible for the high incidence of Keshan disease in central China (Guangi-Qi, 1987).

Typically, deficiency syndromes occur with high frequency among those with very low intake and rarely or never occur among those not so exposed. In addition, these deficiency diseases often have short latent periods; symptoms are usually manifested within months of starting a deficient diet and can typically be reversed within days or weeks. Hence, research has moved rapidly from observations to experiments in both animals and humans.

Deficiency states for essential nutrients, such as scurvy and rickets, differ from most issues confronting nutritional epidemiologists today. The primary focus of contemporary nutritional epidemiology has been the major diseases of Western civilization, particularly heart disease and cancer. More recently, osteoporosis, cataracts, stroke, diabetes, and congenital malformations also have been the objects of such research. Unlike nutritional deficiencies, these diseases almost always have multiple causes, potentially including not only diet but also genetic, occupational, psychosocial, and infectious factors; level of physical activity; behavioral characteristics such as cigarette use; and other influences. These multiple potential determinants may act alone or in combination. Also, many of these diseases have long latent periods; they may sometimes result from cumulative exposure over many years and in other instances from a relatively short exposure occurring many years before diagnosis. For most of these diseases, the relevant period of exposure is unknown. It is possible that exposures with short latent periods are also important for some of these diseases. For example, it is conceivable that smoking a cigarette or consuming large amounts of a certain food could, within hours, precipitate an acute myocardial infarction or thrombotic stroke by altering blood coagulability even though the underlying atherosclerosis has accumulated over decades. A third characteristic of these diseases is that they occur with relatively low frequency despite a substantial cumulative lifetime risk. In addition, these conditions are not readily reversible and may result from excessive, as well as insufficient, intake of dietary factors. All these features have important implications for the design of studies to elucidate their etiologies.

The traditional methods of nutritionists, such as basic biochemistry, animal experimentation, and metabolic studies in humans, contribute substantially but do not address directly the relation between diet and occurrence of major diseases of our civilization. These issues should fall naturally within the realm of epidemiology, a discipline whose focus is the occurrence of human disease. Although epidemiologic efforts originally concentrated primarily on infectious diseases, during the last 40 years attention has largely shifted to the etiology of chronic diseases. Thus contemporary epidemiologists are accustomed to the study of diseases with low frequencies, long latency periods, and multiple causes. For example, hypertension, hypercholesterolemia, and cigarette smoking have been identified as major determinants of coronary heart disease; this knowledge has contributed to a major decline in this cause of death during recent years.

Although epidemiology is logically equipped to address the dietary causes of disease, the complex nature of diet has posed an unusually difficult challenge to this discipline (Willett, 1987). Cigarette smoking is more typical of exposures studied by epidemiologists: With a high degree of accuracy, subjects or their spouses can report whether they smoke cigarettes. Furthermore, individuals can readily provide quantitative information on the number of cigarettes they smoke per day, their usual brand of cigarettes, the age at which they started smoking, and changes in their pattern of use. The ease with which relatively accurate information on cigarette smoking can be obtained has contributed to the rapid accumulation of an enormous and remarkably consistent literature on the health effects of this habit. Diet, in contrast, represents an unusually complex set of exposures that are strongly intercorrelated. With few exceptions, all individuals are exposed to hypothesized causal factors; everyone eats fat, fiber, and vitamin A, for instance. Thus, exposures cannot be characterized as present or absent; rather, they are continuous variables, often with a rather limited range of variation. Furthermore, individuals rarely make clear changes in their diet at identifiable points in time; more typically, eating patterns evolve over periods of years. Finally, individuals are generally not aware of the content of the foods that they eat; therefore, the consumption of nutrients is usually determined indirectly based on the reported use of foods or on the level of biochemical measurements.

Thus, the most serious limitation to research in nutritional epidemiology has been the lack of practical methods to measure diet. Because such epidemiologic studies usually involve at least several hundred and sometimes tens of thousands of subjects, dietary assessment methods must be not only reasonably accurate but also relatively inexpensive.

The difficulties in assessing diet have led some epidemiologists to believe that it is unlikely that useful measurements of the diets of individual subjects within free-living populations can be collected at all (Wynder, 1976). In addition, some have believed that the diets of persons within one country are too homogeneous to detect relationships with disease (Hebert and Wynder, 1987). Much of this skepticism arose from the intense interest in dietary lipids, serum cholesterol, and coronary heart disease beginning in the 1950s. Although it has been demonstrated in controlled metabolic studies that increases in saturated fat and cholesterol or decreases in polyunsaturated fat raise serum cholesterol, no correlation between intake of these lipids and serum cholesterol was found in many cross-sectional studies within the United States (Jacobs et al., 1979). Many concluded that, as an association clearly did exist, the measurement of diet was so inaccurate that the relationship was obscured. In retrospect, it is apparent that any expectation of a strong correlation is unrealistic and that a lack of correlation has several explanations. Most importantly, serum cholesterol is relatively insensitive to dietary lipid intake; metabolic studies clearly show that substantial changes in dietary intake produce rather modest changes in serum cholesterol (see Chapter 17). The expected correlation between cholesterol intake and serum cholesterol in the populations studied would be only on the order of 0.10, even with a perfect measure of dietary intake, because

many factors, including genetic determinants, influence serum cholesterol.

Example: In the data of Shekelle et al. (1981), the standard deviation (SD) for dietary cholesterol is 68 mg/1,000 kcal, and the standard deviation for serum cholesterol is 54 mg/dl. From metabolic ward studies of Mattson et al. (1972), a 10 mg/1,000-kcal change in dietary cholesterol causes 1.2 mg/dl change in serum cholesterol; thus the expected SD of serum cholesterol variation due to dietary cholesterol variation is 8.2 mg/dl. The theoretically expected correlation between cholesterol intake and serum cholesterol is therefore

$$r = \frac{\text{Expected SD due to diet}}{\text{Total SD for serum cholesterol}}$$
$$= \frac{8.2}{54} = 0.15$$

The standard deviation in this example for dietary cholesterol is, in reality, overstated because it included measurement error as well as true variation. Indeed, Shekelle et al. (1981) found that the relationship (using regression analysis) between dietary lipid intake based on carefully conducted interviews and serum cholesterol was similar to that obtained from metabolic studies. Because of other determinants of serum cholesterol, however, the correlation between dietary lipid intake and serum cholesterol was only 0.08; as the study population was large, this small correlation was highly statistically significant. Furthermore, some factors are associated with both reduced cholesterol intake and higher serum cholesterol, such as low levels of physical activity and knowledge of hypercholesterolemia. These tend to distort the true relationship between diet and serum levels toward an inverse association in cross-sectional studies (Shekelle et al., 1981). In studies that examined the relationships between change in diet and change in serum cholesterol using simple questionnaires, it has been possible to demonstrate rather strong correlations (see Chapter 6). The methods of dietary intake measurement in many of the early studies were very inadequate; most commonly these investigations used 24-hour recall methods, which provide a poor assessment of usual intake (see Chapter 3). Nevertheless, it is clear that the use of serum cholesterol as a criterion for the validity of a dietary measurement method is inappropriate. From the standpoint of the development of the field of nutritional epidemiology, the early focus on serum cholesterol was unfortunate. If beta-carotene had been of major interest at that time, the attitude toward the possibility of measuring diet in epidemiologic studies might have been different, as it is easy to demonstrate an association between intake measured by simple questionnaires and blood levels (see Chapter 6).

The resurgent interest in dietary etiologies of disease, particularly cancer, has stimulated the development and evaluation of methods for dietary assessment in epidemiologic applications. Many, although not all, aspects of diet can now be measured readily and inexpensively with sufficient accuracy to provide useful information. These methods, consisting of food intake and biochemical and anthropometric measurements, are discussed in detail in later chapters. Equally important, for most nutrients that have been studied, biologically meaningful between-person variation has been documented to exist within populations; without such variation, observational studies of individuals would not be feasible.

EPIDEMIOLOGIC APPROACHES TO DIET AND DISEASE

The concepts, hypotheses, and techniques of nutritional epidemiology are derived from many sources. Biochemistry, for example, has provided findings that certain nutrients function as antioxidants that may protect critical cell components from damage, potentially reducing the incidence of cancer (Ames, 1983; Ames et al., 1995). Cell culture methods have been used to identify compounds, such as preformed vitamin A, that regulate growth and differentiation of cells and that may, therefore, influence the risk of cancer in humans. Experiments in laboratory animals have provided much information regarding the effects of diet on the occurrence of disease and mechanisms of action. Metabolic and biochemical studies among human subjects have yielded essential information on the physiologic effects of dietary factors. Findings from in vitro studies and animal experiments, however, cannot be extrapolated directly to humans (Ames et al., 1987), and physiologic and metabolic changes are several steps removed from the actual occurrence of disease in humans; thus, epidemiologic approaches are needed to address diet and disease relationships directly. Nevertheless, these basic science areas provide critical direction for epidemiologists, information that can aid in the interpretation of their epidemiologic findings, and new methods for measuring genetic and environmental exposures that can be applied in epidemiologic studies.

Correlation Studies

Until recently, epidemiologic investigations of diet and disease consisted largely of ecologic or correlation studies, that is, comparisons of disease rates in populations with the population per capita consumption of specific dietary factors. Usually the dietary information in such studies is based on *disappearance data,* meaning the national figures for food produced and imported minus the food that is exported, fed to animals, or otherwise not available for humans. Many of the correlations based on such information are remarkably strong; for example, the correlation between meat intake and incidence of colon cancer is 0.85 for men and 0.89 for women (Armstrong and Doll, 1975) (Fig. 1–1).

The use of international correlational studies to evaluate the relationships between diet and disease has several strengths. Most importantly, the contrasts in dietary intake are typically very large. For example,

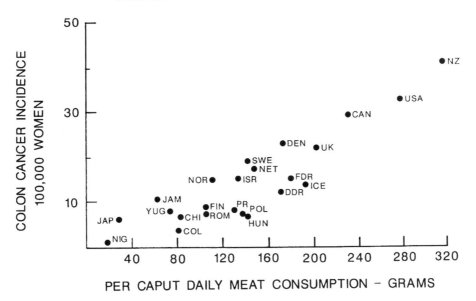

Figure 1–1. Correlation between per capita meat intake and incidence of colon cancer in women in 23 countries. (From Armstrong and Doll, 1975; reproduced with permission.)

within the United States, most individuals consume between 25% and 45% of their calories from fat, whereas the mean fat intake for populations in different countries varies from 11% to 42% of calories (Hebert and Wynder, 1987). Second, the average of diets for persons residing in a country are likely to be more stable over time than are the diets of individual persons within the country; for most countries the changes in per capita dietary intakes over a decade or two are relatively small. Finally, the cancer rates on which international studies are based are usually derived from relatively large populations and are, therefore, subject to only small random errors.

The primary problem of such correlational studies is that many potential determinants of disease other than the dietary factor under consideration may vary between areas with a high and low incidence of disease. Such confounding factors can include genetic predisposition; other dietary factors, including the availability of total energy intake; and other environmental or lifestyle practices. For example, with few exceptions, countries with a low incidence of colon cancer tend to be economically

underdeveloped. Therefore, any variable related to industrialization will be similarly correlated with the incidence of colon cancer. Indeed, the correlation between gross national product and colon cancer mortality rate is 0.77 for men and 0.69 for women (Armstrong and Doll, 1975). More complex analyses can be conducted of such ecologic data that control for some of the potentially confounding factors. For example, McKeown-Eyssen and Bright-See (1985) have found that an inverse association of per capita dietary fiber intake and national colon cancer mortality rates persists after adjustment for fat intake. Rose (1982) and Kromhout (1989) have also emphasized the importance of the temporal relation in correlational studies; for at least some diseases, rates may be most appropriately related to dietary data many years earlier.

Most correlational studies are also limited by the use of food "disappearance" data that are only indirectly related to intake and are likely to be of variable quality. For example, the higher "disappearance" of calories per capita for the United States compared with most countries is probably related in part to wasted food in addition to higher actual intake. Furthermore, aggregate data for a geographic unit as a whole may be only weakly related to the diets of those individuals at risk of disease. As an extreme example, the interpretation of correlational data regarding alcohol intake and breast cancer is complicated because, in some cultures, most of the alcohol is consumed by men, but it is the women who develop breast cancer. These issues of data quality can potentially be addressed by collecting information on actual dietary intake in a uniform manner from the population subgroups of interest. This is currently being done in a study conducted in 65 geographic areas within China that are characterized by an unusually large variation in the rates of many cancers (Chen et al., 1990).

Another serious limitation of the international correlational studies is that they cannot be independently reproduced, which is an important part of the scientific process. Although the dietary information can be improved and the analyses can be refined, the resulting data will really not be independent; the populations, their diets, and the confounding variables are the same. Thus, it is not likely that many new insights will be obtained from further ecologic studies among countries. For this reason, the methodologic aspects of correlational studies are not discussed further in this book.

The role of correlational studies in nutritional epidemiology is controversial. Clearly these analyses have stimulated much of the current research on diet and cancer, and in particular they have emphasized the major differences in cancer rates among countries. Traditionally, such studies have been considered the weakest form of evidence, primarily due to the potential for confounding by factors that are difficult to measure and control (Kinlen, 1983). More recently, some have thought that such studies provide the strongest form of evidence for evaluating hypotheses relating diet to cancer (Hebert and Wynder, 1987; Prentice et al., 1988). On balance, ecologic studies have unquestionably been useful, but are not sufficient to provide conclusions regarding the relationships between dietary factors and disease and may sometimes be completely misleading.

Special Exposure Groups

Groups within a population that consume unusual diets provide an additional opportunity to learn about the relation of dietary factors and disease (Zaridze et al., 1985). These groups are often defined by religious or ethnic characteristics and provide many of the same strengths as ecologic studies. In addition, the special populations often live in the same general environment as the comparison group, which may somewhat reduce the number of alternative explanations for any differences that might be observed. For example, the observation that colon cancer mortality in the largely vegetarian Seventh-day Adventists is only about half that expected (Phillips et al., 1980) has been used to support the hypothesis that meat consumption is a cause of colon cancer.

Findings based on special exposure groups are subject to many of the same limitations as ecologic studies. Many factors, both dietary and nondietary, are likely to distinguish these special groups from the comparison population. Thus, other possible explanations for the lower colon cancer incidence and mortality among the Seventh-day Adventist population are that differences in rates are attributable to a lower intake of alcohol or a higher vegetable consumption. Given the many possible alternative explanations, such studies may be particularly useful when a hypothesis is *not* supported. For example, the finding that the breast cancer mortality rate among the Seventh-day Adventists is not appreciably different from the rate among the general U.S. population provides fairly strong evidence that meat eating does not cause a major increase in the risk of breast cancer (see Chapter 16).

Migrant Studies and Secular Trends

Migrant studies have been particularly useful in addressing the possibility that the correlations observed in the ecologic studies are due to genetic factors. For most cancers, populations migrating from an area with its own pattern of cancer incidence rates acquire rates characteristic of their new location (Staszewski and Haenszel, 1965; Adelstein et al., 1979; McMichael and Giles, 1988; Shimizu et al., 1991; Ziegler et al., 1993), although, for a few tumor sites, this change occurs only in later generations (Haenszel et al., 1972; Buell, 1973). Therefore, genetic factors cannot be primarily responsible for the large differences in cancer rates among these countries. Migrant studies are also useful to examine the latency or relevant time of exposure (see Chapter 16).

Major changes in the rates of a disease within a population over time provide evidence that nongenetic factors play an important role in the etiology of that disease. In the United States, for example, rates of coronary heart disease rose dramatically over the first half of this century, and then subsequently declined (Working Group on Arteriosclerosis, 1981). These secular changes clearly demonstrate that environmental factors, possibly including diet, are primary causes of this disease, even though genetic factors may still influence who becomes affected given an adverse environment.

Case–Control and Cohort Studies

Many of the weaknesses of correlational studies are potentially avoidable in case–control studies (in which information about previous diet is obtained from diseased patients and compared with that from subjects without the disease) or cohort investigations (in which information on diet is obtained from disease-free subjects who are then followed to determine disease rates according to levels of dietary factors). In such studies, the confounding effects of other factors can be controlled either in the design (by matching subjects to be compared on the basis of known risk factors or by restriction) or in the analysis (by any of a variety of multivariate methods) if information has been collected on the confounding variables. Furthermore, dietary information can be obtained for the

individuals actually affected by disease, rather than using the average intake of the population as a whole.

Case–control studies generally provide information more efficiently and rapidly than cohort studies because the number of subjects is typically far smaller and no follow-up is necessary. However, consistently valid results may be difficult to obtain from case–control studies of dietary factors and disease because of the inherent potential for methodologic bias. This potential for bias is not unique for diet but is likely to be unusually serious for several reasons. Due to the limited range of variation in diet within most populations and some inevitable error in measuring intake, realistic relative risks in most studies of diet and disease are likely to be modest, say on the order of 0.5–2.0. These relative risks may seem small, but would be quite important because the prevalence of exposure is high. Given typical distributions of dietary intake, these relative risks are usually based on differences in means for cases and controls (or those who become cases and those who remain noncases in prospective studies) of only about 5% (see Chapters 3 and 12). Thus, a systematic error of even 3% or 4% can seriously distort such a relationship. In case–control studies it is easy to imagine that biases (due to selection or recall) of this magnitude could often occur, and it is extremely difficult to exclude the possibility that this degree of bias has not occurred in any specific study. Hence, it would not be surprising if case–control studies of dietary factors lead to inconsistent findings.

The selection of an appropriate control group for a study of diet and disease is also usually problematic. One common practice is to use patients with another disease as a control group, with the assumption that the exposure under study is unrelated to the condition of this control group. Because diet may well affect many diseases, it is often difficult to identify disease groups that are definitely unrelated to the aspect of diet under investigation. A common alternative is to use a sample of persons from the general population as the control group. In many areas, particularly large cities, participation rates are low; it is common for only 60%–70% of eligible population controls to complete an interview (Hartge et al., 1984). Because diet is particularly associated with the level of general health consciousness, the diets of those who participate may differ substantially from those who do not; unfortunately, little information is available that directly bears on this issue.

The many potential opportunities for methodologic bias in case–control studies of diet raise a concern that incorrect associations may frequently occur. Even if many studies arrive at correct conclusions, distortion of true associations in a substantial percentage produces an inconsistent body of published data, making a coherent synthesis difficult or impossible for a specific diet and disease relationship. Methodologic sources of inconsistency may be particularly troublesome in nutritional epidemiology due to the inherent biologic complexity of nutrient–nutrient interactions. As the effect of one nutrient may depend on the level of another (which can differ between studies and may not have even been measured), such interactions may result in apparently inconsistent findings in the context of epidemiologic studies. Thus, compounding biologic complexity with methodologic inconsistency may result in an uninterpretable literature. Data accumulated in the last several years suggest that case–control studies, even when consistent, can be biased. For example, highly consistent positive associations between total energy intake and risk of colon cancer have been seen in case–control studies (Jain et al., 1980; Bristol et al., 1985; Potter and McMichael, 1986; Lyon et al., 1987; Graham et al., 1988; West et al., 1989; Peters et al., 1992), which seemed biologically implausible (see Chapter 11). However, in prospective studies, either no or inverse associations have been found (Garland and Garland, 1980; Phillips and Snowdon, 1983; Stemmermann et al., 1984; Hiray-

ama, 1986; Willett et al., 1990; Bostick et al., 1994; Giovannucci et al., 1994; Goldbohm et al., 1994). As discussed in detail in Chapter 16, case–control and cohort studies have provided somewhat different perspectives of the relation between dietary fat and breast cancer. On the other hand, in both case–control and cohort studies of green and yellow vegetable intake in relation to lung cancer, remarkably consistent inverse associations have been found (see Chapter 15).

Prospective cohort studies avoid most of the potential sources of methodologic bias associated with case–control investigations. Because the dietary information is collected before the diagnosis of disease, illness cannot affect the recall of diet. Distributions of dietary factors in the study population may be affected by selective participation in the cohort; however, low participation rates at enrollment will not distort the relationships between dietary factors and disease. Although losses to follow-up that vary by level of dietary factors can result in distorted associations in a cohort study, follow-up rates tend to be rather high as participants have already provided evidence of willingness to participate and they may also be followed passively by means of disease registries and vital record listings (Stampfer et al., 1984). In addition to being less susceptible to bias, prospective cohort studies provide the opportunity to obtain repeated assessments of diet over time and to examine the effects of diet on a wide variety of diseases, including total mortality, simultaneously.

The primary constraints on prospective studies of diet are practical. Even for common diseases, such as myocardial infarction or cancers of the lung, breast, or colon, it is necessary to enroll tens of thousands of subjects. The use of structured, self-administered questionnaires has made studies of this size possible, although still expensive. For diseases of somewhat lower frequency, however, even very large cohorts will not accumulate a sufficient number of cases within a reasonable amount of time. Case–control studies, therefore, continue to play an important role in nutritional epidemiology.

Controlled Trials

The most rigorous evaluation of a dietary hypothesis is the randomized trial, optimally conducted as a double-blind experiment. The principal strength of a randomized trial is that potentially distorting variables should be distributed at random between the treatment and control groups, thus minimizing the possibility of confounding by these extraneous factors. In addition, it is sometimes possible to create a larger contrast between the groups being compared by use of an active intervention. Such experiments among humans, however, are best justified after considerable nonexperimental data have been collected to ensure that benefit is reasonably probable and that an adverse outcome is unlikely. Experimental studies are particularly practical for evaluating hypotheses that minor components of the diet, such as trace elements or vitamins, can prevent disease because these nutrients can be formulated into pills or capsules (Stampfer et al., 1985).

Even if feasible, randomized trials of dietary factors and disease are likely to encounter several limitations. The time between change in the level of a dietary factor and any expected change in the incidence of disease is typically uncertain. Therefore, trials must be of long duration, and usually one cannot eliminate the possibility that any lack of difference between treatment groups may be due to insufficient duration. Compliance with the treatment diet is likely to decrease during an extended trial, particularly if treatment involves a real change in food intake, and the control group may well adopt the dietary behavior of the treatment group if the treatment diet is thought to be beneficial. Such trends, which were found in the Multiple Risk Factor Intervention Trial of coronary disease prevention (Multiple Risk Factor Intervention Trial Research Group, 1982), may obscure a real benefit of dietary change.

A related potential limitation of trials is that participants who enroll in such studies tend to be highly selected on the basis of health consciousness and motivation. It is possible, therefore, that the subjects at highest potential risk on the basis of their dietary intake, and thus susceptible to intervention, are seriously underrepresented. For example, if low folic acid intake is thought to be a risk factor for lung cancer and a trial of folic acid supplementation is conducted among a health conscious population that includes few individuals with low folic acid intake, one might see no effect simply because the study population was already receiving the maximal benefit of this nutrient through its usual diet. In such an instance, it would be useful to measure dietary intake of folic acid before starting the trial. Because the effect of supplementation is likely to be greatest among those with low dietary intakes, it would be possible either to exclude those with high intakes (the potentially nonsusceptibles) either before randomization or in subanalyses at the conclusion of the study. This requires, of course, a reasonable measurement of dietary intake.

It is sometimes said that trials provide a better quantitative measurement of the effect of an exposure or treatment because the difference in exposure between groups is better measured than in an observational study. Although this contrast may at times be better defined in a trial (it is usually clouded by some degree of noncompliance), trials still usually produce an imprecise measure of the effect of exposure due to marginally adequate sample sizes and ethical considerations that require stopping soon after a statistically significant effect is seen. For example, with a p value close to 0.05, as was found in the Lipid Research Clinics Coronary Primary Prevention Trial (Lipid Research Clinics Program, 1984), the 95% confidence interval extends from no effect to an implausibly strong effect. In an observational study, an ethical imperative to stop does not exist when statistical significance occurs; continued accumula-

tion of data can provide increasing precision regarding the relation between exposure and disease. A trial can provide unique
information on the latent period between
change in an exposure and change in disease; because spontaneous changes in diet
are typically not clearly demarcated in
time, the estimation of latent periods for
dietary effects is usually difficult in observational studies.

Although all hypotheses would ideally be
evaluated in randomized trials, this is sometimes impossible for practical or ethical reasons. For example, our knowledge of the effects of cigarette smoking on risk of lung
cancer is based on observational studies,
and it is similarly unlikely that randomized
trials could be conducted to examine the effect of alcohol use on human breast cancer
risk. It remains unclear whether trials of sufficient size, duration, and degree of compliance can be conducted to evaluate many hypotheses that involve major changes in
eating patterns, such as a reduction in fat intake.

INTERPRETATION OF
EPIDEMIOLOGIC DATA

The interpretation of positive (or inverse)
associations in epidemiologic studies has
received considerable attention; however,
the evaluation of null or statistically nonsignificant findings has received less. Because either finding is potentially important, both are considered here.

If an association is observed in an epidemiologic study, we are usually concerned
whether it represents a true cause-and-
effect relationship; that is, if we actively
changed the exposure, would that influence
the frequency of disease? Hill (1965) has
discussed factors that have frequently been
considered as criteria for causality. These
have included the strength of association,
the consistency of a finding in various studies and populations, the presence of a
dose–response gradient, the appropriate
temporal relationship, the biologic plausibility, and the coherence with existing data.

As has been pointed out by Rothman
(1986), these cannot be considered as criteria because exceptions are likely to be frequent; this is particularly true in nutritional
epidemiology. In this field, true associations are not likely to be strong, although
relative risks of 0.7 or 1.5 could potentially
be important because the dietary exposures
are common. The consistent finding of an
association that cannot be explained by
other factors in various populations markedly reduces the possibility that chance
explains the findings and increases the likelihood of causality. Although the reproducibility of findings is extremely important,
null findings should sometimes be expected
in nutritional epidemiology as noted above,
even when a causal relationship may exist;
thus, absolute consistency is not a realistic
expectation. Dose–response relationships
are likely to be nonlinear and may be of
almost any shape, depending on the starting point on a hypothetical spectrum of exposure (Fig. 1–2). Moreover, apparently
clear dose–response relationships can easily
be the result of bias or confounding. Although compatibility of a finding with an
established mechanism of disease causation
supports causality, post hoc biologic explanations should be viewed cautiously because they can usually be developed for
most observations, including those that are
later refuted. Moreover, the pathophysiology of most cancers and many other
chronic diseases is poorly understood so
that lack of a well-defined mechanism
should not be construed as evidence against
causality.

Knowledge that an association exists,
even if deemed causal, is not sufficient to
make public or personal decisions. Such actions require some knowledge of the shape
and quantitative aspects of the dose–
response relationship. For instance, knowledge that total fat intake is associated with
risk of colon cancer would not provide a
sufficient basis to recommend a universal
reduction in fat intake. It would be much
more useful to know, for example, the
change in risk associated with a decrease in

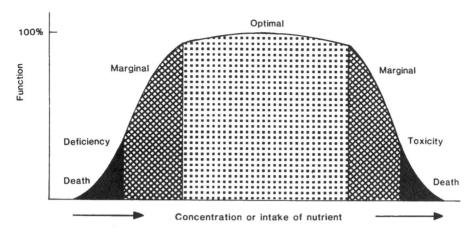

Figure 1–2. Hypothetical relationship between intake of an essential dietary factor and health. If two points on the ascending part of the curve are compared, it might be concluded that the nutrient was beneficial; if points on the horizontal portion were compared, it might be concluded that the nutrient had no effect; if points on the descending segment were contrasted, it might be reported that the nutrient was deleterious. The health effects of the nutrient can only be fully appreciated by an examination of the dose–response relationship over the full range of exposures, which may not be possible within any single study. (From Mertz, 1981; reproduced with permission.)

fat intake from 40% to 30% of total energy intake, which has been considered realistic for the U.S. population (Committee on Diet, Nutrition and Cancer, 1982), as well as the effect of a change from 30% to 20% of calories, which probably represents a limit of feasibility for the United States. It is entirely possible that a strong relation between fat intake and colon cancer risk exists below 20% of calories, but that above that level the relationship is nonlinear, flat, or too weak to be of importance (McMichael and Potter, 1985). In addition to this information, knowledge of the approximate latent period between alteration in diet and change in disease incidence would be important. If this were several decades, older individuals might rationally ignore the association in making decisions regarding their diet.

Interpretation of Null Associations

In a study of diet and disease, failure to observe a statistically significant association when such an association truly exists can occur in several circumstances, alluded to earlier. One possibility is that the variation in diet is insufficient; in the extreme, no associations can occur if everyone in the study population eats the same diet. Second, variation may exist for the study population, but only within a "flat" portion of the total dose–response relationship. A third possibility is that the method of measuring dietary intake is not sufficiently precise to measure differences that truly exist. Fourth, an association may be missed because of low statistical power due to an inadequate number of diseased and nondiseased subjects. Fifth, a relationship could be undetected because the temporal relationship between the measured exposure and the occurrence of disease did not encompass the true latent period; this could easily happen if the critical dietary exposure occurred during childhood and the disease was diagnosed during adulthood. Sixth, an association could be undetected because some unmeasured third variable was related to exposure and disease in opposite directions; in other words, negative confounding existed. In addition to these six largely biologic reasons for failure to observe an association, methodologic sources of bias could obscure a relationship.

It is obviously not informative to describe a study as null or nonsignificant unless the possible explanations noted previously have been addressed. Clearly, no single study can fully encompass the total possible range of human diets, measure all aspects of diet with absolute precision, assess all potential latent periods, and control for all potentially confounding variables. What must be done, then, is to describe the conditions and limitations of the null findings. First, it is critical to demonstrate that true variation in diet exists within the study population and that the method of measuring diet provides useful discrimination among subjects (see Chapter 6). It is not adequate to demonstrate that dietary variation exists on the basis of measurements using the study instrument alone because this variation could merely represent error. On the other hand, demonstration that measurements made using the study instrument correlate with measurements made using another method with independent sources of error provides evidence both that diet does vary within the population and that the study instrument is capable of detecting this variation.

Although confidence intervals are important for reporting positive associations, they are even more critical for results that are near the null (e.g., relative risk = 1.0) or not statistically significant because they provide a sense of the range of values that are still consistent with the data. Although it has only recently been done in practice, confidence limits should ideally be adjusted for measurement error; measurement error tends to make the true confidence intervals wider than those usually calculated, assuming no such error (Rosner et al., 1989). It has become fashionable, and even required by some editors, to include a priori power calculations in reports of study results. Because confidence intervals are determined by the observed data as well as the influence of chance, a priori power estimates add little once the study is completed. (The use of power estimates to interpret nonsignificant findings can easily be misleading; it is quite possible for a study to have low a priori power to detect a positive association but have confidence limits that widely exclude that positive association if the association is in the opposite direction.) The range of latent periods encompassed by the study should also be described; in dietary studies usually this is possible only crudely. If the study is a prospective cohort, or data are available in retrospect for several points in time, analyses can be conducted to evaluate associations separately for different latent periods (Rothman, 1986). Finally, it will be important to describe the dietary and nondietary correlates of the primary exposure that have been evaluated as potential confounding variables.

Because it is rare that all aspects of a hypothesis can be addressed in one study, it is important to describe which aspects have or have not been evaluated. For example, it is of limited use to conclude simply that a given study of dietary vitamin C intake and colon cancer was negative. It would be much more informative to say, for example, "Vitamin C intake determined by a detailed quantitative method was 40 mg per day for the 10th percentile and 200 mg per day for the 90th percentile. During a 5-year follow-up period the observed relative risk was 1.0 with a 95% confidence interval of 0.8–1.3 after adjusting for exposure measurement error for a difference of 50 mg per day of vitamin C intake, which corresponds to a 50% increase for the average subject. Finally, adjustment for parental history of colon cancer and intakes of dietary fiber and calcium did not alter the findings." It is thus clear from this description that the effects of very low and very high vitamin C intakes and the influence of childhood diet, are not being evaluated and that a 10%, but not a 30%, reduction in risk by a 50% increase in vitamin C intake later in life is still quite possible.

Multivariate Relationships of Diet and Disease

Relationships between dietary factors and disease are likely to be extremely complex for both biologic and behavioral reasons. Types and amounts of food eaten may be related to important nondietary determinants of disease, such as age, smoking, exercise, and occupation, which may both distort or confound and modify relationships with diet. As discussed in Chapter 2, intakes of specific nutrients tend to be intercorrelated so that associations with one nutrient may be confounded by other aspects of the diet. Furthermore, the intake of one nutrient may modify the absorption, metabolism, or requirement for another nutrient, thus creating a biologic interaction. Due to these complexities, it is generally unsatisfactory to examine the relationship between a single dietary factor and disease in isolation. In practice, it is almost always necessary to employ multivariate techniques, including both stratified analyses and statistical models, to adjust for potentially confounding variables and examine interactions. These strategies are discussed further in Chapter 13.

The use of multivariate methods in any particular analysis requires a careful consideration of the precise question that is being posed and whether potential covariates are true confounders as opposed to effects of the primary exposure. Confusion resulting from the inappropriate application of multivariate methods is illustrated by the controversy surrounding the relation of body fat and risk of coronary heart disease (Manson et al., 1987). In a number of reports, blood pressure, glucose tolerance, and serum lipid levels were included in multivariate models along with a measure of body fat. Because these other risk factors are strongly influenced by obesity and are thus in the causal pathway relating relative weight with coronary heart disease, their inclusion substantially diminishes the apparent effect of relative weight. Conclusions based on such analyses that obesity has little relationship with coronary heart disease are misleading because obesity cannot be stripped of its metabolic consequences by sophisticated statistical methods. The application of multivariate methods in nutritional epidemiology necessitates maximal use of existing knowledge regarding the effects of dietary factors to avoid similar problems in the future.

SUMMARY

Although growing rapidly, our knowledge is still largely incomplete regarding the relationships between dietary factors and the major illnesses of our culture. These illnesses include not only cancer and heart disease, which have received the most attention, but also congenital malformations, degenerative conditions of the eye, fractures, and many infectious diseases that are hypothesized to be influenced by the nutritional status of the host. Randomized trials may eventually provide definitive answers to some of these questions. However, in the near future, our knowledge of many of these relationships will depend largely on observational epidemiologic data, and for many relationships this may be indefinitely. For this reason, it is crucial to refine maximally our methods of data collection, analytic procedures, and interpretation of findings. The ensuing chapters are intended to further our progress in this direction.

REFERENCES

Adelstein, A. M., J. Staszewski, and C. S. Muir (1979). Cancer mortality in 1970–1972 among Polish-born migrants to England and Wales. *Br J Cancer 40*, 464–475.

Ames, B. N. (1983). Dietary carcinogens and anticarcinogens. Oxygen radicals and degenerative diseases. *Science 221*, 1256–1264.

Ames, B. N., L. S. Gold, and W. C. Willett (1995). The causes and prevention of cancer. *Proc Natl Acad Sci USA 92*, 5258–5265.

Ames, B. N., R. Magaw, and L. S. Gold (1987). Ranking possible carcinogenic hazards. *Science 236*, 271–280.

Armstrong, B., and R. Doll (1975). Environmental factors and cancer incidence and mortality in different countries, with special reference to dietary practices. *Int J Cancer 15*, 617–631.

Bostick, R. M., J. D. Potter, L. H. Kushi, T. A. Sellers, K. A. Steinmetz, D. R. McKenzie, S. M. Gapstur, and A. R. Folsom (1994). Sugar, meat, and fat intake, and nondietary risk factors for colon cancer incidence in Iowa women (United States). *Cancer Causes Control 5*, 38–52.

Bristol, J. B., P. M. Emmett, K. W. Heaton, and R. C. Williamson (1985). Sugar, fat, and the risk of colorectal cancer. *Br Med J Clin Res Ed 291*, 1467–1470.

Buell, P. (1973). Changing incidence of breast cancer in Japanese-American women. *JNCI 51*, 1479–1483.

Chen, J., T. C. Campbell, L. Junyao, and R. Peto (1990). *Diet, Life-style and Mortality in China: A Study of the Characteristics of 65 Chinese Counties.* Oxford, England: Oxford University Press.

Committee on Diet, Nutrition and Cancer, Assembly of Life Sciences, National Research Council (1982). *Diet, Nutrition, and Cancer.* Washington, D.C.: National Academy Press.

Davidson, S., R. Passmore, and J. F. Brock (1973). *Human Nutrition and Dietetics.* Edinburgh: Churchill Livingstone.

Garland, C. F., and F. C. Garland (1980). Do sunlight and vitamin D reduce the likelihood of colon cancer? *Int J Epidemiol 9*, 227–231.

Giovannucci, E., E. B. Rimm, M. J. Stampfer, G. A. Colditz, A. Ascherio, and W. C. Willett (1994). Intake of fat, meat, and fiber in relation to risk of colon cancer in men. *Cancer Res 54*, 2390–2397.

Goldberger, J. E. (1964). *Goldberger on Pellagra.* Baton Rouge: Louisiana State University Press.

Goldbohm, R. A., P. A. van den Brandt, P. van't Veer, H. A. M. Brants, E. Dorant, F. Sturmans, and R. J. J. Hermus (1994). A prospective cohort study on the relation between meat consumption and the risk of colon cancer. *Cancer Res 54*, 718–723.

Graham, S., J. Marshall, B. Haughey, A. Mittelman, M. Swanson, M. Zielezny, T. Byers, G. Wilkinson, and D. West (1988). Dietary epidemiology of cancer of the colon in western New York. *Am J Epidemiol 128*, 490–503.

Guangi-Qi, Y. (1987). Research on selenium-related problems in human health in China. In Combs, G. F., Spallholz, J. E., Levander, O. R., and Oldfield, J. E., (eds): *Sele-nium in Biology and Medicine, Part A.* New York: Van Nostrand Reinhold, pp 9–32.

Haenszel, W., M. Kurihara, M. Segi, and R. K. Lee (1972). Stomach cancer among Japanese in Hawaii. *JNCI 49*, 969–988.

Hartge, P., L. A. Brinton, J. F. A. Rosenthal, J. I. Cahill, R. N. Hoover, and J. Waksberg (1984). Random digit dialing in selecting a population-based control group. *Am J Epidemiol 120*, 825–833.

Hebert, J. R., and E. L. Wynder (1987). Dietary fat and the risk of breast cancer (letter). *N Engl J Med 317*, 165.

Hill, A. B. (1965). The environment and disease: Association or causation? *Proc R Soc Med 58*, 295–300.

Hirayama, T. (1986). A large-scale study on cancer risks by diet—with special reference to the risk reducing effects of green-yellow vegetable consumption. In Hayashi, Y., Magao, M., and Sugimura, T., et al (eds): *Diet, Nutrition, and Cancer.* Tokyo: Japan Scientific Societies Press, pp 41–53.

Jacobs, D. R., Jr., J. T. Anderson, and H. Blackburn (1979). Diet and serum cholesterol: Do zero correlations negate the relationship? *Am J Epidemiol 110*, 77–87.

Jain, M., G. M. Cook, F. G. Davis, M. G. Grace, G. R. Howe, and A. B. Miller (1980). A case–control study of diet and colorectal cancer. *Int J Cancer 26*, 757–768.

Kinlen, L. J. (1983). Fat and Cancer. *Br Med J Clin Res Ed 286*, 1081–1082.

Kromhout, D. (1989). *Diet and Mortality: Strengthening Cross-Cultural Correlations With Time.* Epidemiology, Nutrition, and Health. Proceedings of the 1st Berlin Meeting on Nutritional Epidemiology, 1988, Berlin, Germany, Smith-Gordon, London.

Lind, J. (1753). *A Treatise on the Scurvy.* Reprinted Edinburgh: Edinburgh University Press, 1953.

Lipid Research Clinics Program (1984). The lipid research clinics coronary primary prevention trial results. Reduction in incidence of coronary heart disease. *JAMA 251*, 351–364.

Lyon, J. L., A. W. Mahoney, D. W. West, J. W. Gardner, K. R. Smith, A. W. Sorenson, and W. Stanish (1987). Energy intake: Its relationship to colon cancer risk. *JNCI 78*, 853–861.

Manson, J. E., M. J. Stampfer, C. H. Hennekens, and W. C. Willett (1987). Body weight and longevity. A reassessment. *JAMA 257*, 353–358.

Mattson, F. H., B. A. Erickson, and A. M. Kligman (1972). Effect of dietary cholesterol on serum cholesterol in man. *Am J Clin Nutr* 25, 589–594.

McKeown-Eyssen, G. E., and E. Bright-See (1985). Dietary factors in colon cancer: International relationships. An update. *Nutr Cancer 7*, 251–253.

McMichael, A. J., and G. G. Giles (1988). Cancer in migrants to Australia: Extending descriptive epidemiological data. *Cancer Res 48*, 751–756.

McMichael, A. J. and J. D. Potter (1985). Diet and colon cancer: integration of the descriptive, analytic, and metabolic epidemiology. *Natl Cancer Inst Monogr 69*, 223–228.

Mertz, W. (1981). The essential trace elements. *Science 213*, 1332–1338.

Multiple Risk Factor Intervention Trial Research Group (1982). Multiple Risk Factor Intervention Trial: Risk factor changes and mortality results. *JAMA 248*, 1465–1477.

Peters, R. K., M. C. Pike, D. Garabrandt, and T. M. Mack (1992). Diet and colon cancer in Los Angeles County, California. *Cancer Causes Control 3*, 457–473.

Phillips, R. L., L. Garfinkel, J. W. Kuzma, W. L. Beeson, T. Lotz, and B. Brin (1980). Mortality among California Seventh-day Adventists for selected cancer sites. *JNCI 65*, 1097–1107.

Phillips, R. L., and D. A. Snowdon (1983). Association of meat and coffee use with cancers of the large bowel, breast, and prostate among Seventh-day Adventists: Preliminary results. *Cancer Res 43(suppl)*, 2403S–2408S.

Potter, J. D., and A. J. McMichael (1986). Diet and cancer of the colon and rectum: A case–control study. *JNCI 76*, 557–569.

Prentice, R. L., F. Kakar, S. Hursting, L. Sheppard, R. Klein, and L. H. Kushi (1988). Aspects of the rationale for the Women's Health Trial. *JNCI 80*, 802–814.

Rose, G. (1982). Incubation period of coronary heart disease. *Br Med J Clin Res Ed 284*, 1600–1601.

Rosner, B., W. C. Willett, and D. Spiegelman (1989). Correction of logistic regression relative risk estimates and confidence intervals for systematic within-person measurement error. *Statistics Med 8*, 1051–1069.

Rothman, K. J. (1986). *Modern Epidemiology*. Boston, MA: Little, Brown and Company.

Shekelle, R. B., A. M. Shryock, O. Paul, M. Lepper, J. Stamler, S. Liu, and W. J. Raynor Jr. (1981). Diet, serum cholesterol, and death from coronary heart disease: The Western Electric Study. *N Engl J Med 304*, 65–70.

Shimizu, H., R. K. Ross, L. Bernstein, R. Ya-

tani, B. E. Henderson, and T. M. Mack (1991). Cancers of the prostate and breast among Japanese and white immigrants in Los Angeles County. *Br J Cancer 63*, 963–966.

Stampfer, M. J., J. E. Buring, W. Willett, B. Rosner, K. Eberlein, and C. H. Hennekens (1985). The 2×2 factorial design: Its application to a randomized trial of aspirin and carotene in US physicians. *Statistics Med 4*, 111–116.

Stampfer, M. J., W. C. Willett, F. E. Speizer, D. C. Dysert, R. Lipnick, B. Rosner, and C. H. Hennekens (1984). Test of the National Death Index. *Am J Epidemiol 119*, 837–839.

Staszewski, J., and W. Haenszel (1965). Cancer mortality among the Polish-born in the United States. *JNCI 35*, 291–297.

Stemmermann, G. N., A. M. Nomura, and L. K. Heilbrun (1984). Dietary fat and the risk of colorectal cancer. *Cancer Res 44*, 4633–4637.

West, D. W., M. L. Slattery, L. M. Robison, K. L. Schuman, M. H. Ford, A. W. Mahoney, J. L. Lyon, and A. W. Sorensen (1989). Dietary intake and colon cancer: Sex and anatomic site-specific associations. *Am J Epidemiol 130*, 883–894.

Willett, W. (1987). Nutritional epidemiology: Issues and challenges. *Int J Epidemiol 16*, 312–317.

Willett, W. C., M. J. Stampfer, G. A. Colditz, B. A. Rosner, and F. E. Speizer (1990). Relation of meat, fat, and fiber intake to the risk of colon cancer in a prospective study among women. *N Engl J Med 323*, 1664–1672.

Williams, R. R. (1961). *Toward the Conquest of Beriberi*. Cambridge, MA: Harvard University Press.

Working Group on Arteriosclerosis of the National Heart, Lung, and Blood Institute (1981). *Decline in Coronary Heart Disease Mortality, 1963–78. Vol. 2.* DHHS Publication No. (NIH) 82–2035. Bethesda, MD: National Institutes of Health, pp 157–258.

Wynder, E. L. (1976). Nutrition and cancer. *Fed Proc 35*, 1309–1315.

Zaridze, D. G., C. S. Muir, and A. J. McMichael (1985). Diet and cancer: Value of different types of epidemiological studies. *Nutr Cancer 7*, 155–166.

Ziegler, R. G., R. N. Hoover, M. C. Pike, A. Hildesheim, A. M. Nomura, D. W. West, A. H. Wu-Williams, L. N. Kolonel, P. L. Horn-Ross, and J. F. Rosenthal (1993). Migration patterns and breast cancer risk in Asian-American women. *JNCI 85*, 1819–1827.

2

Foods and Nutrients

WALTER C. WILLETT AND I. MARILYN BUZZARD

The complexity of the human diet represents a daunting challenge to anyone contemplating a study of its relation to disease. The foods we consume each day contain literally thousands of specific chemicals, some known and well quantified, some characterized only poorly, and others completely undescribed and presently unmeasurable. The chemicals that comprise our food can be described by the following nonmutually exclusive categories:

1. *Essential nutrients.* The essential nutrients, which include minerals, vitamins, lipids, and amino acids, have little in common except that insufficient intake results in predictable clinical signs and symptoms of deficiency. Although it is likely that additional essential micronutrients remain to be identified, most are already well characterized; this represents the remarkable achievement of twentieth-century nutritional scientists.

2. *Major energy sources.* Most foods contain one or more of the major sources of energy: proteins, carbohydrates, fats, and alcohol. Proteins, carbohydrates, and fats are, of course, very heterogeneous, and the mix of these fuels may influence the long-term function of the human organism.

3. *Additives.* These substances are consciously added to our food for purposes such as preservation (e.g., nitrates, butylated hydroxy-toluene, and salt), coloring, and enhancement of consistency or flavor. Although such additives have elicited great public concern, they represent only a small fraction of the substances in our food and are among the best characterized and most closely regulated. Apart from salt intake, the health effects of these additives have been minimally studied epidemiologically; however, evidence does not presently exist that they contribute importantly to disease in the United States (Doll and Peto, 1981).

4. *Agricultural chemical contaminants.* These products include pesticides, her-

bicides, fungicides, and growth hormones for both plants and animals.

5. *Microbial toxin contamination.* Aflatoxins produced by the mold *Aspergillus flavus* are a classic example of this class of substances. The contamination of grains and other plant products by this mold is widespread, particularly where storage conditions are poor. Although aflatoxins are likely to contribute to the high rates of liver cancer in many developing countries (Busby and Wogan, 1984), there is presently little direct evidence that they are responsible for disease in the industrialized countries.

6. *Inorganic contaminants.* A wide variety of other chemicals inadvertently enter our food supply, including metals such as cadmium and lead and synthetic compounds such as polychlorinated biphenyls.

7. *Chemicals formed in the cooking or processing of food.* In vitro testing systems have shown that burning or charring food creates many substances that are mutagenic. Even heating meat products without burning can create a series of substances that are mutagenic (Sugimura, 1986; Ames et al., 1987; Gerhardsson de Verdier et al., 1991; Adamson and Thorgeirsson, 1995). The relevance of these substances to human health remains unknown.

8. *Natural toxins.* Many plants have, through evolution, developed the capacity to produce chemicals that are toxic to the insects or other animals that might attack them. Although many plants are recognized as poisonous to humans, the foods we eat also contain natural pesticides even though they do not consistently produce acute symptoms (Ames et al., 1987).

9. *Other natural compounds.* In the process of eating plant and animal products, we consume the countless substances that are vital for maintaining the structure and function of these living cells. For example, we consume DNA and RNA, the specialized lipids of cell membranes, and thousands of enzymes and enzyme inhibitors. Although some of these compounds provide essential nutrients for humans, most are thought of as incidental to the human diet. It is likely, however, that many of these compounds influence the occurrence of chronic human diseases (Steinmetz and Potter, 1991). For example, cholesterol has an important structural role in the membranes of animal tissues; however, the consumption of excessive cholesterol in the form of animal products is likely to contribute to the occurrence of coronary heart disease. More recently, accumulating evidence suggests that protease inhibitors and anti-estrogenic compounds contained in certain plant products may reduce the risk of some cancers (Troll et al., 1984; Adlercreutz, 1990; Herman et al., 1995; Kennedy, 1995; Watanabe et al., 1995).

The complex array of dietary chemicals outlined above creates obvious challenges for investigators seeking to understand the relationships of diet with human disease. In particular, it is difficult to know where to begin the search and how to set priorities for investigation along the way. Up to this point, most research has focused on the first two categories: the essential nutrients and major energy sources. This has some justification as a starting point. In general, living organisms do not respond in either a linear or an all-or-nothing manner to increasing levels of an external exposure. This principle has been depicted graphically for essential nutrients by Mertz (1981) (Fig. 1–2). Given that low intake of an essential nutrient produces clinical dysfunction in the short run, it is reasonable to hypothesize that less extreme levels of intake might produce subclinical dysfunction that affects the probability of developing chronic disease over a period of decades.

The additional focus on the major energy sources has justification in the simple fact that they are quantitatively important in our diets. Furthermore, gross and obvious differences exist in the mix of these energy sources among human populations. As noted in Chapter 1, these differences are correlated with striking variation in rates of many diseases; the temptation to invoke a causal interpretation of these associations has been strong. Tradition, based on the focus of nutritionists earlier in this century, and convenience have also probably contributed to the research emphasis on essential nutrients and energy sources. Many of us have become accustomed to think first of nutrients when the topic of diet is raised. Moreover, decades of work have been invested in improving available data on the nutrient content of foods so that much better information is available for this group of dietary chemicals than for the other categories of substances. However, data on dietary components not considered to be nutrients are beginning to be available; for example, the values for lycopene and lutein, two types of carotenoids in foods, have been added to many databases (Chug-Ahuja et al., 1993; Mangels et al., 1993).

Apart from essential nutrients and energy sources, the immense variety of other dietary substances confronts investigators with the need to establish research priorities. Additives and agricultural chemicals deserve attention because they may be controlled and because accidents can lead to high local concentrations. Ames and coworkers (1987) have provided an extensive review of dietary chemicals with respect to their potential for causing cancer. They pointed out that many of the naturally occurring substances are both more potent toxins or mutagens and far more abundant in food than the man-made chemicals that have been consciously or accidentally added to food. Although there is good reason for the research emphasis to date, it is important that tradition and convenience do not deter us from consideration that other aspects of diet may be important influences on the risk of human disease.

NUTRIENTS VERSUS FOODS

Throughout the nutrition literature in general and in the preceding discussion, diet has usually been described in terms of its chemical composition, for example, its nutrient content. Alternatively, diet can be described in terms of foods or food groups. It is useful to consider the advantages and disadvantages of representing diet in these ways.

The primary advantage of representing diets as specific compounds or groups of compounds is that such information can be directly related to our fundamental knowledge of biology. From a practical perspective, the exact structure of a compound must usually be known if it is to be synthesized and used for supplementation. In epidemiologic studies, calculation or measurement of the total intake of a nutrient (as opposed to using the contribution of only one food at a time) provides the most powerful test of a hypothesis, particularly if a number of foods each contribute only modestly to intake of that nutrient. For example, in a particular study, it is quite possible that total fat intake could be clearly associated with risk of disease, whereas none of the contributions to fat intake by individual foods would, on their own, be significantly related to disease.

The use of foods to represent diet has several practical advantages when examining relationships with disease. Particularly when suspicion exists that some aspect of diet is associated with risk but a specific hypothesis has not been formulated, an examination of the relations of foods and food groups with risk of disease provides a means to explore the data. Associations observed with specific foods may lead to a hypothesis relating to a defined chemical substance. For example, the finding by Graham and coworkers (1978) that intake of cruciferous vegetables was inversely related to risk of colon cancer supported the suggestion that indole compounds contained in these vegetables may be protective (Wattenberg and Loub,

1978). Similarly, lower rates of coronary heart disease among Eskimos and individuals who consume higher amounts of fish has generated the hypothesis that omega-3 fatty acids reduce the risk of this disease, perhaps by inhibiting the formation of thromboxane and thus the propensity for intracoronary thrombus formation (Lands, 1986). More recently, the observation that spinach, but not other sources of beta-carotene, was associated with lower risk of macular degeneration of the eye (Seddon et al., 1994) suggested that lutein, a carotenoid preferentially incorporated in the retina, might protect against this condition.

Even more seriously, premature focus on a specific nutrient that turns out to have no relation with disease may lead to the erroneous conclusion that diet has no effect. Mertz (1984) has pointed out that foods are not fully represented by their nutrient composition, noting as an example that milk and yogurt produce different physiologic effects despite a similar nutrient content. Furthermore, the valid calculation of a nutrient intake from data on food consumption requires that reasonably accurate food composition information be available, which markedly constrains the scope of dietary chemicals that may be investigated, as such information exists for only several dozen commonly studied nutrients.

Epidemiologic analyses based on foods, as opposed to nutrients, are generally most directly related to dietary recommendations because individuals and institutions ultimately manipulate nutrient intake largely by their choice of foods. Even if the intake of a specific nutrient is convincingly shown to be related to risk of disease, this is not sufficient information on which to make dietary recommendations. Because foods are an extremely complex mixture of chemicals that may compete with, antagonize, or alter the bioavailability of any single nutrient contained in that food, it is not possible to predict with certainty the health effects of any food solely on the basis of its content of one specific factor. For example, there is concern that high intake of nitrates may be deleterious, particularly with respect to gastrointestinal cancer. The primary sources of nitrates in our diets, however, are green, leafy vegetables, which, if anything, appear to be associated with reduced risk of cancer at several sites. Similarly, because of the high cholesterol content of eggs, their avoidance has received particular attention in diets aimed at reducing the risk of coronary heart disease; per capita consumption of eggs declined by 25% in the United States between 1948 and 1980 (Welsh and Marston, 1982). Eggs, however, are more than cholesterol capsules; they provide a rich source of essential amino acids and micronutrients and are relatively low in saturated fat. It is thus difficult to predict the net effect of egg consumption on risk of coronary heart disease, much less the effect on overall health. At present there are few data indicating that individuals who consume more eggs have a higher risk of coronary heart disease.

On the other hand, dietary recommendations can be made regarding the consumption of particular foods, even when the beneficial factors remain unknown. As discussed in Chapter 15, the observations that higher intakes of green and yellow vegetables were associated with reduced rates of lung cancer led to the hypothesis that beta-carotene might protect DNA from damage due to free radicals and singlet oxygen (Peto et al., 1981). Although trials of beta-carotene supplementation have not supported the hypothesis that this is the responsible factor, there is enough evidence from epidemiologic studies to recommend the frequent consumption of green and yellow vegetables.

Given the strengths and weaknesses of using nutrients or foods to represent diet, it appears that an optimal approach to epidemiologic analyses employs both. In this way, a potentially important finding is least likely to be missed. Moreover, the case for causality is strengthened when an association is observed with overall intake of a nutrient and also with more than one food source of that nutrient, particularly when the food sources are otherwise different. This provides, in some sense, multiple assessments of the potential for confounding by other nutrients; if an association was observed for only one food source of the nutrient, other factors contained in that food would tend to be similarly associated with disease. As an example, the hypothesis that alcohol intake causes breast cancer was strengthened by observing not only an overall association between alcohol intake and breast cancer risk but also by independent associations between both beer and liquor intake and risk of breast cancer, thus making it less likely, but not impossible, that some factor other than alcohol in these beverages was responsible for the increased risk. As another example, Kolonel et al. (1988) initially reported that intake of beta-carotene was positively associated with risk of prostate cancer. However, in a subsequent analysis of foods, intake of carrots, the largest source of beta-carotene, was not associated with risk of prostate cancer; the entire association was due to consumption of papaya (Le Marchand et al., 1991). Thus, the analysis of foods provided evidence against an effect of beta-carotene and suggested that some factors specific to papaya, or perhaps chance, were responsible for the original finding.

One practical drawback to the use of foods to represent diet is their large number and complex, often reciprocal, interrelationships that are largely due to individual behavioral patterns. For example, in one unpublished analysis, we found that potato chips were the food most strongly associated (inversely) with blood carotene levels, presumably because potato chip consumers tend to avoid vegetables and fruits in general. If carotene intake was truly protective for a certain disease, the resulting positive association between potato chip intake and disease could be misleading, as the relationship would have been indirect. Many other reciprocal relationships emerge upon perusal of typical datasets; for example, dark bread eaters tend not to eat white bread, margarine users tend not to eat butter, and skim milk users tend not to use whole milk. This complexity is, of course, one of the reasons to compute nutrient intakes that summarize the contributions of all foods.

An intermediate solution to the problem posed by the complex interrelationships among foods is to use food groups or to compute the contribution of nutrient intake from various food groups. For example, Manousos and coworkers (1983) combined the intakes of foods from several predefined groups to study the relation of diet with risk of colon cancer; they observed increased risk among subjects with high meat intake and with low consumption of vegetables. The computation of nutrient intakes from different food groups is illustrated by a prospective study among British bank clerks conducted by Morris and coworkers (1977), who observed an inverse relation between overall fiber intake and risk of coronary heart disease. It is well recognized that fiber is an extremely heterogeneous collection of substances and that the available food composition data for specific types of fiber are incomplete. Therefore, these authors computed fiber intake separately from various food groups and found that the entire protective effect was attributable to fiber from grains; fiber from fruits or vegetables was not associated with risk of disease. This analysis both circumvents the inadequacy of food composition databases and provides information in a form that is directly useful to individuals faced with decisions regarding choices of foods. Similarly, Witteman and colleagues (1989) found an inverse relation between overall intake of calcium and incidence of hypertension, as well as independent associations between calcium from dairy products, from grains, and from other sources. Because these various sources of calcium differed widely with respect to other factors, this added information provided further support for the overall finding.

Another approach for dealing with the complex intercorrelations of many foods is to use "pattern analysis" as suggested by Jacobson and Stanton (1986). This basically employs factor analysis or cluster analysis, which are both well-developed statistical techniques, to aggregate empirically individuals with similar diets based on their reported intake of foods rather than according to predefined scales as is done in the calculation of nutrient intakes. These methods may be most useful when well-developed hypotheses do not exist or when associations with specific nutrients have not been found, possibly because they do not represent the relevant aspects of diet. A limitation of these approaches is the need to provide a post hoc interpretation for the factors or clusters that evolve from the data. Although their utility has not been established in nutritional research, such approaches deserve consideration, particularly in situations where our understanding of disease etiology is limited (Randall et al., 1992; McCann et al., 1994).

In summary, a single optimal representation of diet does not exist for epidemiologic analyses. The choices depend on the nature and refinement of the hypotheses being addressed, the availability of food composition data, and the form of the dietary data that are available. In general, maximal information is obtained when analyses are conducted at the levels of nutrients, foods, and food groups.

FOOD COMPOSITION DATA SOURCES AND COMPUTATION SYSTEMS

To calculate the total intake of a nutrient for each subject in a study, information is required on the content of each food that has been reported. In some instances, existing databases and computer software can be used, particularly for standard summaries from diet records or 24-hour recalls (see Chapter 4). In other situations, such as when a structured questionnaire has been created for a specific application, it is necessary to assemble a special database for this purpose. Because the size of many

databases is formidable and they are frequently updated, it is not the objective of this section to provide primary information on food composition. Rather, existing options and considerations in selecting sources of data are discussed.

Before computing intake of a nutrient from information on the use of foods, it is important to consider whether such a calculation is appropriate. The fundamental assumption underlying such a calculation is that the nutrient content of a specific food is approximately constant, for example, that each carrot eaten by every subject has the same beta-carotene content. We know that this assumption is never completely correct; the beta-carotene content of a carrot will vary with its size, growing and harvesting conditions, degree of maturity, processing, storage, and cooking. Moreover, plant geneticists have selectively increased the carotene content of this vegetable in the United States because marketing experts have found that Americans prefer dark orange carrots. In other parts of the world, however, pale yellow carrots are especially valued and plants are selected for this attribute; thus substantial genetic variability contributes to differences in the carotenoid content of carrots. Although all these sources of variation contribute to errors in the estimation of calculated nutrient intake, the real question is whether these sources of variation are quantitatively large enough to distort calculations seriously. Although the carotenoid content of carrots may vary by a factor of three or four, someone who eats carrots regularly will still, on average, consume more beta-carotene than someone who does not. Moreover, if long-term beta-carotene intake is of interest, much of the error due to sample-to-sample variation in nutrient composition will be reduced because the average beta-carotene content of carrots eaten by individuals is likely to vary substantially less between persons than the beta-carotene content of carrots eaten by a person from one time to another. The finding that calculated beta-carotene intake is correlated with plasma beta-carotene level provides direct evidence that the calculations are providing informative data.

Whereas the assumption of constant nutrient content in foods does not appear to be seriously violated in the case of beta-carotene, selenium provides an example where this assumption is sufficiently incorrect so as to preclude useful calculations of intake. The underlying reason for variation in the selenium content of foods is that the selenium content of soil can vary tremendously—from areas in South Dakota where animals grazing on fields will die within days of selenium toxicity to areas in New Zealand where animals will die of deficiency unless supplemented. Even within the United States, the selenium content of corn can vary by as much as 200-fold due to differences in soil levels (Ullrey, 1981). This, in turn, is reflected in an approximately 50-fold variation in selenium content of swine muscle. Because of the complexities of the food distribution system within most countries, it is extremely difficult to know the ultimate source of any particular slice of bread or cut of meat. Hunter and colleagues (1990) have provided evidence that the calculation of selenium intake is unlikely to provide useful information on intake of this element; calculations of dietary selenium intake (based on a version of the questionnaire used to estimate beta-carotene intake in the example noted previously) were not correlated with nail selenium levels even though the use of selenium supplements within the range of normal dietary intakes exhibited a clear dose–response relationship with nail levels.

Beta-carotene and selenium provide clear contrasts of nutrients for which the assumption of constant nutrient content of foods is and is not reasonable; it is not entirely clear where other nutrients lie on this spectrum. For many of the major constituents of foods that are reasonably stable under typical preservation, storage, and cooking conditions, such as the primary dietary fats, carbohydrate fractions, and calcium, the assumption of constant nutrient content is probably not seriously violated.

Recognizing that all specimens or examples of any particular food do not necessarily have the same nutrient content, the designers of major food composition databases have attempted to provide increasingly specific information. For example, values are provided for specific cuts of meat, specific methods of food preparation, and specific manufacturers of prepared food. In some cases, this provides improved calculations of nutrient intake; if detailed food information is available, this would usually require data on a meal-by-meal basis. Unfortunately, a high degree of specificity is often not obtainable in epidemiologic applications in which food intake data represent extended periods of time. In the context of validation studies (see Chapter 6), however, the maximal degree of specificity is generally desirable.

Uncertainty regarding the constancy of the nutrient content of food raises the issue of how this assumption can be evaluated. One classic method of evaluating assumptions used in the calculation of nutrient intake is to collect replicate food samples for single meals or 24-hour periods, meaning that for each food eaten an identical serving is placed in a container for analysis. Nutrient intake is then estimated by calculation from the foods that were recorded as eaten and also by chemical analysis of a homogenate of the duplicate meals consumed by each subject. For example, Moser and Allen (1984) compared zinc analyses of three 24-hour duplicate meals with calculated intakes among 36 lactating or nonlactating postpartum women; calculated and analyzed mean values were nearly identical. Although this method can be very useful for identifying serious problems, the correlations between calculated and chemically analyzed intakes are likely to be overly optimistic as the differences between subjects based on single 24-hour periods will be much larger than the true long-term differences between subjects (see Chapter 3). Some of the differences in nutrient intake between subjects are due to differences in total food intake, and thus adjustment for total caloric intake reduces between-subject variation and, therefore, correlation coefficients even further. For example, it is possible that identical mean values and positive correlations would be seen for selenium using this method due to large intakes of meat, dairy products, or overall food intake on some days, even though other evidence indicates that calculated intakes are unlikely to be useful in realistic epidemiologic settings.

A second and more rigorous method of evaluating the assumption of constant nutrient composition of foods is to examine the correlation of calculated nutrient intakes with a biochemical indicator of nutrient intake, such as for beta-carotene as discussed in the previous example. For a calculated intake and biochemical indicator to be correlated requires that intake of foods be accurately reported, the nutrient content of the foods be known accurately and be constant within specific foods, the nutrients be similarly bioavailable from the different foods, and the level of the biochemical indicator be responsive to nutrient intake over the range and time frame being studied. Thus, the demonstration of a positive correlation provides evidence that the nutrient composition is reasonably accurate and constant within foods. Failure to observe a correlation, however, does not imply that composition data are faulty because any of the other assumptions may not have been met. As discussed later, responsive biochemical indicators of intake do not exist for most nutrients of major interest, thus seriously limiting the application of this approach.

Given the lack of more direct information, judgments about the appropriateness of calculated intakes often needs to be made indirectly based on knowledge about the stability of nutrients and their variability in foods. For example, folic acid tends to be less stable during preservation, processing, and cooking than many nutrients, thus raising uncertainty about the validity of calculated values. Without additional data about validity, the findings of epidemiologic studies of folic acid intake would need to be interpreted cautiously because absence of an association with disease could be due to large variation in the nutrient content of specific foods.

The calculation of nutrient intakes from information on food consumption requires two resources: the food composition data and the computer software to perform the calculations (hand calculation now being obsolete). These are discussed separately.

Food composition information is needed for two general purposes in epidemiologic studies. The first is for the analysis of traditional open-ended dietary data collected by short-term recall or meal-by-meal recording methods (see Chapter 4). This requires an extensive and comprehensive database because nutrient values are needed for all foods that might be reported by subjects. In contrast, most epidemiologic studies employ a structured questionnaire consisting of not more than 100 or 200 food items (see Chapter 5). To compute nutrient intakes based on information obtained with such a questionnaire, a customized nutrient database must be created to provide values for each nutrient to be computed for every food on the questionnaire. Investigators need to compile this information, often by using an available comprehensive database supplemented with other sources of information as needed. Whether an existing comprehensive or a custom database is used, several features need to be considered:

1. Most fundamentally, food composition data should be as accurate and as up to date as possible. Not only are technologic advances making improved chemical analyses possible, but also food composition itself changes over time due to selective plant and animal breeding and alterations in preservation and processing techniques. New foods and formulations are constantly being added to the market. Nutrient calculation for long-term studies requires the use of procedures for ongoing database maintenance and time-specific codes (Buz-

zard et al., 1995) that takes into consideration changes in the marketplace and food preparation.

2. Uniformity in the determination of nutrient composition is desirable as it is important that, for any one nutrient, the same method is used to determine the nutrient values for all foods.

3. Comprehensiveness in the scope of foods is particularly important when the database is used to analyze open-ended data on food intake, as all foods reported must be assigned nutrient values.

4. Specificity may be especially important for some nutrients that are affected by manufacturing or processing. For example, if sodium intake is of particular interest when analyzing open-ended food intake information, considerable specificity may be needed regarding brands and types of processed foods that differ with respect to sodium content.

5. Completeness in nutrient values is of extreme importance when a database is used to compute nutrient intakes; no food should have a blank value because this will effectively be counted as zero when summarizing intake of that nutrient for a person. This issue represents a continuing challenge for persons maintaining a database because, even for a single nutrient, food analysis laboratories rarely conduct measurements of all foods that are listed in any single database. For example, cholesterol measurements may well not be made on both fried eggs and poached eggs, although these may be listed as separate items in the database. Some database systems have not been willing to make the reasonable assumption that cholesterol content is the same in both these items, even though only one has been analyzed directly. Although blank values may be perfectly appropriate for listings of food composition that are purely for reference purposes, this is not tolerable in the case of computerized databases that are used to calculate intakes. An intelligently imputed value based on analy-

ses of similar foods is almost always a better approximation to truth than a zero value.

6. Comprehensiveness in the nutrients for which values are provided is a highly desirable feature. No database can be truly complete because technology continually provides additional ways to subdivide and characterize the components of our food supply. Because it is rarely appropriate to examine only a few nutrients in isolation in epidemiologic studies, a database should provide the ability to calculate simultaneously at least the major components of our food, in addition to any minor components of particular research interest.

The use of quality-control procedures is essential for reducing the potential for error and identifying errors that occur inadvertently in maintaining a comprehensive nutrient database (Buzzard et al., 1995). Every nutrient value and other data elements in the database should be carefully documented so that the source of information can be verified whenever desired.

Specific Sources of Food Composition Data

In constructing a food composition database for a specific application, it is typically necessary to use multiple sources of information (Schakel et al., 1988). For example, to compile values for the questionnaire used in a prospective study among U.S. nurses (Willett et al., 1987), nutrient information was obtained from several governmental and commercial sources, approximately 15 different manufacturers, and 27 journal articles; this list continues to grow as the scope of nutrients computed increases. Available sources of food composition data include the following:

1. *United States Department of Agriculture (USDA) publications.* The USDA provides comprehensive and up-to-date information on food composition. This resource is almost always the starting point for any specific database in the United States; an outline of available

documents is included in Table 2–1. The central publication is *Composition of Foods—Raw, Processed, Prepared*, Agricultural Handbook No. 8 (U.S. Department of Agriculture, 1963). This is published as a series of revised sections with updated values for one or two food groups released annually. This information is also available in electronic format (e.g., Nutrient Data Base for Standard Reference, Release 11, 1997; available from the National Technical Information Service, U.S. Department of Commerce, Springfield, VA 22161, or on the internet at http://www. ars.usda.gov). A current listing of publications and datasets of food composition available from the USDA can be obtained from the USDA Bulletin Board on the Internet: http://www.inform. umd.edu/EdRes/Topic/AgrEnv/USDA. The USDA has also made most data sources accessible on the World Wide Web: http://www.nal.usda.gov/fnic/ foodcomp.

2. *Non-USDA and international food composition tables* (see Table 2–2). A variety of food composition databases have been published by other U.S. governmental units or commercial establishments, but many may not be regularly updated. Bowes and Church's Food Values for Portions Commonly Consumed (Bowes et al., 1994) is regularly maintained. Relatively few countries have food composition data resources that are as extensive as those provided by the USDA. Particularly for small or developing countries, resources may not be adequate to maintain a comprehensive local database, and it may often be necessary to import values from other sources, such as the USDA or regional databases. In many cases, this may be reasonable; for example, there is little reason to believe that an apple in India that looks like an apple from the United States will have substantially different nutrient composition. However, a typical portion of beef in East Africa is likely to be much leaner

Table 2–1. Sources of food composition data in the United States published by the USDA[a]

1. Composition of Foods—Raw, Processed, and Prepared. Agricultural Handbook No. 8, 1963. (Revised sections for several specific food groups are published annually.)
2. Computerized Nutrient Data Set: Nutrient Data Base for Standard Reference, Release 11, 1997. (Available from the National Technical Information Service, U.S. Department of Commerce, Springfield, VA 22161, or on the internet at http://www.ars.usda.gov.)
3. Computerized Data Sets Used To Create Release 7 of the USDA Nutrient Data Base for Individual Food Intake Surveys. (Includes Primary Nutrient Data Set for USDA Nationwide Food Consumption Surveys; USDA Table of Nutrient Retention Factors; Recipe File; Documentation for Data Sets. Available from the National Technical Information Service.)
4. Nutritive value of American foods in common units. Agriculture Handbook No. 456, 1975. (The nutrient values are out of date, but information on common units may be useful.)
5. Nutritive value of foods. Home and Garden Bulletin No. 72, revised, 1985
6. Iron content of food. Home Economics Research Report No. 45, 1983
7. Pantothenic acid, vitamin B_6, and vitamin B_{12} in foods. Home Economics Research Report No. 36, 1969
8. Sugar content of selected foods: individual and total sugars. Home Economics Research Report No. 48, 1987
9. Supplement to Provisional Table, Folacin Content of Foods, 1979
10. Table of Amino Acids in Fruits and Vegetables, 1983
11. The Fortification of Foods: A Review Agriculture Handbook No. 598, 1982
12. The Sodium Content of Your Food. Home and Garden Bulletin No. 233, 1980
13. Trans fatty acid data (available on the USDA Bulletin Board)
14. USDA-NCI Carotenoid Food Composition Data Base: Version I, 1993
15. Provisional tables on the food contents of specific nutrients are published periodically. These include omega-3 fatty acids, dietary fiber, fatty acids and cholesterol, selenium, sugar, vitamin D, and vitamin K.

[a]Available from Superintendent of Documents, U.S. Government Printing Office, Washington, DC 20402.

For current listing of specific documents, see http://www. nal.usda.gov/fnic/usda.

Table 2–2. Examples of sources of food composition data in other countries

Country/region	Reference
Australia	Cashel, K., R. English, J. Lewis. (1989). Composition of Foods Australia. Canberra: Nutrition Section, Department of Community Services and Health, Australian Government Publishing Service. In English
Canada	Health and Welfare Canada. Canadian nutrient file. Canadian Government Publishing Centre, Ottawa K1A 0S9, 1992
China	Ershow, A. G., and K. Wong-Chen (1990). Chinese food composition tables. An annotated translation of the 1981 edition, published by the Institute of Nutrition and Food Hygiene, Chinese Academy of Preventive Medicine, Beijing. J Food Composition 3:191–434. In English
France	Ostrowske, Z. L., and M. C. Josse (1985). Les Aliments—Tables des valeurs nutritives. Paris: ADE et Ville de Paris. In French
Germany	Souci, S. W., W. Fachmann, and H. Kraut (1989). Food Composition and Nutrition Tables, 1989/90. Stuttgart: Wissenschaftliche Verlagsgesellschaft mgH. In English
Japan	Resources Council, Science and Technology Agency. Standard tables of food composition in Japan. 1992. In Japanese with English translation
Mexico	Hernandez, M., A. Chavez, and H. Bourges (1980). Valor nutritivo de los alimentos Mexicanos—Tablas de uso practico. Publication L-12, 8th ed. Nutrition Division, National Institute of Nutrition. In Spanish
Near East	Polacchi, W. et al. (1982). Food composition tables for the Near East. FAO, Rome, and USDA, Washington, DC
The Netherlands	Kommissie Uniforme Codering Voedingsenquetes (UCV). UCV Tabel: Uitgebreide voedingsmiddelentabel 1985 [extended food composition tables]. Voorlichtingsbureau voor de Voeding, 's-Gravenhage, 1985. In Dutch
Pacific Islands	Dignan, C. A., B. A. Burlingame, J. M. Arthur, R. J. Quigley, and G. C. Milligan (1994). The Pacific Islands Food Composition Tables. South Pacific Commission, New Zealand Institute for Crop & Food Research Ltd—A Crown Research Institute, Nd International Network of Food Data Systems. Programme Leader, New Zealand Institute for Crop & Food Research Limited, Private Bag 11030, Palmerston North, New Zealand. In English
South Africa	Gouws, E., and M. L. Langenhoven (1986). NRIND Food Composition Tables, 2nd edition. National Research Institute for Nutritional Diseases Publications Unit, Medical Research Council, P.O. Box 70, Tygerberg 7505, South Africa. In English
United Kingdom	Holland, B., A. A. Welch, I. D. Unwin, D. H. Buss, A. A. Paul, and D. A. T. Southgate (1991). McCance and Widdowson's The Composition of Foods, 5th edition. Ministry of Agriculture, Fisheries and Food and The Royal Society of Chemistry, The Royal Society of Chemists, Distribution Centre, Letchworth, Herts SG6 1HN, England

than in the United States, so that careful judgment must be exercised when using external data. INFOODS, through United Nations support, has available on the Internet the International Directory of Food Composition Tables (http://www.crop.cri.nz/foodinfo/infoods/infoods. html), which lists several hundred publications related to food composition around the world. Some examples are included in Table 2–2.

3. *Manufacturers' data.* In some instances information obtained from food manufacturers is useful. Data on specific brands of breakfast cereals may be particularly important because of extensive fortification with vitamins and minerals and because of their regular use by many persons. Names and addresses of U.S. food manufacturers are published periodically (*Thomas Grocery Register*, published by Thomas Publishing Co., New York, NY).

4. *Professional journals.* For some nutrients that have not yet been incorporated into the major databases, it may be nec-

essary to use primary published sources of food analyses.

Nutrient Computation Systems

The computation of nutrient intakes from food consumption information requires both a computerized food composition database and the software to perform these calculations. The coding and entry of open-ended food information, such as that obtained from a short-term recall, has been an extremely tedious and expensive process requiring a highly trained person, preferably a dietitian. In the past, every food was looked up in a book or list to obtain a code number, which was then entered into a computer. A unit, such an ounce or cup, was then designated and a multiplier was entered. Such time-consuming and error-prone procedures have rapidly become archaic with the availability of inexpensive computing resources. A large number of automated coding systems have been developed that allow direct entry of foods by name, avoiding the manual entering of numerical codes by the user (see Chapter 4).

The available choices in food composition databases and nutrient calculation systems are presently in a state of rapid evolution. Features of several of the larger and more commonly used systems that include both a database and some form of analysis software are included in Table 2–3. Some systems provide a software "shell" for nutrient calculations that can be used with other databases, which may be particularly useful internationally. The Nutrient Databank Directory provides extensive information about nutrient databank systems, including software programs (Smith, 1993). The 9th edition lists 38 software program and nutrient databases and is available for purchase.* Also, the Food and Nutrition Information Center (FNIC) of the U.S. Department of Agriculture's National Agricultural Library maintains an updated database of nutrition software, including many nutrient calculation programs. The contents of the FNIC database are available electronically and on disk. Users can request custom searches of the database at no charge.*

In choosing a nutrient computation system, all of the points noted previously regarding the database employed should be considered; Buzzard et al. (1991) have described these issues in detail. In addition, several factors related to the software should be considered:

1. The manual entry of coding numbers for foods should be avoided if possible; as discussed, coding should be provided as an automated feature, allowing the user to enter foods by name.
2. If the researcher intends to make modifications to the database, the system should have the capacity to add foods or nutrients of particular interest for a specific study and to update existing values.
3. The system should provide flexibility for different portion units so that the user does not have to convert manually various measures of volume or weight. Inclusion of food-specific units, such as a "slice" of bread or "medium" apple is helpful.
4. The system should provide an option to display nutrients calculated for each food as well as summaries for each meal or day.
5. The system should allow common recipes to be compiled and entered as a single item rather than re-entering each of the components of the recipe separately.
6. Transfer of data to other computers where the information will ultimately be used should be easily accommodated.

Although efficient systems for the analysis of open-ended dietary data are increas-

---

*Nutrient Databank Directory (9th edition, 1993), Alison Hall, Department of Nutrition and Dietetics, University of Delaware, Newark, DE 19715-3360.

*Food and Nutrition Information Center (FNIC), Room 304, 10301 Baltimore Blvd, Beltsville, MD 20705-2351; tel: 301-504-5719; tty 301-504-6856; fax: 301-504-6409; Internet: http://www.nal.usda.gov/fnic.

Table 2–3. Examples of nutrient computation systems

System name	Number of foods	Number of components per food	Special feature	Vendor
DINE Healthy	10,000	26	Software available for Macintosh, as well as for DOS and Windows operating systems	DINE Systems, Inc., Amherst, NY; tel: 800-688-1848; fax: 716-688-2505
Food Intake Analysis System (FIAS)	7,200	30	Uses the USDA Survey Database & Recipe Calculation methodology	University of Texas, Houston: tel: 713-500-9775; fax: 713-500-9329
Food Processor	14,000	100	800 telephone no. available for no-cost technical support	ESHA Research, Salem, OR; tel: 503-585-6242 or 800-659-3742; fax: 503-585-5543
Minnesota Nutrition Data System (NDS)	19,000	93	System prompts for required level of food description detail for each food item	University of Minnesota, Minneapolis; tel: 612-626-9450; fax: 612-626-9444
Nutritional Software Library (NSL III)	4,500	24	800 telephone no. available for no-cost technical support	Computrition, Inc., Chatsworth, CA; tel: 818-701-5544 or 800-222-4488; fax: 818-701-1702
Nutritionist IV	15,500	74	System allows users to customize their own reports	First DataBank, San Bruno, CA; tel: 800-633-3453; fax: 415-588-4003
WorldFood	1,816	49	Database of basic foods for worldwide use, especially for developing countries	University of California, Berkeley; tel: 510-643-7201; fax: 510-642-4566

ingly available, this does not reduce the need for careful training and monitoring of the personnel who collect and process the data.

SUMMARY

Diets of human populations are extremely complex. They can be viewed in several ways, including as intake of constituent chemicals (such as essential nutrients, nonnutritive components of foods, and contaminants) or as foods or food groups. Maximal insight into the relation between diet and disease will usually be obtained by examining diet both as constituents and as foods. Calculation of nutrients and other constituents requires a food composition database that should include a wide range of nutrients and that is complete and current.

REFERENCES

Adamson, R. H., and U. P. Thorgeirsson (1995). Carcinogens in foods: Heterocyclic amines and cancer and heart disease. *Adv Exp Med Biol 369*, 211–220.

Adlercreutz, H. (1990). Western diet and western diseases: Some hormonal and biochemical mechanisms and associations. *Scand J Clin Lab Invest 50 (suppl 201)*, 3–23.

Ames, B. N., R. Magaw, and L. S. Gold (1987). Ranking possible carcinogenic hazards. *Science 236*, 271–280.

Bowes, A., H. N. Church, and J. A. T. Pennington (1994). *Bowes and Church's Food Values of Portions Commonly Used*. Philadelphia, PA: J. B. Lippincott.

Busby, W. F., Jr., and G. N. Wogan (1984). Aflatoxins. In Searle, C. E. (ed). *Chemical Carcinogens*, 2nd edition, vol 2. Washington, DC: ACS Monograph 182, American Chemical Society, pp 945–1136.

Buzzard, I. M., K. S. Price, and R. A. Warren (1991). Considerations for selecting nutrient-calculation software: Evaluation of the nutrient database (editorial). *Am J Clin Nutr 54*, 7–9.

Buzzard, I. M., S. F. Schakel, and J. Ditter-Johnson (1995). Quality control in the use of food and nutrient databases for epidemiologic studies. In Greenfield, R. (ed): *Quality and Accessibility of Food-Related Data*. Arlington, VA: AOAC International, pp 241–252.

Chug-Ahuja, J. K., J. M. Holden, M. R. Forman, A. R. Mangels, G. R. Beecher, and E. Lanza (1993). The development and application of a carotenoid database for fruits, vegetables, and selected multicomponent foods. *J Am Dietet Assoc 93*, 318–323.

Doll, R., and R. Peto (1981). The causes of cancer: Quantitative estimates of avoidable risks of cancer in the United States today. *JNCI 66*, 1191–1308.

Gerhardsson de Verdier, M., U. Hagman, R. K. Peters, and G. Steineck (1991). Meat, cooking methods and colorectal cancer: A case-referent study in Stockholm. *Int J Cancer 49*, 520–525.

Graham, S., H. Dayal, M. Swanson, A. Mittelman, and G. Wilkinson (1978). Diet in the epidemiology of cancer of the colon and rectum. *JNCI 61*, 709–714.

Herman, C., T. Adlercreutz, B. R. Goldin, S. L. Gorbach, K. A. Hockerstedt, S. Watanabe, E. K. Hamalainen, M. H. Markkanen, T. H. Makela, and K. T. Wahala (1995). Soybean phytoestrogen intake and cancer risk. *J Nutr 125 (suppl)*, 757S–770S.

Hunter, D. J., J. S. Morris, C. G. Chute, E. Kushner, G. A. Colditz, M. J. Stampfer, F. E. Speizer, and W. C. Willett (1990). Predictors of selenium concentration in human toenails. *Am J Epidemiol 132*, 114–122.

Jacobson, H. N., and J. L. Stanton (1986). Pattern analysis in nutrition research. *Clin Nutr 5*, 249–253.

Kennedy, A. R. (1995). The evidence for soybean products as cancer preventive agents. *J Nutr 125 (suppl)*, 733S–743S.

Kolonel, L. N., C. N. Yoshizawa, and J. H. Hankin (1988). Diet and prostatic cancer: A case–control study in Hawaii. *Am J Epidemiol 127*, 999–1012.

Lands, W. E. M. (1986). *Fish and Human Health*. Orlando: Academic Press, Inc.

Le Marchand, L., J. H. Hankin, L. N. Kolonel, and L. R. Wilkins (1991). Vegetable and fruit consumption in relation to prostate cancer risk in Hawaii: A reevaluation of the effect of dietary beta-carotene. *Am J Epidemiol 133*, 215–219.

Mangels, A. R., J. M. Holden, G. R. Beecher, M. R. Forman, and E. Lanza (1993). Carotenoid content of fruits and vegetables: An evaluation of analytic data. *J Am Dietet Assoc 93*, 284–296.

Manousos, O., N. E. Day, D. Trichopoulos, F. Gerovassilis, A. Tzanou, and A. Polychronopoulou (1983). Diet and colorectal cancer: A case–control study in Greece. *Int J Cancer 32*, 1–5.

McCann, S. E., E. Randall, J. R. Marshall, S. Graham, M. Zielezny, and J. L. Freudenheim (1994). Diet and diversity and risk of colon cancer in western New York. *Nutri Cancer 21*, 133–141.

Mertz, W. (1981). The essential trace elements. *Science 213*, 1332–1338.

Mertz, W. (1984). Food and nutrients. *J Am Dietet Assoc 84*, 769–770.

Morris, J. N., J. W. Marr, and D. G. Clayton (1977). Diet and heart: A postscript. *Br Med J 2*, 1307–1314.

Moser, P. B., and D. Allen (1984). Zinc intakes of lactating and non-lactating women. Analyzed vs. calculated values. *J Am Diet Assoc 84*, 42–46.

Peto, R., R. Doll, J. D. Buckley, and M. B. Sporn (1981). Can dietary beta-carotene materially reduce human cancer rates? *Nature 290*, 201–208.

Randall, E., J. R. Marshall, J. Brasure, and S. Graham (1992). Dietary patterns and colon cancer in western New York. *Nutr and Cancer 18*, 265–276.

Schakel, S. F., Y. A. Sievert, and I. M. Buzzard (1988). Sources of data for developing and maintaining a nutrient database. *J Am Diet Assoc 88*, 1268–1271.

Seddon, J. M., U. A. Ajani, R. D. Sperduto, R. Hiller, N. Blair, T. C. Burton, M. D. Farber, E. S. Gragoudas, J. Haller, D. T. Miller, L. A. Yannuzzi, and W. C. Willett for the Eye Disease Case–Control Study Group (1994). Dietary carotenoids, vitamins A, C, and E, and advanced age-related macular degeneration. *JAMA 272*, 1413–1420.

Smith, J. L. (1993). *Nutrient Databank Directory*. Newark, DE: University of Delaware.

Steinmetz, K. A., and J. D. Potter (1991). Vegetables, fruit, and cancer. II. Mechanisms. *Cancer Causes Control 2*, 427–442.

Sugimura, T. (1986). Studies on environmental chemical carcinogenesis in Japan. *Science 233*, 312–318.

Troll, W., K. Frenkel, and R. Wiesner (1984). Protease inhibitors as anticarcinogens. *JNCI 73*, 1245–1250.

U.S. Department of Agriculture (1963). *Composition of Foods—Raw, Processed, and Prepared*. Agricultural Handbook No. 8, Washington, DC: U.S. Government Printing Office.

Ullrey, D. E. (1981). Selenium in the soil-plant-food chain. In Spallhotz, J. E., et al. (eds): *Selenium in Biology and Medicine*. Westport, CT: AVI Publishing, pp 176–191.

Watanabe, S., E. K. Hamalainen, M. H. Markkanen, T. H. Makela, and K. T. Wahala et al. (1995). Soybean phytoestrogen intake and cancer risk. *J Nutr 125 (suppl)*, 757S–770S.

Wattenberg, L. W., and W. D. Loub (1978). Inhibition of polycyclic aromatic hydrocarbon-induced neoplasia by naturally occurring indoles. *Cancer Res 38*, 1410–1413.

Welsh, S. O., and R. M. Marston (1982). Review of trends in food use in the United States, 1909 to 1980. *J Am Dietet Assoc 81*, 120–128.

Willett, W. C., M. J. Stampfer, G. A. Colditz, B. A. Rosner, C. H. Hennekens, and F. E. Speizer (1987). Dietary fat and the risk of breast cancer. *N Engl J Med 316*, 22–28.

Witteman, J. C., W. C. Willett, M. J. Stampfer, G. A. Colditz, F. M. Sacks, F. E. Speizer, B. Rosner, and C. H. Hennekens (1989). A prospective study of nutritional factors and hypertension among U.S. women. *Circulation 80*, 1320–1327.

3

Nature of Variation in Diet

For most epidemiologic applications, long-term diet, rather than intake on any specific day or small number of days, is the conceptually relevant exposure parameter. The period of time may be years in studies of factors that affect atherogenesis or cancer, or it may be a critical period of a few weeks in studies of nutrients that influence fetal malformation. In studies of physiologic intermediates, such as plasma lipids or endogenous hormone excretion, dietary intake during several days, weeks, or months may be of interest. Because we are usually interested in long-term diet, an understanding of day-to-day variation in dietary intake is essential in choosing an appropriate method to assess diet and to interpret data collected by various approaches.

A central feature of the dietary intake of free-living individuals is variation from day to day superimposed on an underlying consistent pattern. (If there were no element of consistency, and daily intake were a completely random event, then there would be no hope of measuring the effects of nutri-

ents epidemiologically.) A number of factors, such as day of the week or season, may contribute to daily variation in dietary intake in a systematic manner. The magnitude of these influences is largely determined by cultural and ecologic factors. For example, it is traditional for many American families to have unusually large meals on Sunday. In countries without extensive food preservation and transportation systems, seasonal effects are relatively strong (Brown et al., 1982); for example, in some parts of the world much of the vitamin A is consumed during a limited portion of the year when certain fruits and vegetables are available. In industrialized societies, seasons make a relatively small contribution to variation in nutrient intake (van Staveren et al., 1986a); however, intakes of some fruits and vegetables may vary substantially according to the time of year (Ziegler et al., 1987). Although there is evidence that total caloric intake varies with the menstrual cycle (Dalvit, 1981), most of the variation in an individual's diet is without an obvious pattern. This apparently random variation is largely due to true variation in the food that is eaten but also has a component of measurement error, meaning error in the measurement of food intake on a given day. Because the topic of measurement error is discussed in detail in other chapters, this source of variation is ignored for the moment.

The degree of random variation differs according to nutrient. Total energy (caloric) intake is quite well regulated by physiologic mechanisms and thus has the least day-to-day variation among nutrients. For macronutrients, because of their large contribution to total caloric intake, there is a somewhat constrained possibility for large degrees of variation. As micronutrients tend to be concentrated in certain foods, intake can be very low or very high, depending on food choices for that day. The daily variation in total fat and total dietary vitamin A intake for three women (one from each of the high, middle, and low quintiles of the 28-day average intakes of these nutrients) is displayed in Figure 3–1. The data for these and the other examples are based on diaries provided by 194 Boston-area women who recorded their daily food intake during four 1-week periods over 1 year (Willett et al., 1985). It can be appreciated that on any single day, the individual intakes overlap considerably, even though on the average they are distinct. It can be seen that variability is greater for vitamin A than for total fat and is also related to the level of intake.

The consumption of a specific nutrient for a single individual can be described as a frequency distribution of daily intakes with a mean and standard deviation (Fig. 3–2); the individual's *true* intake can be considered as the mean for a large number of days. In most epidemiologic investigations we are interested in measuring these true intakes for individual subjects. Collectively, these true individual intakes define a frequency distribution for the study population as a whole; this distribution characterizes the true population mean and stan-

dard deviation. Distributions for mean daily intakes of total calories, total fat, and vitamin A for the group of 194 women are shown in Figure 3–3. This figure closely describes the true between-person variation for this population as the day-to-day fluctuations will be dampened or canceled out by averaging many days for each person, in this example 28 days.

In reality, it is rarely possible to measure a large number of days of dietary intake for an individual subject; therefore, intakes during a sample of one or several days are usually measured. The effect of this sampling on the apparent distribution of intakes for individual subjects will be to artificially increase the standard deviation (i.e., to broaden the tails of the distribution). This effect can be appreciated by considering that individuals with the highest true intakes have some days when their intake is higher than their long-term average, and individuals with the lowest true intake have days when their intake is below their long-term mean. Thus, the observed distribution has extreme values that are higher and lower than any of the true long-term averages for any subject. To graphically demonstrate the effect of sampling a small number of days for an individual on the apparent between-person distribution of dietary intake, data from the 194 Boston-area women who each recorded daily food intake during four 1-week periods are shown in Figure 3–4.

The effect is fairly dramatic. In data based on a single day per subject, those at the 90th percentile were consuming 3.0 times as much fat and 6.4 times as much total vitamin A (excluding supplements) as were those at the 10th percentile. Using data based on 1 week of intake, these ratios were 2.2 for fat and 3.0 for vitamin A. The change observed using a 4-week sample was less striking; the ratios were 1.9 for fat and 2.5 for vitamin A, suggesting that a further increase in the number of days per subject would have a minimal effect on the distribution. The distortion of true between-person variation in dietary

A

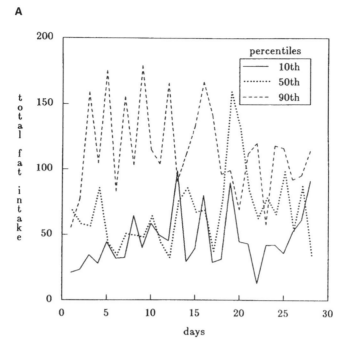

B

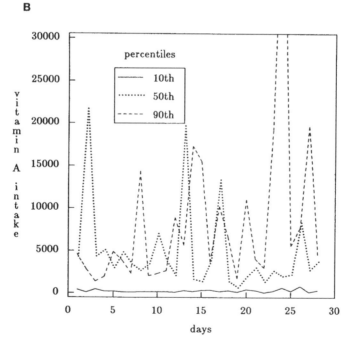

Figure 3–1. Daily intakes for three women at the 10th, 50th, and 90th percentiles of distribution for total fat intake in grams (A) and vitamin A intake in international units (B). See text for details.

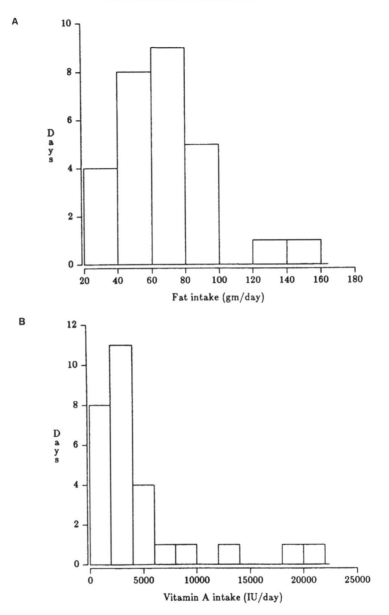

Figure 3–2. Frequency distribution of daily intakes of total fat (A) and vitamin A (B) for one woman (the women at the 50th percentile in Fig. 3–1). For this person, 28 days of intake are displayed; the mean of these days can be considered as the true intake for that person.

intake resulting from the use of a single day of dietary intake per subject is not purely an academic matter. National nutrition surveys have traditionally employed only a single 24-hour recall per subject; thus many major reports of the distributions of dietary intake are extremely misleading. For example, it is not really plausible that 5% of U.S. men aged 25–34 years consume less than 1,250 calories per day and that 10% consume more than 4,000 calories per day, as suggested by a publication based on the first National Health and Nutrition Survey (NHANES I)

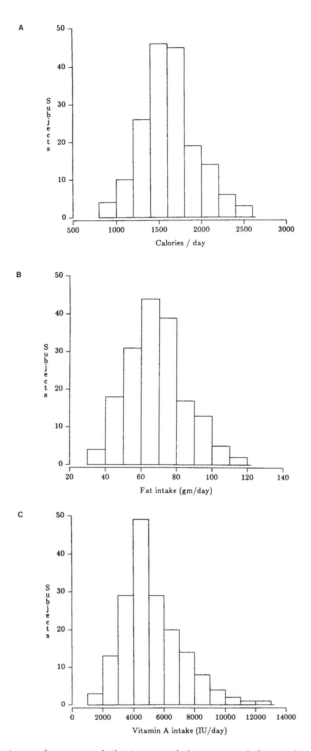

Figure 3–3. Distributions of average daily intakes (based on 28 days per person) for calories (A), total fat (B), and vitamin A (C) for 194 women. Because the average of a large number of days is used for each woman, these distributions closely approximate the true between-person variation for this group of women.

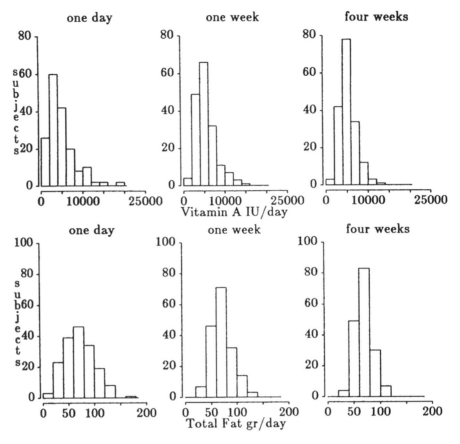

Figure 3–4. Effect of sampling 1 day, 7 days, or 28 days per subject on the observed distribution of fat and vitamin A intakes. Data are based on diet records provided by 194 women.

(U.S. Department of Health, 1979). Distributions for micronutrients tend to be even more seriously distorted due to their greater day-to-day variation.

The variation in daily intake of specific nutrients has been studied formally by Beaton and colleagues (1979, 1983), Liu and colleagues (1978), Rush and Kristal (1982), Sempos and colleagues (1985), Hunt and colleagues (1983), and Tarasuk and Beaton (1991) using analysis of variance techniques. In this approach, the daily nutrient intake is the dependent (outcome) variable, and explanatory variables are the independent variables. Because within-person intake is being examined, at least 2 days of information is needed for each person. The data are arrayed as shown in Table 3–1, with repeated measurements for persons considered as separate "records."

Data are analyzed using a random effects (repeated measures) model of the form:

$$\text{Nutrient } Y_{ijk} = \mu + \text{subject}_i + \text{factor } X_{ij} + \text{day of week}_{ijk} + \varepsilon_{ijk}. \quad (3\text{-}1)$$

In this model, the long-term average intake can vary between subjects, but within subjects daily diet can be influenced by specific identifiable variables denoted by factor X_{ij} such as season and day of the week. The error term (ε_{ijk}) represents the random within-person variance, that is, the day-to-day variance within a person not explained by the other independent variables.

Among a group of adult men and

Table 3–1. Data arrayed for analysis of variance (ANOVA) using the model described in Equation (3-1)

Nutrient (Y)	Person	Factor X	Day of week
Value 1	1	1	1
Value 2	1	1	2
Value 3	1	2	1
Value 4	1	2	2
Value 5	2	1	1
Value 6	2	1	2
Value 7	2	2	1
Value 8	2	2	2
Value 9	3	1	1
Value 10	3	1	2

women, Beaton and colleagues (1979) found that the within-person (residual) and between-person factors were the major contributors to variance for all nutrients examined (Tables 3–2 and 3–3). Days of the week (with intakes higher for Sundays) explained a small portion of variance for women but not for men. Different interviewers and sequence of days of data collection, however, made negligible contributions. Thus, dietary intake could be reasonably well expressed by the simple model where ε represents the day-to-day variation:

$$\text{Nutrient } Y = \mu + \text{subject}_i + \varepsilon. \quad (3\text{-}2)$$

For total caloric intake, the within-person variance was approximately equal to the between-person variance, but for specific nutrients the ratio of within-person to between-person variance was greater than 1; for polyunsaturated fat, cholesterol, and most micronutrients the within-person variance was much greater. When nutrient intakes were considered in relation to total energy intake, expressed as a percentage of total calories, the differences between persons decreased so that the relative importance of the within-person component of variance was even larger, ranging from approximately 30%

to 90% of total variance for the nutrients examined.

As pointed out by Beaton and coworkers, the pattern of high within-person variation in nutrient intakes is largely cultural, and these findings may not necessarily apply to other populations. In other U.S. studies, however, similarly high within-person variation has been observed (Table 3–4). Similar degrees of within-person variation were also seen across age and gender groupings in a large representative sample of the U.S. population (Table 3–5).

The contribution of variable intervals of time between repeated measurements to the variation in dietary intake deserves further consideration. In one unpublished analysis among postmenopausal women, subsequently analyzed in more detail by Freedman et al. (1991), we observed less within-person variation when the days were consecutive than when separated by several months. This could have important implications for study design, as misleading estimates of within-person variation may be obtained using consecutively collected diet recalls or records. In addition, the seasonal contribution to variance has not been explored carefully. As mentioned previously, seasonal variation in diet may not be large within the United States and other industrialized countries. In one study, the correlations between 1-week diet records did not vary appreciably when they were collected at intervals of 3, 6, 9, or 12 months (Willett et al., 1985). Year-to-year variation was examined by Hunt and colleagues (1983); for most nutrients the contribution was minor at a 1-year interval in comparison with day-to-day variation.

A basic assumption underlying the analytic methods described previously is that the within-person component of variation is random, that is, for one person, the deviation from that person's long-term average intake on 1 day is independent from the deviation on the previous day. This assumption has been questioned by el Lozy (1983), who pointed out that humans are subject to homeostatic mechanisms (prob-

Table 3–2. Relative sources of variation for daily nutrient intake, not adjusted for energy intake (subjects, between-person variation; residual, within-person variation)

Component of variance	Energy	Protein	Carbohydrate	Fat	SFA	MFA	PFA	Cholesterol
			Men					
Subjects	51.8%	39.2%	42.0%	48.6%	52.0%	42.8%	27.0%	25.7%
Sequence	0.4%	0	0	1.2%	0.4%	1.3%	1.1%	0.6%
Interviewer	0	0	0.5%	0	0	0	0	0
Day of week	0	0	0	0	0	0	0	0.6%
Residual	47.7%	60.8%	57.5%	50.2%	47.6%	55.9%	72.0%	73.2%
			Women					
Subjects	41.9%	38.9%	44.3%	38.3%	41.3%	37.4%	21.2%	19.1%
Sequence	0	0	0	0.3%	0	1.4%	1.3%	0
Interviewer	0	0	0	0	0	0	0	0.6%
Day of week	9.4%	5.3%	4.5%	5.7%	4.2%	5.2%	3.2%	4.6%
Residual	49.4%	55.7%	51.2%	55.7%	54.6%	56.1%	74.3%	75.8%

SFA, saturated fatty acid; MFA, monounsaturated fatty acids; PFA, polyunsaturated fatty acids.

From Beaton et al., 1979.

ably both physiologic and cultural) such that overeating on 1 day is likely to be followed by undereating the next. Morgan and colleagues (1987) formally explored the assumption of independence for consecutive days of dietary intake of energy, fat, vitamin A, and iron among 100 women. They found autocorrelations for many subjects, meaning that intake on 1 day added to the prediction of intake on the next above and beyond the mean intake for a person. A simple pattern, however, was not evident as persons with positive autocorrelations, indicating high intake on 1 day was associated with high intake on the next, were similar in number to those with negative autocorrelations, indicating that high intake on 1 day was associated

Table 3–3. Relative sources of variation for daily nutrient intake divided by energy intake (subjects, between-person variation; residual, within-person variation)

Component of variance	Protein	Carbo-hydrate	Fat	SFA	MFA	PFA	P:S ratio	Cholesterol mg/1,000 kcal	mg/1,000 g fat
				Men					
Subjects	13.7%	31.3%	20.8%	23.2%	19.8%	16.4%	20.2%	10.5%	6.2%
Sequence	0	0	0.5%	0	0	1.7%	0.6%	0	0
Interviewer	0.3%	0	0	0	0	0.8%	0	0	0
Day of week	0	0	0	0	0	0	0	0	0
Residual	86.0%	68.7%	78.7%	76.8%	80.2%	81.1%	79.2%	89.5%	93.8%
				Women					
Subjects	18.5%	37.2%	30.0%	33.9%	24.7%	8.8%	11.3%	12.8%	18.3%
Sequence	0	0	0	0	0	2.1%	1.7%	0.8%	0.8%
Interviewer	0	0.7%	1.3%	0	2.2%	0	0	1.4%	3.3%
Day of week	0	0	0	0	0	0.4%	0	0	0
Residual	81.5%	62.1%	68.7%	66.1%	73.1%	88.8%	87.0%	85.0%	77.6%

SPA, saturated fatty acids, MFA, monounsaturated fatty acids; PFA, polyunsaturated fatty acids.

From Beaton et al., 1979.

Table 3–4. Ratios of the within-person and between-person components of variance (S_w^2/S_b^2) for nutrient intakes observed in several North American studies

| Nutrient | Beaton et al. (1983) | | Liu et al. (1978) | | Hunt et al. (1983) | | Sempos et al. (1985) | NHS[c] | Rush et al. (1982) |
	20 Men	30 Women	181 Men[a]	318 Men[b]	25 Men	25 Women	151 Women	173 Women	225 Pregnant women
Energy (calories)	1.0	1.4	1.8	2.2	1.0	0.8	1.6	1.9	1.1
Protein	1.4	1.4	—	—	1.2	1.3	2.1	3.9	1.4
(% of calories)	5.8	4.0	—	—	2.3	1.9	—	2.7	—
Carbohydrate	1.7	1.4	—	—	2.0	1.2	—	1.2	1.2
(% of calories)	2.3	1.7	—	—	1.9	1.6	—	1.9	—
Total fat	1.2	1.7	—	—	1.2	0.9	—	2.8	1.2
(% of calories)	4.8	2.6	2.3	1.3	1.5	1.5	—	4.1	—
Saturated fat	1.0	1.4	—	—	2.2	1.7	—	2.8	—
(% of calories)	3.2	2.0	2.6	3.9	—	—	—	4.1	—
Polyunsaturated fat	2.9	4.0	—	—	3.5	2.2	5.0	5.0	—
(% of calories)	5.3	7.8	—	—	—	—	6.2	6.2	—
Cholesterol	3.6	4.4	3.8	1.8	5.6	4.2	6.8	6.8	—
per 1,000 calories	3.6	2.7	—	—	—	—	5.7	5.7	—
Vitamin C	4.0	2.3	—	—	2.3	2.8	2.3	2.0	—
Vitamin B$_6$	—	—	—	—	2.1	3.1	1.9	2.7	—
Folic acid	—	—	—	—	1.6	2.0	1.7	6.5	—
Vitamin A	>100	47.6	—	—	1.6	2.5	3.8	11.7	—
Iron	3.6	2.6	—	—	1.8	1.5	2.7	3.1	—
Calcium	2.6	2.3	—	—	1.1	1.7	1.1	2.2	1.0
Potassium	—	—	—	—	0.9	1.2	1.9	1.9	—
Zinc	—	—	—	—	2.7	1.7	2.2	11.7	—

[a] Japanese men in Japan.

[b] Japanese men in Hawaii.

[c] Unpublished data from analyses of diet records collected as part of the Nurses Health Study questionnaire validation study (Willet et al., 1985).

with lower intake on the next. Morgan and coworkers also observed, as suggested in Figure 3–1B, that those with higher mean intakes have greater within-person variation. For this reason, it may be useful to transform data, such as by taking the natural logarithm, before proceeding with analyses. Further investigation of the influence of 1 day's diet on intake on the following day may eventually refine our understanding of dietary variation, but is not likely to affect substantially the implications of data already published. The possible nonindependence of intake on

consecutive days, however, argues for sampling days at random intervals whenever possible.

NUMBER OF DAYS NECESSARY TO ESTIMATE TRUE INTAKE

A single day provides a poor estimate of a person's true long-term nutrient intake, but this estimate can be improved by using the average of multiple days of data for that person. The number of days needed has been discussed by Liu and coworkers (1978) and el Lozy (1983). Obviously, this

Table 3–5. U.S. mean nutrient intakes and within- and between-person coefficients of variation (CV %) in 1994

| | Children 1–5 years (n=1,065) | | | Children 6–11 years (n=629) | | | Men 20 + years (n=1,547) | | | Women 20+years (n=1,541) | | |
| | | CV (%) | | | CV (%) | | | CV (%) | | | CV (%) | |
	Mean	Within	Between	Mean	Within	Between	Mean	Within	Between	Mean	Within	Between
Energy (kcal)	1,434	28	26	1,687	30	35	2,403	33	31	1,587	31	28
Protein (g)	52	33	29	59	35	40	95	42	30	62	39	27
Total fat (g)	53	38	30	63	40	34	91	45	33	59	45	33
Saturated fat (g)	20	41	31	23	42	36	30	48	37	20	49	38
Monounsaturated fat (g)	20	41	33	24	44	37	35	48	33	22	47	38
Polyunsaturated fat (g)	9	50	37	11	54	29	18	63	33	12	63	34
Cholesterol (mg)	183	68	38	192	65	56	332	68	39	217	77	38
Carbohydrate (g)	192	29	28	228	32	38	288	35	34	202	33	30
Fiber (g)	10	43	35	11	49	47	18	46	39	13	46	37
Vitamin A (re)	774	102	50	870	76	41	1,131	108	59	957	179	53
Carotenes (re)	260	156	61	289	149	82	536	149	69	480	165	66
Vitamin E (α-te)	5	66	40	7	52	48	10	70	78	7	75	51
Vitamin C (mg)	92	67	48	94	69	50	107	94	68	87	78	59
Thiamin (mg)	1	37	27	1	40	38	2	45	36	1	46	33
Riboflavin (mg)	2	35	32	2	35	40	2	47	37	1	55	33
Niacin (mg)	14	37	33	17	41	36	28	46	35	18	47	29
Vitamin B$_6$ (mg)	1	43	30	1	45	46	2	48	44	1	52	33
Folate (μg)	195	52	34	228	51	51	298	59	53	215	63	41
Vitamin B$_{12}$ (μg)	4	200	50	4	95	45	6	162	36	4	368	41
Iron (mg)	11	47	33	13	46	44	18	48	43	12	53	35
Magnesium (mg)	187	31	28	206	35	41	321	37	32	224	35	29
Calcium (mg)	785	39	36	856	39	44	863	52	42	622	49	41
Potassium (mg)	1,942	34	28	2,063	35	40	3,138	35	31	2,258	34	28
Phosphorus (mg)	966	31	29	1,078	33	40	1,449	37	29	993	36	28
Zinc (mg)	7	44	31	9	43	40	14	62	39	9	56	32
Copper (mg)	1	52	30	1	40	31	1	50	33	1	71	27

Unpublished results of the USDA 1994 Continuing Survey of Food Intakes by Individuals (CSFII), U.S. Department of Agriculture, Agricultural Research Service, 1996, 1994 Continuing Survey of Food Intakes by Individuals and 1994 Diet and Health Knowledge Survey. CD-ROM, accession no. PB96-501010. National Technical Information Service, 5285 Port Royal Road, Springfield, VA 22161.

number depends on both the degree of accuracy that is needed and the variability of the nutrient in question.

Beaton and colleagues (1979) have provided a simple formula that can be rearranged to calculate the number of days needed to estimate a person's true intake with a specified degree of error:

$$n = (Z_\alpha CV_w/D_0)^2 \qquad (3\text{--}3)$$

where:

n = the number of days needed per person

Z_α = the normal deviate for the percentage of times the measured value should be within a specified limit

CV_w = the within-person coefficient of variation

D_0 = the specified limit (as a percentage of long-term true intake)

The within-person coefficient of variation (CV_w) can be obtained from the analysis of variance on repeated days of dietary intake; the square root of the within-person variance is the within-person standard deviation, and this value divided by the mean ($s/x \times 100\%$) is the within-person coefficient of variation. Values for x and the within-person and between-person coefficients of variation for a variety of nutrients are shown in Table 3–6, based on data provided by the 194 Boston-area women (Willett et al., 1985). Although these coefficients of variation may vary among different populations, they are remarkably similar to those reported for both men and women by Beaton and colleagues (1979) and thus probably are reasonable approximations for the general U.S. population.

Example: Suppose we wish to calculate the number of days needed to estimate a person's cholesterol intake to within 20% of their true mean 95% of the time. Thus $Z_\alpha = 1.96$ and CV_w from Table 3–6 is 62%:

$$n = (1.96 \times 62\%/20\%)^2 = 37 \text{ days}$$

Using such calculations, the number of days needed for the observed estimate of a person's intake to lie within a specified percentage of their true mean 95% of the time is given in Table 3–7. As can be appreciated, the days needed differ greatly for various nutrients. For many nutrients, obtaining a highly accurate estimate of individual intake by using repeated measurements is simply beyond practical possibilities in an epidemiologic study.

IMPLICATIONS FOR DEVELOPING COUNTRIES

The overwhelming importance of day-to-day variation in dietary intake has been described formally in affluent countries. Conventional wisdom suggests that diets of poor populations in nonindustrialized areas are homogeneous, so that within-person variation may not be a serious consideration for epidemiologic studies. This issue deserves examination, as 24-hour recalls and direct observations for a limited number of days are commonly employed in developing countries.

Despite conventional wisdom, it seems likely that important sources of variation in daily dietary intake do exist in the developing world, even though the number of foods available may be limited. Where economic resources are severely restricted, food intake is strongly linked to income so that even small economic differences are directly reflected in diet. This linkage would tend to increase between-person variation. As in industrialized countries, individual preferences and cultural taboos also contribute to between-person differences in diet. Day-to-day variation may be particularly large in developing countries if expensive foods can be afforded only irregularly. For example, if meat is only eaten twice per week and caloric intake on other days is primarily obtained from a carbohydrate staple, then protein intake may appear high

Table 3–6. Means and within-person and between-person coefficients of variation for daily intake of selected nutrients

| Nutrient | Mean | Coefficient of variation (%) | | | |
| | | Unadjusted nutrients | | Calorie-adjusted nutrients[a] | |
		Within	Between	Within	Between
Energy (kcal)	1,620	27.0	19.3		
Protein (g)	68.3	32.9	16.4	25.0	14.0
Total fat (g)	68.6	38.4	22.6	27.3	14.1
Monounsaturated fat (g)	24.2	42.5	23.6	27.8	13.1
Polyunsaturated fat (g)	11.1	64.2	28.3	47.3	20.2
Cholesterol (mg)	311	62.2	23.8	61.5	24.1
Carbohydrate (g)	169.8	29.9	26.5	18.7	13.5
Sucrose (g)	46.9	60.3	45.3	50.1	29.1
Crude fiber (g)	3.27	44.3	31.5	31.0	23.0
Vitamin B_1 (mg)	1.08	40.8	23.3	36.6	17.5
Vitamin B_2 (mg)	1.43	39.1	23.1	35.3	18.4
Vitamin B_6 (mg)	0.85	51.9	31.1	21.4	12.8
Vitamin C (mg)	106.5	55.3	38.6	54.9	37.6
Vitamin A (IU)	5,252	105.0	30.7	104.7	31.9
Iron (mg)	11.6	34.1	19.6	28.7	16.0
Calcium (mg)	616.9	41.9	28.3	36.1	21.7
Potassium (mg)	252.1	30.5	21.9	27.0	19.9

[a] Adjusted for caloric intake using regression analysis (see Chapter 11).

Data are based on four 1-week diet records completed by 194 U.S. women (Willett et al., 1985).

on some days and inadequate on others; that is, the within-person variance may be large. Within developing countries, lower economic status has been shown to be associated with higher within-person variability in energy and protein intake because poorer families are less able to adapt to temporary short-falls in income (Bhargava, 1992). If preservation and transportation facilities are lacking, the influence of season may be much stronger than in industrialized countries, again increasing within-

Table 3–7. Number of repeated days needed per person for 95% of observed values to lie within specified percent of true mean

| Nutrient | Within-person coefficient of variation | Number of days needed to lie within specified % of true means | | | |
		10%	20%	30%	40%
Total fat	38.4	57	14	6	4
Calorie-adjusted[a]	19.8	15	4	2	1
Cholesterol	62.2	149	37	17	9
Calorie-adjusted[a]	61.5	145	36	16	9
Sucrose	60.3	140	35	16	9
Calorie-adjusted[a]	50.1	96	24	11	6
Vitamin A	105.0	424	106	47	26
Calorie-adjusted[a]	104.7	424	106	47	26

[a] Adjusted for total caloric intake using regression analysis.

person variation. The components of variation in dietary factors have been formally examined in several recent studies in developing countries, and major within-person variation was observed (Torres et al., 1990; Bhargava, 1992; Romieu et al., 1997). After adjusting for age and sex, within-person variation in energy and protein intake in Indian and Filipino populations accounted for a substantially greater proportion of total variance than in the populations of affluent countries (Bhargava, 1992).

Data from a national nutrition survey in Bangladesh that included over 25,000 persons (Schaefer, 1981) provided a striking example of seasonal variation (Fig. 3–5). From November through March the intake of leafy green vegetables and ripe fruits is very low and is temporally associated with a striking rise in the percentage of the population with low or deficient serum vitamin A levels (less than 20 μg/dl). A single measurement of diet in June would obviously provide a very misleading representation of usual carotene intake for the population, as well as for most individuals.

The potentially large sources of between-person variation in diet in nonindustrialized countries may provide excellent opportunities for epidemiologic studies of the relation between diet and health. The similarly large potential for day-to-day variation means that careful, formal studies must be undertaken in such populations to measure the important components of variation, including seasonality, before embarking on any study based on a short-term measure of dietary intake.

EFFECTS OF RANDOM WITHIN-PERSON VARIATION ON MEASURES OF ASSOCIATIONS IN EPIDEMIOLOGIC STUDIES

Day-to-day variation in individual dietary intake has important implications for common measures of association in epidemiologic studies. If only one or a few days are measured, a subject's true long-term intake is likely to be misrepresented, that is, his or her dietary intake may be misclassified. This within-person variation, which may be regarded as random fluctuation above and below a person's true long-term average, can substantially distort correlation coefficients, regression coefficients, and relative risks. The general effect is to reduce the strength of associations.

The effect of within-person variation on the correlation between two normally distributed variables, x and y, has been discussed by Beaton and coworkers (1979), Liu and coworkers (1978), and Madonsky (1959). Within-person variation (i.e., random error) in either x or y will cause the observed correlation between these variables to be attenuated, meaning lower than the true correlation between x and y. Specifically, let us consider the classic error model

$$x = \mu_x + \varepsilon_x$$
$$y = \mu_y + \varepsilon_y$$

where $\varepsilon_x \sim N(0, \sigma^2)$, $\varepsilon_y \sim N(0, \sigma^2)$. In this model, x and y represent observed values for one person based on one or more (n_x, n_y) repeated measurements. The underlying mean values are μ_x and μ_y, that is, the mean values that would be observed if no measurement error were present (referred to as the true mean values), and ε_x and ε_y represent measurement error about the true mean values. If only a small number of measurements are made of x and y per individual, then the observed correlation (r_0, the correlation between x and y) is smaller than the true correlation (r_1, the correlation between μ_x and μ_y). The true correlation can also be interpreted as the correlation that would be observed if the average of many measurements were used to compute x and y for each person.

To estimate r_1 (the true correlation), two methods have been proposed. The first is to collect a large number of replicate measurements for each individual and use the

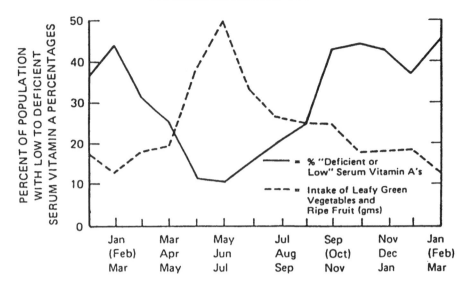

Figure 3–5. Seasonal variation of intake of leafy green vegetables and ripe fruit and in serum vitamin A levels in Bangladesh. (From Schaefer, 1981; reproduced with permission.)

average of these to approximate the true value of x and y for that subject in computing the correlation coefficient. For example, Liu and colleagues (1979) have demonstrated that 14 24-hour collections of urine per subject are necessary to obtain an observed correlation between sodium excretion and another variable (say blood pressure) that is within 10% of the true correlation. Similarly, Beaton and coworkers (1979) and Sempos and coworkers (1985) have shown that, for most nutrients, many days of dietary intakes are necessary to avoid a major attenuation in the correlation between a nutrient and another factor. An alternative way to estimate the true correlation (r_1) is to make a small number of repeated measurements per subject and use knowledge of the within-person variance of x and/or y to estimate the true correlation. This approach is discussed in Chapter 12.

van Staveren and colleagues (1986b) have provided an example of the degree to which the use of a single 24-hour recall can reduce the true correlation between dietary intake and another variable. They first used the average of 19 24-hour recalls per person to compute the correlation between lin-

oleic acid intake (expressed as the ratio of linoleic acid to saturated fatty acid intake) and the linoleic acid content of adipose tissue among 59 Dutch women. This correlation was 0.62. They then correlated each of the single days of linoleic acid intake alone, that is, one per person with the adipose linoleic acid levels; these correlations using individual 24-hour recalls were substantially lower, ranging from 0.14 to 0.50, with a median of 0.28.

Regression coefficients are attenuated by within-person variation in the independent variable. In an experimental feeding study, for example, it has been found that serum cholesterol increases 12 mg/100 ml for each increase of 100 mg/1,000 kcal in dietary cholesterol (Mattson et al., 1972). That is to say, the slope of the regression line relating these variables is about 0.12 mg/100 ml change in serum cholesterol per milligram per 1,000 kcal change in dietary cholesterol. By contrast, Beaton and colleagues (1979) used their data on the within-person variation of cholesterol intake to estimate that the observed regression coefficient would be only about 0.01, rather than 0.12, if a single day of cholesterol intake data were used to describe each subject's diet. The statistical relationship between the true and observed regression coefficients is discussed further in Chapter 12. In contrast with the effects of within-person error in the independent variable, random variation in the dependent variable does not systematically bias (i.e., attenuate) the regression coefficient. Within-person error in the dependent variable, however, increases the standard error of the regression coefficient.

The effect of random within-person variation on relative risk estimates is perhaps less obvious but no less important. Dietary factors are usually continuous variables; thus, in epidemiologic studies we are fundamentally comparing the distribution of a continuous variable among persons with a disease and without the disease. (In a prospective cohort study, the previous diets of subjects who became diseased would be compared with the previous diets of the total group or of those who remained free of disease.)

These distributions can be portrayed as in Figure 3–6A, where it is assumed that diet is measured without random error, that is, there is no within-person variation. To compute a relative risk, we need to specify a cut-point to define high and low intakes. This point is sometimes rather arbitrary, and often several cut-points are used. For simplicity, in this example we have used a cut-point (x_n) corresponding to 1 standard deviation (SD) above the mean of the noncases. Let us assume that the distributions for both groups are normal and that the mean nutrient intake for cases is 0.5 SD above the control value.

The proportions of subjects in each of the cells of a 2 × 2 table are then described as the areas defined by these distributions, these values being obtained from a table of normal deviates:

	High nutrient intake	Low nutrient intake
Cases	$a = 0.31$	$b = 0.69$
Noncases	$c = 0.16$	$d = 0.84$

where:

a = area proportional to the number of cases above cut-point (x_n)
b = area proportional to the number of cases below cut-point (x_n)
c = area proportional to the number of noncases above cut-point (x_n)
d = area proportional to the number of noncases below cut-point (x_n)

The odds ratio is then computed as

$$\frac{a/b}{c/d} = \frac{0.31/0.69}{0.16/0.84} = 2.36$$

Now let us assume that the single measurement of intake is subject to random error. As described previously, the distributions for both cases and noncases are wider: The standard deviations are increased. In this example, assume that the ratio of within-person to between-person variance is 3.0, which is realistic for many nutrients (see Table 3–4). Because the between-person variance is unchanged, as the subjects are the same, this implies that the observed standard deviation is twice as large as the true standard deviation, s_b:

$$\text{Observed SD} = (s_b^2 + 3s_b^2)^{1/2} = 2s_b$$

These broader observed distributions are shown in Figure 3–6B; it is obvious that the case and noncase distributions are now less distinct. The observed areas corresponding to the cells of a 2 × 2 table can be recalculated from a table of normal deviates (note that the same change in nutrient intake corresponding to 1 normal deviate for the true distribution is now 0.5 of a normal deviate for the observed distribution): It is apparent that the observed odds ratio has been attenuated, as it is now considerably closer to the null value of 1.0.

	High nutrient intake	Low nutrient intake
Cases	$a' = 0.40$	$b' = 0.59$
Noncases	$c' = 0.31$	$d' = 0.69$

Odds ratio = 1.51

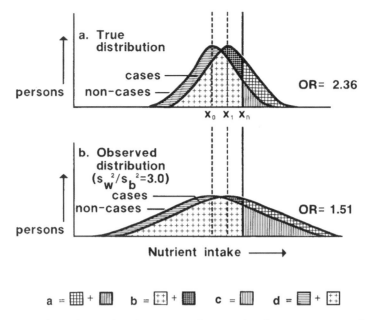

Figure 3–6. (A) Hypothetical true distributions for noncases (mean nutrient = x_1, which is 0.5 standard deviation (SD) larger than x_o). X_n is an arbitrary cut-point 1.0 SD above x_o: values higher than x_n are considered high; values below x_n are considered low. (B) Observed distributions for the same cases and noncases based on a single observation per subject when the within-to-between variance ratio for the nutrient = 3.0. The observed SD is now twice the true SD.

SUMMARY

The day-to-day variation in nutrient intake among free-living subjects has consistently proved to be large, although the magnitude varies according to nutrient. Measurements of dietary intake based on a single or small number of 24-hour recalls per subject may provide a reasonable (unbiased) estimate of the mean for a group, but the standard deviation will be greatly overestimated. Furthermore, measurements of association in epidemiologic studies, such as correlation and regression coefficients and relative risks, are substantially weakened, possibly to the point of being undetectable.

REFERENCES

Beaton, G. H., J. Milner, P. Corey, V. McGuire, M. Cousins, E. Stewart, M. de Ramos, D. Hewitt, P. V. Grambsch, N. Kassim, and J. A. Little (1979). Sources of variance in 24-hour dietary recall data: Implications for nutrition study design and interpretation. *Am J Clin Nutr 32,* 2546–2549.

Beaton, G. H., J. Milner, V. McGuire, T. E. Feather, and J. A. Little (1983). Source of variance in 24-hour dietary recall data: Implications for nutrition study design and interpretation. Carbohydrate sources, vitamins, and minerals. *Am J Clin Nutr 37,* 986–995.

Bhargava, A. (1992). Malnutrition and the role of individual variation with evidence from India and the Phillipines. *J R Statist Soc A 155 (part 2),* 221–231.

Brown, K. H., R. E. Black, and S. Backer (1982). Seasonal changes in nutritional status and the prevalence of malnutrition in a longitudinal study of young children in rural Bangladesh. *Am J Clin Nutr 36,* 303–313.

Dalvit, S. P. (1981). The effect of the menstrual cycle on patterns of food intake. *Am J Clin Nutr 34,* 1811–1815.

el Lozy, M. (1983). Dietary variability and its impact on nutritional epidemiology. *J Chronic Dis 36,* 237–249.

Freedman, L. S., R. J. Carroll, and Y. Wax (1991). Estimating the relation between dietary intake obtained from a food frequency questionnaire and true average intake. *Am J Epidemiol 134*, 310–320.

Hunt, W. C., A. G. Leonard, P. J. Garry, and J. S. Goodwin (1983). Components of variation in dietary data for an elderly population. *Nutr Res 3*, 433–444.

Liu, K., R. Cooper, J. McKeever, P. McKeever, R. Byington, I. Soltero, R. Stamler, F. Gosch, E. Stevens, and J. Stamler (1979). Assessment of the association between habitual salt intake and high blood pressure: Methodological problems. *Am J Epidemiol 110*, 219–226.

Liu, K., J. Stamler, A. Dyer, J. McKeever, and P. McKeever (1978). Statistical methods to assess and minimize the role of intra-individual variability in obscuring the relationship between dietary lipids and serum cholesterol. *J Chronic Dis 31*, 399–418.

Madonsky, A. (1959). The fitting of straight lines when both variables are subject to error. *J Am Statis Assoc 54*, 173.

Mattson, F. H., B. A. Erickson, and A. M. Kligman (1972). Effect of dietary cholesterol on serum cholesterol in man. *Am J Clin Nutr 25*, 589–594.

Morgan, K. J., S. R. Johnson, and B. Goungetas (1987). Variability of food intakes. An analysis of a 12-day data series using persistence measures. *Am J Epidemiol 126*, 326–335.

Romieu, I., M. Hernandez, S. Parra, J. Hernandez, H. Madrigal, and W. Willett (1998). Validity and reproducibility of a semiquantitative food frequency questionnaire to assess antioxidants and retinol intake in a Mexican population. Submitted.

Rush, D., and A. R. Kristal (1982). Methodologic studies during pregnancy: The reliability of the 24-hour dietary recall. *Am J Clin Nutr 35(suppl)*, 1259–1268.

Schaefer, A. E. (1981). Can nutritional status be determined from consumption or other measures? In National Academy of Sciences: *Assessing Changing Food Consumption Patterns*. Washington, DC: National Academy Press, pp. 207–219.

Sempos, C. T., N. E. Johnson, E. L. Smith, and C. Gilligan (1985). Effects of intraindividual and interindividual variation in repeated dietary records. *Am J Epidemiol 121*, 120–130.

Tarasuk, V., and G. H. Beaton (1991). The nature and individuality of within-subject variation in energy intake. *Am J Clin Nutr 54*, 464–470.

Torres, A., W. Willett, J. Orav, L. Chen, and E. Huq (1990). Variability of total energy and protein intake in rural Bangladesh: Implications for epidemiological studies of diet in developing countries. *Food Nutr Bull 12*, 220–228.

U.S. Department of Health, Education, and Welfare, Public Health Service, National Center for Health Statistics (1979). *Dietary Intake Source Data, United States, 1971–74* (DHEW Pub No. [PHS] 79–1221). Washington, DC: U.S. Department of Health, Education, and Welfare.

van Staveren, W. A., P. Deurenberg, J. Burema, L. C. de Groot, and J. G. Hautvast (1986a). Seasonal variation in food intake, pattern of physical activity and change in body weight in a group of young adult Dutch women consuming self-selected diets. *Int J Obesity 10*, 133–145.

van Staveren, W. A., P. Deurenberg, M. B. Katan, J. Burema, L. C. de Groot, and M. D. Hoffmans (1986b). Validity of the fatty acid composition of subcutaneous fat tissue microbiopsies as an estimate of the long-term average fatty acid composition of the diet of separate individuals. *Am J Epidemiol 123*, 455–463.

Willett, W. C., L. Sampson, M. J. Stampfer, B. Rosner, C. Bain, J. Witschi, C. H. Hennekens, and F. E. Speizer (1985). Reproducibility and validity of a semiquantitative food frequency questionnaire. *Am J Epidemiol 122*, 51–65.

Ziegler, R. G., H. B. 3rd. Wilcox, T. J. Mason, J. S. Bill, and P. W. Virgo (1987). Seasonal variation in intake of carotenoids and vegetables and fruits among white men in New Jersey. *Am J Clin Nutr 45*, 107–114.

4

24-Hour Dietary Recall and Food Record Methods

MARILYN BUZZARD

The two methods described in this chapter, the 24-hour dietary recall and the food record method, are based on foods and amounts actually consumed by an individual on one or more specific days. Thus, these methods differ from food frequency questionnaires (FFQ) and diet histories, which are based on an individual's perceptions of usual intake over a less precisely defined period of time (see Chapter 5). If a suitable number of recalls or records are collected over a long period (e.g., six recalls or records per individual spaced over a 12-month period), these methods may also be used to estimate usual intake in prospective studies. The number of days required depends on the day-to-day variability of the nutrients of interest and on the precision desired. These issues are discussed in Chapter 3 and are further elaborated in this chapter. For practical reasons, collection of multiple days of intake is not feasible for most epidemiologic studies involving large numbers of individuals.

The most common current use of recall and record methods in nutritional epidemiology is to assess the validity of a food-frequency questionnaire that is used as the primary dietary data collection instrument. The validity of the food-frequency questionnaire is evaluated by collecting one or more recalls or records from a representative subsample of the study population. The results of the validation study may then be used as a basis for adjusting associations between nutrient intake, as assessed by the food-frequency questionnaire, and risk of disease (see Chapter 12).

For most epidemiologic investigations of dietary intake and disease, relative rankings of food and nutrient intakes are adequate for determination of correlations or relative risks. However, in some situations, such as when comparing nutrient intakes with specific dietary recommendations, estimates of the absolute energy and macronutrient intakes may be required. In such cases, records or recalls are generally the methods of choice.

Because dietary recalls and food record

methods are completely open ended, they can accommodate any level of food description detail necessary for addressing the questions of research interest. They can also accommodate any extent of diversity in the study population, which may be critical for obtaining a representative sample. Finally, the use of recall or record methods permits considerable flexibility for data analysis, since data can be analyzed by nutrients, as well as by individual foods, by any food grouping scheme desired or by meals.

DATA COLLECTION METHODS

24-Hour Dietary Recall Method

The 24-hour dietary recall method is based on an in-depth interview conducted by a trained dietary interviewer. The method has been described in detail by many others (Pekkarinen, 1970; Burk and Pao, 1976; Bingham, 1987; Gibson, 1990). In most situations, the interviewees are the subjects themselves; however, in the case of young children or mentally incapacitated adults, the interviewee may be a parent or other caretaker. The dietary interviewer solicits detailed information about everything the subject had to eat and drink from midnight to midnight of the previous day or over the past 24-hour period. Thus, the accuracy of the dietary intake data is dependent on the subject's short-term memory.

Although it is possible to have subjects self-administer their own recall by listing all the foods and amounts consumed during the 24-hour period, this approach is seldom used in a research setting due to the importance of having a skilled interviewer probe for additional foods and food preparation methods. A skilled interviewer asks questions in a manner designed to put the respondent at ease and to facilitate his or her ability to recall the previous day's intake. Collecting a brief history of the previous day's activities prior to beginning to ask questions about food intake may facilitate memory and set the stage for later questions, such as, "Did you have anything to eat or drink when you were at your friend's house?"

The interviewer generally proceeds forward in time beginning with the first thing the subject had to eat or drink on the previous day. This chronologic approach focusing on a single day of intake is generally the preferred procedure. However, if the subject has difficulty remembering what was eaten on the previous day, it may be preferable to begin with the present and work backward over the past 24-hour period. An alternative approach is to begin with the first thing eaten on the day of the interview and proceed forward to the present, then go back exactly 24 hours and collect intake details from that point on the preceding day until the subject awoke on the day of the interview. A recall interview typically requires 20 to 30 minutes to complete, but it may be considerably longer if many different foods or mixed dishes with many ingredients were consumed.

Intensive training of the dietary interviewer is critical for obtaining accurate and complete dietary recalls. Detailed information about food preparation methods, recipe ingredients, and brand name identification of commercial products is often required. If the respondent does not provide adequate information about a food item, the interviewer must probe further for the necessary level of detail. Information on the use of vitamins, minerals, and other dietary supplements may also be collected. The interviewer's ability to ask questions in a nonjudgmental manner, to maintain a neutral attitude toward all responses, to use open-ended questions in probing for foods and food descriptive detail, and to avoid asking questions in a manner that might influence the subject's responses are important factors in obtaining complete and accurate information (Dennis et al., 1980; Snetselaar, 1989; Westat, 1992).

Accurate quantification of amounts of foods consumed is a critical component of data collection for the 24-hour recall

(Guthrie, 1984; Bolland et al., 1988; Yuhas et al., 1989; Brown et al., 1990; Wein et al., 1990; Faggiano et al., 1992). Because respondents may have difficulty expressing amounts in standard units of weight or volume (e.g., the number of ounces of coffee consumed), various amount estimation tools may be used to help estimate portion sizes from memory (Kirkcaldy-Hargreaves and Lynch, 1980; Westat, 1992). Examples of amount estimation tools include: common sizes of mugs, glasses, and bowls; standard measuring cups and spoons; a ruler or two-dimensional grid for estimating dimensions; a container of dried beans for measuring handfuls; three-dimensional food models; photographs or drawings of foods; and geometric shapes. The tools for estimating amounts should be representative of measures commonly used in the communities in which the subjects reside.

Respondents often describe amounts in terms of food-specific quantities, such as a "large" muffin, a "pat" of butter, or a "small package" of a particular brand of candy. Such descriptions are often more accurate than trying to estimate amounts using standard units of weight or volume. Food-specific amounts must then be converted to weights for nutrient calculation. Identification of commercial products by brand name often facilitates quantification of the amount consumed. For example, most brands of cookies come in a specified size per cookie, so indicating the number of cookies and the brand is sufficient for determining the amount consumed.

Dietary recalls may now be obtained interactively using computer software that prompts the interviewer to collect all of the necessary information about a food consumed by the subject. The Minnesota Nutrition Data System (NDS) was developed specifically for this purpose (Feskanich et al., 1988, 1989). When a food name is entered into the system, the computer guides the interviewer through a series of menus that capture descriptive information, such as the type or brand name of the food,

methods used in food preparation, specification of key ingredients in recipes, whether fat and/or salt was added to the food, and whether the food was prepared commercially or at home. To facilitate quantification of amounts, the system provides a large number of options for describing portion sizes. All of the options are specific for the particular food item. Numerous edit checks, such as flagging amounts that exceed established maxima, are built into the system to reduce data entry errors. Once the foods have been completely described and quantified, the coding and nutrient calculations are done automatically. Use of such an automated system standardizes the data collection process and ensures that the appropriate level of detail is obtained for every food consumed. In addition, it eliminates the need for manual coding, which has traditionally been the most labor intensive step in dietary data processing.

The 24-hour recall method is currently the most commonly used method for dietary surveys in the United States. This method is used by the National Center for Health Statistics for collecting dietary data for the National Health and Nutrition Examination Surveys (Briefel, 1994) and also by the U.S. Department of Agriculture for their Nationwide Food Consumption Surveys and the Continuing Surveys of Food Intakes by Individuals (Guenther, 1994). The recall method is also frequently used for nutrition-related clinical trials such as the Multiple Risk Factor Intervention Trial (Dolecek et al., 1997), the Lipid Research Clinics Coronary Primary Prevention Trial (Dennis et al., 1980), the Dietary Intervention Study in Children (van Horn et al., 1993), and the Child and Adolescent Trial for Cardiovascular Health (Lytle et al., 1993), to name a few.

Although the 24-hour dietary recall has traditionally consisted of a face-to-face interview with the respondent, recalls conducted by telephone interview have become increasingly common (Krantzler et al., 1982; Posner et al., 1982; Schucker, 1982;

Dubois and Boivin, 1990; Fox et al., 1992; Galasso et al., 1994; Andersson and Rossner, 1996). There are two major advantages of using the telephone for conducting recall interviews. First, it eliminates the need for the respondent and/or the interviewer to travel to a common location. This is especially advantageous when multiple days of intake are to be collected. Second, collection of recalls by telephone makes it possible to conduct the interview without the subject knowing in advance exactly when the interview will take place. This "surprise" aspect of the unannounced telephone recall is especially important in situations such as a diet intervention study in which the subjects in the intervention group are likely to modify their food selections to more closely adhere to the intervention protocol as a result of knowing when the interview is to be conducted (Buzzard et al., 1996).

Food Record Method

The food record or food diary method consists of a detailed listing of all foods consumed by an individual on one or more days (Pekkarinen, 1970; Block, 1982; Bingham et al., 1988; Thompson and Byers, 1994). Food intake is recorded by the subject (or observer) at the time the foods are eaten to minimize reliance on memory. Subjects should be trained in advance in methods of keeping complete and accurate food records. Face-to-face training is preferable and should include a discussion of the significance of the research and the importance of the dietary information. Special forms and instructions are provided to guide subjects in recording the appropriate level of food description detail. In some situations, particularly in developing countries, a skilled field worker keeps food records based on observation of food preparation and consumption in the home (Pekkarinen, 1970; Bingham et al., 1988). The field worker weighs the raw ingredients, as well as the individual portions of the cooked dishes. This information is then used to determine individual food intakes.

Food records are quantified either by weighing or by determining volumes using household measuring tools such as standard measuring cups and spoons and a ruler for measuring dimensions. In European countries, where foods are typically quantified by gram weight, weighed records are most common. In the United States, amounts are more often quantified by volume or by food-specific units, such as a "medium" apple, a "small bag" of potato chips, or a "can" of soda. Some studies provide subjects with food-weighing scales to be used along with the volumetric measuring tools (Buzzard et al., 1990). Various electronic devices are available to facilitate weighing and describing foods (Stockley et al., 1986; Bingham et al., 1988; Kretsch and Fong, 1990). One such device developed in the United Kingdom automatically records weights along with a spoken description of the food item (Cherlyn Electronics, Cambridge, England). Use of such devices for large-scale studies may be prohibitive due to the expense of the equipment and the training required. Unquantified food records, which include listings of the foods eaten but not the amounts, may be used for determining frequency of consumption by individual foods and food groups or for analysis by meal pattern.

Food records should be carefully reviewed by a trained nutritionist immediately after completion to ensure an adequate level of detail in describing foods and food preparation methods. If this cannot be done in a face-to-face interview, subjects may be contacted by telephone to obtain additional detail or to clarify ambiguous information.

STRENGTHS AND LIMITATIONS OF THE 24-HOUR DIETARY RECALL AND FOOD RECORD METHODS

The 24-hour recall and food record methods have several strengths in common. Both methods are based on actual intake and may be used to estimate absolute rather than relative intake of energy and other food components such as the macronutrients and some vitamins and minerals that are broadly distributed within the food supply. Also, because both methods are completely open ended, they can accommodate any food or food combination reported by the subject, and they allow an unlimited level of specificity regarding type of food, food source, food processing method, food preparation, and other detail related to describing foods and amounts. This high level of specificity may be required for addressing certain research questions, such as assessing dietary change in nutrition intervention studies. This higher level of specificity may not be obtainable using a limited number of food items in a structured questionnaire (Briefel et al., 1992). Also, recalls and records are especially useful for estimating intakes in culturally diverse populations representing a wide range of foods and eating habits. Recall interviews may be individualized to be sensitive to cultural differences, rather than enforcing a level of standardization that could result in obtaining less accurate information (Buzzard and Sievert, 1994; Cassidy, 1994).

A major strength of the recall method compared with food records is that it does not require literacy. This may be a critical factor in obtaining a representative sample of a population. The literacy requirement for the food record method may be circumvented by permitting subjects to use tape recorders or telephones for reporting food intakes, but these alternative approaches demand additional resources and present other practical and logistical problems. Another strength of the recall compared with the food record is that it is less likely to alter eating behavior, since the information is collected after the fact. An additional advantage of the recall method is its relatively minimal respondent burden. The interview generally requires less than 30 minutes to complete, and no record keeping is necessary. The major limitations of the 24-hour recall method include its reliance on memory, both for identification of foods eaten and for quantification of portion sizes, and the need for a highly trained dietary interviewer.

A major strength of the food record method is that it does not rely on memory. If subjects comply with the instructions, foods and amounts are recorded at the time they are eaten. Another major advantage of food records compared with recalls is that portion sizes can be directly measured rather than estimated from memory. The most accurate approach is to provide subjects with food-weighing scales so that all foods (or at least those eaten at home) can be weighed before eating. Because keeping food records places substantial burden on subjects, this method requires a high level of subject motivation. This can lead to a poor response rate in situations in which subjects are not highly motivated.

Both the recall and the record methods are limited by the fact that a single day of intake is unlikely to be representative of usual individual intake. As discussed in Chapter 3, day-to-day intake is highly variable for many individuals. Use of either method for estimation of usual individual intake requires the collection of multiple days of intake, the number of days depending on the day-to-day variability of the nutrient(s) of interest.

NUMBER OF DAYS AND WHICH DAYS

If food records or 24-hour dietary recalls are to be used as the data collection method, issues regarding the number of days and which days to include must be considered. A single food record or 24-hour recall per individual may be adequate if estimates of group means are sufficient for answering the questions that the study is designed to answer (National Research Council, National Academy of Sciences, Subcommittee on Criteria for Dietary Evaluation, Coordinating Committee on Evaluation of Food Consumption Surveys, 1986). For example, if sample sizes are sufficiently large, a single day of intake may be used to determine the average intake of total fat in defined subgroups of a population. Ideally, all 7 days of the week should be equally represented within the subgroups, since there may be systematic differences in dietary intake on different days of the week (Beaton et al., 1983; Thompson et al., 1986; Tarasuk and Beaton, 1992; Bhargava et al., 1994 Maisey, 1995; Guenther, 1997) If that is not possible, an appropriate balance of the types of days that are likely to differ with respect to food intake (e.g., work days vs. weekend days) should be reflected within the groups. The design of the study determines the relative importance of balancing the days of the week. For example, if the purpose of the study is to determine the effectiveness of an intervention program, it may be less important to include a balance of days as long as the same combination of days is used for data collection both before and after the intervention. However, if the purpose is to estimate changes in absolute nutrient intakes, an appropriate balance of the days of the week is likely to be of greater importance.

If the purpose of the study requires estimating the distribution of individual intakes within the group, it is necessary to collect more than one recall or record per individual in the study population or in a random subsample of the population (National Research Council, 1986; Guenther, 1997). Estimating the distribution of individual intakes would be necessary, for example, if one wished to determine the proportion of individuals at risk of inadequate intake of a particular nutrient. To estimate within-person day-to-day variability, it is usually statistically most efficient to increase the number of individuals in the sample rather than to increase the number of days beyond 2 days per individual (see Chapter 12). In the case of food records, however, it may be more cost effective to train fewer people in methods of record keeping and increase the number of days per individual. When multiple days of intake are collected to permit

estimation of within-person variability, the combination of days of the week for each individual should be randomly assigned and nonconsecutive. Several studies suggest that consecutive days may not be independent of one another (Morgan et al., 1987; Hartman et al., 1990; Larkin et al., 1991) (see also Chapter 3).

If an estimate of usual individual intake is needed for investigating relationships between dietary intake and various biochemical, clinical, or other indicators of health status, or for assessing individual adherence to dietary recommendations, multiple days of intake must be collected. The number of days needed depends on the within-person variability for the nutrient(s) of interest and the level of precision desired (see Chapter 3). Numerous studies have investigated the number of days required at various levels of precision for various nutrients in different populations (Balogh et al., 1971; Liu et al., 1978; Beaton et al., 1979; Bingham et al., 1981; Marr, 1981; Jackson et al., 1986; Marr and Heady, 1986; Basiotis et al., 1987; Nelson et al., 1989; Hartman et al., 1990; Miller et al., 1991). In general, these studies suggest that the minimum number of days of intake required for gross characterization of usual individual intake of energy and the macronutrients ranges from 3 to 10 days. For food components with large day-to-day variability, such as cholesterol and vitamins A and C, the number of days required may range from 20 to more than 50 days, which becomes impractical in most research settings. Decisions must be made based on what is practical and feasible in a given situation with limited resources. It has been suggested that participant motivation falls off with increasing number of days of data collection, especially if the days are consecutive (Gersovitz et al., 1978). If the days are nonconsecutive, the logistics of data collection for multiple days and timely review of food records may become a limiting factor. Four to 5 days of intake are often selected as a reasonable compromise for assessing current individual intake of energy and the macronutrients (Rush and Kristal, 1982; Jackson et al., 1986; Marr and Heady, 1986; Nelson et al., 1989; Miller et al., 1991). If an estimate of long-term usual intake is required, collection of 3 to 4 days of records or recalls in each of four seasons of the year is ideal, resulting in a total of 12 to 16 days of intake per individual. For micronutrients such as vitamins A and C, which have very high within-person variability and are contributed by relatively few food sources, a food-frequency questionnaire designed specifically to assess the selected nutrients is likely to provide the most accurate estimates of usual individual intake.

REDUCING ERROR IN
DATA COLLECTION

A major source of error in collecting dietary data using the 24-hour dietary recall method is its reliance on the subject's memory. Krall and coworkers (1988) found that one's ability to recall food intake was associated with a number of factors including age, gender, intelligence, mood, attention, and consistency of eating pattern. Studies that have compared mean energy intake of 24-hour dietary recalls with food records collected in the same population and the same general time frame report energy intakes ranging from 0% to 16% lower for the recalls (Table 4–1). Memory limitations can be minimized by using well-trained interviewers who are skilled in the art of asking questions that help subjects remember what they ate. Providing a relaxed and unhurried atmosphere gives the subject a chance to carefully reflect on his or her eating behavior. Asking about the previous day's activities and relating these activities to food intake may also help subjects recall their food intake. Providing a list of foods commonly forgotten can help jog the subject's memory of items inadvertently omitted, such as snack items, beverages, and desserts. Campbell and Dodds (1967) found that extensive probing substantially increased estimates of energy intake ob-

tained by 24-hour recall in both elderly and younger respondents.

In theory, memory limitation should not be a source of error for the food record method; however, subjects who keep food records sometimes delay recording their intakes for several hours or more, in which case they are relying to some extent on short-term memory. Black and colleagues (1993) reviewed studies comparing weighed food records with the doubly labeled water method of assessing energy expenditure. They reported that highly motivated subjects can keep accurate records but that randomly selected men and women underreport their intakes by approximately 20% on average. Other investigators, using estimated rather than weighed procedures for quantification of amounts, reported underestimation of energy intake by more than 20% in highly motivated volunteer subjects (Howat et al., 1994). Procedures for reducing the extent of underreporting in food records include careful training of subjects in methods of keeping accurate records, providing written as well as verbal instructions for record keeping, emphasizing the importance of the subject's contribution to the research, stressing the need for timely recording of food intake, and encouraging subjects to maintain usual eating habits during the recording period. Underreporting of energy intake is further addressed in a later section of this chapter dealing with validation issues.

Another source of error in collecting food intake data is the lack of adequate food descriptive detail. With respect to the 24-hour recall, the interviewer must remember to ask all of the appropriate probing questions to obtain the necessary level of specificity for meeting the study objectives. To do this well may require considerable training and practice. One approach to reducing this type of error is to use an automated system for collecting the data in which the computer provides all of the prompts for describing foods at the appropriate level of detail (Feskanich et al.,

Table 4–1. Comparison of mean energy intakes calculated from 24-hour dietary recalls and food records obtained from the same population

Source	Population	24-hour recall method		Food record method		Recall/record ratio
		No. days[a]	Energy (kcal)	No. days	Energy (kcal)	
Morgan et al. (1978)	Healthy women in four areas of Canada n=400 recalls n=347 records	1	1,615 ± 880[b]	4	1,780 ± 578	0.91
Bull and Wheeler (1986)	British civil servants n=30	2[c]	2,127 ± 478	7[d]	2,533 ± 574	0.84
Fanelli and Stevenhagen (1986)	Older adults, aged 65–74 years, in USDA nationwide survey (1977–78)					
	n=1057 women	1	1,430 ± 542	1	1,439 ± 555	0.99
	n=686 men	1	1,929 ± 735	1	1,924 ± 739	1.00
Borelli et al. (1989)	Elderly Italians, aged 65–95 years n=230	1	4,039 ± 1482	3	4,111 ± 1243	0.98
Mullenbach et al. (1992)	Minnesota adolescents, aged 11–16 years n=40	1[e]	1,835 ± 143	3	2,097 ± 136	0.88
Howat et al. (1994)	Adult women	2[f]	1,820 ± 635	14	1,918 ± 567	0.95

[a] All multiple records were consecutive days.

[b] Mean ± SD.

[c] Approximately 17 months apart.

[d] Portion sizes were weighed.

[e] Obtained by telephone interview.

[f] Four days apart.

1988). The use of such a system considerably reduces the burden on the interviewer. In the case of food records, training of subjects regarding the level of detail needed and providing written examples can help to minimize this type of error. It is also helpful to review the food records with the subject as soon as possible after data collection. This review should include probing for beverages and between-meal snacks that may have been inadvertently omitted and asking about possible additions such as butter or margarine added to vegetables. Meals that are eaten away from home often lack an adequate level of descriptive detail. Because eating out is becoming an increasingly common practice, efforts should be made to obtain the necessary level of detail on these occasions. Study participants should be instructed to ask about ingredients and preparation methods at the time they place their orders, since it is often difficult to obtain this information from eating establishments at a later date.

Quantification of portion sizes is another source of error in collecting food intake data. This is of particular concern for the 24-hour recall method, since amounts consumed must be recalled from memory. Guthrie (1984) found that the ability of men and women to estimate portion sizes was poor without the aid of measuring devices. Bird and Elwood (1983) reported that the use of photographs for estimating portion sizes compared favorably with weighed-food records. When using photographs or food models, it is preferable to present more than one portion size option so that subjects can relate their portion to a variety of sizes. Otherwise, there is a tendency to report whatever amount is represented by the model. Using models of geometric shapes, such as cubes, rectangles, spheres, circles, mounds, and wedges, may be preferable to using models of actual foods because they are less suggestive and can be provided in multiple sizes. Training of subjects in the use of food models has been found to improve the accuracy of estimating amounts (Yuhas et al., 1989; Bolland et al., 1990). Bolland and colleagues (1990) conducted brief small-group sessions to train subjects how to estimate portion sizes of 10 food models. When tested on the day of training and 1 week later, the trained subjects made significantly less error than untrained subjects in estimating portion sizes for six real foods (Table 4–2). By week 4, the training effects had disappeared for three of the six foods.

Estimating portion sizes in interviews conducted by telephone is somewhat more difficult because the subject does not have access to all the food models and other amount estimation tools typically available at a face-to-face interviewing site. Some tools such as a ruler and standard measuring cups and spoons, or a notebook of photographs of different portion sizes for selected foods, can be provided to each subject to keep at home and/or at work to facilitate comparison with recollected amounts at the time of the telephone interview. Use of two-dimensional visuals portraying various sizes of geometric shapes, mounds, and beverage containers may further facilitate amount estimation during the interview (Posner et al., 1992).

An especially serious type of error is the error introduced by the measuring instrument itself. The food record method is particularly prone to this type of error because

the process of writing down the foods one eats may lead to a change in eating behavior. Thus, the record may be accurate as to the foods actually eaten, but those foods may not be representative of what one would normally have eaten. A suggested explanation for changes in eating behavior while keeping food records has to do with the burden associated with recording mixed dishes containing many ingredients. For ease of recording, subjects may choose simple foods that are easy to record. Another reason might be related to the social desirability factor—when one becomes more conscious of what one is eating, there may be a tendency to select foods that are more socially acceptable or considered to be healthier. One approach to reducing this type of bias is to caution subjects in advance of this potential source of error and ask them to make an effort to avoid any changes in the foods they would ordinarily select. The tendency to eat differently when recording one's intake is of particular concern in assessing nutrient intakes in nutrition intervention studies, because individuals in the diet intervention group are likely to adhere more closely to the intervention protocol while keeping food records. Buzzard et al. (1996) compared 4-day food records with unannounced 24-hour recalls collected by telephone interview to determine differences in fat intake between intervention and control groups in a low-fat diet intervention study (Table 4–3). Compared with the unannounced telephone recall method, the food record overestimated the difference in fat intake between the study groups by approximately 40% at 6 months ($p = 0.08$) and by 25% at 12 months ($p = 0.62$). Although these differences were not statistically significant, they were consistent in direction and magnitude at the two time periods, suggesting some cause for concern regarding bias in using the food record method in diet intervention studies.

Finally, lack of motivation is a potential source of error for both subjects and interviewers. Social science researchers have

Table 4–2. Mean[a] percentage errors in estimating portion size by food item and by time lapse between training and testing

| Food item | Untrained | Trained | | | p Value |
		Tested same day	Tested 1 week later	Tested 4 weeks later	
Meat loaf	39.8 ± 37.1	22.5 ± 17.9	31.5 ± 27.9	40.6 ± 54.9	0.0456
Fish	68.6 ± 63.7	43.8 ± 39.7	36.7 ± 33.7	70.1 ± 87.7	0.0079
Milk	66.5 ± 42.2	48.6 ± 38.0	55.1 ± 64.3	57.8 ± 39.8	0.2403
Soup	108.8 ± 60.6	46.7 ± 41.4	57.4 ± 35.9	54.6 ± 45.8	0.0001
Spaghetti	134.7 ± 134.6	84.1 ± 81.0	94.3 ± 66.1	97.5 ± 82.1	0.0340
Applesauce	145.5 ± 209.5	106.5 ± 122.9	94.2 ± 80.3	140.8 ± 196.6	0.3039
All foods combined	94.0 ± 116.1	58.7 ± 71.9	61.5 ± 60.0	76.9 ± 104.5	≤0.0001

[a] Mean ± standard deviation.
Adapted from Bolland et al., 1990.

suggested that subject motivation to provide complete and accurate information is affected by the perceived importance and applicability of the study results (Bureau of Social Science Research, 1980). It is critical that the interviewers and/or others who introduce the study to the subjects be enthusiastic about the study and able to convey this enthusiasm to the participants. Taking time to explain the purpose and importance of the research and to establish a friendly and relaxed but business-like rapport with the participants creates an atmosphere of trust and motivates the participants to provide accurate information.

Monetary or other types of incentives are sometimes used to increase participant motivation, but such incentives cannot substitute for convincing participants of the importance of the research and the critical role they play in making it possible to answer questions about the role of diet in health and disease.

ANALYSIS OF FOOD INTAKE DATA

Data obtained from food records and 24-hour dietary recalls may be analyzed at the individual food level, by food group, or by meal pattern, and nutrient intakes may be

Table 4–3. Comparison of the 4-day food record (4DFR) and the unannounced telephone recall (TR) in estimating differences in fat intake between study groups

	Fat intake (g) in control group (C) (mean ± SD)	Fat intake (g) in low-fat group (LF) (mean ± SD)	Difference in fat intake (g) (C−LF)	Ratio of 4DFR to TR in estimating difference in fat intake (C−LF)
6 months	n=103	n=101		
4DFR	56.9 ± 21.3	33.1 ± 14.0	23.8[a]	
TR	51.7 ± 27.2	34.8 ± 21.4	16.9[a]	
4DFR−TR	5.2	−1.7	6.9[b]	1.41
12 months	n=94	n=93		
4DFR	56.3 ± 22.6	32.7 ± 11.7	23.6[a]	
TR	51.4 ± 27.2	32.5 ± 21.1	18.9[a]	
4DFR−TR	4.9	0.2	4.7[c]	1.25

[a] $p < 0.0001$.
[b] $p = 0.08$.
[c] $p = 0.62$.
From Buzzard et al., 1996.

analyzed by meal or by food group, as well as by total daily intake. Thus, there is considerable flexibility in terms of analysis options with food intake data obtained from food records or recalls. The ability to group foods in an unlimited variety of ways enables the investigator to address many different research questions using the same data set. This is especially important in exploratory research in which one may suspect that certain categories of foods confer health-or disease-enhancing properties, but the beneficial or harmful component(s) have not yet been identified. Advantages and limitations of using foods rather than nutrients for investigating diet–disease relationships are discussed in detail in Chapter 2. Analysis by meals permits the investigation of the effects of foods when eaten together, such as the increased absorption of vitamins A and E when eaten with fat-containing foods or the reduced absorption of minerals such as calcium or zinc when eaten with foods containing phytates.

The most common method of analyzing food records or recalls is the calculation of nutrient intakes. The major components of a nutrient calculation system include a database of food composition, a coding system for matching foods listed on records or recalls with entries in the food composition database, and program software for calculating the nutrients. A recipe database containing ingredients and amounts, preparation methods, and yields for commonly consumed mixed dishes may also be used to facilitate nutrient calculation and database maintenance. The food composition database must contain the foods consumed by the study population as well as values for all of the nutrients of interest to the study. Identification of foods by brand name is becoming increasingly important as the consumption of processed foods continues to increase. In 1990, Gorman reported that the rate of introduction of new products in the U.S. marketplace was approximately 1,000 per month. Within some product categories, different brands may have substantially different nutrient compositions. For example, the content of saturated fat ranges from 5% to 35% among the available brand name margarines in the U.S. marketplace (Buzzard et al., 1991a).

Because manual food coding and nutrient calculation are labor intensive and subject to error, automated systems for nutrient calculation are now universally available. Most of these systems also automate, to a greater or lesser extent, the coding process by allowing the user to enter the name of a food and the computer automatically assigns it to the appropriate entry in the food composition database. Nutrient calculation software packages should be carefully evaluated, both for program features, such as ease of data entry, reporting capabilities, and hardware requirements, and for the quality of the nutrient database (Buzzard et al., 1991b; Orta, 1991; Lee and Nieman, 1993; Smith, 1993). (See Chapter 2 for a listing of the sources of food composition data and some of the factors to be considered in selecting a food composition database and nutrient calculation software.)

The researcher must keep in mind that the degree of specificity of food description detail required at the data collection level must be reflected at the level of coding and nutrient calculation (Buzzard et al., 1991a). For example, it would be of little use to collect information regarding brands of ready-to-eat cereal if the entries for cereals in the food composition database were not brand specific. On the other hand, it would be useless to require brand-specific entries in the food composition database if this level of detail was not being collected from subjects.

SOURCES OF ERROR IN NUTRIENT CALCULATION

Converting food intakes to nutrient intakes involves a number of sources of error. Inaccuracies in the coding of food intake data are a major source of error in nutrient calculation (Dennis et al., 1980). Although many of the errors associated with manual coding have been eliminated through the use of on-line data entry systems and incorporation of edit checks at the point of data entry, there is always some potential for error when entering data into the computer. Errors related to selecting incorrect matches for items listed on records or recalls are more difficult to control. Intensive training and certification of coders prior to coding study data is essential (Dennis et al., 1980; Dolecek et al., 1997). Coding errors can be reduced by having the records or recalls coded by more than one coder. However, since coding is highly labor intensive, most studies cannot afford 100% duplicate coding. Duplicate coding of a sample of 10% or 20% of a study's records may be sufficient to identify coders who are having difficulty with the matching process. Duplicate coding also provides a vehicle for ongoing continuing education of coders.

By automating the coding process, software now available for interactive collection of 24-hour recall data eliminates errors due to coding (Feskanich et al., 1988). The computer prompts for all of the detail needed for matching a food with the entries in the food composition database. Such a system greatly improves the accuracy and standardization of both the data collection and the coding process, as well as resulting in considerable savings in time and effort, because coding has traditionally been the most labor intensive part of processing dietary data.

As discussed in Chapter 2, the use of food composition data for calculating nutrient intakes assumes that the nutrient values for a given food are representative of the available food consumed by the study subject. Such an assumption is usually violated to a greater or lesser extent even if the nutrient values are, on average, representative of the overall food supply. Nutrient values appearing in food composition databases are often based on an exceedingly small numbers of samples. The U.S.

Department of Agriculture, the major compiler of food composition data for the United States, uses whatever data are available and of acceptable quality for estimating nutrient values, even though such data may have been drawn from convenience rather than from representative samples. Food composition errors can also result from procedures for compiling and weighting available data to derive single representative values to include in the database (Rand et al., 1991). Other sources of error in calculating nutrient intakes include the error associated with analytical methodology and the use of outdated nutrient data. The importance of using a complete and updated database of nutrient values is addressed in Chapter 2.

VALIDATION OF 24-HOUR RECALLS AND FOOD RECORDS

Three major aspects of assessing the validity of dietary recalls and food records for estimating usual individual intakes are (1) how accurately individuals can record or recall their intakes on a given day in terms of both identification of foods eaten and estimation of portion sizes, (2) how well the food composition database and the coding and nutrient calculation system reflect the overall composition of the actual foods eaten, and 3) how well the selected days of intake represent usual individual intake.

Reporting Accuracy

Investigators have attempted to shed light on issues related to the accuracy of recording or recalling by unobtrusively observing what subjects eat and comparing observed with self-reported intakes. When foods are compared on an item by item basis, agreement between items observed and items recalled ranges from about 70% to 80% (Emmons and Hayes, 1973; Schnakenberg et al., 1981; Krantzler et al., 1982). Omissions (forgotten foods) are considerably more common than additions (foods recalled but not observed) (Linusson et al., 1974; Greger and Etnyre, 1978; Schnakenberg et al., 1981; Krantzler et al., 1982; Karvetti and Knuts, 1985). Karvetti and Knuts (1985) assessed the validity of 24-hour recalls by comparing recalled with observed intakes of 140 adults in a rehabilitation center in Finland. They found that certain foods, such as cooked vegetables, were more frequently omitted in the recall, and some food items were erroneously recalled that were not actually eaten. The proportions of omitted and erroneously recalled foods are shown in Figure 4–1. Omitted foods tend to be those less frequently consumed or those used as "add-ons" to major foods or as side dishes. It should be noted that these observations are based only on food item identification, not portion size.

Studies investigating differences between actual and recalled portion sizes have found that certain types of foods are more likely to be overestimated than others but that, in general, overestimation appears to be more frequent than underestimation (Lansky and Brownell, 1982; Guthrie, 1984; Webb and Yuhas, 1988; Wein et al., 1990; Faggiano et al., 1992). Guthrie (1984) investigated the ability of young adults to estimate portion sizes of 12 common foods without the aid of food models or interviewer assistance. The results are shown in Table 4–4. Beverages (milk and orange juice) were most accurately reported, and add-ons such as butter and salad dressing were least accurately reported. Overestimation was more common that underestimation. It was concluded that there is a need to provide assistance to respondents in estimating portion sizes.

Wein et al. (1990) compared recalled estimates of portion sizes with portions observed in a cafeteria for 61 Canadian college students. Recalled estimates were within 10% of observed portions for half of the foods and within 20% for three-fourths of the foods. Only 6 of the 39 foods were underestimated compared with

33 that were overestimated. These results suggest that the underreporting of energy intake observed in validation studies of records and recalls is more likely due to omissions in reporting foods than to underestimates of portion sizes. Wein and colleagues also found that the greatest difficulty in estimating amounts was associated with items that could not be separately visualized, such as milk in coffee or tea and condiments such as gravy, salad dressing, ketchup, jam, margarine, and whipped topping added to other foods.

Faggiano et al. (1992) compared weighed serving sizes with recalled estimates based on graduated photographs for 17 Italian dishes. The pictures included seven portion sizes for each dish. Differences ranged from 50% underestimation of rice to 89% overestimation of fresh cheese. Overestimation tended to be greater among those who ate smaller portions and underestimation by those who ate larger portions. Yuhas and coworkers (1989) reported that solid food items appeared to be more accurately estimated than liquids, and shapeless items such as spaghetti and applesauce were estimated with the least accuracy. Webb and Yuhas (1988) observed that portion estimates expressed by weight (e.g., ounces of meat), tended to be less accurate than estimates expressed by volume among participants in the Women, Infants and Children (WIC) program. Lansky and Brownell (1982) reported that subjects had a tendency to make larger errors for foods with higher caloric density. Some studies have reported that women estimate portion sizes more accurately than men (Karvetti and Knuts, 1985; Yuhas et al., 1989), but other investigators have found no difference between the sexes (Young et al., 1953; Wein et al., 1990).

Reported differences in mean energy intakes calculated from 24-hour recalls compared with calculations from observed intakes range from no significant difference (Gersovitz et al., 1978; Greger and Etnyre, 1978; Karvetti and Knuts, 1985) to 19% less for recalled intakes (Carter et al.,

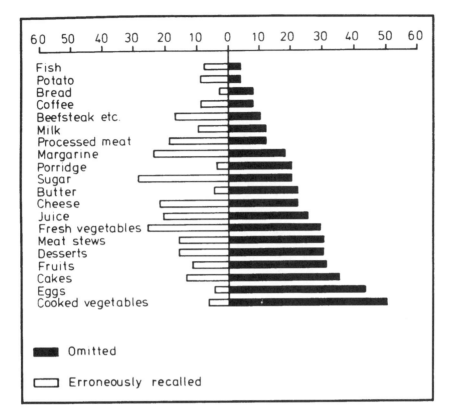

Figure 4–1. Percentage of omissions (failing to report a food) or additions (erroneously reporting a food) when 24-hour recalls were compared with observed intake. (From Karvetti and Knuts, 1985; reproduced with permission.)

1981). Overall, recalls tend to underestimate intake by about 10% compared with observed intake. The extent of underreporting appears to vary considerably among individuals. In general, those who consume considerably less than the average are more likely to overreport their intakes, while those who eat considerably more than the average tend to underreport. This phenomenon, sometimes referred to as the *flat slope syndrome*, has been reported in a number of studies based on observed intake (Linusson et al., 1974; Madden et al., 1976; Gersovitz et al., 1978; Carter et al., 1981; Faggiano et al., 1992). Correlations between nutrient intakes calculated from recalls and those calculated from observations vary greatly among nutrients, and there is little consistency in the correlations

for specific nutrients among different studies and different populations.

Few studies of observed intake have involved the use of food records. A 10% underestimation of energy intake was reported by Schnakenberg et al. (1981), who compared 3- and 4-day diaries kept by military personnel with observed intakes in a dining hall setting. Karvetti and Knuts (1992) compared 2-day estimated records with observed intakes of adults in a rehabilitation center in Finland. They reported no significant difference between the two methods in terms of the calculated intakes of energy and most nutrients.

There are a number of difficulties associated with studies of observed intake that must be considered when interpreting the results. One is that nearly all of these stud-

Table 4–4. Comparison of estimated serving size with actual serving size

Food item	Reporting n	%[a]	Percentage of respondents in each category of error in estimation of actual serving size				
			≤−51%	−26% to −50%	±25%	26% to 50%	>51%
Breakfast							
Orange juice	48	92	0	8	73	19	0
Corn flakes	53	100	4	4	41	8	43
Milk on cereal	44	83	5	11	36	14	34
Sugar on cereal	18	64	11	28	28	11	22
Milk—beverage	7	47	0	0	58	28	14
Butter on toast	36	78	8	6	8	11	67
Lunch							
Tuna salad	91	95	10	10	25	16	39
Tossed salad	90	96	10	14	49	8	19
Salad dressing	66	80	25	6	13	10	46
Fruit salad	89	91	2	6	34	7	51
Milk—beverage	78	86	1	3	68	23	5
Butter	11	79	14	0	22	0	64

[a] Percentage of those using a food who remembered to report it.
Adapted from Guthrie, 1984.

ies are conducted in institutional settings (e.g., congregate meal sites, school cafeterias, hospitals). Generalizing the results of such studies to noninstitutionalized populations is problematic, since the availability of food choices may be quite different in a free-living population. Eating in a cafeteria is likely to affect one's level of consciousness of the foods selected and thus his or her ability to recall, or even record, what and how much was eaten.

An alternative approach to assessing the accuracy of reported intakes is to ask the subject to collect duplicate portions of all foods consumed. The investigator then identifies and carefully weighs each food item for comparison with the self-reported foods and amounts. A problem with studies of this nature is that the procedures are burdensome for both the subject and the researcher, and subjects tend to eat less during periods of collecting duplicate portions (Gibson and Scythes, 1982; Kim et al., 1984; Stockley, 1985). However, because subjects are more conscious of what they are eating when preparing duplicate

portions, they may record their intakes more accurately than they would otherwise.

Accuracy of Nutrient Calculations

The accuracy of a nutrient calculation system, including the representativeness of the food composition database and coding procedures, as well as the accuracy of the calculation software, may be assessed by comparing calculated nutrient intakes with chemical analysis of food composites (Marshall et al., 1975; Ahrens and Boucher, 1978; Bingham et al., 1982; Marshall and Judd, 1982; Brennan et al., 1983; Miles et al., 1984; Persson and Carlgren, 1984; Pietinen et al., 1984; Bingham and Cummings, 1985; Petersen et al., 1986; Giovannetti, 1987; Lee-Han et al., 1988; Obarzanek et al., 1993; Alberti-Fidanza et al., 1994). For example, Brennan et al. (1983) compared calculated nutrient values with chemically analyzed values of 1-day composites of 22 pregnant women. The results are presented in Table 4–5. In general, such studies indicate that calculated intakes

Table 4–5. Comparison of nutrient calculations with chemically analyzed values of 24-hour diet composites of 22 pregnant women

Food component	Calculated mean (SD)		Chemically analyzed mean (SD)		Percent difference[a]	Correlation coefficient
Energy (kcal)	1,873	(529)	1,722	(531)	8.8	0.87
Protein (g)	74.2	(25.0)	67.9	(22.1)	9.3	0.83
Total fat (g)	82.1	(27.8)	78.3	(27.8)	4.9	0.80
Carbohydrate (g)	211.9	(76.0)	193.5	(80.1)	9.5	0.74
Calcuim (mg)	790	(376)	931	(493)	−15.1	0.50
Phosphorus (mg)	1,147	(397)	1,365	(417)	−16.0	0.68
Iron (mg)	11.0	(4.0)	14.4	(5.4)	−23.6	0.55
Sodium (mg)	2,761	(970)	3,848	(1,147)	−28.2	0.45
Potassium (mg)	1,951	(710)	1,736	(749)	12.4	0.83
Magnesium (mg)	204	(88)	200	(85)	2.0	0.87
Zinc (mg)	8.7	(4.1)	8.4	(2.8)	3.6	0.81
Vitamin A (IU)	5,083	(4,458)	5,550	(4,582)	−8.4	0.29
Thiamin (mg)	1.22 (0.45)		1.19 (0.52)		2.5	0.37
Riboflavin (mg)	1.80 (0.75)		1.85 (0.69)		−2.7	0.64
Niacin (mg)	15.1	(6.3)	16.7	(7.1)	−9.6	0.65
Vitamin C (mg)	87	(79)	48	(39)	81.3	0.56
Folacin (mcg)	175	(78)	168	(102)	4.2	0.54

[a] Percent difference: (calculated mean − chemically analyzed mean)/chemically analyzed mean × 100.
Adapted from Brennan et al., 1983.

for energy and the macronutrients fall within 5% to 10% of the chemically analyzed values. In general, the greater the number of days of intake included in the composite, the better the agreement between the analyzed and calculated values. Calculated values tend to be higher than the analyzed values. This may be partly due to systematic error in collecting duplicate food samples (e.g., a tendency to collect less food than was consumed); however, similar results have been found in studies based on composites that are prepared by the investigators according to specifications of well-defined menus (Marshall et al., 1975; Marshall and Judd, 1982). Differences may be due to systematic error in the food composition database or in the coding or calculation procedures or to systematic error in sample preparation and handling or the analytic method used. For nutrients such as vitamins A and C, calcium, iron, sodium, potassium, and cholesterol, differences between calculated and analyzed values vary widely and are often greater than

20% (Ahrens and Boucher, 1978; Bingham et al., 1982; Marshall and Judd, 1982; Brennan et al., 1983). One must keep in mind that the food composition database provides single "representative" values for each nutrient in each food in the database. The greater the sample-to-sample variability of nutrient content within a food and the smaller the number of foods contributing to the nutrient content of the composite, the greater the expected deviation of the analyzed value from the calculated value. (Refer to Chapter 2 for a discussion of sources of nutrient variability.)

Accuracy of Assessing Usual Intake

For most epidemiologic investigations the measurement of primary interest is usual individual intake rather than intake on any single day. Unfortunately, the "truth" against which to judge validity of usual individual intake is difficult, if not impossible, to obtain. Thus, the best we can do is either compare the results of one method of dietary assessment with another method designed to measure the same thing or compare the calculated intakes of individual nutrients with biochemical indicators or "biomarkers" that reflect in a predictable manner the average intake of the related dietary component, such as urinary nitrogen as an indicator of protein intake (Bingham and Cummings, 1985; Snetselaar et al., 1995). A major advantage of using a biochemical indicator to assess the validity of self-reported methods of dietary assessment is the fact that it is independent of self-reporting. However, there are a number of problems associated with the use of biomarkers for validation of nutrient intakes. First of all, there are many food components for which no suitable biomarker has yet been identified. Second, all biochemical indicators of dietary intake are subject to influences of nondietary factors that can alter their relationship with the dietary component of interest. Chapter 9 presents a detailed discussion of the use of biochemical indicators for assessing dietary intake of specific nutrients.

Multiple days of weighed records are often considered to provide the most accurate estimate of absolute usual individual intake (Gibson, 1990). However, a growing volume of literature comparing energy intakes calculated from self-reports with measured energy expenditure indicate that energy intake calculated from food records may be significantly underestimated. The availability of the doubly labeled water technique for measuring energy expenditure is largely responsible for the increase in studies of this nature (International Dietary Energy Consultative Group, 1990; Schoeller et al., 1990). Underestimation of energy intake compared with energy expenditure is attributed mainly to underreporting, although there is evidence that undereating also occurs during record-keeping periods, particularly if subjects are simultaneously making duplicate food collections (Kim et al., 1984; Schoeller et al., 1990). Kim et al. (1984) reported a 13% reduction in energy intake in both men and women during food collection periods compared with

noncollection periods in the 1-year Beltsville dietary intake study. Underestimations of mean energy intakes calculated from food records range from 8% to 30%, averaging about 20% (Prentice et al., 1986; Bandini et al., 1990; Livingstone et al., 1990; 1992; Black et al., 1993). Some studies, however, using highly motivated, well-educated, nonobese subjects have found no significant differences between energy intake and expenditure (Prentice et al., 1989; Schulz et al., 1989; Goldberg et al., 1991; Black et al., 1992; Diaz et al., 1992).

The extent of underreporting of total energy intake varies among individuals. A number of studies have shown that obese individuals tend to underreport to a greater extent than lean individuals (Kromhout, 1983; Avons and James, 1986; Prentice et al., 1986; Schulz et al., 1989; Bandini et al., 1990; Schoeller et al., 1990; Black et al., 1991b; Fricker et al., 1992; Welle et al., 1992; Westerterp et al., 1992; Johnson et al., 1994; Andersson and Rossner, 1996). Lichtman et al. (1992) observed a 47% underestimation of energy intake in young obese subjects whose reported intakes were less than 1,200 kcal per day, and Lansky and Brownell (1982) noted a 53% underestimation of energy intake among obese patients. Underreporting of intake has also been noted among female athletes (Westerterp et al., 1986), as well as among male athletes (Haggarty et al., 1988). These observations led Schoeller and colleagues (1990) to hypothesize that individuals tend to report intakes that are closer to perceived population and cultural norms of intake than to actual intake. Thus, obese individuals are likely to report intakes more similar to those of nonobese individuals, and highly physically active individuals tend to report intakes closer to those of less active individuals. Some studies have reported significantly greater underreporting by women than men (Hallfrisch et al., 1982; Schoeller et al., 1990; Black et al., 1991a; Goran and Poehlman, 1992; de Vries et al., 1994; Johnson et al., 1994), but other investigators found no significant differences between the sexes (Livingstone et al., 1990). The extent of underreporting tends to be greater in adolescent populations (Bandini et al., 1990; Jorgensen, 1992; Livingstone et al., 1992) and in the elderly (Pannemans and Westerterp, 1993; Reilly et al., 1993; Sawaya et al., 1996). Some studies suggest that the degree of underreporting increases with increasing energy intake (Schoeller et al., 1990); Livingstone, 1995), but others have found no relationship between underreporting and level of intake (de Vries et al., 1994; Sawaya et al., 1996). Thus, it is clear that there is considerable variability in the accuracy of self-reported intakes. The presence of systematic error is a serious problem that must be taken into consideration in analyzing and interpreting all self-reported dietary intake data. However, as discussed in Chapter 11, nutrient intakes expressed as a percentage of total energy intake have not been found to be biased, even when energy intake itself was underreported.

Reproducibility (also referred to as *reliability, repeatability*, or *precision*) is the extent to which one is able to obtain the same results when the method is repeated under the same conditions. If a method does not give consistent results on repeated similar occasions, it cannot be valid. Reproducibility studies of food records and recalls are difficult to design. If the time between repeated assessments is brief, there is greater possibility of a learning effect that can bias the results. However, if the time between administrations of the instrument is long, there is increased probability that eating habits will have changed in some individuals. Lack of reproducibility may also occur if the assessments are conducted during different times of the year, which can reflect seasonal differences in food availability and consumption. Single days of intake for a single individual have low reproducibility due to day-to-day variability in food intake (see Chapter 3). At the group level, however, the mean of a single day of intake is highly reproducible (Gersovitz et al., 1978; Rasanen, 1979). Good reproducibility at the individual level requires the averaging of multiple days of intake.

Limitations in our ability to validate dietary recalls and food records must be kept in mind when using these methods to validate food-frequency questionnaires or diet histories designed for estimating long-term usual dietary intake. (see Chapter 6.) Our expectations regarding the extent of agreement between the methods must be reasonably conservative when we keep in mind their many limitations and potential sources of error.

SUMMARY

Food records and 24-hour recalls, which consist of specific foods consumed by an individual on one or more days, differ from food-frequency questionnaires, which are designed to estimate usual intake over a longer period of time. The short-term methods allow greater specificity for describing foods and food preparation methods, and they permit greater flexibility for analyzing the data. However, due to the large amount of effort required to collect and process multiple days of food records or recalls, these methods are seldom used as the primary method for estimating usual intake in large-scale epidemiologic research. Nevertheless, these short-term methods serve important functions in describing mean values for groups and in validating food frequency questionnaires, which are now the most commonly used method for measuring dietary exposures in epidemiologic studies.

REFERENCES

Ahrens, E. H., Jr., and C. A. Boucher (1978). The composition of a simulated American diet. Comparison of chemical analyses and estimates from food composition tables. *J Am Diet Assoc 73*, 613–620.

Alberti-Fidanza, A., C. A. Paolacci, M. P. Chiuchiu, R. Coli, M. G. Parretta, G. Verducci, and F. Fidanza (1994). Dietary studies on two rural Italian population groups of the Seven Countries Study. 2. Concurrent validation of protein, fat and carbohydrate intake. *Eur J Clin Nutr 48,* 92–96.

Andersson, I., and S. Rossner (1996). The Gustaf Study: Repeated, telephone-administered 24-hour dietary recalls of obese and normal-weight men—Energy and macronutrient intake and distribution over the days of the week. *J Am Diet Assoc 96,* 686–692.

Avons, P., and W. P. James (1986). Energy-expenditure of young men from obese and non-obese families. *Hum Nutr Clin Nutr 40,* 259–270.

Balogh, M., H. A. Kahn, and J. H. Medalie (1971). Random repeat 24-hour dietary recalls. *Am J Clin Nutr 24,* 304–310.

Bandini, L. G., D. A. Schoeller, H. N. Cyr, and W. H. Dietz (1990). Validity of reported energy intake in obese and nonobese adolescents. *Am J Clin Nutr 52,* 421–425.

Basiotis, P. P., S. O. Welsh, F. J. Cronin, J. L. Kelsay, and W. Mertz (1987). Number of days of food intake records required to estimate individual and group nutrient intakes with defined confidence. *J Nutr 117,* 1638–1641.

Beaton, G. H., J. Milner, P. Corey, V. McGuire, M. Cousins, E. Stewart, M. de Ramos, D. Hewitt, P. V. Grambsch, N. Kassim, and J. A. Little (1979). Sources of variance in 24-hour dietary recall data: Implications for nutrition study design and interpretation. *Am J Clin Nutr 32,* 2546–2549.

Beaton, G. H., J. Milner, V. McGuire, T. E. Feather, and J. A. Little (1983). Source of variance in 24-hour dietary recall data: Implications for nutrition study design and interpretation. Carbohydrate sources, vitamins, and minerals. *Am J Clin Nutr 37,* 986–995.

Bhargava, A., R. Forthofer, S. McPherson, and M. Nichaman (1994). Estimating the variations and autocorrelations in dietary intakes on weekdays and weekends. *Statist Med 13,* 113–126.

Bingham, S., N. I. McNeil, and J. H. Cummings (1981). The diet of individuals: A study of a randomly-chosen cross section of British adults in a Cambridgeshire village. *Br J Nutr 45,* 23–35.

Bingham, S., H. S. Wiggins, H. Englyst, R. Seppanen, P. Helms, R. Strand, R. Burton, I. M. Jorgensen, L. Poulsen, A. Paerregaard, L. Bjerrum, and W. P. James (1982). Methods and validity of dietary assessments in four Scandinavian populations. *Nutr Cancer 4,* 23–33.

Bingham, S. A. (1987). The dietary assessment of individuals; methods, accuracy, new techniques and recommendations. *Nutr Abstr Rev 57,* 705–743.

Bingham, S. A., and J. H. Cummings (1985). Urine nitrogen as an independent validatory measure of dietary intake: A study of nitrogen balance in individuals consuming their normal diet. *Am J Clin Nutr 42,* 1276–1289.

Bingham, S. A., M. Nelson, A. Paul, J. Haraldsdottir, E. B. Loken, and W. A. van Staveren (1988). Methods for data collection at an individual level. In Cameron, M. E. and van Staveren, W. A. (eds.): *Manual on Methodology for Food Consumption Studies.* New York: Oxford University Press, pp 53–106.

Bird, G., and P. C. Elwood (1983). The dietary intakes of subjects estimated from photographs compared with a weighed record. *Hum Nutr Appl Nutr 37,* 470–473.

Black, A. E., G. R. Goldberg, S. A. Jebb, S. A. Bingham, M. B. E. Livingstone, and A. M. Prentice (1992). Validations of dietary assessment using doubly labelled water (abstract). *Proc Nutr Soc 51,* 72.

Black, A. E., G. R. Goldberg, S. A. Jebb, M. B. E. Livingstone, T. J. Cole, and A. M. Prentice (1991a). Critical evaluation of energy intake data using fundamental principles of energy physiology: 2. Evaluating the results of published surveys. *Eur J Clin Nutr 45,* 583–599.

Black, A. E., S. A. Jebb, and S. A. Bingham (1991b). Validation of energy and protein intakes assessed by diet history and weighed records against energy expenditure and 24 hr urinary nitrogen excretion (abstract). *Proc Nutr Soc 50,* 108.

Black, A. E., A. M. Prentice, G. R. Goldberg, S. A. Jebb, S. A. Bingham, M. B. E. Livingstone, and W. A. Coward (1993). Measurements of total energy expenditure provide insights into the validity of dietary measurement of energy intake. *J Am Diet Assoc 93,* 572–579.

Block, G. (1982). A review of validations of dietary assessment methods. *Am J Epidemiol 115,* 492–505.

Bolland, J. E., J. Y. Ward, and T. W. Bolland (1990). Improved accuracy of estimating food quantaties up to 4 weeks after training. *J Am Diet Assoc 90,* 1402–1404, 1407.

Bolland, J. E., J. A. Yuhas, and T. W. Bolland (1988). Estimation of food portion sizes: Effectiveness of training. *J Am Diet Assoc 88,* 817–821.

Borrelli, R., T. J. Cole, G. Di Biase, and F. Contaldo (1989). Some statistical considerations on dietary assessment methods. *Eur J Clin Nutr 43*, 453–463.

Brennan, R. E., M. B. Kohrs, J. W. Nordstrom, J. P. Sauvage, and R. E. Shank (1983). Composition of diets of low-income pregnant women: Comparison of analyzed with calculated values. *J Am Diet Assoc 83*, 538–545.

Briefel, R. R. (1994). Assessment of the U.S. diet in national nutrition surveys: National collaborative efforts and NHANES. *Am J Clin Nutr 59(suppl)*, 164S–167S.

Briefel, R. R., K. M. Flegal, D. M. Winn, C. M. Loria, C. L. Johnson, and C. T. Sempos (1992). Assessing the nation's diet: Limitations of the food frequency questionnaire. *J Am Diet Assoc 92*, 959–962.

Brown, J. E., T. M. Tharp, E. M. Dahlberg-Luby, D. A. Snowdon, S. K. Ostwald, I. M. Buzzard, S. M. Rysavy, and S. M. Wieser (1990). Videotape dietary assessment: Validity, reliability, and comparison of results with 24-hour dietary recalls from elderly women in a retirement home. *J Am Diet Assoc 90*, 1675–1679.

Bull, N. L., and E. F. Wheeler (1986). A study of different dietary survey methods among 30 civil servants. *Hum Nutr Appl Nutr 40*, 60–66.

Bureau of Social Science Research (1980). Long interviews are not main cause of refusals. *BSSR Newslett Fall*, 1–2.

Burk, M. C., and E. M. Pao (1976). *Methodology for Large-Scale Surveys of Household and Individual Diets*. Home Economics Research Report No. 40. Washington, DC: Agricultural Research Service, U.S. Department of Agriculture.

Buzzard, I. M., E. H. Asp, R. T. Chlebowski, A. P. Boyar, R. W. Jeffery, D. W. Nixon, G. L. Blackburn, P. R. Jochimsen, E. F. Scanlon, W. Insull, Jr., R. M. Elashoff, R. Butrum, and E. L. Wynder (1990). Diet intervention methods to reduce fat intake: Nutrient and food group composition of self-selected low-fat diets. *J Am Diet Assoc 90*, 42–50.

Buzzard, I. M., C. L. Faucett, R. W. Jeffery, L. McBane, P. McGovern, J. S. Baxter, A. C. Shapiro, G. L. Blackburn, R. T. Chlebowski, R. M. Elashoff, and E. L. Wynder (1996). Monitoring dietary change in a low-fat diet intervention study: Advantages of using 24-hour dietary recalls vs food records. *J Am Diet Assoc 96*, 574–579.

Buzzard, I. M., K. S. Price, and D. Feskanich (1991a). Preparation for data analysis: How the structure of the database influences data collection and analysis, and vice versa. In Kohlmeier, L. (ed.): *The Diet His-tory Method*. London: Smith-Gordon, pp 39–51.

Buzzard, I. M., K. S. Price, and R. A. Warren (1991b). Considerations for selecting nutrient-calculation software: Evaluation of the nutrient database (editorial). *Am J Clin Nutr 54*, 7–9.

Buzzard, I. M., and Y. A. Sievert (1994). Research priorities and recommendations for dietary assessment methodology: First International Conference on Dietary Assessment Methods. *Am J Clin Nutr 59(suppl)*, 275S–280S.

Campbell, V. A., and M. L. Dodds (1967). Collecting dietary information from groups of older people. *J Am Diet Assoc 51*, 29–33.

Carter, R. L., C. O. Sharbaugh, and C. A. Stapell (1981). Reliability and validity of the 24-hour recall. *J Am Diet Assoc 79*, 542–547.

Cassidy, C. M. (1994). Walk a mile in my shoes: Culturally sensitive food-habit research. *Am J Clin Nutr 59(suppl)*, 190S–197S.

de Vries, J. H., P. L. Zock, R. P. Mensink, and M. B. Katan (1994). Underestimation of energy intake by 3-d records compared with energy intake to maintain body weight in 269 nonobese adults. *Am J Clin Nutr 60*, 855–860.

Dennis, B., N. Ernst, M. Hjortland, J. Tillotson, and V. Grambsch (1980). The NHLBI nutrition data system. *J Am Diet Assoc 77*, 641–647.

Diaz, E. O., A. M. Prentice, G. R. Goldberg, P. R. Murgatroyd, and W. A. Coward (1992). Metabolic response to experimental overfeeding in lean and overweight healthy volunteers. *Am J Clin Nutr 56*, 641–655.

Dolecek, T. A., J. Stamler, A. W. Caggiula, J. L. Tillotson, and I. M. Buzzard (1997). Methods of dietary and nutritional assessment and intervention and other methods in the Multiple Risk Factor Intervention Trial. *Am J Clin Nutr 65(suppl)*, 196S–210S.

Dubois, S., and J. F. Boivin (1990). Accuracy of telephone dietary recalls in elderly subjects. *J Am Diet Assoc 90*, 1680–1687.

Emmons, L., and M. Hayes (1973). Accuracy of 24-hour recalls of young children. *J Am Diet Assoc 62*, 409–415.

Faggiano, F., P. Vineis, D. Cravanzola, P. Pisani, G. Xompero, E. Riboli, and R. Kaaks (1992). Validation of a method for the estimation of food portion size. *Epidemiology 3*, 379–382.

Fanelli, M. T., and K. J. Stevenhagen (1986). Consistency of energy and nutrient intakes of older adults: 24-hour recall vs. 1-day food record. *J Am Diet Assoc 86*, 665–667.

Feskanich, D., I. M. Buzzard, B. T. Welch, E. H. Asp, L. S. Dieleman, K. R. Chong, and G. E. Bartsch (1988). Comparison of a computerized and a manual method of food coding for nutrient intake studies. *J Am Diet Assoc 88, 1263–1267.* 1263–1267.

Feskanich, D., B. H. Sielaff, K. Chong, and I. M. Buzzard (1989). Computerized collection and analysis of dietary intake information. *Comput Methods Programs Biomed 30*, 47–57.

Fox, T. A., J. Heimendinger, and G. Block (1992). Telephone surveys as a method for obtaining dietary information: A review. *J Am Diet Assoc 92*, 729–732.

Fricker, J., D. Baelde, L. Igoin-Apfelbaum, J. M. Huet, and M. Apfelbaum (1992). Underreporting of food intake in obese "small-eaters." *Appetite 19*, 273–283.

Galasso, R. S. Panico, E. Celentano, and M. Del Pezzo (1994). Relative validity of multiple telephone versus face-to-face 24-hour dietary recalls. *Ann Epidemiol 4*, 332–336.

Gersovitz, M., J. P. Madden, and H. Smiciklas-Wright (1978). Validity of the 24-hour dietary recall and seven-day record for group comparisons. *J Am Diet Assoc 73*, 48–55.

Gibson, R. S. (1990). Food consumption of individuals. In Gibson, R. S. (ed.): *Principles of nutritional assessment*. New York: Oxford University Press. pp. 37–54.

Gibson, R. S., and C. A. Scythes (1982). Trace element intakes of women. *Br J Nutr 48*, 241–248.

Giovannetti, P. M. (1987). Calculated versus analytical nutrient values of diets in research studies. *J Can Diet Assoc 48*, 95–102.

Goldberg, G. R., A. M. Prentice, W. A. Coward, H. L. Davies, P. R. Murgatroyd, M. B. Sawyer, J. Ashford, and A. E. Black (1991). Longitudinal assessment of the components of energy balance in well-nourished lactating women. *Am J Clin Nutr 54*, 788–798.

Goran, M. I., and E. T. Poehlman (1992). Total energy expenditure and energy requirements in healthy elderly persons. *Metab Clin Exp 41*, 744–753.

Gorman, B. (1990). New products for a new century. *Prep Foods New Prod Ann 159*, 16–18, 47–52.

Greger, J. L., and G. M. Etnyre (1978). Validity of 24-hour dietary recalls by adolescent females. *Am J Public Health 68*, 70–72.

Guenther, P. M. (1994). Research needs for dietary assessment and monitoring in the United States. *Am J Clin Nutr 59(suppl)*, 168S–170S.

Guenther, P. M., P. S. Kott, and A. L. Carriquiry (1997). Development of an approach for estimating usual nutrient intake distributions at the population level. *J Nutr 127*, 1106–1112.

Guthrie, H. A. (1984). Selection and quantification of typical food portions by young adults. *J Am Diet Assoc 84*, 1440–1444.

Haggarty, P., B. A. McGaw, R. J. Maughan, and C. Fenn (1988). Energy expenditure of elite female athletes measured by the doubly-labelled water method (abstract). *Proc Nutr Soc 47*, 35.

Hallfrisch, J. J., P. Steele, and L. Cohen (1982). Comparison of seven-day diet record with measured food intake of twenty-four subjects. *Nutr Res 2*, 263–273.

Hartman, A. M., C. C. Brown, J. Palmgren, P. Pietinen, M. Verkasalo, D. Myer, and J. Virtamo (1990). Variability in nutrient and food intakes among older middle-aged men. Implications for design of epidemiologic and validation studies using food recording. *Am J Epidemiol 132*, 999–1012.

Howat, P. M., R. Mohan, C. Champagne, C. Monlezun, P. Wozniak, and G. A. Bray (1994). Validity and reliability of reported dietary intake data. *J Am Diet Assoc 94*, 169–173.

International Dietary Energy Consultative Group (1990). *The Doubly-Labeled Water Method for Measuring Energy Expenditure: Technical Recommendations for Use in Humans*. No. IAEA NAHRES-4. Vienna A consensus report by IDECG. A. M. Prentice, ed.

Jackson, B., C. A. Dujovne, S. DeCoursey, P. Beyer, E. F. Brown, and K. Hassanein (1986). Methods to assess relative reliability of diet records: Minimum records for monitoring lipid and caloric intake. *J Am Diet Assoc 86*, 1531–1535.

Johnson, R. K., M. I. Goran, and E. T. Poehlman (1994). Correlates of over- and underreporting of energy intake in healthy older men and women. *Am J Clin Nutr 59*, 1286–1290.

Jorgensen, L. M. (1992). Who completes seven-day food records? *Eur J Clin Nutr 46*, 735–741.

Karvetti, R. -L., and L. R. Knuts (1985). Validity of the 24-hour dietary recall. *J Am Diet Assoc 85*, 1437–1442.

Karvetti, R.-L., and L. R. Knuts (1992). Validity of the estimated food diary: Comparison of 2-day recorded and observed food and nutrient intakes. *J Am Diet Assoc 92*, 580–584.

Kim, W. W., W. Mertz, J. T. Judd, M. W. Marshall, J. L. Kelsay, and E. S. Prather (1984). Effect of making duplicate food collections on nutrient intakes calculated from diet records. *Am J Clin Nutr 40*, 1333–1337.

Kirkcaldy-Hargreaves, M., and G. W. Lynch (1980). Assessment of the validity of four food models. *J Can Diet Assoc 41*, 102–110.

Krall, E. A., J. T. Dwyer, and K. A. Coleman (1988). Factors influencing accuracy of dietary recall. *Nutr Res 8*, 829–841.

Krantzler, N. J., B. J. Mullen, H. G. Schutz, L. E. Grevetti, C. A. Holden, and H. L. Meiselman (1982). Validity of telephoned diet recalls and records for assessment of individual food intake. *Am J Clin Nutr 36*, 1234–1242.

Kretsch, M. J., and A. K. H. Fong (1990). Validation of a new computerized technique for quantitating individual dietary intake: The Nutrition Evaluation Scale System (NESSy) vs the weighed food record. *Am J Clin Nutr 51*, 477–484.

Kromhout, D. (1983). Energy and macronutrient intake in lean and obese middle-aged men (The Zutphen Study). *Am J Clin Nutr 37*, 295–299.

Lansky, D., and K. D. Brownell (1982). Estimates of food quantity and calories: Errors in self-report among obese patients. *Am J Clin Nutr 35*, 727–732.

Larkin, F. A., H. L. Metzner, and K. E. Guire (1991). Comparison of three consecutive-day and three random-day records of dietary intake. *J Am Diet Assoc 91*, 1538–1542.

Lee, R. D., and D. C. Nieman (1993). Computerized dietary analysis systems. In Lee, R. D. and Nieman, D.C. (eds.): *Nutritional Assessment*. Oxford: Brown & Benchmark, pp 103–119.

Lee-Han, H., M. Cousins, M. Beaton, V. McGuire, V. Kriukov, M. Chipman, and N. Boyd (1988). Compliance in a randomized clinical trial of dietary fat reduction in patients with breast dysplasia. *Am J Clin Nutr 48*, 575–586.

Lichtman, S. W., K. Pisarska, E. R. Berman, M. Pestone, H. Dowling, E. Offenbacher, H. Weisel, S. Heshka, D. E. Mathews, and S. B. Heymsfield (1992). Discrepancy between self-reported and actual caloric intake and exercise in obese subjects. *N Engl J Med 327*, 1893–1898.

Linusson, E., E. I. D. Sanjur, and E. C. Erickson (1974). Validating the 24-hour recall methods as a dietary survey tool. *Arch Latinoam Nutr 24*, 277–281.

Liu, K., J. Stamler, A. Dyer, J. McKeever, and P. McKeever (1978). Statistical methods to assess and minimize the role of intra-individual variability in obscuring the relationship between dietary lipids and serum cholesterol. *J Chronic Dis 31*, 399–418.

Livingstone, M. B., A. M. Prentice, J. J. Strain, W. A. Coward, A. E. Black, M. E. Barker, P. G. McKenna, and R. G. Whitehead (1990). Accuracy of weighed dietary records in studies of diet and health. *BMJ 300*, 708–712.

Livingstone, M. B. E. (1995). Assessment of food intakes—are we measuring what people eat? *Br J Biomed Sci 52*, 58–67.

Livingstone, M. B. E., A. M. Prentice, W. A. Coward, J. J. Strain, A. E. Black, P. S. W. Davies, C. M. Stewart, P. G. McKenna, and R. G. Whitehead (1992). Validation of estimates of energy intake by weighed dietary record and diet history in children and adolescents. *Am J Clin Nutr 56*, 29–35.

Lytle, L. A., M. Z. Nichaman, E. Obarzanek, E. Glovsky, D. Montgomery, T. Nicklas, M. Zive, and H. Feldman (1993). Validation of 24-hour recalls assisted by food records in third-grade children. The CATCH Collaborative Group. *J Am Diet Assoc 93*, 1431–1436.

Madden, J. P., S. J. Goodman, and H. A. Guthrie (1976). Validity of the 24-hour recall. Analysis of data obtained from elderly subjects. *J Am Diet Assoc 68*, 143–147.

Maisey S., J. Loughridge, S. Southon, and R. Fulcher (1995). Variation in food group and nutrient intake with day of the week in an elderly population. *Brit J Nutr 73*, 359–373.

Marr, J. W. (1981). Individual variation in dietary intake. In Turner, M. (ed.): *Preventive Nutrition and Society*. London: Academic Press.

Marr, J. W., and J. A. Heady (1986). Within- and between-person variation in dietary surveys: Number of days needed to classify individuals. *Hum Nutr Appl Nutr 40A*, 347–364.

Marshall, M. W., J. M. Iacono, C. W. Young, Jr., V. A. Washington, H. T. Slover, and P. M. Leapley (1975). Composition of diets containing 25 and 35 percent calories from fat: Analyzed vs. calculated values. *J Am Diet Assoc 66*, 470–481.

Marshall, M. W., and J. T. Judd (1982). Calculated vs. analyzed composition of four modified fat diets. Formulated to study effects in human subjects of kind and amount of dietary fat. *J Am Diet Assoc 80*, 537–549.

Miles, C. W., B. Brooks, R. Barnes, W. Marcus, E. S. Prather, and C. E. Bodwell (1984).

Calorie and protein intake and balance of men and women consuming self-selected diets. *Am J Clin Nutr 40(s)*, 1361–7.

Miller, J. Z., T. Kimes, S. Hui, M. B. Andon, and C. C. Johnston, Jr. (1991). Nutrient intake variability in a pediatric population: Implications for study design. *J Nutr 121*, 265–274.

Morgan, K. J., S. R. Johnson, B., and Goungetas (1987). Variability of food intakes. An analysis of a 12-day data series using persistence measures. *Am J Epidemiol 126*, 326–335.

Morgan, R. W., M. Jain, A. B. Miller, N. W. Choi, V. Matthews, L. Munan, J. D. Burch, J. Feather, G. R. Howe, and A. Kelly (1978). A comparison of dietary methods in epidemiologic studies. *Am J Epidemiol 107*, 488–498.

Mullenbach, V., L. H. Kushi, C. Jacobson, O. Gomez-Marin, R. J. Prineas, L. Roth-Yousey, and A. R. Sinaiko (1992). Comparison of 3-day food record and 24-hour recall by telephone for dietary evaluation in adolescents. *J Am Diet Assoc 92*, 743–745.

National Research Council, National Academy of Sciences, Subcommittee on Criteria for Dietary Evaluation, Coordinating Committee on Evaluation of Food Consumption Surveys (1986). *Nutrient Adequacy: Assessment Using Food Consumption Surveys*. Washington, DC: National Academy Press.

Nelson, M., A. E. Black, J. A. Morris, and T. J. Cole (1989). Between- and within-subject variation in nutrient intake from infancy to old age: Estimating the number of days required to rank dietary intakes with desired precision. *Am J Clin Nutr 50*, 155–167.

Obarzanek, E., D. B. Reed, C. Bigelow, E. Glovsky, R. Pobocik, T. Nicklas, A. Clesi, M. Zive, L. A. Lytle, and E. Lakatos (1993). Fat and sodium content of school lunch foods: Calculated values and chemical analysis. *Int J Food Sci Nutr 44*, 155–165.

Orta, J. (1991). Software scan: Scanning recent nutrition computer software. *Food Nutr News 63*, 10.

Pannemans, D. L., and K. R. Westerterp (1993). Estimation of energy intake to feed subjects at energy balance as verified with doubly labelled water: A study in the elderly. *Eur J Clin Nutr 47*, 490–496.

Pekkarinen, M. (1970). Methodology in the collection of food consumption data. *World Rev Nutr Dietetics 12*, 145–171.

Persson, L. A., and G. Carlgren (1984). Measuring children's diets: Evaluation of dietary assessment techniques in infancy and childhood. *Int J Epidemiol 13*, 506–517.

Petersen, R., W. H. Kaye, and H. E. Gwirtsman (1986). Comparison of calculated estimates and laboratory analysis of food offered to hospitalized eating disorder patients. *J Am Diet Assoc 86*, 490–492.

Pietinen, P., R. Dougherty, M. Mutanen, U. Leino, S. Moisio, J. Iacono, and P. Puska (1984). Dietary intervention study among 30 free-living families in Finland. *J Am Diet Assoc 84*, 313–318.

Posner, B. M., C. L. Borman, J. L. Morgan, W. S. Borden, and J. C. Ohls (1982). The validity of a telephone-administered 24-hour dietary recall methodology. *Am J Clin Nutr 36*, 546–553.

Posner, B. M., C. Smigelski, A. Duggal, J. L. Morgan, J. Cobb, and L. A. Cupples (1992). Validation of two-dimensional models for estimation of portion size in nutrition research. *J Am Diet Assoc 92*, 738–741.

Prentice, A. M., A. E. Black, W. A. Coward, H. L. Davies, G. R. Goldberg, P. R. Murgatroyd, J. Ashford, M. Sawyer, and R. G. Whitehead (1986). High levels of energy expenditure in obese women. *Br Med J Clin Res 292*, 983–987.

Prentice, A. M., K. Leavesley, P. R. Murgatroyd, W. A. Coward, C. J. Schorah, P. T. Bladon, and R. P. Hullin (1989). Is severe wasting in elderly mental patients caused by an excessive energy requirement? *Age Aging 18*, 158–167.

Rand, W. M., J. A. T. Pennington, S. P. Murphy, and J. C. Klensin (1991). *Compiling Data for Food Composition Data Bases*. Tokyo: United Nations University Press.

Rasanen, L. (1979). Nutrition survey of Finnish rural children. VI. Methodological study comparing the 24-hour recall and the dietary history interview. *Am J Clin Nutr 32*, 2560–2567.

Reilly, J. J., A. Lord, V. W. Bunker, A. M. Prentice, W. A. Coward, A. J. Thomas, and R. S. Briggs (1993). Energy balance in healthy elderly women. *Br J Nutr 69*, 21–27.

Rush, D., and A. R. Kristal (1982). Methodologic studies during pregnancy: The reliability of the 24-hour dietary recall. *Am J Clin Nutr 35(suppl)*, 1259–1268.

Sawaya, A. L., K. Tucker, R. Tsay, W. Willett, E. Saltzman, G. E. Dallal, and S. B. Roberts (1996). Evaluation of four methods for determining energy intake in young and older women: Comparison with doubly labeled water measurements of total energy expenditure. *Am J Clin Nutr 63*, 491–499.

Schnakenberg, D. D., T. M. Hill, M. J. Kretsch, and B. S. Morris (1981). Diary-interview technique to assess food consumption patterns of individual military personnel. In National Research Council, Committee on Food Consumption Patterns: *Assessing Changing Food Consumption Patterns.* Washington, DC: National Academy Press, pp 187–197.

Schoeller, D. A., L. G. Bandini, and W. H. Dietz (1990). Inaccuracies in self-reported intake identified by comparison with the doubly labelled water method. *Can J Physiol Pharmacol 68,* 941–949.

Schucker, R. E. (1982). Alternative approaches to classic food consumption measurement methods: Telephone interviewing and market data bases. *Am J Clin Nut 35(suppl),* 1306–1309.

Schulz, S., K. R. Westerterp, and K. Bruck (1989). Comparison of energy expenditure by the doubly labeled water technique with energy intake, heart rate, and activity recording in man. *Am J Clin Nutr 49,* 1146–1154.

Smith, J. L. (1993). *Nutrient Databank Directory.* Newark, DE: University of Delaware.

Snetselaar, L. G. (1989). *Nutrition Counseling Skills.* Rockville, MD: Aspen Publishers, Inc.

Snetselaar, L. G., C. A. Chenard, L. G. Hunsicker, and P. J. Stumbo (1995). Protein calculation from food diaries of adult humans underestimates values determined using a biological marker. *J Nutr 125,* 2333–2340.

Stockley, L. (1985). Changes in habitual food intake during weighed inventory surveys and duplication diet collections. A short review. *Ecol Food Nutr 17,* 263–269.

Stockley, L., R. I. Chapman, M. L. Holley, F. A. Jones, E. H. Prescott, and A. J. Broadhurst (1986). Description of a food recording electronic device for use in dietary surveys. *Hum Nutr Appl Nutr 40,* 13–18.

Tarasuk, V., and G. H. Beaton (1992). Day-to-day variation in energy and nutrient intake: Evidence of individuality in eating behavior? *Appetite 18,* 43–54.

Thompson, F. E., and T. Byers (1994). Dietary assessment resource manual. *J Nutr 124 (suppl),* 2245S–2317S.

Thompson, R. E., F. A. Larkin, and M. B. Brown (1986). Weekend–weekday differences in reported dietary intake. The Nationwide Food Consumption Survey. *Nutr Res 6,* 647–662.

van Horn, L. V., P. Stumbo, A. Moag-Stahlberg, E. Obarzanek, V. W. Hartmuller, R. P. Farris, S. Y. Kimm, M. Frederick, L. Snetselaar, and K. Liu (1993). The Dietary Intervention Study in Children (DISC): Dietary assessment methods for 8- to 10-year-olds. *J Am Diet Assoc 93,* 1396–1403.

Webb, C. A., and J. A. Yuhas (1988). Ability of WIC clientele to estimate food quantities. *J Am Diet Assoc 88,* 601–602.

Wein, E. E., J. H. Sabry, and F. T. Evers (1990). Recalled estimates of food portion size. *J Can Diet Assoc 51,* 400–403.

Welle, S., G. B. Forbes, M. Statt, R. R. Barnard, and J. M. Amatruda (1992). Energy expenditure under free-living conditions in normal-weight and overweight women. *Am J Clin Nutr 55,* 14–21.

Westat, Inc. (1992). *NHANES-III Dietary Interviewer's Manual.* Hyattsville, MD: National Center for Health Statistics.

Westerterp, K. R., W. H. Saris, M. van Es, and F. ten Hoor (1986). Use of the doubly labeled water technique in humans during heavy sustained exercise. *J Appl Physiol 61,* 2162–2167.

Westerterp, K. R., W. P. H. Verboeket-van de Venne, G. A. L. Meijer, and F. ten Hoor (1992). Self-reported intake as a measure for energy intake. A validation against doubly-labelled water. In Ailhaud, G., Guy-Grand, B., Lafontan, M., and Riquier, D. (eds.): *Obesity in Europe.* London: John Libbey, pp 17–22.

Young, C. M., F. W. Chalmers, H. N. Church, M. M. Clayton, G. C. Murphy, and R. E. Tucker (1953). Subjects' estimation of food intakes and calculated nutritive value of the diet. *J Am Diet Assoc 29,* 1216–1220.

Yuhas, J. A., J. E. Bolland, and T. W. Bolland (1989). The impact of training, food type, gender, and container size on the estimation of food portion sizes. *J Am Diet Assoc 89,* 1473–1477.

5

Food-Frequency Methods

Because short-term recall and diet record methods are generally expensive, unrepresentative of usual intake if only a few days are assessed, and inappropriate for assessment of past diet, investigators have sought alternative methods for measuring long-term dietary intake. Burke (1947) developed a detailed dietary history interview that attempted to assess an individual's usual diet; this included a 24-hour recall, a menu recorded for 3 days, and a checklist of foods consumed over the preceding month. This method was time consuming and expensive, and a highly skilled professional was needed for both the interview and the processing of the information. The checklist, however, was the forerunner of the more structured dietary questionnaires in use today. During the 1950s, Stephanik and Trulson (1962), Heady (1961), Wiehl and Reed (1960), and Marr (1971) developed food-frequency questionnaires and evaluated their role in dietary assessment. Stephanik and Trulson (1962) found that a food-frequency questionnaire discrimi-

nated between groups of subjects defined by ethnicity, but did not consider that such a questionnaire could be useful in computing nutrient intakes. Heady (1961), using diet records collected by British bank clerks, demonstrated that the *frequencies* that foods were used correlated highly with the total *weights* of the same foods consumed over a several-day period. He then designed a self-administered questionnaire for use in large populations based strictly on the frequencies that foods were eaten; unfortunately, this questionnaire was apparently never employed for its intended use. Nichols and coworkers (1976) used a food-frequency questionnaire in the Tecumseh Heart Study population and failed to find an association between intake of fat, sugar, or starch-containing foods and level of serum cholesterol. Perhaps in part because of this failure to observe correlations with serum cholesterol, interest in food-frequency questionnaires (and nutritional epidemiology in general) waned during the early 1970s, but has greatly increased more recently. (In retrospect, correlation with serum cholesterol was an unfortunate criterion for validity as it is only moderately sensitive to changes in diet; see Chapters 1 and 6.) Multiple investigators have converged, apparently independently, toward the use of food-frequency questionnaires as the method of dietary assessment best suited for most epidemiologic applications. During the 1980s and 1990s, substantial refinement, modification, and evaluation of food-frequency questionnaires has occurred so that data derived from their use have become considerably more interpretable.

RATIONALE AND CONCEPTUAL BASIS

The underlying principle of the food-frequency approach is that average long-term diet, for example, intake over weeks, months, or years, is the conceptually important exposure rather than intake on a few specific days. Therefore, it may be advantageous to sacrifice precise intake measurements obtainable on 1 or a few days in exchange for more crude information relating to an extended period of time. Moreover, it is typically easier to describe one's usual frequency of consuming a food than to describe what foods were eaten at any specific meal in the past. This concept, often referred to as *generic* as opposed to *episodic* memory, is supported by cognitive research (Bradburn et al., 1987; Smith et al., 1991b; Smith, 1993) and has long been used by infectious disease epidemiologists investigating food-borne outbreaks; even when interest is focused on a specific meal, subjects find it difficult to recall their food intake at that time. Therefore, general questions are often posed as to whether a specified food is almost never eaten or whether it is usually eaten, if available.

The basic food-frequency questionnaire consists of two components: a food list and a frequency response section for subjects to report how often each food was eaten. Questions related to further details of quantity and composition may be appended. In the following sections, considerations for the design of such questionnaires are discussed.

THE FOOD LIST

A basic decision in designing a questionnaire is whether the objective is to measure intake of a few specific foods or nutrients or whether a comprehensive assessment of dietary intake is desired. A comprehensive assessment is generally desirable whenever possible for several reasons. First, it is often impossible to anticipate at the beginning all the questions regarding diet that will appear important at the end of a study; a highly restricted food list may not have included an item that is, in retrospect, important. Furthermore, as discussed in Chapter 11, total food intake, represented by energy consumption, may be related to disease outcome and thus confound the effects of specific nutrients or foods. Even if total energy intake is not related to a disease outcome, adjustment for total intake may increase the precision of specific nutrient measurements (discussed in Chapter 11). Nevertheless, epidemiologic practice is usually a compromise between ideal and reality, and it may simply not be possible to include a comprehensive diet assessment in a particular interview or questionnaire, especially if diet is not the primary focus of the study. When the number of questions is severely constrained and the focus is on one or a few nutrients only, it may be reasonable to select a list of foods identified by other investigators as important predictors of these nutrients if the general cultural background of the study population is similar. Brief food frequency questionnaires have also been developed to screen for eligibility in dietary trials, to monitor compliance with dietary interventions, and to identify individuals in clinical settings for more detailed dietary assessments (Guthrie and Scheer, 1981; Heller et al., 1981; Knapp et al., 1988; Block et al., 1989; Hopkins et al., 1989; Kristal et al., 1990a–

c; Ammerman et al., 1991; Kinlay et al., 1991; Beresford et al., 1992; Connor et al., 1992; van Assema et al., 1992; Serdula et al., 1993).

A second questionnaire design issue is whether the primary objective is to rank individuals (i.e., to discriminate among subjects according to dietary intake) or to provide a measure of absolute intake. In most epidemiologic applications ranking is the primary objective, and conversion to absolute intake may even be done by post hoc statistical methods (see Chapter 12). In either circumstance, it is important to select carefully the most informative items for the food list because an excessively long questionnaire can lead to fatigue and boredom, which can impair concentration and accuracy. We have been impressed that individuals are willing to complete relatively long dietary questionnaires, probably because of strong general interest in food. Our current questionnaires, however, which include approximately 130 food items, may be approaching the limit. Even in a highly motivated cohort (Willett et al., 1987), approximately 5% of women willing to complete a two-page, health-related mailed questionnaire did not complete an additional 61-item dietary questionnaire (unpublished data).

For a food item to be informative it must have three general characteristics. First, the food must be used reasonably often by an appreciable number of individuals. Second, the food must have a substantial content of the nutrient(s) of interest. Third, to be discriminating, the use of the food must vary from person to person. To illustrate the last point, a question about carrots would not help to rank subjects according to carotene intake if everyone ate one carrot a day. On the other hand, an item about spinach, which is often either avoided or is enjoyed and eaten frequently, may provide much more information even though it has a somewhat lower carotene content and lower average frequency of use. In theory, if the intake of two foods are very highly correlated, it would not be necessary to in-

clude them both; however, we have yet to observe a good example of this situation. These three characteristics can be summarized by calculating the contribution of each food to the between-person variance in the intake of specific nutrients; an application of this approach using stepwise regression analysis is described later. Apart from considerations of nutrient intake, foods may be included on a questionnaire on the basis of prior information, epidemiologic or otherwise, that an association might exist. For example, we have included mushrooms in a study of diet and cancer on the basis of a strong effect on stomach cancer in animals (Toth et al., 1982).

Several approaches can be used to compile a food list. The simplest is to examine published food composition tables and identify the foods that contain substantial amounts of the nutrient(s) of interest. Although rapid and simple, this strategy would lead to the inclusion of foods that have high nutrient concentration, such as brains, which are exceedingly rich in cholesterol, but that are not eaten with sufficient frequency to be important.

Another approach is to start with a long list of foods that are potentially important nutrient sources and systematically reduce this list. The original list may be derived from food composition tables or informally with the help of an experienced dietitian. Reduction of the list can be accomplished by pilot testing of the questionnaire. The easiest method is simply to delete items that are infrequently used. This process, however, ignores the fact that foods with high between-person variation in their use are more informative than those that are of similar average use, but used uniformly by all persons. A more sophisticated approach is to use stepwise regression analysis of pilot study data to identify the most discriminating food items (Heady, 1961).

We used stepwise regression to develop a questionnaire used in a cohort of over 100,000 women (Willett et al., 1985). The objective was to measure a fairly comprehensive list of 18 nutrients, but the space and the cost of data entry constrained the form to approximately two pages. A four-page pilot questionnaire including approximately 120 items was developed by consultation with an experienced dietitian and we conducted small-scale pilot studies to eliminate very infrequently used items. A four-page form consisting of about 100 food items was then mailed to a sample of 2,000 cohort members and returned by 86%. For every individual we computed a total intake score for each of the 18 nutrients (computation detailed later). We then conducted a separate stepwise multiple regression analysis for each nutrient with the total nutrient intake as the dependent variable. In this process the computer algorithm identifies the food that explains the most between-person variance in nutrient intake as the first independent variable, the food that explains the most variance not accounted for by the first food as the second independent variable, and so on. The contribution a food makes is reflected in the change in cumulative R^2. This analysis thus identifies the foods that most discriminate between individuals rather than those that contribute most to absolute intake. Results for animal fat, vegetable fat, cholesterol, and vitamin C are shown as examples in Table 5–1. It will be appreciated that R^2 values accumulate much more rapidly for those nutrients that are highly concentrated in a few foods (e.g., vitamin C) than those that are dispersed through many foods (e.g., protein). We were able to account for at least an R^2 of 80% (and often much more than 80%) for each of the 18 nutrients using only a modest number of foods. Several foods, such as meat, were important contributors to more than one nutrient. By selecting the most discriminating foods, and by combining several nutritionally similar items into single items, we constructed a 61-item questionnaire, which was then mailed to over 120,000 cohort members (see Appendix 5–1). Mark and coworkers (1996) have suggested another empirical approach for selecting informative foods from a longer list. For a fixed

Table 5–1. Foods most predictive of between-person variation in animal and vegetable fat, cholesterol, and vitamin C intake

Food	Cumulative R^{2a}
Animal fat	
Beef, main dish	0.31
Whole milk	0.41
Hard cheese	0.52
Beef, mixed dish	0.60
Chicken, with skin	0.67
Butter	0.71
Eggs	0.74
Hot dogs	0.76
Ice cream	0.78
Chicken, no skin	0.80
Processed meats	0.81
Hamburger, regular	0.82
Hamburger, lean	0.83
Vegetable fat	
Margarine	0.18
Cookies, ready made	0.36
Nuts	0.49
Peanut butter	0.60
Chocolate candy	0.65
Potato, corn chips	0.69
Pie, homemade	0.72
Home fried foods	0.74
Pie, ready-made	0.76
White bread	0.77
Cake, homemade	0.78
French fries	0.79
Dark bread	0.79
Cholesterol	
Eggs	0.53
Beef, main dish	0.61
Lean hamburger	0.68
Corn	0.71
Chicken, with skin	0.73
Chicken, no skin	0.76
Beef, mixed dish	0.78
Whole milk	0.80
Hard cheese	0.81
Liver	0.82
Butter	0.83
Custard	0.84
Cookies, ready made	0.85
Vitamin C	
Supplement	0.91
Orange juice	0.93
Multi vitamins	0.94
Fruit punch	0.96
Spinach, greens	0.96
Berries	0.96
Brussel sprouts	0.96

[a]Data are based on cumulative R^2 values in stepwise regression analysis of a semiquantitative food-frequency questionnaire pilot-tested among 1,742 U.S. women.
From Willett et al., 1981.

number of foods to be selected, they developed a computer algorithm to select all possible combinations of foods, calculate nutrient intakes from each combination, and pick the combination having the highest correlation with intakes calculated from the full list This gave results generally similar to the stepwise procedure.

Some caution should be entertained in using regression analysis to design a form. Because several hundred food variables may be included in an original long list of potential foods, some will enter as "statistically significant" predictors on the basis of chance alone. Therefore, the sample should be large, probably on the order of 1,000 to 2,000 rather than a few hundred. With this sample size, even unimportant contributors to cumulative R^2 may be statistically significant, but can be ignored. Even with a large sample, a few foods may occasionally make a modest contribution to R^2, but not make sense in terms of containing the nutrient being predicted or having an obvious association with a food rich in that nutrient. For example, in Table 5–1, corn entered as a modest predictor of cholesterol intake even though it contains none; this is presumably the result of correlation between the use of corn and another food, perhaps butter. It must be appreciated that this type of analysis used to identify items for inclusion on a questionnaire is in no sense a test of validity. Even though a high cumulative R^2 is obtained, the dependent variable, total nutrient score, is calculated using the same food items so that the cumulative R^2 would be 1.00 if all food items are entered as predictors.

A third approach to constructing a questionnaire is to use open-ended data, such as those obtained by diet records or 24-hour recalls, to identify the foods that contribute most importantly to the total absolute intake of a nutrient by the group as a whole. In this type of analysis, which has been used by Block and coworkers (1986), who employed 24-hour recall data from

the National Health and Nutrition Examination Surveys (NHANES) study, individuals are ignored; only the pooled information is examined (by necessity when using NHANES data, as only one 24-hour collection was available per subject). Howe and colleagues (1986) have used this strategy, based on data from a comprehensive diet history, to identify a short list of foods contributing the most to intake of N-nitrosamines or their precursors. Similarly, Stryker and colleagues (1991) used data from the 28 days of diet recording by 194 women in the Nurses' Health Study validation study to compile lists of foods that contributed to the intake of 18 nutrients.

An advantage of this open-ended approach is that important contributors to nutrient intake are unlikely to be missed. Many arbitrary decisions, however, must be made regarding the collapsing of variables as the open-ended methods are typically coded in much finer detail than would be appropriate for items on a questionnaire. For example, in conducting this type of analysis using diet record data (Willett et al., 1988), over 300 codes for beef, pork, and lamb were collapsed into two categories on meat consumption that corresponded to our questionnaire. In addition, carefully collected open-ended methods often include mixed dishes, baked goods, and prepared foods that have been "dissected" and coded into ingredients (e.g., flour and shortening) that would not be included on a questionnaire, even though the final product (e.g., bread or cake) would be listed. Thus, the use of open-ended dietary data to identify foods for a questionnaire can require a major investment of time and still be subject to arbitrary groupings of foods that may not correspond to the perception of persons completing the final questionnaire.

A modification of the open-ended approach would be to tally the foods from diet recalls or records collected from a sample of the study population without calculating nutrients. This might be particularly useful in situations when the size of the study or available resources would not justify a major investment in questionnaire development. An advantage of this approach is that information will be gained regarding the familiar names and descriptions of foods, which may be useful for studies among migrants or ethnic minority groups. At the same time, a tally of portion sizes of foods could be made; the use of such information is discussed later.

Byers and colleagues (1985) analyzed data to determine the relative contribution of 20 foods to absolute intake and to between-person variance expressed as cumulative R^2 (Fig. 5–1 gives an example). These investigators observed that a relatively small list of foods, identified by stepwise regression, was able to explain a substantially higher percentage of between-person variance than the percentage of absolute total intake. Stryker and coworkers (1991) conducted similar analyses, based on 4-week diet records collected by 194 women, that supported the observation that a relatively short list of foods selected by stepwise regression could account for a high portion of between-person variation. Some foods, such as meat, which was eaten regularly by nearly all persons and was the most important single contributor to absolute intake of calories and total fat, contributed less impressively to between-person variance in these nutrients than did foods such as cake and cookies, which were eaten frequently by some participants but avoided by others. The contribution of supplements to between-person variance was particularly striking, although not unexpected, as their use is an all-or-nothing phenomenon. These data, as well as the work of Mark and coworkers (1996) that compared various methods of food selection, suggest that the method of identifying foods simply on the basis of their contribution to absolute intake is not likely to lead to the optimal questionnaire when the number of items is constrained by cost, space, or time. Furthermore, foods or groups of foods that are most discriminating among persons should probably be asked about with greater detail than those that are less discriminating.

Assembling a selected list of foods into a clear and unambiguous questionnaire is critical. To some extent this is a process of trial and error, but the following considerations may be helpful. The organization and structure of a food list is important because one item can change the interpretation of another. For this reason, related items should be clustered together, such as by traditional food groups. For closely related foods, more specific items should precede general items (e.g., "low calorie salad dressing" should appear first, then "other salad dressing"). It is tempting to maximize the comprehensiveness of a questionnaire while maintaining brevity by combining or collapsing several foods into single questions. Our experience and that of Subar et al. (1995) suggest that this should be avoided; multiple simple, clear questions are preferable to a single longer, complex question. For example, on our original questionnaire we asked how often "peaches, apricots, or plums" were eaten over the past year. If more than one of these fruits are eaten, it is a very challenging task for respondents to consider each separately, integrate information over a year, and then describe a summary frequency. It would probably be better to ask three separate questions or drop one or two of the fruits entirely. In a related example, we found that the deletion of a clarifying item can alter the response to another item. In the stepwise regression analysis described previously, we found that lettuce did not contribute importantly to variance for any nutrient, so we dropped this item. We had, however, included another item, "spinach and other greens," that was an important predictor of carotene intake. With the lettuce item deleted, we discovered that reporting of "spinach and other greens" increased, apparently because some may have interpreted this to in-

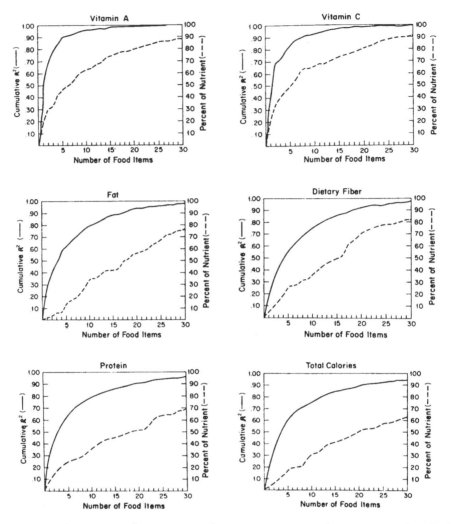

Figure 5–1. Cumulative R^2 and percentage of nutrients accounted for according to the number of food items included in the nutrient index.

(From Byers et al., 1985; reproduced with permission.)

clude lettuce. Although we thought we may have been gaining information on possible use of kale, collard, and mustard greens with our more comprehensive question, we probably gained statistical noise instead; it would have been better simply to ask about "spinach." Arriving at the optimal balance between splitting foods into many detailed separate questions or collapsing (combining) items into a few broad questions is extremely important. Because it is critical that

the person completing the questionnaire has the same mental picture of the foods as intended by the investigator, simplicity and clarity are paramount. Cognitive research indicates that subjects often decompose a question into several steps when they are unable to retrieve and count separate incidents, such as the repeated use of a food (Bradburn et al., 1987). Thus, much may be learned from focus groups and pilot studies that include informal or structured interviewing of participants as to their interpretation of questionnaire items (Subar et al., 1995).

Instead of using a food list that encompasses foods eaten at any time of the day, a meal-by-meal assessment of usual diet has been proposed (Kohlmeier, 1994). However, the function and validity of such a method in populations, such as in the United States, where food intake is increasingly less confined to formal meals, remains to be established.

An alternative to designing a questionnaire de novo is to use or modify an existing questionnaire.* This will be particularly attractive when time (often years) and resources are not available for a major investment in questionnaire development. There appears to be general willingness on the part of epidemiologists to share their questionnaires for scientific purposes. If the hypotheses are adequately addressed by an existing questionnaire and the form is reasonably appropriate for the cultural background of the study population, using an existing questionnaire may be the best approach.

If the population is somewhat different,

*Existing food-frequency questionnaires are described in detail in the Dietary Assessment Resource Manual by Thompson and Byers, published as a special edition of the *Journal of Nutrition* (Thompson and Byers, 1994). Specific questionnaires that have been used in a wide variety of applications include the Harvard Semiquantitative Food Frequency Questionnaire, available in several lengths and formats including for children (for further information, contact Ms. Laura Sampson, R. D., Department of Nutrition, Harvard School of Public Health, 677 Huntington Ave, Boston, MA 02115 or [978] 777-0744); the NCI/Block Health Habits and History Questionnaire (HHHQ), also available in several formats and lengths (for further information, contact Gladys Block, Ph.D., Professor of Epidemiology and Public Health Nutrition, University of California–Berkeley, School of Public Health, 419 Warren Hall, Berkeley, CA 94720), and The University of Texas Human Nutrition Center – Food Frequency Questionnaire (UT-HNC FFQ) (R. Sue McPherson, Ph.D., Associate Professor of Epidemiology and Nutrition, Human Nutrition Center, University of Texas, Houston School of Public Health, 1200 Herman Pressler Drive, Houston, TX 77030, [713] 500-9317).

such as an ethnic subgroup of a general population for which an existing questionnaire was designed, the addition of some foods to the existing questionnaire may be desirable. The methods described above may be used to identify such foods. The appropriate threshold for making changes to an existing questionnaire when the population is somewhat different is not clear. However, Borrud et al. (1989) found that the important foods in the diets of African-Americans and Mexican-Americans living in Texas were largely similar to those of white Americans. Thus, even though the frequency distributions of foods used by ethnic subgroups may differ substantially, it is likely that a reasonably comprehensive questionnaire may function across a wide spectrum of subgroups. This is particularly likely if the questions have been framed generically, such as by asking about meat included in mixed dishes (perhaps with some examples) rather than about meat in only a few of the many hundreds of possible ethnic mixed dishes. When a food-frequency questionnaire is being developed for a population with a substantially different cultural background from the investigator, considerable effort will be needed to learn about dietary patterns and the description and preparation of foods (Cassidy, 1994; Forsythe and Gage, 1994; Hankin and Wilkens, 1994). If possible, confirmation of the validity of a questionnaire in a new population would be desirable, as discussed in Chapter 6.

FREQUENCY RESPONSE SECTION

For most epidemiologic purposes, dietary intake over a number of years is the exposure of conceptual interest. Because diets tend to be reasonably correlated from year to year, we and most others have asked subjects to describe their frequencies of using foods in reference to the preceding year. This provides a full cycle of seasons so that, in theory, the responses should be independent of the time of year. For other purposes, the time frame could be a period 5 years previously (such as in a case–control study of colon cancer), the first 2 months of pregnancy (in a study of congenital malformations), or the preceding month (in a study of plasma high-density lipoprotein cholesterol). The relevant reference period is a function of both the physiology or the pathophysiology of the outcome being studied and the metabolism of the dietary factor under investigation. In the case of congenital malformations, the occurrence of the critical event, such as the closing of the neural tube, can be identified with precision to within several days. Because most nutrients (e.g., vitamin A) have long half-lives in the body, however, the nutritional status at the time of neural tube closure will depend on intake over the preceding weeks or months.

Response formats to frequency questions may appear to be a simple issue, but opportunities exist for serious pitfalls. Most investigators have provided a multiple-choice response format, with the number of options usually ranging from 5 to 10. If the same options are to be used for all food questions, however, five choices are likely to be too few and will usually result in serious loss of information. This can be appreciated by examining the frequency distributions for selected items in our pilot study of 1,742 women (Table 5–2). For some items (such as butter), most of the information on between-person variation is captured at the high end of the scale, but for other items (e.g., liver), most of the information is at the low end. Broadening the response categories to reduce their number would decrease the discrimination capacity of questions. For example, Gray and colleagues (1984) compared a food-frequency questionnaire having a small number of response options with a detailed dietary interview and observed a poor correlation. They attributed this to the limited response options, because, for many items, most subjects fell into a single category that encompassed a possible fourfold variation of intake. In an early questionnaire, Stephanik

and Trulson (1962) perceptively created 10 categories so that the range of intake within a category was no more than two-fold:

Never
Once a month or less
2–3 times per month
once per week
2–4 times per week
5–7 times per week
over one, under two times a day
2–3 times per day
4–6 times per day
over 6 times per day

This produces a scale with greater detail at the high frequency end, which is appropriate because a food consumed less than once per week makes relatively little contribution to nutrient intake. We have modified these categories slightly (see Appendices 5–1 and 5–2), collapsing two low-frequency responses into one, thus more efficiently using contemporary data-processing facilities (because nine possible responses plus "blank" use a single column of data storage). For an occasional food that contains an extremely high amount of a particular nutrient but that is used infrequently, such as liver, which is uniquely high in vitamin A, additional categories for use at low frequencies may be important (see Appendix 5–2).

An alternate format to the grid lay-out shown in Appendices 5–1 and 5–2 is to list the frequency choices vertically under each food item (see Appendix 5–3). This format was found to be easier for children and is also likely to be easier for populations with lower educational levels and the elderly. The number of frequency choices for each question can be limited to those that are actually used in the population (for example, broccoli is almost never eaten more than once per day), which reduces erroneous and extreme responses. The main disadvantage is that the same questionnaire will require several times more space, which is only an issue in very large studies.

Another approach is to use an open-

Table 5–2. Frequency distributions of responses to selected foods

Food	Responses of women, by percent[a]								
	Almost never	1–3/mo	1/wk	2–4/wk	5–6/wk	1/day	2–3/day	4–6/day	6+day
Skim/low fat milk	45	6	4	9	5	19	12	0	0
Whole milk	51	8	7	6	2	14	6	1	0
Yogurt	61	17	9	6	1	2	0	1	0
Ice cream	22	29	23	19	3	3	0	0	0
Butter	56	4	6	7	3	8	12	1	0
Apples or pears	14	18	19	27	4	13	4	0	0
Fish	9	34	39	15	3	0	0	0	0
Cabbage, cauliflower	15	36	34	12	1	1	0	0	0
Liver	33	64	3	0	0	0	0	0	0
Coffee	23	2	1	3	2	11	33	17	8
Low-calorie carbonated beverage	49	9	7	11	5	10	7	1	0

[a]Data are based on a pilot study conducted among 1,742 women. See Appendix 5–1 for data on additional foods.
From Willett et al., 1981.

ended format and provide subjects the option of answering in terms of frequency per day, week, or month (Block et al., 1986). In theory, an open-ended frequency response format might provide for some enhanced precision in reporting as the frequency of use is truly a continuous rather than a categorical variable. It is unlikely, however, that the overall increment in precision is large because the estimation of the frequency a food is used is inherently an approximation. In a detailed examination of questionnaire comprehension, Subar et al. (1995) found that using multiple-choice frequency response categories increased clarity and reduced errors compared with open-ended frequency responses.

Block (personal communication) has examined the relative validity of multiple choice compared with open-ended frequency response by calculating intakes first using open-ended frequency responses and then collapsing these open-ended responses into the nine frequency categories used in the form in Appendices 5–1 and 5–2. Intakes calculated using the two approaches were then correlated with an independent assessment of intake based on dietary records; these correlations were similar, indicating little if any loss of information due to the categorization of variables. Tylavsky

and Sharp (1995) simply compared nutrient intakes based on open-ended and collapsed frequency responses (without an independent assessment of true intakes) and concluded that categorization resulted in appreciable loss of information. However, such an analysis is uninformative as it assumes that the open-ended questions provide exact truth; a comparison with an independent assessment of intake is needed to evaluate relative validity.

OPTIONS FOR PORTION SIZE INFORMATION

Whether to collect additional data on portion sizes has been a controversial topic; but some relevant data are now becoming available. Several options exist. The first is to collect no additional information on portion sizes, that is, to use a simple frequency questionnaire. A second possibility is to specify a portion size as part of the question on frequency, that is, to ask how often a glass of milk is consumed rather than only how often milk is consumed. This has been termed a semiquantitative food-frequency questionnaire. For foods that come in natural units (such as a slice of bread, one egg, a cup of coffee) this additional specification can add clarity to the question. For example, if we just ask about "milk," a thoughtful subject will not know if we are asking about the milk added to coffee and breakfast cereal or whether three glasses consumed at one meal should count as one or as three. Because the specification of unit size does not require an additional question and should provide additional information and clarity, there is little reason not to pose questions in this way. The issue is less clear for foods that do not come in natural or typical units, such as meat or rice. It is possible to specify a typical portion (e.g., 4 to 6 ounces for a serving of meat or half a cup of rice); if a subject's usual portion is twice that amount, they would be expected to double their reported frequency of use. We have informally evaluated whether participants in the Nurses' Health Study cohort responded in this way by providing them with a hypothetical eating pattern and asking them to complete questions describing the diet. Although items about foods with natural units were consistently interpreted correctly, the portion size specification for foods without natural units, such as meat, was sometimes ignored. Whether it is advantageous to include a portion size specifically for these foods deserves further investigation (discussed later).

A third alternative is to include an additional item for each food to describe the usual portion size. This may involve describing a medium portion size in words and asking subjects to describe their usual portion as small, medium, or large (Block et al., 1986); using a realistic food model or a simple shape as a unit of reference (Morgan et al., 1978); or providing pictures of different portion sizes as a multiple-choice question (Hankin et al., 1983). The descriptions of usual serving sizes can also be left as completely open-ended items, although this will be expensive to code and process. Subar et al. (1995) have observed that providing ranges for categories of serving sizes (e.g., for peas, less than ¼ cup, ¼ to ¾ cup, and more than

¾ cup) improves clarity compared with asking subjects to report their usual serving size as small, medium, or large in relation to a specified medium serving size. However, they also found that subjects frequently ignored either type of portion size question when questionnaires were self-administered.

To provide useful information on serving sizes, subjects must be able to conceptualize the unit clearly and relate this to their own habits. Guthrie (1984) has observed, however, that individuals are generally unable to accurately describe their portion sizes. When subjects were asked, immediately after a meal, to describe the portions of foods they had just consumed, for most of the foods evaluated, fewer than half of the participants were accurate to within 25%. Smith et al. (1991a) also found that subjects had difficulty conceptualizing specified serving sizes, particularly when expressed as small, medium, or large. Furthermore, substantial within-person variation exists in portion sizes for most foods (Hunter et al., 1988). For example, beef is eaten in a variety of forms and circumstances in which the portion size may vary substantially.

In Table 5–3 the within-person and between-person coefficients of variation for portion sizes of several commonly eaten foods are provided. Among a total of 66 foods examined, the average ratio of the within-person to between-person variance was approximately four (Hunter et al., 1988). This large within-person variation raises doubt about the concept of "usual" portion size. Indeed, in some situations we would not really be interested in the mode serving size for an individual if it was substantially smaller than another commonly used serving size. For example, a common serving size reported for yogurt is one tablespoon. Even if yogurt is consumed as a tablespoon serving size at, say, three times the frequency as a cup, we would still be more interested in learning about the frequency that the cup serving was used as it will provide a greater source of nutrients.

Table 5–3. Within-person and between-person coefficients of variation in portion sizes (CV_w and CV_b) of selected commonly consumed foods among 194 women

Food item	Portion	Mean	Median	CV_w (%)	CV_b (%)	Variance ratio[a]	Variance ratio (ln)[b]
			Dairy foods				
Yogurt	cup	0.5	0.5	39.8	61.9	0.4	0.8
Ice cream	cup	0.6	0.5	43.1	23.1	3.5	3.7
Cottage cheese	cup	0.5	0.4	75.6	45.4	2.8	3.1
Hard cheese	oz	1.0	1.0	73.3	24.1	9.3	9.5
Butter	tsp	1.9	1.2	78.3	33.1	5.6	5.3
			Meats				
Processed meat	oz	2.0	1.8	62.0	23.0	7.2	4.9
Hamburgers	oz	2.9	2.6	54.7	33.0	2.7	3.1
Chicken	100 g	0.9	0.8	53.9	24.5	4.9	5.4
Red meat	100 g	1.0	0.9	60.2	22.0	7.5	11.3
			Vegetables				
Broccoli	cup	0.4	0.5	54.7	25.0	4.8	4.3
Cabbage/cauliflower	cup	0.6	0.5	63.0	25.3	6.2	7.1
Carrots	cup/one	0.5	0.4	75.3	33.6	5.0	6.0
Corn	cup/one	1.0	0.5	85.8	56.1	2.3	3.3
Spinach	cup	0.6	0.5	79.0	28.2	7.9	2.6
Peas	cup	0.4	0.5	44.5	25.3	3.1	4.5
Potatoes, mashed/baked	cup	0.7	0.8	36.2	19.6	3.4	5.7
Lettuce	cup	0.9	0.7	61.6	36.0	2.9	3.0
Tomatoes	raw, one	0.4	0.4	63.4	28.4	5.0	5.1
			Fruit				
Peaches	cup	0.5	0.5	45.9	25.0	3.4	2.0
Raisins	oz	0.4	0.3	95.0	48.5	3.8	1.9
Canteloupe	cup	0.7	0.7	49.3	31.0	2.5	2.5
			Fish				
Tuna fish, canned	100 g	0.7	0.6	37.2	27.2	1.9	1.6
Dark fish	100 g	1.1	1.0	47.4	32.1	2.2	2.5
White fish	100 g	1.3	1.1	37.9	21.7	3.1	4.4
			Breads, cereals, starches				
Cake	oz	2.3	1.9	61.2	26.0	5.5	6.1
Pizza	⅛	2.1	2.0	55.1	11.7	22.4	93.2
Pasta/spaghetti noodles	cup	1.0	1.0	54.5	24.9	4.8	4.8
Cold cereal	cup	0.8	0.8	43.3	52.2	0.7	0.5
Cooked cereal	cup	0.7	0.8	22.9	25.6	0.8	0.8
Potato/corn chips	oz	1.0	0.8	57.4	36.6	2.5	1.7
Popcorn	cup	2.7	2.0	81.4	58.1	2.0	1.9
Crackers	one	4.4	4.0	100.8	47.9	4.4	3.5
Pancakes/waffles	one	2.4	2.0	40.4	41.2	1.0	0.4
Bagel/muffins	one	1.1	1.0	40.8	23.4	3.1	3.0

[a]Variance ratio = Within-person variance/Between-person variance = s_u^2/s_b^2.

[b]Based on $\log_e$ transformed data.

From Hunter et al., 1988

One possibility is to ask separate questions when foods are used in different ways. For example, we have asked separately about cooked spinach (½ cup) and spinach leaves in salad; the amount of spinach consumed when cooked is typically much larger.

Samet and colleagues (1984) have addressed the contribution of portion-size questions to the ranking of individuals. They calculated intake of vitamin A in two ways; the first was based on simple frequency questions alone and the second by weighting frequency responses by "usual" portion sizes obtained for the same foods during an in-person interview that employed food models. The correlation between the methods was 0.86 for controls and 0.91 for cases, indicating that the portion-size questions provided little additional information. Furthermore, vitamin A intake calculated with and without portion sizes was similarly related to a reduced risk of lung cancer (Humble et al., 1987).

We have conducted similar analyses using data collected as part of a case–control study of coronary heart disease (Hernandez-Avila et al., 1988). Participants completed a mailed, self-administered food-frequency questionnaire that specified units for foods commonly consumed in "natural" units but did not specify portions for items such as meat, cooked vegetables, rice, and mashed potatoes. After completing the questionnaire, subjects were interviewed by a dietitian who used realistic food models to estimate usual portion sizes. Nutrient intakes were then calculated in two ways: first, assuming common portion sizes for all subjects and, second, using the portion size data obtained at the interview. For each nutrient examined, the correlation between these methods of computation was greater than 0.90 (Table 5–4). Ninety-eight male control subjects in this study also collected a 1-week diet record after completing the questionnaire. Nutrients calculated with and without the additional portion-size data correlated equally well with those estimated by the diet record (Hernandez-Avila, 1988). Although it remains

Table 5–4. Spearman correlation coefficients[a] comparing semiquantitative food-frequency questionnaire nutrient intakes with and without data on portion sizes

Nutrient	Cases (n=115)	Controls (n=114)	Cases + controls (n=229)
Protein	0.94	0.94	0.94
Animal fat	0.94	0.93	0.93
Vegetable fat	0.99	0.99	0.99
Saturated fat	0.97	0.96	0.97
Oleic acid	0.95	0.96	0.96
Linoleic acid	0.98	0.98	0.98
Crude fiber	0.93	0.94	0.94
Dietary fiber	0.93	0.95	0.94
Preformed vitamin A	0.99	0.95	0.99
Carotene	0.90	0.91	0.91
Cholesterol	0.96	0.96	0.96
Vitamin C	0.97	0.98	0.97
Vitamin B_6	0.93	0.95	0.94
Vitamin E	0.98	0.99	0.99
Sucrose	0.99	0.99	0.99
Total carbohydrate	0.97	0.98	0.98
Total calories	0.97	0.97	0.97

[a]Calculated assuming common portion sizes for all subjects and using data for individual portion sizes collected during an interview.

Unpublished data derived from a case–control study of myocardial infarction.

possible that a more detailed assessment of usual portion sizes would slightly improve measurements of nutrient intake, it is apparent that the data collected (at considerable expense) during the personal interview added little to the assessment of nutrient intake. In a study among 37 postmenopausal women, Cummings and coworkers (1987) found that calcium intake calculated from a questionnaire, which included ratings of portion sizes as small, medium, and large, correlated only somewhat and nonsignificantly more with calculations from a diet record ($r = 0.76$) than did the questionnaire without added information on serving sizes ($r = 0.64$). A questionnaire completed by the same women that asked for portion sizes in ounces or cups performed less well; the correlation with diet records was 0.49. Although Hankin and colleagues (1975) have suggested that additional questions on portion sizes may be important, they found that the use of data obtained with color photographs of different portion sizes only slightly increased correlations between intake of foods assessed by a questionnaire completed at an interview and by a 1-week diet record. For 30 food items examined, the average Spearman correlation only increased from 0.55 to 0.59. Among women in the control group of a randomized trial, Block and colleagues (1990) also found that the inclusion of portion size data had a minimal effect on correlations with dietary records. Among participants in the fat reduction group of the trial, whose intervention focused on portion sizes, questions on portion sizes did increase correlations. In a similar analysis, (Block et al., 1992) inclusion of portion size data increased average correlations from 0.43 to 0.57; however, the population was heterogeneous in both gender and age, and no account was taken of these factors. Thus, it is not clear whether the higher correlation was simply the result of accounting for variations due to sex, age, and total energy intake. As age and gender would be controlled in any epidemiologic application of a questionnaire, only increments in validity independent of these variables will be useful. Tjonneland and coworkers (1992) computed nutrient intakes using portion sizes estimated from pictures and also assuming a standard portion size. Correlations with diet records were slightly lower using the pictures (for women 0.39 vs. 0.40 and for men 0.49 vs. 0.51).

As pointed out by Samet and colleagues (1984) and Pickle and Hartman (1985), for most foods, portion sizes vary less among individuals than do frequencies of use. Because most of the variation in intake of any food is explained by frequency of use (Heady, 1961), it is not surprising that portion size data are relatively unimportant. Furthermore, these investigators found that portion sizes were positively correlated with frequency of use (Heady, 1961), meaning that some of the information on portion size was already accounted for by

frequency of use. The finding by Hunter and coworkers (1988) that, for most foods, portion sizes vary considerably more within a person over time than between persons of similar age and sex, means that the concept of usual portion size is inherently complex and unlikely to be reported precisely. Although it may be tempting to add portion size questions because there is "nothing to lose," this is not necessarily true. If the amount of variation due to error exceeds the amount of information gained on true variation in portion sizes, validity can actually be reduced.

The potential contribution of additional questions on portion size deserves further investigation; however, available data suggest that such questions do not add substantially to the assessment of dietary intake. This has important implications for study design as the cost of data collection by mail or telephone is far less than the cost of personal interviews, which are necessary if food models are to be used for assessing portion sizes. It should be noted that the relative importance of portion sizes are, in part, culturally based. It is possible to conceive of other situations: for instance, a culture in which meat is usually eaten once a week, but the amount eaten on that day varies substantially between persons; in this case, a question focused on the amount of meat eaten could be quite informative.

COMPUTATION OF NUTRIENT INTAKES

Although the data on frequency of food use obtained from a questionnaire is intrinsically useful, most investigators also want to examine the relationships between nutrient intakes and health outcomes. A nutrient database and analysis program must be compiled to calculate these intakes. In constructing the database, a value for each nutrient being computed must be assigned to each food. If portion sizes have been specified on the questionnaire, the nutrient values relate to that portion size. If no portion sizes have been specified, the nutrient content for a typical or average portion size should be used. Sources of nutrient composition data and their limitations are discussed in Chapter 2; because most published databases are incomplete, it is often necessary to use more than one source for less common nutrients when compiling the database for a specific study. If open-ended questions are included, such as for types and brands of breakfast cereal or multiple vitamins, it is necessary to obtain specific data for each possible response.

Total intake of a nutrient can be calculated as the sum of the products of the frequency weight and the nutrient content for each food, that is, Σ (frequency weight $\times$ nutrient content). For frequency weights, it is simplest to assign a weight of 1.0 to once a day and proportional weights to the other responses, that is, "2–3 times a day" = 2.5. The calculation of intake based on a section of a semiquantitative food-frequency questionnaire is shown in Figure 5–2. If separate portion size questions were asked, the product for each food would also be multiplied by a weight proportional to the usual serving size.

In more complex questionnaires, the nutrient content of some foods may be modified by responses to other questions. For example, the composition of the cold breakfast cereal item could be modified by the brand and type of cereal, or the values of margarine might be modified by whether stick or tub margarines are usually used. Similarly, the nutrient values for baked goods made at home may be modified by the type of fat used (e.g., margarine vs. butter), which, in turn, can be modified by the type of margarine.

Because open-ended questions relating to specific types or brands of foods, such as for cold breakfast cereal or margarine, require an additional coding step, they add appreciably to the cost of processing a questionnaire. We therefore examined the increment in validity provided by open-ended questions for types of breakfast ce-

real, multiple vitamins, and cooking oil. Nutrient intakes computed with and without them (assuming a common value for all breakfast cereals, multiple vitamins, and cooking oil) were compared with intakes measured by diet records (Willett et al., 1988). In the case of breakfast cereals and cooking oil, correlations for each nutrient examined were essentially unchanged; the type of multiple vitamin did contribute to the estimation of vitamins and iron (e.g., the correlation for iron was 0.55 with the brand and type of multiple vitamin and 0.42 when a common type of vitamin was assumed for all subjects). The added costs of open-ended questions related to details of foods and supplements thus appear to provide only a small increment to the estimation of nutrient intake if the basic questionnaire is reasonably complete. This issue, however, deserves further examination as it might not apply to other populations and for all nutrients.

USE OF EMPIRICAL PREDICTOR SCORES

An alternative to the calculation of nutrient intakes from food-frequency questionnaires using values from published food composition tables is to employ empirically derived weights for each food item. The rationale for such a procedure is that the importance of a food item should reflect not only the nutrient content of the food but also the validity of the responses to that particular item. Calculation of empirical weights require that an external measurement of intake be available for a group of subjects who completed the questionnaire; this independent measurement could be based on either diet records or a biochemical parameter, such as plasma beta-carotene. Weights for the questionnaire food items can be obtained by fitting a multiple regression model with the external measurement as the dependent variable and the food items as the independent var-

	FOODS AND AMOUNTS	Never or less than once per mo	1-3 per mo	1 per wk	2-4 per wk	5-6 per wk	1 per day	2-3 per day	4-5 per day	6+ per day
A	Eggs (1)	○	○	Ⓦ	○	○	●	○	○	○
B	Whole milk (8 oz glass)	○	○	Ⓦ	○	○	Ⓓ	●	○	○
C	Ice cream (½ cup)	○	○	Ⓦ	○	●	Ⓓ	○	○	○

Figure 5–2. Example of calculation of daily cholesterol intake. From a food composition table the cholesterol contents are 1 egg = 274 mg, 1 glass of milk = 33 mg, ½ cup of ice cream = 29.5 mg. Thus, the average daily cholesterol intake for the person completing this abbreviated questionnaire would be: 274 mg × 1 + 33 mg × 2.5 + 29.5 mg × 0.8 = 380.1 mg/day. (From Sampson, 1985; reproduced with permission.)

iables. The coefficients for the food items would serve as weights that could then be applied to questionnaire responses in other studies.

This empirical approach has the advantage that it avoids many assumptions regarding portion sizes, nutrient composition, and bioavailability. Furthermore, questions that are unclear and thus improperly answered tend to receive low weights, thereby reducing error as persons who might have been erroneously assigned extreme values will be given a more average value. The use of empirical weights is limited largely by practical considerations. For their computation, the regression coefficients for individual foods must be estimated with considerable precision; it is of minimal use simply to know whether they are significantly different from zero. When many foods contribute to intake of a nutrient, the coefficient for any single food is relatively small and a number of variables are likely to be statistically significant on the basis of chance alone. For these reasons the generation of reasonably precise empirical predictor weights requires a large sample, probably many hundreds or several thousand subjects. Unless a large sample is used, weights corresponding to values from food composition tables will probably be more accurate than the empirical weights.

In an exploratory analysis, we found that empirical weights provided a better prediction of plasma vitamin E (alpha-tocopherol) levels when tested in an independent dataset than did weights from a food composition table (unpublished data). The appropriate role for empirical weights is not yet clear and deserves examination in other settings (see Chapter 13 for further discussion).

OVERALL QUESTIONNAIRE DESIGN AND ADMINISTRATION

Basic principles of survey research (Worsley, 1981; Rossi and Wright, 1985; Bradburn et al., 1987) are likely to apply to the collection of food frequency data; however, dietary assessment has received limited formal investigation from this perspective (Krall et al., 1988; Friedenreich, 1994). Although a detailed discussion of these principles is beyond the scope of this book, Babor and colleagues (1987) have provided an outline of sources of bias and solutions (Table 5–5).

The accurate collection of dietary data requires a motivated subject; thus, emphasizing the scientific importance of the information and assuring confidentiality is basic. Clear instructions are essential,

Table 5–5. Procedures for minimizing response bias and enhancing validity

Source of bias	Solution
Ambiguous role requirements or task definition	Guarantee anonymity/confidentiality Give clear instructions/examples Emphasize scientific role
Specificity of desired responses	Question wording Multiple questions Probe questions
Interviewer bias and unreliability	Interviewer training Standardized protocols Interview techniques
Forgetting, telescoping	Increase question length Better instructions Aided recall Memory aids Bounded recall
Response distortion	Alert subject to problem Recognition questions Diaries/calendars/time-line
Motivation	Commitment agreement Clear instructions Bounded recall Prompts/encouragement/reinforcement Session feedback Bogus pipeline

From Babor et al., 1987.

which can usually be enhanced by the use of relevant examples. As already discussed, clarity of questions is paramount; they can often be improved by feedback from subjects during questionnaire development.

If a questionnaire is to be used in an interview format, standardized procedures are essential. Interestingly, Babor and co-workers (1987) suggest that longer questions may be helpful in an interview as this may provide subjects with a longer time to think about their response. The use of memory aides and prompts, perhaps related to well-known events, has been used for many types of surveys, but their utility for the recall of dietary data remains to be documented. Among the recall aides, Babor and colleagues note that fixed response

choices, as we have employed for frequency-of-use, can reduce memory errors.

A number of the other suggestions offered by Babor and colleagues have not been used or evaluated in the collection of food-frequency data. One interesting approach, which they have called *bogus pipeline,* is to ask subjects to provide information under conditions where they are led to believe that objective, external validation of their responses, such as by blood test, will also be available to the investigator. This technique has been proven to enhance the validity of reporting of alcohol intake. Although conveying "bogus" information to study participants would trouble most epidemiologists, circumstances may actually exist in dietary studies where blood or other tissues are being collected, frequently to assess a limited number of nutrients; explicitly linking these sources of data when describing the study might be useful. Although most of the general principles of survey research are already incorporated into standard epidemiologic practice, some of the methods developed to enhance recall of past information deserve consideration and evaluation in the context of food-frequency questionnaires.

Food-frequency questionnaires can be administered by personal interview or by telephone or can be self-administered, including by mail (Caan et al., 1991). The widespread availability of computers is also creating new opportunities for interactive, self-administered dietary assessment that can include a wide range of branching questions to extract greater details of foods consumed. The cost can vary dramatically among methods, as much as 100-fold between an interview administered at home by a professional compared with a mailed self-administered form, with telephone interviews being intermediate (Fox et al., 1992). In survey research in general, response rates are usually higher for telephone interviews than mailed questionnaires. Also, we have found a greater willingness of population-based controls to participate in telephone than in at-home interviews. Thus in situations where participation rate is critical, as in case–control studies or surveys meant to provide a representative sample, telephone interviews may have distinct advantages. The relative validity of the various methods of administration is unclear; in principle, in-person interviews have the potential for the most assistance to the participant, but the relative anonymity of the other approaches may reduce biases induced by the environment of the interview. In one study, responses to a mailed food-frequency questionnaire appeared less valid than those obtained by interview administration (Sobell et al., 1989), but this is likely to depend on the specific instructions, questionnaire formats, and populations that are used. Indeed, Jain and coworkers (1996) found that a mailed, self-administered questionnaire and a detailed interviewer-administered questionnaire provided similar correlations with diet records.

SUMMARY

Food-frequency questionnaires have become the primary method for measuring dietary intake in epidemiologic studies. Such questionnaires are directed to the dietary exposure of conceptual interest in most applications, which is average intake over an extended period of time. Food-frequency questionnaires are extremely practical in epidemiologic applications as they are easy for subjects to complete, often as a self-administered form. Processing is readily computerized and inexpensive so that even prospective studies involving tens of thousands of subjects are feasible. In constructing food-frequency questionnaires, careful attention must be given to the choice of foods, the clarity of the questions, and the format of the frequency response section. The actual performance of such questionnaires in terms of reproducibility and validity is considered in the next chapter.

REFERENCES

Ammerman, A. S., P. S. Haines, R. F. DeVellis, D. S. Strogatz, T. C. Keyserling, R. J. J. Simpson, and D. S. Siscovick (1991). A brief dietary assessment to guide cholesterol reduction in low-income individuals: Design and validation. *J Am Diet Assoc 91*, 1385–1390.

Babor, T. F., R. S. Stephens, and G. A. Marlatt (1987). Verbal report methods in clinical research on alcoholism: Response bias and its minimization. *J Stud Alcohol 48*, 410–424.

Beresford, S. A., E. M. Farmer, L. Feingold, K. L. Graves, S. K. Sumner, and R. M. Baker (1992). Evaluation of a self-help dietary intervention in a primary care setting. *Am J Public Health 82*, 79–84.

Block, G., C. Clifford, M. D. Naughton, M. Henderson, and M. McAdams (1989). A brief dietary screen for high fat intake. *J Nutr Educ 21*, 199–207.

Block, G., A. M. Hartman, C. M. Dresser, M. D. Carroll, J. Gannon, and L. Gardner (1986). A data-based approach to diet questionnaire design and testing. *Am J Epidemiol 124*, 453–469.

Block, G., F. E. Thompson, A. M. Hartman, F. A. Larkin and K. E. Guire (1992). Comparison of two dietary questionnaires validated against multiple dietary records collected during a 1-year period. *J Am Diet Assoc 92*, 686–693.

Block, G., M. Woods, A. Potosky, and C. Clifford (1990). Validation of a self-administered diet history questionnaire using multiple diet records. *J Clin Epidemiol 43*, 1327–1335.

Borrud, L. G., R. S. McPherson, M. Z. Nichaman, P. C. Pillow, and G. R. Newell (1989). Development of a food frequency instrument: Ethnic differences in food sources. *Nutr Cancer 12*, 201–211.

Bradburn, N. M., L. J. Rips, and S. K. Shevell (1987). Answering autobiographical questions: The impact of memory and inference on surveys. *Science 236*, 157–161.

Burke, B. S. (1947). The dietary history as a tool in research. *J Am Diet Assoc 23*, 1041–1046.

Byers, T., J. Marshall, R. Fiedler, M. Zielezny, and S. Graham (1985). Assessing nutrient intake with an abbreviated dietary interview. *Am J Epidemiol 122*, 41–50.

Caan, B., R. A. Hiatt, and A. M. Owen (1991). Mailed dietary surveys: Response rates, error rates, and the effect of omitted food items on nutrient values. *Epidemiology 2,* 430–436.

Cassidy, C. M. (1994). Walk a mile in my shoes: Culturally sensitive food-habit research. *Am J Clin Nutr 59(suppl),* 190S–197S.

Connor, S. L., J. R. Gustafson, G. Sexton, N. Becker, W. Artaud-Wild, and W. E. Connor (1992). The Diet Habit Survey: A new method of dietary assessment that relates to plasma cholesterol changes. *J Am Diet Assoc 92,* 41–47.

Cummings, S. R., G. Block, K. McHenry, and R. B. Baron (1987). Evaluation of two food frequency methods of measuring dietary calcium intake. *Am J Epidemiol 126,* 796–802.

Forsythe, H. E., and B. Gage (1994). Use of multicultural food-frequency questionnaire with pregnant and lactating women. *Am J Clin Nutr 59(suppl),* 203S–206S.

Fox, T. A., J. Heimendinger, and G. Block (1992). Telephone surveys as a method for obtaining dietary information: A review. *J Am Diet Assoc 92,* 729–732.

Friedenreich, C. M. (1994). Improving long-term recall in epidemiologic studies. *Epidemiology 5,* 1–4.

Gray, G. E., A. Paganini-Hill, R. K. Ross, and B. E. Henderson (1984). Assessment of three brief methods of estimation of vitamin A and C intakes for a prospective study of cancer: Comparison with dietary history. *Am J Epidemiol 119,* 581–590.

Guthrie, H. A. (1984). Selection and quantification of typical food portions by young adults. *J Am Diet Assoc 84,* 1440–1444.

Guthrie, H. A., and J. C. Scheer (1981). Validity of a dietary score for assessing nutrient adequacy. *J Am Diet Assoc 78,* 240–245.

Hankin, J. H., A. M. Nomura, J. Lee, T. Hirohata, and L. N. Kolonel (1983). Reproducibility of a dietary history questionnaire in a case–control study of breast cancer. *Am J Clin Nutr 37,* 981–985.

Hankin, J. H., G. G. Rhoads, and G. A. Glober (1975). A dietary method for an epidemiologic study of gastrointestinal cancer. *Am J Clin Nutr 28,* 1055–1060.

Hankin, J. H., and L. R. Wilkens (1994). Development and validation of dietary assessment methods for culturally diverse populations. *Am J Clin Nutr 59(suppl),* 198S–200S.

Heady, J. A. (1961). Diets of bank clerks. Development of a method of classifying the diets of individuals for use in epidemiologic studies. *J R Statist Soc 124,* 336–361.

Heller, R. F., H. D. Pedoe, and G. Rose (1981). A simple method of assessing the effect of dietary advice to reduce plasma cholesterol. *Prev Med 10,* 364–370.

Hernandez-Avila, M., C. Master, D. J. Hunter, J. Buring, J. Philips, W. C. Willett, and C. H. Hennekens (1988). Influence of additional portion size data on the validity of a semi-quantitative food frequency questionnaire (abstract). *Am J Epidemiol 128,* 891.

Hopkins, P. N., R. R. Williams, H. Kuida, B. M. Stults, S. C. Hunt, G. K. Barlow, and K. O. Ash (1989). Predictive value of a short dietary questionnaire for changes in serum lipids in high-risk Utah families. *Am J Clin Nutr 50,* 292–300.

Howe, G. R., L. Harrison, and M. Jain (1986). A short diet history for assessing dietary exposure to N-nitrosamines in epidemiologic studies. *Am J Epidemiol 124,* 595–602.

Humble, C. G., J. M. Samet, and B. E. Skipper (1987). Use of quantified and frequency indices of vitamin A intake in a case–control study of lung cancer. *Int J Epidemiol 16,* 341–346.

Hunter, D. J., L. Sampson, M. J. Stampfer, G. A. Colditz, B. Rosner, and W. C. Willett (1988). Variability in portion sizes of commonly consumed foods among a population of women in the United States. *Am J Epidemiol 127,* 1240–1249.

Jain, M., G. R. Howe and T. Rohan (1996). Dietary assessment in epidemiology: Comparison of a food frequency and a diet history questionnaire with a 7-day food record. *Am J Epidemiol 143,* 953–960.

Kinlay, S., R. F. Heller, and J. A. Halliday (1991). A simple score and questionnaire to measure group changes in dietary fat intake. *Prev Med 20,* 378–388.

Knapp, J. A., H. P. Hazuda, S. M. Haffner, E. A. Young, and M. P. Stern (1988). A saturated fat/cholesterol avoidance scale: Sex and ethnic differences in a biethnic population. *J Am Diet Assoc 88,* 172–177.

Kohlmeier, L. (1994). Gaps in dietary assessment methodology: Meal- vs list-based methods. *Am J Clin Nutr 59(suppl),* 175S–179S.

Krall, E. A., J. T. Dwyer, and K. A. Coleman (1988). Factors influencing accuracy of dietary recall. *Nutr Res 8,* 829–841.

Kristal, A. R., B. F. Abrams, M. D. Thornquist, L. Disogra, R. T. Croyle, A. L. Shattuck, and H. J. Henry (1990a). Development and validation of a food use checklist for evaluation of community nutrition interventions. *Am J Public Health 80,* 1318–1322.

Kristal, A. R., A. L. Shattuck, and H. J. Henry (1990b). Patterns of dietary behavior associated with selecting diets low in fat: Reliability and validity of a behavioral approach to dietary assessment. *J Am Diet Assoc 90*, 214–220.

Kristal, A. R., A. L. Shattuck, H. J. Henry, and A. S. Fowler (1990c). Rapid assessment of dietary intake of fat, fiber, and saturated fat: Validity of an instrument suitable for community intervention research and nutritional surveillance. *Am J Health Promotion 4*, 288–295.

Mark, S. D., D. G. Thomas, and A. Decarli (1996). Measurement of exposure to nutrients: An approach to the selection of informative foods. *Am J Epidemiol 143*, 514–521.

Marr, J. W. (1971). Individual dietary surveys: Purposes and methods. *World Rev Nutr Diet 13*, 105–164.

Morgan, R. W., M. Jain, A. B. Miller, N. W. Choi, V. Matthews, L. Munan, J. D. Burch, J. Feather, G. R. Howe, and A. Kelly (1978). A comparison of dietary methods in epidemiologic studies. *Am J Epidemiol 107*, 488–498.

Nichols, A. B., C. Ravenscroft, D. E. Lamphiear, and L. D. Ostrander Jr. (1976). Independence of serum lipid levels and dietary habits. The Tecumseh Study. *J Am Med Assoc 236*, 1948–1953.

Pickle, L. W., and A. M. Hartman (1985). Indicator foods for vitamin A assessment. *Nutr Cancer 7*, 3–23.

Rossi, P. H., and J. D. Wright (eds.) (1985). *Handbook of Survey Research*. New York: Academic Press.

Samet, J. M., C. G. Humble, and B. E. Skipper (1984). Alternatives in the collection and analysis of food frequency interview data. *Am J Epidemiol 120*, 572–581.

Sampson, L. (1985). Food frequency questionnaires as a research instrument. *Clin Nutr 4*, 171–178.

Serdula, M., R. Coates, T. Byers, A. Mokdad, S. Jewell, N. Chavez, J. Mares-Perlman, P. Newcomb, C. Ritenbaugh, F. Treiber, and G. Block (1993). Evaluation of a brief telephone questionnaire to estimate fruit and vegetable consumption in diverse study populations. *Epidemiology 4*, 455–463.

Smith, A. F. (1993). Cognitive psychological issues of relevance to the validity of dietary reports. *Eur J Clin Nutr 47(suppl)*, S6–S18.

Smith, A. F., J. B. Jobe, and D. J. Mingay (1991a). Question-induced cognitive biases in reports of dietary intake by college men and women. *Health Psych 10*, 244–251.

Smith, A. F., J. B. Jobe, and D. J. Mingay (1991b). Retrieval from memory of dietary information. *Appl Cognitive Psychol 5*, 269–296.

Sobell, J., G. Block, P. Koslowe, J. Tobin, and R. Andres (1989). Vaildation of a retrospective questionnaire assessing diet 10–15 years ago. *Am J Epidemiol 130*, 173–187.

Stefanik, P. A., and M. F. Trulson (1962). Determining the frequency of foods in large group studies. *Am J Clin Nutr 11*, 335–343.

Stryker, W. S., S. Salvini, M. J. Stampfer, L. Sampson, G. A. Colditz, and W. C. Willett (1991). Contributions of specific foods to absolute intake and between-person variation of nutrient consumption. *J Am Diet Assoc 91*, 172–8.

Subar, A. F., F. E. Thompson, A. F. Smith, J. B. Jobe, R. G. Ziegler, N. Potischman, A. Schatzkin, A. Hartman, C. Swanson, L. Kruse, R. B. Hayes, D. R. Lewis, and L. C. Harlan (1995). Improving food frequency questionnaires: A qualitative approach using cognitive interviewing. *J Am Diet Assoc 95*, 781–788.

Thompson, F. E., and T. Byers (1994). Dietary assessment resource manual. *J Nutr 124 (suppl)*, 2245S–2317S.

Tjonneland, A., J. Haraldsdottir, K. Overvad, C. Stripp, M. Ewertz, and O. M. Jensen (1992). Influence of individually estimated portion size data on the validity of a semiquantitative food frequency questionnaire. *Int J Epidemiol 21*, 770–777.

Toth, B., D. Nagel, and A. Ross (1982). Gastric tumorigenesis by a single dose of 4-(hydroxymethyl) benzenediazonium ion of *Agaricus bisporus*. *Br J Cancer 46*, 417–422.

Tylavsky, F. A., and G. B. Sharp (1995). Misclassification of nutrient and energy intake from use of closed-ended questions in epidemiologic research. *Am J Epidemiol 142*, 342–352.

van Assema, P., J. Brug, G. Kok, and H. Brants (1992). The reliability and validity of a Dutch questionnaire on fat consumption as a means to rank subjects according to individual fat intake. *Eur J Cancer Prev 1*, 375–380.

Wiehl, D. G., and R. Reed (1960). Development of new or improved dietary methods for epidemiological investigations. *Am J Public Health 50*, 824–828.

Willett, W., L. Sampson, C. Bain, B. Rosner, C. H. Hennekens, J. Witschi, and F. E. Speizer (1981). Vitamin supplement use among registered nurses. *Am J Clin Nutr 34*, 1121–1125.

Willett, W. C., L. Sampson, M. L. Browne, M. J. Stampfer, B. Rosner, C. H. Hennekens, and F. E. Speizer (1988). The use of a self-administered questionnaire to assess diet four years in the past. *Am J Epidemiol 127*, 188–199.

Willett, W. C., L. Sampson, M. J. Stampfer, B. Rosner, C. Bain, J. Witschi, C. H. Hennekens, and F. E. Speizer (1985). Reproducibility and validity of a semiquantitative food frequency questionnaire. *Am J Epidemiol 122*, 51–65.

Willett, W. C., M. J. Stampfer, G. A. Colditz, B. A. Rosner, C. H. Hennekens, and F. E. Speizer (1987). Dietary fat and the risk of breast cancer. *N Engl J Med 316*, 22–28.

Worsley, T. (1981). Psychometric aspects of language dependent techniques in dietary assessment. *Trans Menzies Found 3*, 161–192.

APPENDIX 5–1
1980 Nurses' Health Study Dietary Questionnaire.

Frequency distributions of responses (%) are also given for this population.

For each food listed, check the box indicating how often, **on average,** you have used the amount specified **during the past year.** If your intake of a food item has greatly increased or decreased during the past 10 years, indicate this in the last 2 columns.

FOOD AND AMOUNTS	Average use last year								
	6+ per day	4–6 per day	2–3 per day	1 per day	5–6 per week	2–4 per week	1 per week	1–3 per month	Almost Never
Dairy Foods Skim or low fat milk (8 oz. glasses)	0	1	12	20	5	12	6	5	39
Whole milk (8 oz. glasses)	0	0	4	10	2	8	7	7	62
Yoghurt, (1 c.)	0	0	0	2	1	8	9	20	61
Ice cream (½-c.)	0	0	0	3	3	18	22	32	22
Cottage cheese (½-c.)	0	0	1	3	3	18	17	29	28
Hard cheese, plain or as part of a dish (slice or servings)	0	0	3	12	13	36	20	11	5
Margarine (pats added to food or bread)	2	4	28	23	9	11	4	3	17
Butter (pats added to food or bread)	1	2	10	10	4	7	4	5	58
Fruits Fresh apples or pears (1)	0	2	3	15	6	27	19	20	11
Oranges (1)	0	0	2	11	4	22	19	23	19
Orange or grapefruit juice (small glass)	4	3	4	35	9	19	10	10	13
Peaches, apricots or plums (fresh, ½-c. canned, or dried)	0	1	1	3	2	14	19	32	30
Bananas (1)	0	0	0	6	4	23	25	27	15
Other fruits (fresh, or ½-c. canned)	0	0	2	9	6	24	23	23	14
Vegetables String beans (½-c.)	0	0	0	2	3	30	46	16	3
Broccoli (½-c.)		0	0	1	1	16	42	29	11
Cabbage, cauliflower, brussels sprouts (½-c.)	0	0	0	1	1	12	34	37	15
Carrots (whole or ½-c. cooked)	0	0	0	3	4	21	39	26	7
Corn (ear or ½-.c)	0	0	0	0	1	13	38	32	15
Spinach or other greens (½-c.)	0	0	2	10	8	21	30	20	10
Peas or lima beans (½-c. fresh, frozen or canned)	0	0	0	1	1	15	39	29	15
Yellow (winter) squash (½-c.)	0	0	0	0	0	4	14	34	48
Sweet potatoes (½-c.)		0	0	0	1	4	29	67	
Beans or lentils, dried (½-c.)	0	0	0	0	0	3	12	36	48
Tomatoes (1) or tomato juice (4 oz.)	0	0	1	11	12	33	24	15	4

FOOD AND AMOUNTS	Average use last year								
	6+ per day	4–6 per day	2–3 per day	1 per day	5–6 per week	2–4 per week	1 per week	1–3 per month	Almost Never
Meats Chicken, without skin (6–8 oz.)	0	0	0	1	2	19	36	16	26
Chicken, with skin (6–8 oz.)		0	0	0	1	11	35	16	37
Hamburgers (1)	0	0	0	0	1	22	52	19	5
Hot dogs (1)	0	0	0	0	0	5	27	37	30
Processed meats (sausage, salami, bologna, etc.) (piece or slice)	0	0	0	2	3	15	20	27	32
Bacon (2 slice servings)	0	0	0	1	1	9	24	33	31
Beef, pork or lamb as a sandwich or mixed dish (stew, casserole, lasagne, etc.)	0	0	0	2	3	25	34	26	9
Beef, pork or lamb as a main dish (steak, roast, ham, etc. 6–8 oz.)	0	0	1	5	10	41	31	10	3
Fish (6–8 oz.)	0	0	0	1	2	15	39	34	9
Eggs (1)	0	0	2	8	9	48	20	9	5
Sweets, Baked Goods, Cereals Chocolate (1 oz.)	0	0	1	4	3	12	18	28	34
Candy without chocolate (1 oz.)	0	0	0	2	1	6	13	26	51
Pie, home made (slice)		0	0	0	0	1	8	40	50
Pie, ready made (slice)		0	0	0	0	1	4	21	74
Cake, (slice)	0	0	0	1	1	7	17	45	30
Cookies (1)	0	1	5	5	9	20	16	24	20
Cold breakfast cereal (½-c.)	0	0	0	10	6	21	13	14	35
White bread (slice)	0	2	17	15	9	17	7	6	27
Dark or whole grain bread (slice)	0	1	14	17	10	20	9	12	17
Miscellaneous Peanut butter (tbsps)	0	0	1	4	4	13	15	23	40
Potato or corn chips (small bag or 1 oz.)	0	0	0	1	2	8	17	28	44
French fried potatoes (4 oz.)	0	0	0	0	0	4	19	36	41
Nuts (1 oz.)	0	0	1	2	2	9	15	36	34
Potatoes, mashed (½-c.) or baked (1)	0	0	0	4	7	35	26	18	9
Rice or pasta (½-c.)	0	0	0	1	2	27	38	23	9
Coffee, not decaffinated (cups)	8	17	33	11	2	3	1	2	23
Tea (cups)	1	4	15	16	4	10	8	11	30
Beer (bottles or cans)	0	0	1	1	1	4	5	9	78
Wine (glasses)	0	0	2	6	3	11	10	23	44
Liquor—whiskey, gin, etc. (drinks)	0	0	2	4	2	8	8	18	56
Coca Cola, Pepsi, other cola (glasses)	0	0	2	5	3	9	9	14	57
Low calorie carbonated drink (glasses)	0	1	7	10	5	11	6	9	50
Other carbonated beverage (root beer, ginger ale, 7-Up, etc.) (glasses)	0	0	1	2	1	6	9	20	62
Fruit-flavored punch or non-carbonated beverage (glasses)	0	0	1	2	2	6	6	12	71
Home-fried food, any type (servings)	0	0	0	2	3	15	18	23	38
Artificial sweetner (packet, tablets, etc.)	2	4	9	6	2	4	2	4	68

How often do you eat liver (3–4 oz servings)   [3] 1 per week   [12] 2–3 per month   [52] 1 per month or less   [33] never

What do you do with the visible fat on your meat?   [4] eat most of it   [20] eat some of it   [76] eat as little as possible

What kind of fat do you usually use for baking?   [4] lard or butter   [27] vegetable oil   [29] vegetable shortening   [27] margarine

What kind of fat do you usually use for frying?   [3] lard or butter   [61] vegetable oil   [15] vegetable shortening   [13] margarine

Do you use a microwave oven?   [27] Yes   [73] No   if yes, for how many years?   [ ]

Are you currently on a special diet?   [17] Yes   [83] No   If yes, for [ ] years   type of diet _____

In what form do you usually use your margarine?   [66] stick form   [34] tub form

Do you currently take any of the following vitamins?

	YES	NO
Multiple vitamins	38	62
Vitamin A	4	96
Vitamin C	19	81
Vitamin E	13	87

APPENDIX 5–2

Optically scannable format for Nurses' Health Study Dietary Questionnaire. Currently includes about 120 food items.

For each food listed, fill in the circle indicating how often <u>on average</u> you have used the amount specified <u>during the past year</u>.

DAIRY FOODS	Never, or less than once per month	1-3 per mo.	1 per week	2-4 per week	5-6 per week	1 per day	2-3 per day	4-5 per day	6+ per day
			AVERAGE USE LAST YEAR						
Skim or low fat milk (8 oz. Glass)	O	O	Ⓦ	O	O	Ⓓ	O	O	O
Whole milk (I oz. Glass)	O	O	Ⓦ	O	O	Ⓓ	O	O	O
Cream, e.g. coffee, whipped (Tbs.)	O	O	Ⓦ	O	O	Ⓓ	O	O	O
Sour cream (Tbs)	O	O	Ⓦ	O	O	Ⓓ	O	O	O
Non-dairy coffee whitener (tsp.)	O	O	Ⓦ	O	O	Ⓓ	O	O	O
Sherbet or ice milk (½ cup)	O	O	Ⓦ	O	O	Ⓓ	O	O	O
Ice cream (½ cup)	O	O	Ⓦ	O	O	Ⓓ	O	O	O
Yogurt (1 cup)	O	O	Ⓦ	O	O	Ⓓ	O	O	O
Cottage or ricotta cheese (½ cup)	O	O	Ⓦ	O	O	Ⓓ	O	O	O
Cream cheese (1 oz.)	O	O	Ⓦ	O	O	Ⓓ	O	O	O
Other cheese, e.g. American, cheddar, etc., plain or as part of a dish (1 slice or 1 oz. Serving)	O	O	Ⓦ	O	O	Ⓓ	O	O	O
Margarine (pat), added to food or bread; exclude use in cooking	O	O	Ⓦ	O	O	Ⓓ	O	O	O
Butter (pat), added to food or bread; exclude use in cooking	O	O	Ⓦ	O	O	Ⓓ	O	O	O

APPENDIX 5–3

Vertical format for food-frequency questionnaire, also optically scannable.

In the following section, please describe how often <u>on average</u> you have used the amount specified in the past year. Please indicate your average <u>total</u> use, taking the portion size into account. For example, if you use ½ a glass of milk twice a week, mark 1 glass per week to represent your average total intake.

3. For each food listed, fill in the circle indicating your <u>average total</u> use of the amount specified <u>during the past year</u>.

Skim milk (8 oz. glass)	**1% or 2% milk (8 oz. glass)**	**Whole milk (8 oz. glass)**
O Never	O Never	O Never
O Less than once per month	O Less than once per month	O Less than once per month
O 1-3 glasses per month	O 1-3 glasses per month	O 1-3 glasses per month
O 1 glass per week	O 1 glass per week	O 1 glass per week
O 2-4 glasses per week	O 2-4 glasses per week	O 2-4 glasses per week
O 5-6 glasses per week	O 5-6 glasses per week	O 5-6 glasses per week
O 1 glass per day	O 1 glass per day	O 1 glass per day
O 2-3 glasses per day	O 2-3 glasses per day	O 2-3 glasses per day
O 4 or more glasses per day	O 4 or more glasses per day	O 4 or more glasses per day

Cream, e.g., in coffee, whipped or sour cream (1 tbs.)	**Non-dairy coffee whitener (tsp.)**	**Frozen yogurt, sherbet or non-fat ice cream (1/2 cup)**
O Never	O Never	O Never
O Less than once per month	O Less than once per month	O Less than once per month
O 1-3 tbs. per month	O 1-3 tbs. per month	O 1-3 tbs. per month
O 1 tbs. per week	O 1 tbs. per week	O 1 tbs. per week
O 2-4 tbs. per week	O 2-4 tbs. per week	O 2-4 tbs. per week
O 5-6 tbs. per week	O 5-6 tbs. per week	O 5-6 tbs. per week
O 1 tbs. per day	O 1 tbs. per day	O 1 tbs. per day
O 2-3 tbs. per day	O 2-3 tbs. per day	O 2-3 tbs. per day
O 4 or more tbs. per day	O 4 or more tbs. per day	O 4 or more tbs. per day

Ice cream (1/2 cup)	**Flavored yogurt, <u>without</u> Nutrasweet (1 cup)**	**Yogurt, plain or with Nutrasweet (1 cup)**
O Never	O Never	O Never
O Less than once per month	O Less than once per month	O Less than once per month
O 1-3 times per month	O 1-3 cups per month	O 1-3 cups per month
O Once per week	O 1 cup per week	O 1 cup per week
O 2-4 times per week	O 2-4 cups per week	O 2-4 cups per week
O 5-6 times per week	O 5-6 cups per week	O 5-6 cups per week
O Once per day	O 1 cup per day	O 1 cup per day
O 2-3 times per day	O 2-3 cups per day	O 2-3 cups per day
O 4 or more times per day	O 4 or more cups per day	O 4 or more cups per day

3. (Continued) Fill in your <u>average</u> total use, <u>during the past year</u>, of each specified food.

What type of yogurt do you usually eat?
- O None
- O Regular
- O Low fat
- O Nonfat

Cottage or ricotta cheese (1/2 cup)
- O Never
- O Less than once per month
- O 1-3 times per month
- O Once per week
- O 2-4 times per week
- O Once per day
- O Once per day
- O 2 or more servings per day

Cream cheese (1 oz.)
- O Never
- O Less than once per month
- O 1-3 times per month
- O Once per week
- O 2-4 times per week
- O Once per day
- O Once per day
- O 2 or more servings per day

Other cheese, e.g., American, cheddar, etc., plain or as part of a dish (1 slice or 1 oz. serving)
- O Never
- O Less than once per month
- O 1-3 slices per month
- O 1 slice per week
- O 2-4 slices per week
- O 5-6 slices per week
- O 1 slice per day
- O 2 or more slices per day

What type of cheese do you usually eat?
- O None
- O Regular
- O Low fat or lite
- O Nonfat

Butter (small pat or tsp.), added to food or bread; exclude use in cooking
- O Never
- O Less than once per month
- O 1-3 pats per month
- O 1 pat per week
- O 2-4 pats per week
- O 5-6 pats per week
- O 1 pat per day
- O 2-3 pats per day
- O 4 or more pats per day

Margarine (small pat or tsp.), added to food or bread; exclude use in cooking
- O Never
- O Less than once per month
- O 1-3 pats per month
- O 1 pat per week
- O 2-4 pats per week
- O 5-6 pats per week
- O 1 pat per day
- O 2-3 pats per day
- O 4 or more pats per day

What form of margarine do you usually use? (Do not include "spray" type margarine)

O None   **Form?**
- O Stick
- O Tub
- O Squeeze (liquid)

Type?
- O Regular
- O Light spread
- O Extra light spread
- O Nonfat

What specific **brand** and **type** (e.g., Land O' Lakes Country Morning Blend Light)?

6

Reproducibility and Validity of Food-Frequency Questionnaires

WALTER WILLETT AND ELIZABETH LENART

For reasons discussed in Chapter 5, the food-frequency questionnaire is usually the most appropriate method for dietary assessment in epidemiologic studies. It is, therefore, crucial to consider in detail the degree to which such questionnaires can measure true dietary intake. This chapter deals with approaches used to evaluate dietary questionnaires, the design of validation studies, and the analysis and presentation of data from validation studies.

In this chapter *reproducibility* refers to consistency of questionnaire measurements on more than one administration to the same persons at different times, realizing that conditions are never identical on repeated administration. Repeatability and reliability are frequently considered to be synonymous with reproducibility; however, the latter term has taken different meanings in other disciplines so that it is not used here. *Validity* refers to the degree to which the questionnaire actually measures the aspect of diet that it was designed to measure. This implies that a comparison

is made with a superior, although always imperfect, standard. A closely related term, *calibration*, refers to a process in which values from one method are quantitatively related to values from a superior, standard method. Reproducibility and validity can be addressed from several aspects. Most common is the relative ordering of subjects by the repeated measurements or different methods, which is typically evaluated by correlation coefficients. Comparisons of absolute levels can also be made, which usually involve examination of means and standard deviations; other methods of comparing measurements are discussed later in the chapter. The quantitative implications of measures of association between different levels of reproducibility and validity are discussed in Chapter 12.

Because even subtle changes in the design of food-frequency questionnaires can affect their performance (see Chapter 5), each instrument should ideally be evaluated separately. Moreover, these structured questionnaires are culture specific; even within a population they can perform differently among various demographic groups and subcultures. Thus, it is important to document the reproducibility and validity of any new questionnaire and to measure the performance of previously tested questionnaires for use in substantially different populations. As discussed in Chapter 2, an examination of dietary associations with disease at the level of individual foods, food groups, and nutrients is frequently useful. Thus, studies of questionnaire reproducibility and validity at these three levels are important.

APPROACHES FOR EVALUATING DIETARY QUESTIONNAIRES

Various approaches that have been used to assess the performance of food-frequency questionnaires, include the following

1. Comparison of means
2. Proportion of total intake accounted for by foods included on the questionnaire
3. Reproducibility
4. Validity (comparison with an independent standard)
5. Comparison with biochemical markers
6. Correlation with a physiologic response
7. The ability to predict disease

Comparison of Means With Data From Other Sources

The comparison of mean nutrient intakes computed from a questionnaire with values derived from another source provides a simple and inexpensive method to assess performance. The comparison data may be external, such as the National Health and Nutrition Examination Surveys (NHANES) study (Centers for Disease Control and Prevention, 1994; Briefel et al., 1995), or internal, based on another dietary assessment method among the same individuals who completed the questionnaire. For example, we have compared mean nutrient intakes based on a semiquantitative food-frequency questionnaire with means calculated from a 1-year diet record completed

by 27 men and women (Willett et al., 1987a) (Table 6–1).

Although simple and inexpensive, a comparison of means provides limited information on validity. Similar mean values provide some reassurance that the questionnaire is reasonably comprehensive. It remains possible, however, that important items were not included on the questionnaire but that the portion sizes assumed in the calculation of nutrient intakes were erroneously high; such compensating errors could produce correct mean values. Most seriously, such comparisons of means provide no information on the ability of the questionnaire to discriminate among persons.

Proportion of Total Intake Accounted for by Food Items Included on the Questionnaire

In developing a food-frequency questionnaire, one approach to the selection of foods for inclusion has been to use an open-ended method, such as 24-hour recall or diet record, to identify those foods that contribute importantly to absolute nutrient intake for a group as a whole (see Chapter 5). Such data have also been used as support for the completeness of the questionnaire.

As an example, we calculated the percentage of total nutrient intakes that were accounted for by food items on a compressed questionnaire (displayed in Appendix 5–1) and on a more comprehensive questionnaire that has been used in a wide variety of studies including, in slightly revised format, the 1984 Nurses' Health Study (Willett et al., 1987b) (Table 6–2). In this analysis, diet records completed by 194 women were used to compute the true total intakes of 26 nutrients. Then we used the diet records to calculate the contribution of foods that were listed on the questionnaires to this true total nutrient intake; if all the foods recorded on the diet records had been listed on the questionnaire, the contribution would be 100%. In performing these calculations it quickly becomes

Table 6–1. Comparison of mean nutrient intakes measured among 27 men and women using a 116-item food-frequency questionnaire and 1-year diet record[a]

Nutrient	Diet record	Questionnaire mean
Total energy (kcal)	2,229 ± 706.9[b]	2,114 ± 1,012
Protein (g)	82.0 ± 24.8	87.0 ± 40.0
Total fat (g)	89.9 ± 30.1	81.9 ± 45.8
Saturated fat (g)	33.5 ± 13.1	31.9 ± 18.0
Linoleic acid (g)	14.0 ± 4.1	13.9 ± 7.8
Total carbohydrate (g)	258 ± 96	263 ± 116
Crude Fiber (g)	4.4 ± 1.6	5.1 ± 2.8
Cholesterol (mg)	362 ± 122	332 ± 151
Oleic acid (g)	30.9 ± 9.85	29.4 ± 17.0
Vitamin A (IU)	6,434 ± 2,679	10,553 ± 6,194[c]
Niacin (mg)	21.9 ± 6.41	27.0 ± 12.2
Vitamin C (mg)	125 ± 87	146 ± 88
Calcium (mg)	894 ± 446	917 ± 586
Phosphorus (mg)	1,384 ± 504	1,420 ± 717
Thiamin (mg)	1.50 ± 0.55	1.30 ± 0.63
Riboflavin (mg)	1.91 ± 0.86	2.19 ± 1.31
Potassium (mg)	2,778 ± 1,045	3,076 ± 1,559
Iron (mg)	14.6 ± 5.92	13.6 ± 5.89

[a]Data were provided by 27 men and women aged 20 to 54 years.
[b]Mean ± standard deviation.
[c]Discrepancy for vitamin A is in part due to use of new USDA tables, which have dramatically changed vitamin A values for several vegetables. Use of older USDA values reduced this value to 8,511 IU.
From Willet et al., 1987a.

apparent that there is not a one-to-one correspondence between foods on the questionnaire and foods reported in the diet record. For example, we had to collapse several hundred different codes for meat items on the diet records to correspond to the two meat items on the questionnaire. In addition, the coding of diet records and 24-hour recalls frequently requires the "dissection" of recipes into the basic ingredients such as the flour, shortening, and eggs used in baking. These basic ingredients would not be reported as such on the questionnaire, but would probably be recognized as the final products, such as cake or muffin. Because calculations like those shown in Table 6–2 include basic ingredients in the denominator (i.e., the total nutrient intakes from the diet records) but not in the numerator (i.e., the foods recorded in the diet records that are also listed on the questionnaire), they will tend to under-

represent the proportions of nutrients accounted for by items on the questionnaire. Thus, the data in Table 6–2 represent a conservative evaluation of the questionnaire by this particular criterion.

As a measure of questionnaire performance, the approach of calculating the percentages of nutrients accounted for by a questionnaire is limited. A low percentage of nutrient intake accounted for would raise concern regarding the comprehensiveness of the form. As discussed in Chapter 5, however, such a questionnaire might still be reasonably discriminating if the foods had been carefully selected so as to explain maximally the between-person variation in nutrient intake. More seriously, a high percentage of nutrients accounted for does not guarantee validity, as the questionnaire may be inadequately interpreted by potential respondents. For example, it is tempting to use broad categories of foods on a

Table 6–2. Percentage of total nutrient intakes accounted for by foods listed on a 61-item compressed food-frequency questionnaire (see Appendix 5–1) and on an expanded 116-item revision of this questionnaire.

Nutrient	Percentage of intake accounted for by foods on questionnaire[a]	
	Compressed questionnaire	Revised questionnaire
Total calories	69	93
Protein	77	95
Total fat	70	96
Saturated fat	75	96
Polyunsaturated fat	51	95
Monounsaturated fat	72	96
Cholesterol	85	97
Total carbohydrate	61	90
Crude fiber	64	86
Sucrose	78	92
Total vitamin A	77	96
without supplements	73	95
Vitamin C	84	93
without supplements	76	90
Vitamin B_1	81	95
without supplements	67	91
Vitamin B_2	85	95
without supplements	75	92
Vitamin B_6	97	99
without supplements	84	95
Calcium	77	94
without supplements	77	94
Phosphorus (no supplements)	77	94
Potassium (no supplements)	73	93
Iron	75	93
without supplements	69	91
Mean	75	94

[a]Percentages are underestimated because ingredients of recipes (e.g., flour, shortening) were included in the denominators but could not be attributed to specific foods. Nutrient intakes are based on four 1-week diet records completed by 194 women in 1980.

Adapted from Willett et al., 1987a.

questionnaire such as "bread, crackers, and other baked goods." Although such questions account for a large percentage of absolute nutrient intake, they are likely to be more difficult to answer than a series of shorter specific questions. A series of more specific questions is thus likely to provide more accurate information, even though they may collectively account for a lower proportion of absolute nutrient intake.

The highest priority in designing a dietary questionnaire is usually to discriminate among persons with respect to their intake rather than to estimate their absolute intake. Thus, it may be useful to employ diet record or short-term recall data to examine the proportion of between-person variance in specific nutrient intake that is accounted for by food items on a questionnaire. Although usually of more conceptual interest than an analysis based on absolute nutrient intakes, this computation requires a dataset with many days of dietary intake for each subject. Stryker and colleagues (1987) have conducted such analyses for purposes of identifying items to be included on questionnaires. This approach, using open-ended dietary data, has apparently not been used to evaluate existing questionnaires.

Reproducibility

The reproducibility of questionnaire measurements made at two points in time can provide a useful first approximation of questionnaire performance. In conducting a reproducibility study, it is unrealistic to administer the questionnaire at a very short interval, such as a few days or weeks, as subjects may simply tend to remember their previous responses. When a longer interval of time is used, true changes in dietary intake, as well as variation in response, contribute to reduced reproducibility. Although it may be viewed as a disadvantage that such a measure of reproducibility reflects both the performance of a questionnaire and the true change in diet, both sources of variation realistically contribute to misclassification of long-term dietary intakes. Therefore, the difficulty in separating variation due to questionnaire performance from true change in diet is not extremely serious from the standpoint of evaluating measurement error. This feature, however, does hinder our capacity to measure the constancy of diet within individuals; the reproducibility correlation provides only an estimate of a lower limit of consistency. Assessment of the reproducibility of a method over several intervals of time may be useful in this respect. If a questionnaire refers to intake over the past year, administrations a few months apart should largely reflect variation associated with completing the questionnaire, whereas further decreases in reproducibility assessed at longer intervals, such as several years, should largely be due to true change in diet.

The reproducibility of food-frequency questionnaires has been examined under a wide variety of conditions (Table 6–3). In these studies, correlations have generally ranged from 0.5 to 0.7 for nutrient intakes measured at periods of 1 to 10 years. A notable exception is the study of Hankin and colleagues (1983) in which correlations for specific nutrients over an interval of only 3 months ranged from 0.12 to 0.41 among healthy whites. As the authors suggested, this low level of reproducibility may be due to the questionnaire format in which the reference period of time was only 1 week. When assessed at an interval of 17 to 25 years, Byers and coworkers (1983) found the Spearman correlation for the reproducibility of a vitamin A index to be 0.29. Relatively few studies of food-frequency questionnaire reproducibility have been conducted among children (Domel et al., 1994; Rockett and Colditz, 1996); parental reports of diets consumed by their preschool children were reasonably reproducible (Treiber et al., 1990; Stein et al., 1992), as were self-reported diets of adolescent children (Rockett et al., 1995).

In a smaller number of studies, the reproducibility of specific food items has been examined (Table 6–4). Correlation coefficients have been considerably more variable than for nutrients. Among 323 U.S. men and women interviewed at an interval of 6 to 10 years, Byers and colleagues (1987) found average correlations of 0.41 for vegetables, 0.41 for fruits, 0.53 for dairy products, and 0.39 for meats. Colditz and coworkers (1987) compared frequencies of foods reported by 1,497 women at an interval of approximately 9 months. Correlations were highest for beverages ($r = 0.70$) and ranged from 0.60 to 0.70 for foods eaten frequently and from 0.34 to 0.45 for foods eaten infrequently. In this study, the reproducibility of food intake did not vary appreciably by age, relative weight, cigarette smoking status, or alcohol intake.

As part of a large Dutch cohort study, Goldbohm and colleagues (1995) examined the reproducibility of the baseline

Table 6-3. Comparison of nutrient intakes measured by repeated food-frequency questionnaires[a]

Source	Population	FFQ design	Time to complete FFQ	Interval	Average (and range) of correlations
Hankin et al. (1983)	Japanese-Hawaiian women; cases, controls (n = 117)	43 items; portions estimated by pictures, interview; focus on fat, cholesterol, and protein	NI	3 mo	0.28 (0.12 for protein to 0.83 for cholesterol)
Byers et al. (1983)	Men and women patients admitted to Roswell Park Memorial, 50–74 yr (n = 175)	12 items, 12 response categories; interview focus on vitamin A intake	15 min	17–25 yr	0.28 (−0.04 for bread to 0.52 for coffee, 0.29 for vitamin A)
Rohan and Potter (1984)	South Australian men and women, 35–78 yr (n = 70)	141 items; standard portions; first questionnaire by interview, second by mail	NI	3 yr	Men: 0.52 (0.25 for protein to 0.78 for calcium) Women: 0.56 (0.43 for calcium to 0.76 for vitamin B_2)
Willett et al. (1985)	Registered nurses from Mass., 34–59 yr (n = 194)	61 items, 9 response categories; standard portions; mailed; focus on nutrients related to cancer	15 min	9–12 mo	0.60 (0.52 for vitamin A without supplements to 0.71 for sucrose)
Byers et al. (1987)	U.S. men and women n = 323)	129 foods plus serving sizes; interview (reinterviewed for 47 foods only)	>60 min	6–10 yr	0.56 (0.50 for fat to 0.61 for vitamin A and fiber)
Colditz et al. (1987)	U.S. nurses (n = 1497)	61-item form vs. 116-item form	15 and 25 min	9 mo	0.57 (0.40 for *trans* fatty acids to 0.71 for vitamin E)
Willett et al. (1988)	Registered nurses from Mass., 39–63 yr (n = 150)	116 items, 9 response categories; standard portions; mailed; focus on nutrients related to cancer	25 min	3 yr	0.53 (0.44 for total carbohydrate to 0.62 for vitamin C)
Pietinen et al. (1988b)	Finnish men (n = 107)	44 foods; frequency only	NI	6 mo	0.73 (0.53 for vitamin A to 0.85 for polyunsaturated fat)
Pietinen et al. (1988a)	Finnish men (n = 121)	276 foods and mixed dishes; pictures for portion review with dietitian	2 hr + ½ hr for review	6 mo	0.66 (0.56 for vitamin A to 0.73 for fiber)
Treiber et al. (1990)	Parents of preschool children (n = 55)	111 items	NI	1 wk	0.62 (0.42 for carbohydrate to 0.74 for sodium)
Engle et al. (1990)	Long Island adults (n = 50)	120 items self-entered into computer	20–70 min	1 mo	0.60 (0.53 for calcium, 0.75 for vitamin A)
Munger et al. (1992)	Older Iowa women (n = 44)	129 items	NI	5 mo to 2.5 yr	0.65 (0.40 for iron to 0.87 for folate from foods)

Reference	Population	FFQ description	Administration time	Recall period	Correlations
Rimm et al. (1992)	Male health professionals (n = 127)	131 items	NI	1 yr	0.59 (0.38 for polyunsaturated fat to 0.79 for vitamin C)
Longnecker et al. (1993)	Ranchers and others in So. Dakota and Wyoming (n = 138)	116 items	NI	6–12 mo	0.58 (0.43 for polyunsaturated fat to 0.69 for monounsaturated fat)
Ajani et al. (1994)	Participants in National Eye Institute study (n = 325)	60 items	NI	12–18 mo	0.62 (0.37 for iron to 0.73 for monounsaturated fat)
Goldbohm et al. (1995)	Dutch men and women (n = 400)	150 items	NI	1–5 yr	0.62 (0.40 for retinol to 0.69 for dietary fiber)
Riley and Blizzard (1995)	Tasmanian diabetics (n = 28)	153 items	NI	7–20 mo	0.68 (0.57 for protein to 0.79 for cholesterol)
Mannisto et al. (1996)	Finnish women (n = 152)	110 items	NI	3 mo	0.68 (0.49 for thiamine with supplements to 0.81 for monosaccharides)
Ocke et al. (1996)	Dutch men (Zutphen study) (n = 561)	Open-ended diet history collection collapsed into 18 food groups	80 min, mostly with spouse	6–12 mo	1960–65: 0.39 (0.36 for beta-carotene to 0.44 for vitamin E) 1960–70: 0.30 (0.25 for vitamin E to 0.33 for beta-carotene)
Elmstahl et al. (1996)	120 Malmo, Sweden, residents	Combination of 2-week record, 130-item questionnaire	NI	1 yr	0.62 (0.33 for folate to 0.83 for tocopherol)
van Liere et al. (1997)	French hospital employees (n = 119)	238 items with some grouped by meal and some by individual foods	NI	1 yr	0.66 (0.54 for vitamin E to 0.73 for lipids, vitamin C)
Ocke et al. (1997a)	Dutch men and women (n = 121)	77 items	NI	6–12 mo	0.71 (0.46 for vitamin E to 0.89 for carbohydrate)
Katsouyanni et al. (1997)	Greek school teachers (n = 80)	190 items	NI	1 yr	0.56 (0.24 for beta carotene to 0.75 for cholesterol)
EPIC Group of Spain (1997b)	Spanish hospital and municipal workers (n = 65)	Diet history questionnaire	50–60 min	1 yr	0.57 (0.14 for cholesterol to 0.84 for carbohydrates)
Pisani et al. (1997)	Italian residents (n = 189)	47 dishes or food items, some with portion size photos	NI	1 yr	0.61 (0.37 for protein to 0.73 for vitamin C)
Bohlscheid-Thomas et al. (1997b)	German men and women from a health insurance co. (n = 104)	158 items	NI	6 mo	0.63 (0.37 for polysaccharides to 0.69 for cholesterol)
Romieu et al. (1997)	Women from Mexico City (n = 110)	116 items	NI	1 yr	0.40 (0.23 for lutein and zeaxanthin to 0.50 for retinol)

aFFQ, food-frequency questionnaire; NI, no information. Correlations do not include alcohol.

Table 6-4. Reproducibility of food intake measured by repeated food-frequency questionnaires[a]

Source	Population	FFQ design	Time required to complete FFQ (min)	Interval between FFQs	Average correlations (and range) or percent agreement
Acheson and Doll (1964)	GI cancer cases; control men and women over 75 yr (n = 63)	56 items, 5 response categories; interviews	NI	3 mo	90% agreement within one category
Graham et al. (1967)	Gastric cancer cases, control subjects (n = 99)	27 items, 4 response categories; interview; focus on Polish-American diets	NI	18 mo	81% agreement for exact category
Nomura et al. (1976)	Japanese-Hawaiian men (n = 109)	33 items; portions estimated by pictures; interview; focus on food associated with GI cancer	15	6 mo to 2 yr	0.29 (−0.08 for dried seaweed paste to 0.71 for coffee)
Byers et al. (1987)	U.S. men and women (n = 323)	129 foods plus serving sizes; interview (reinterview for 47 foods only)	>60	6–10 yr	0.48 (0.18 for roast beef to 0.71 for coffee)
Colditz et al. (1987)	U.S. nurses (n = 1497)	61-item form vs. 116-item form	15 and 25	9 mo	0.55 (0.34 for pie to 0.76 for tea)
Thompson et al. (1987)	U.S. men and women (n = 1,184)	83 items, 8 response categories with "card sort" response	NI	15 yr	0.34 (0.05 for liquid diet foods to 0.53 for fried eggs)
Feskanich et al. (1993)	Male health professionals (n = 127)	131 items	NI	1 yr	0.59 (0.31 for pie to 0.92 for coffee)

Reference	Population	FFQ description		Time interval	Correlation (range)[a]
Ajani et al. (1994)	Participants in National Eye Institute study (n = 325)	60 items	NI	12–18 mo	0.57 (0.29 for beef, pork, lamb as a main dish to 0.81 for artificial sweetener)
Mannisto et al. (1996)	Finnish women (n = 152)	110 items and mixed dishes	NI	3 mo	0.67 (0.52 for poultry to 0.82 for cream)
Elmstahl et al. (1996)	Swedish men and women of Malmo (n = 241)	2-week food record and 130-item questionnaire	NI	1 yr	0.61 (0.23 for rice in women to 0.96 for meat products in men)
Bohlscheid-Thomas et al. (1997a)	German men and women from a health insurance co. (n = 104)	158 items and 87 photos	NI	6 mo	0.67 (0.49 for bread to 0.77 for meat)
EPIC Group of Spain (1997a)	Spanish men and owmen (n = 91)	Open-ended with food suggestions; portion size photos; interview	NI	Up to 1 yr	0.63 (0.11 for eggs to 0.88 for cereals other than breads)
Ocke et al. (1997b)	Dutch men and women (n = 121)	77 items with photos for portion sizes	NI	6 mo, 12 mo	0.49 (0.45 for fish to 0.90 for bread)
Pisani et al. (1997)	Italian men and women (n = 189	47 items	NI	1 yr	0.66 (0.31 for bread to 0.76 for legumes)
van Liere et al. (1997)	French hospital employees (n = 119)	66 foods or groups of foods with photos; detailed secondary frequency questions	NI	1 yr	0.61 (0.40 for seasonings to 0.73 for dairy products)

[a]FFQ, food-frequency questionnaire; GI, gastrointestinal; NI, no information.

food frequency questionnaire at 1-year intervals for 5 years, using independent samples of 400 participants (see Fig. 6–1). As expected, correlation coefficients with the baseline questionnaire declined with time, but the decline was slight; the average reduction for the nutrients examined was 0.07 over the 5-year period. This provides evidence that, at least in this population, dietary changes over time were not substantial, and frequent readministrations of the questionnaire were not necessary. As noted above, in the usual reproducibility study, true changes in diet cannot be separated from errors in measurement. However, the repeated measurements of reproducibility in this study allowed the authors to assess the effect of elapsed time on the correlation coefficient and thus estimate the reproducibility correlation with no change in diet; this is represented as the *y*-intercept in Figure 6–1. In another Dutch population of men, reproducibility correlations for intake of fruits, vegetables, and nutrients contained in these foods averaged 0.37 at an interval of 5 years and only decreased to 0.30 at an interval of 10 years (Ocke et al., 1996). A much larger decrease in reproducibility correlation with time was observed among rural Japanese men (Tsubono et al., 1995); median correlation declined steadily from 0.62 at 2 weeks to 0.28 at 5 years for questionnaires administered in the same season. The contrast with the Dutch study presumably reflects differences in the stability of diets and the fact that long-term reproducibility in one population cannot be generalized to others.

Correlation coefficients on the order of 0.5 to 0.7, which appear to be typical for the reproducibility of nutrient intakes, may seem disappointingly low for those accustomed to the reproducibility of laboratory measurements made under highly controlled conditions. Nevertheless, this level of reproducibility is comparable with that of many biological measurements made among free-living subjects over a period of months or years. For example, measurements of serum cholesterol level and blood pressure have similar degrees of reproducibility (Table 6–5) and yet are strong and consistent predictors of disease in epidemiologic studies.

The interpretation of reproducibility studies should be somewhat asymmetric: A low degree of reproducibility is a definite indication that the questionnaire does not provide a valid measure of long-term intake. On the other hand, a high degree of reproducibility does not ensure validity because high correlation can be simply the result of correlated error (i.e., systematic within-person error). For example, a questionnaire that has omitted important sources of a nutrient or that includes questions that are consistently misinterpreted may be highly reproducible, but fail to provide a true measure of intake for that nutrient (for a careful illustration, see Goldbohm and colleagues, 1995). Because reproducibility studies are usually quick and inexpensive to conduct, they are an appropriate part of the questionnaire evaluation, but cannot substitute for studies of validity.

Validity: Comparison of Individual Values With an Independent Measure of Diet

The ability of a questionnaire to discriminate among individuals is most directly evaluated by comparing individual estimates of nutrient intake based on the questionnaire with those measured by a more accurate method, that is, a gold standard. It has been frequently said that there is no perfect measure of dietary intake, with the implication that validation studies are not possible. Lack of a perfect standard is, however, not unique to dietary intake; all measurements have error, although these errors differ in their magnitude. Thus, validation studies never compare an operational method with absolute truth; rather, they compare one method with another method that is judged to be superior. Given that neither method is perfect, it is crucial that the errors of both methods be as independent (i.e., uncorrelated) as possible to avoid spuriously high estimates of validity.

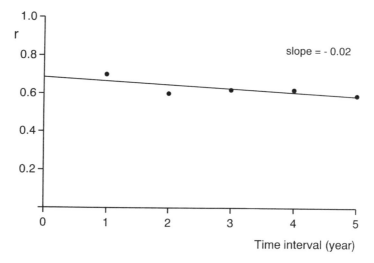

Figure 6–1. Correlations for calcium intake between baseline questionnaire and successive annual repeated questionnaires in women. A regression line is fit through the data points to estimate the correlation coefficient at time zero (the y-intercept). (From Goldbohm et al., 1995; reproduced with permission.)

For example, in some studies a dietary questionnaire has been compared with a detailed diet history interview. This provides a very limited assessment of validity because the major sources of error in the questionnaires (e.g., memory, interpretation of questions, and perception of serving sizes) are likely to be replicated in this diet history. To the extent that errors in the comparison method are uncorrelated with error in the questionnaire being evaluated, the correlation between the two tends to be underestimated. The lack of a perfect comparison method also indicates a continued need to search for better gold standards.

Among the available and feasible comparison methods for validating a food-frequency questionnaire, diet records are likely to have the least correlated errors. Major sources of error associated with

Table 6–5. Reproducibility of commonly used epidemiologic variables

Study	Variables	Population	Interval	Correlation
Shekelle et al. (1981)	Serum cholesterol	1,900 men	1 yr	0.65
Rosner et al. (1977)	Systolic blood pressure, diastolic blood pressure	863 men and women	4 yr	0.64 0.60
Willett et al. (1983)	Plasma retinol, plasma total carotenoid, plasma alpha-tocopherol	15 men and women	8wk 8wk 8wk	0.58 0.60 0.50
Gordon and Shurtleff (1973)	Blood glucose	1,597 men 1,841 women	2 yr	0.58 0.52
	Vital capacity	2,085 men 2,603 women	2 yr	0.79 0.77
	Pulse rate	2,008 men 2,529 women	2 yr	0.52 0.49

food-frequency questionnaires are due to the restrictions imposed by a fixed list of foods, memory, perception of portion sizes, and interpretation of questions. These sources of error are minimally shared by diet records because diet records are open-ended, they do not depend on memory (foods are recorded on a meal-by-meal basis), they allow direct assessment of portion sizes by measurement of weight or dimensions, and errors related to interpretation are largely at the level of the dietitian coding the records rather than the subject. Because errors associated with food-frequency questionnaires and diet records are largely independent, validity, if anything, tends to be understated. When used as a standard to assess questionnaire validity, diet records should, in principle, be kept for a sufficient number of days to represent average intake and cover the interval of time corresponding to the questionnaire, typically 1 year.

One source of error that is likely to remain correlated when comparing nutrient intakes measured by a food-frequency questionnaire with diet records is the food composition data. Nutrient intakes calculated from the two methods are usually based on a similar body of published data. Thus, for nutrients that vary greatly for different examples of the same food, the calculated values from the diet record may be incorrect, but still correlated with the questionnaire. For example, intakes of selenium (which can vary widely depending on the soil content where the food was produced) or folic acid intake (which is sensitive to processing, cooking, and storage) may appear to be measured well as judged by comparison of a questionnaire with a diet record, but both methods may be incorrect due to the nutrient composition tables being unrepresentative of the foods that were actually consumed. Thus, knowledge about the variation of a nutrient among different samples of the same food should be used when interpreting correlations calculated by two different methods. As discussed below, comparisons with biochemical indicators of intake can be helpful when there is uncertainty about the validity of calculated intakes.

As noted in Chapter 4, the process of keeping a diet record may alter food intake; to the extent that this is a departure from usual food habits (which are the focus of a food-frequency questionnaire), this will tend to reduce the correlation between the questionnaire and the record. On the other hand, keeping a diet record will heighten awareness of food and thus might increase the accuracy in completing the food-frequency questionnaire.

The primary alternative to the use of diet records as a standard for evaluating a food-frequency questionnaire is the collection of multiple 24-hour recalls. Because errors are more likely to be correlated with use of this method (both rely on memory and perception of serving sizes), it is probably suboptimal. In many situations, however, such as when subjects are illiterate or less than highly motivated, multiple 24-hour recalls may be the only reasonable option.

The validity of food-frequency questionnaires has now been examined in many studies (Table 6–6). In several early investigations, usually based on a relatively small number of subjects, impressively high correlations for both food and nutrients were observed between simple dietary questionnaires and diet histories (Abramson et al., 1963; Browe et al., 1966; Balogh et al., 1968; Epstein et al., 1970). Stefanik and Trulson (1962) found that a simple food-frequency questionnaire could reasonably characterize cultural differences in eating habits between Irish-born and Italian-born American men.

Subsequently, Jain and colleagues (1982) compared a simple, mailed questionnaire with a detailed diet history interview conducted after an interval of 3 months among 50 women. Reasonably high correlations were observed, ranging from 0.47 for cholesterol to 0.72 for vegetable protein. Lower correlations were observed by Gray and coworkers (1984) for intake of vitamins C ($r = 0.29$) and A ($r = 0.03$) when the diet history was completed at an interval of 15 months. The authors attributed these low correlations to the broad response categories that were used. In this study, the majority of important food sources of these vitamins were used one to several times a week; however, the questionnaire required subjects to describe these frequencies as either "a few times a week" or "daily or almost daily." The apparently carefully conducted study by Stuff and co-workers (1983) is a clear contrast to the generally encouraging findings of others. Among 40 lactating women, these investigators found essentially no correlation between nutrients measured by a food-frequency questionnaire and a 1-week diet record completed the following week. There is no obvious explanation for this discrepant finding, although it might possibly relate to unusual variation in diet during lactation.

Among the early detailed studies was our validation assessment of a 61-item food-frequency questionnaire used in 1980 as part of the Nurses' Health Study (Willett et al., 1985). In this study, women aged 34 to 59 years and living in the greater Boston area were randomly selected from among the respondents to the 1980 Nurses' Health Study questionnaire. Approximately 3 months after completing the questionnaire, each participant was provided with a dietetic scale and instructed by a research dietitian in recording food intake for 1 week. The process of keeping a 1-week diet record was repeated at 3-month intervals to obtain a total of 4 1-week records. At the end of either the third or fourth week's record, a second food-frequency questionnaire, identical to the first, was completed (Fig. 6–2).

Because we inquired on the dietary questionnaire about the average intake of foods over the past year, the Nurses' Health Study validation study was designed to measure optimally food over a 1-year period using diet records. Thus, the repeated diet record measurements at 3-month intervals should have accounted for seasonal changes and medium-term drifts in food habits over this period of time. Because day-to-day variability in intake of many nutrients is large, we collected 4 weeks of intake data per person to provide a reasonably stable estimate of true long-term intake for nearly all nutrients. Beaton and colleagues (1983), however, have suggested that even this number of days of diet recording may be insufficient to measure accurately intake of some nutrients such as vitamin A; our analyses have indeed indicated that the correlations for highly variable nutrients (e.g., cholesterol intake) based on 4 weeks of data are still somewhat attenuated due to within-person variability (see Chapter 12).

In designing the Nurses' Health Study food-frequency questionnaire validation study, we chose to administer the questionnaire before and at the end of the diet record collection out of concern that the process of recording diet might alter awareness of food intake and thus artificially improve accuracy in completing the questionnaire. Although this possibility is avoided by comparing the initial questionnaire with the diet records collected during the subsequent year, this comparison would tend to underestimate validity because the initial questionnaire asked about diet during the year before recording. The use of a questionnaire both before and after recording provides, in some sense, minimal and maximal estimates of true validity. An added benefit of administering the questionnaire before and after the diet record collection is the opportunity to access the reproducibility of the questionnaire over that 1-year period. Reassuringly, correlations between the initial food-frequency questionnaire and the mean diet record intake were only slightly lower than those between the repeat questionnaire and the diet record mean, which represents the conceptually appropriate time sequence (Table 6–7). In these data we found that adjustment for total caloric intake improved the correlations for macronutrients, presumably due to "canceling" of correlated errors (see Chapter 11 for a more detailed discussion). After

Table 6–6. Comparison of food-frequency questionnaires with other dietary assessment methods[a]

Source	Population	Comparison methods	Interval between methods	Reference period	Average (and range) of correlations	Comments
Abramson et al. (1963)	Pregnant Israeli women (n = 60)	30-min inteview	0	Usual diet for previous 3 mo	0.82 (0.42 for bread and rolls to 0.99 for herring)	Correlations are between frequency of consumption and quantity of consumption
Browe et al. (1966)	Albany Cardiovascular Health Study (n = 29 men)	Diet history	4 wk	Usual monthly meal patterns	0.74 (0.66 for vegetable protein to 0.79 for cholesterol)	
Balogh et al. (1968)	Israeli men (n = 48)	Diet history	A few hours	Usual diet	0.82 (0.78 for polyunsaturated fatty acids to 0.95 for animal protein)	
	Israeli men (n = 14)	Food record		Week after FFQ	0.80 (0.69 for polyunsaturated fatty acids to 0.94 for total fat)	
Epstein et al. (1970)	Heterogenous Israeli adults (n = 161)	Diet history	4–30 days	Usual diet	0.53 (0.14 for linoleic acid to 0.76 for total protein)	
Hankin et al. (1975)	Japanese-Hawaiian men (n = 50)	Food record	0	1 wk, FFQ recalled previous 1-wk record	0.73 (0.47 for beef to 0.88 for shrimp, raw fish, and coffee)	
Hunt et al. (1979)	California adults (n = 46)	24-hr recall	1–5 wk	Usual diet	0.43 (0.04 for vitamin A to 0.61 for carbohydrate)	Unusually large portion sizes for vitamin C foods were used in FFQ
Jain et al. (1982)	Canadian women n = 50)	Diet history	3 mo	Usual diet for previous 2 mo, FFQ reports usual diet	0.62 (0.47 for cholesterol to 0.72 for vegetable protein)	
Stuff et al. (1983)	Lactating Texan women (n = 40)	Food record	0	FFQ reports usual diet	0.1 (0.00 for iron and phosphorus to 0.24 for calcium)	FFQ requested usual intake during a time that diet might be changing
Jensen et al. (1984)	Danish men and women (n = 79)	Dietary household suvey	15–25 yr	15–25 yr	0.31 (0.13 for fresh vegetables to 0.42 for energy)	Correlations similar for present vs. remote diet

Reference	Population	Reference method	Time	Recall period	Correlation	Comments
Gray et al. (1984)	Southern California elderly (n = 50)	Diet history	15 mo	Usual diet	0.39 (0.16 for vitamin A to 0.63 for vitamin C)	Very broad response categories were used in FFQ
Willett et al. (1985)	Registered nurses (n = 194)	Diet record	1 mo to 1 yr	Previous year	0.56 (0.36 for vitamin A without supplements to 0.75 for vitamin C)	
Willett et al. (1988)	U.S. registered nurses, 39–63 yr (n = 150)	Four 1-wk diet records	3–4 yr	1 yr (3–4 yr earlier)	0.50 (0.28 for iron to 0.61 for carbohydrate)	Correlations were higher after adjustment for energy
Pietinen et al. (1988b)	Finnish men (n = 189)	Twelve 2-day diet records (vs. 44-item questionnaire)	1–6 mo	1 yr	0.58 (0.36 for vitamin A to 0.77 for polyunsaturated fat)	Adjustment for energy increased correlations for most nutrients
Pietinen et al. (1988a)	Finnish men (n = 189)	Twelve 2-day diet records (vs. 273-item questionnaire)	1–6 mo	1 yr	0.61 (0.43 for monounsaturated fat to 0.76 for polyunsaturated fat)	Adjustment for energy had little effect on correlations
Larkin et al. (1989)	White and black men and women (n = 228)	16 days of food record	3 mo to 1 yr	Previous year	0.36 (0.09 for iron in black men to 0.62 for calcium in white men)	Race and sex group differences were much greater in the food records than the FFQ
Stiggelbout et al. (1989)	Dutch women (n = 82)	Diet history	25 days	Previous year	0.59 (0.54 to 0.64 for retinol, beta-carotene, and vitamin A)	FFQ and validation was specifically designed for classifying by retinol and beta-carotene intake
Block et al. (1990a)	Middle-aged women (n = 260), older men (n = 83)	Diet records	Women: 3 mo to 1 yr Men: 10–15 yr in the past	Usual diet	0.54 (0.38 vitamin A to 0.66 percentage calories from fat for women) 0.49 (0.37 calcium to 0.67 for cholesterol)	Validation of a reduced item questionnaire utilizing 60 of 98 items from original questionnaire
Block et al. (1990b)	Middle-aged women (n = 260)	Diet records	3 mo to 1 yr	Past 6 mo	0.54 (0.37 for vitamin A to 0.74 for vitamin C including supplements)	Feasibility trial comparing diets of women on low-fat or usual diet
Horwath and Worsley (1990)	Adelaide men and women (n = 40)	Direct observation of foods in home	2 wk	Usual diet	0.65 (0.42 for vegetable consumption to 0.86 for total variety and number of foods)	Reference standard was food item observation and checklist

Table 6–6. Comparison of food-frequency questionnaires with other dietary assessment methods (continued)

Source	Population	Comparison methods	Interval between methods	Reference period	Average (and range) of correlations	Comments
Treiber et al. (1990)	Parents of preschool children (n = 55)	24-hr recall	1 wk	Usual diet for previous 3 mo	0.48 (0.40 potassium to 0.62 for cholesterol)	Usual diet for 3 mo was chosen due to concern that children's diet changes quickly during this time. FFQ was designed for 1-year assessment. Only significant correlations were reported
Engle et al. (1990)	Long Island adults (n = 50)	7-day diet record	1–2 mo	Usual diet for previous 3 mo	0.44 (0.16 vitamin C to 0.62 for % calories from fat)	Computerized, self-administered FFQ
Tjonneland et al. (1991)	Danish men and women (n = 144)	7-day diet record	2 mo	Previous year	0.45 (0.26 for protein to 0.71 for calcium)	Photographs were used to assist in accurate portion size estimation
Block et al. (1992)	Michigan men and women (n = 85)	24-hr recall plus 3-day dietary record	3 mo	Previous year	0.48 (0.31 for potassium to 0.60 for oleic acid)	Recalls and diet records were pooled; correlations for University of Michigan FFQ
Rimm (1992)	Male health professionals (n = 12)	Diet record	6 mo	Previous year	0.59 (0.28 for iron without supplements to 0.86 for vitamin C)	
Stein et al. (1992)	Parents of preschool children (n = 224)	24-hr recall	Up to 2 mo	Usual diet for past 6 mo	0.34 (−0.14 for polyunsaturated fat to 0.59 for calories)	Adjustment for energy and intraindividual variability raised most correlations
Munger et al. (1992)	Older Iowa women (n = 44)	5 recalls of 24 hrs each	Up to 4 mo	Previous year	0.48 (−0.01 for iron to 0.76 for vitamin C)	Recalls were administered by telephone
Horwath (1993)	Older New Zealand men and women (n = 53)	2-day diet records	2 wk	Previous year	0.56 (0.37 for protein to 0.77 for zinc)	Unadjusted for energy intake
Callmer et al. (1993)	Swedish men and women (n = 206)	3-day diet records	Up to 1 yr	Usual diet	0.58 (0.28 for energy to 0.80 for ascorbic acid) (long FFQ)	250-question FFQ plus photos, or 130-question FFQ and 2-wk record were measured against 3-day diet records

Reference	Population	Reference method	Duration	Period	Correlations	Comments
Goldbohm et al. (1994)	Dutch men and women (n = 109)	3-day diet records	3-mo	Previous year	0.71 (0.53 for fat to 0.84 for polysaccharides)	
Bingham et al. (1994)	British women (n = 160)	Weighed food records	A few weeks to several months	Previous year	Cambridge 0.31, Oxford 0.51 (0.13 for protein to 0.57 for nonstarch polysaccharides)	Two FFQs were completed. "Cambridge" completed as part of recruitment in season one had lower correlations than "Oxford" completed later in season three
Riley and Blizzard (1995)	Tasmanian diabetics (n = 84)	Weighed dietary records	1 day to several months	Previous year	0.42 (0.23 for protein to 0.49 for cholesterol)	Energy estimate decreased significantly at the second administration of FFQ
Johansson and Hallmans (1995)	Swedish men and women (n = 195)	24-hr recall by telephone	1 mo	Previous year	0.46 (0.25 for retinol to 0.61 for vitamin E and sucrose)	Use of portion size photos helped only marginally. Correlations not adjusted for energy
Jain et al., (1996)	Canadian men and women (n = 203)	Food record	1 mo	Previous year	0.51 (0.26 for thiamin to 0.72 for calcium in men)	
Rockett et al. (1996)	Adolescents (n = 260)	24-hr recall by telephone	1 mo	Previous year	0.62 (0.25 for sodium to 0.77 for calcium without supplements)	
Mannisto et al. (1996)	Finnish women (n = 152)	7-day diet records	3 mo	Previous year	0.55, 0.62 (0.24 for thiamine, 0.37 for organ meats to 0.70 for total N-6 fatty acids and 0.84 for soft margarine)	
Katsouyanni et al. (1997)	Greek school teachers (n = 80)	24-hr recall	1 mo	Previous year	0.4 (0.1 for beta-carotene in women to 0.73 for phosphorus in men)	
EPIC Group of Spain (1997a,b)	Spanish men and women (n = 64)	24-hr recall	1 mo to 1 yr	Typical week in the previous year	0.66, 0.71 (0.14 for legumes, 0.28 for retinol to 0.90 for other dairy products, 0.89 for mono, poly, and total fat)	Diet history questionnaire developed from Burke diet history

Table 6-6. Comparison of food-frequency questionnaires with other dietary assessment methods (continued)

Source	Population	Comparison methods	Interval between methods	Reference period	Average (and range) of correlations	Comments
van Liere et al. (1997)	French hospital employees (n = 119)	24-hr recall	1 mo	Previous year	0.44, 0.59 (0.12 for mixed dishes, 0.29 for retinol to 0.67 for dairy foods, 0.81 for beta-carotene)	First part of questionnaire assessed consumption of food groups, second captured specific foods within groups. Portion sizes were estimated with use of photos
Ocke et al. (1997a)	Dutch men and women (n = 121)	24-hr recall	1 mo	Previous year	0.55, 0.59 (0.31 for vegetables, 0.29 for retinol to 0.79 for milk products, 0.76 for carbohydrates)	
Pisani et al. (1997)	Italian men and women (n = 197)	24-hr recall	1 mo to several mo	Usual diet	0.45 (0.31 for fat to 0.60 for cholesterol)	
Bohlscheid-Thomas et al. (1997a)	German men and women from a health insurance co. (n = 104)	24-hr recall	1 mo	Previous year	0.60, 0.60 (0.48 for vegetables, 0.43 for polyunsaturated fat to 0.77 for bread, 0.75 for saturated fat)	A short questionnaire was used to correct food consumption frequencies for the second FFQ. 24-hour recalls did not include meals eaten on Friday or Saturday
Wolk et al. (1997)	Swedish women (n = 184)	7-day dietary records	A few months	Previous year	0.50 (0.24 for alpha-linolenic to 0.59 for saturated fat)	Additional questions were added to Modified FFQ to test validity of fat estimates.
Romieu et al. (1997)	Mexican women (n = 110)	Four 4-day 24-hr recall	Up to 1 yr	Previous year	0.32 (0.11 for lutein to 0.53 for vitamin C)	FFQ reflected seasonal availability of fruits and vegetables
Smith-Warner (1997)	U.S. men and women (n = 101)	3-day diet records	Up to 1 yr	Previous year	0.53 (0.32 for vegetables to 0.82 for juice)	Specifically designed to compare methods of capturing consumption of fruits and vegetables

[a] Extension of data compiled by Sampson (1985). Correlations do not include alcohol. FFQ, food-frequency questionnaire.

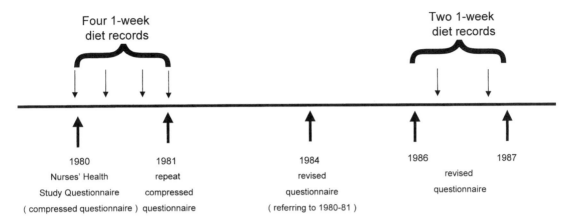

Figure 6–2. Design of Nurses' Health Study food-frequency questionnaire validation study.

Table 6–7. Pearson correlation coefficients for comparison of semiquantitative food-frequency questionnaire scores with the means of four 1-week diet reocrds, both unadjusted and adjusted for total caloric intake[a]

Nutrient[b]	Questionnaire 1 vs. means of 4 records		Questionnaire 2 vs. means of 4 records	
	Unadjusted	Adjusted[c]	Unadjusted	Adjusted[c]
Protein	0.18	0.37	0.33	0.47
Total fat	0.27	0.48	0.39	0.53
Saturated fat	0.31	0.49	0.44	0.59
Polyunsaturated fat	0.31	0.42	0.40	0.48
Cholesterol	0.46	0.61	0.52	0.61
Total carbohydrate	0.48	0.44	0.53	0.45
Sucrose	0.52	0.41	0.60[c]	0.54[d]
Crude fiber	0.43	0.51	0.46	0.58
Total vitamin A	0.37	0.43	0.41	0.49
without supplements	0.21	0.28	0.26	0.36
Vitamin B$_6$	0.44	0.47	0.54[d]	0.58[d]
without supplements	0.32	0.43	0.43[d]	0.54[d]
Vitamin C	0.53	0.56	0.73[d]	0.75[d]
without supplements	0.46	0.52	0.63[d]	0.66

[a] Data based on information provided by 173 female registered nurses aged 34–59 years and residing in the Boston area, 1980–1981.

[b] Nutrient intakes transformed using log$_e$ to improve normality.

[c] Intakes adjusted using the residuals from regression models with caloric intake as the independent variable and nutrient intakes as the dependent variables.

[d] $p < 0.05$ for comparison of Pearson r for questionnaire 2 vs. means of four records with Pearson r for questionnaire 1 vs. means of four records.

From Willett et al., 1985.

adjustment for caloric intake, correlations ranged from 0.35 for vitamin A without supplements to 0.75 for vitamin C with supplements. As noted earlier, correlation coefficients of 0.5 to 0.7 typically seen in validation studies may seem low to scientists accustomed to comparisons of laboratory methods, but these are similar to the validities of other epidemiologic measurements in populations, including physical activity (Wolf et al., 1994; Chasan-Taber et al., 1996), that have well-established associations with disease risk. The impact of this degree of error on disease relationships is discussed quantitatively in Chapter 12.

The Nurses' Health Study validation study also provided the opportunity to compare the relative capacities of the simple questionnaire or a 1-week diet record to represent long-term intake (Table 6–8). The correlations of both a single 1-week (week 4) diet record and the second questionnaire with the mean of the first 3 weeks of diet recording were examined. Although the correlations were slightly higher between the fourth diet record and the first three diet records than between the questionnaire and the first three diet records, the differences were generally small, indicating that the simple questionnaire captured nearly as much information on individual dietary intakes as the considerably more expensive diet record.

A large number of food frequency questionnaire validation studies have been conducted, more recently using designs similar to that employed in the 1980 Nurses' Health Study investigation. (A register of published and ongoing validation or calibration studies has been developed and is now established as an Internet resource [Thompson et al., 1997].*) Although the nature of the study populations has varied widely, similar results have been seen in most of the more recent studies (see Table 6–6). In recent validation studies using quite comprehensive questionnaires (generally over 100 items), average correlations

for energy-adjusted nutrients have generally been from 0.6 to 0.7 (Block et al., 1990a,b; Rimm et al., 1992; Goldbohm et al., 1994; Mannisto et al., 1996). Thus far, validation studies in children have been few, but in one recent analysis among children aged 9 to 18 years, adjusted correlations comparing a self-administered food-frequency questionnaire with multiple telephone-administered 24-hour recalls were similar to those that have been observed in adult populations (Rockett et al., 1996). Thus, the food-frequency approach appears to be robust across a wide range of applications.

The large study conducted in Finland by Pietinen and coworkers (1988a,b) provided the opportunity to compare the relative validities of an extremely short questionnaire and an extremely detailed questionnaire, which were both self-administered. The short questionnaire consisted of 44 foods, and only information on simple frequency-of-use was obtained. The detailed questionnaire contained 273 foods and mixed dishes and a corresponding 63-page book of portion sizes; this required 2 hours to complete and ½ hour to review with a nutritionist. When compared with the mean of 12 2-day diet records, reasonable correlations were seen with both methods (Table 6–6); after adjustment for total energy intake, the correlations with the diet record were on average only 0.07 higher for the detailed questionnaire compared with the extremely short form. Because few study populations would tolerate a more extensive questionnaire than the detailed one used in this study, these data provide an indication of the limits of the food-frequency methodology and demonstrate the rapidly decreasing marginal gain in information obtained with increasingly detailed questionnaires.

In a probing analysis of reasons for differences between intakes assessed by a food-frequency questionnaire and by diet records, Flegal and Larkin (1990) examined the relative contributions of differences in nutrient composition, servings

*http://www-dacv.ims.nci.nih.gov/.

Table 6–8. Comparison of the second semiquantitative food-frequency questionnaire and diet record 4 nutrient scores with mean nutrient scores from diet records 1 to 3[a]

| | Pearson correlation coefficients for calorie-adjusted intakes | |
Nutrient[b]	Questionnaire 2 vs. records 1–3	Record 4 vs. records 1–3
Protein	0.48	0.66[c]
Total fat	0.52	0.64
Saturated fat	0.58	0.64
Polyunsaturated fat	0.46	0.60[c]
Cholesterol	0.58	0.56
Total carbohydrate	0.42	0.76[c]
Sucrose	0.56	0.63
Crude fiber	0.56	0.78[c]
Total vitamin A	0.49	0.63[c]
without supplements	0.36	0.49
Vitamin B_6	0.59	0.80[c]
without supplements	0.51	0.62[c]
Vitamin C	0.76	0.75
without supplements	0.64	0.72

[a]Data based on information provided by 173 female registered nurses aged 34–59 years and residing in the Boston area, 1980–1981.

[b]Nutrients transformed using log_e to improve normality.

[c]$p < 0.05$ for comparison of Pearson r for record 4 v. records 1 to 3 with Pearson r for questionnaire 2 versus records 1 to 3.

From Willett et al., 1985.

sizes, and frequency of reporting foods. Differences in nutrient composition contributed only slightly to error, and errors in serving sizes contributed modestly to differences in group means between methods. However, differences in reported frequencies of foods were by far the most important source of error both for group means and for relative ranking of subjects. This observation is consistent with earlier work indicating that frequency of food consumption is the most important determinant of between-person variation in nutrient intakes.

Most validation studies have been analyzed on the basis of nutrient intakes; however, it is also possible to compare methods at the level of individual foods or food groups. Such comparisons may be particularly helpful in focusing attention on the questionnaire items that are performing poorly, thus suggesting specific areas that

could be improved in subsequent questionnaires. Data from the 1980 Nurses' Health Study dietary questionnaire validation analysis were also used to examine the validity of specific food items (Salvini et al., 1989). As noted earlier, such an analysis is complex because foods are usually recorded in much more detail in the diet records and these need to be combined to correspond to items on the food-frequency questionnaire. Furthermore, day-to-day variation in intake of most specific foods is substantially greater than variation in nutrients. Thus, even 28 days of diet recording did not adequately represent usual intake of many foods. For this reason, correlation coefficients were corrected for within-person variation in the diet record (see Chapter 12).

Data for selected foods analyzed in this manner using the 1980–1981 repeat questionnaire (Fig. 6–2) are presented in Table

6–9. Correlations for most foods were similar in magnitude to those observed for nutrient intakes, indicating that the questionnaire performed reasonably well. The questionnaire, however, substantially overestimated intake of "spinach and other greens" and correlated poorly with the diet record for this item. We suspected that this problem arose because of deletion of lettuce from the questionnaire in the process of compressing the forms so that individuals variably considered lettuce as "other greens." This was addressed in subsequent questionnaires by deleting the phrase "other greens" (which leaves much to individual interpretation) and adding back items on lettuce to the questionnaire. When responses by the same women to the 1982 and 1984 Nurses' Health Study questionnaire were compared with the diet records collected in 1980, the correlations for spinach were substantially higher and similar to those for other foods, indicating that the altered wording had corrected the problem in the original questionnaire. Similar findings for the validity of individual food items were observed among a population of men (Feskanich et al., 1994).

The existence of the four 1-week diet records collected in 1980 and 1981 in the Nurses' Health Study also provided the opportunity to examine the validity of the food-frequency questionnaire for assessing diet several years in the past (Willett et al., 1988). In 1984 we mailed a revised and expanded (116-item) version of the semiquantitative food-frequency questionnaire to the women who had recorded their diet in 1980 to 1981; the questionnaire was worded to ask about food intake 3 to 4 years earlier. This expanded questionnaire included additional foods that had been eliminated during the development of the 1980 questionnaire due to their small independent contribution to between-person variance in nutrient intakes (see Chapter 5). The revised form thus accounted for a larger absolute intake of nutrients (see Table 6–2). In addition, a number of foods

that had been previously asked about as a single broad item were separated into discrete items. Mean nutrient intakes assessed by the revised questionnaire were similar to those measured by the diet record (see Table 6–1). Correlations with intake measured by diet records again tended to be higher after adjustment for total caloric intake in the case of macronutrients and were, overall, quite similar to correlations observed for the questionnaire completed at the end of the diet recording in 1980 to 1981 (Tables 6–9 and 6–10). Because memory inevitably tends to fade with time (Bradburn et al., 1987), this similarity in correlations was interpreted as meaning that the revised questionnaire represented an improvement that was sufficient to compensate for an increased interval of time. These data also provide evidence that the semiquantitative food-frequency questionnaire method can reasonably measure dietary intake several years earlier, as would typically be done in a case–control study. To some extent, the recall of past diet may be a function of some consistency in diet over time and the tendency of recent food intake to influence the recall of past diet (see Chapter 7).

The Nurses' Health Study assessment of questionnaire validity has been further extended in time, which provided an opportunity to evaluate the degree to which the questionnaire characterizes dietary intake over a multiyear period. In 1986, we sent a slight modification of the expanded questionnaire, consisting of 136 items, to the entire cohort population. We then conducted another validation study among 191 participants using a similar design as in 1980 except that 2 rather than 4 weeks of diet records were used. The de-attenuated correlations between the repeat 1986 questionnaire and the 1986 diet records (mean $r = 0.62$; see Table 6–11) were appreciably higher than between the 1980 questionnaire and 1980 diet records (see Table 6–7), providing additional evidence for an enhanced performance. In the sec-

Table 6–9. Comparison of average intake of selected specific foods reported on a compressed 61-item questionnaire with intake measured by 28 days of dietary record among 173 U.S. women[a]

	Diet record mean	Questionnaire mean	Records vs. questionnaire (Pearson correlation)	
			Crude	Adjusted
Low-fat milk (cups)	0.28	0.53	0.79	0.81
Whole milk (cups)	0.27	0.22	0.62	0.62
Margarine (pats)	1.24	1.50	0.71	0.76
Butter (pats)	0.97	0.64	0.79	0.85
Spinach, other greens (½ cup)	0.06	0.28	0.08	0.17
Broccoli (½ cup)	0.07	0.17	0.49	0.69
Apples (1 fruit)	0.20	0.33	0.66	0.80

[a] Variables transformed by $\log_e$ to improve normality. Adjusted correlations are corrected for within-person variation in dietary record intake (see Chapter 12).

From Salvini et al., 1989

ond validation study, approximately half of the participants were selected at random from among those in the 1980 study (n = 92) (see Fig. 6–2). For this group, we examined the correlations between nutrients measured by the 1986 questionnaire and the 1980 diet records, as well as the mean of intakes obtained by diet records in 1980 and 1986. The correlations with the mean intakes assessed by the 1980 plus 1986 diet records were similar to those for 1986 only, providing evidence that questionnaires focused on diet during the previous year are actually providing information about diet during a more extended period of time, which is a critically important assumption for the investigation of conditions such as heart disease and cancer. We also evaluated the degree to which change in diet over a 6-year period assessed by food-frequency questionnaire correlated with change assessed by diet records. For the seven nutrients that could be evaluated, the average de-attenuated correlation was 0.54 (see Table 6–12). These provide documentation that changes in diet can be assessed by food-frequency questionnaire, but the correlation is probably underesti-

mated because the questionnaire format had changed appreciably between 1980 and 1986 and had more than doubled in length.

Although the design of the 1980 to 1981 Nurses' Health Study questionnaire validation study had many attractive features, it was an expensive process. The full-time efforts of a research dietitian were required for over 2 years in addition to the support of programmers and data-entry personnel. Although improved computer-based systems for the coding of diet records enhance efficiency to some extent, the cost of such a study may sometimes be difficult to justify when evaluating further versions of a dietary questionnaire or applications in different populations. In such instances, most of the useful information appears to be obtainable with a substantially smaller number of days of diet recording or 24-hour recalls and the use of de-attenuated procedures to account for the smaller number of days (discussed later and in Chapter 12).

In principle, the use of direct observation of food intake would provide an excellent gold standard for validation of a dietary questionnaire. Unfortunately, this ap-

Table 6–10. Correlations between nutrients estimated by a 116-item semiquantitative food-frequency questionnaire and the average of four 1-week diet records collected 3–4 years earlier[a]

Nutrient	1984 revised questionnaire vs. 1980 diet records	
	Crude	Adjusted
Total calories	0.37	—
Protein	0.29	0.52
Total fat	0.37	0.54
Saturated fat	0.38	0.52
Polyunsaturated fat	0.43	0.58
Monounsaturated fat	0.37	0.48
Cholesterol	0.50	0.57
Total carbohydrate	0.47	0.61
Crude fiber	0.43	0.56
Sucrose	0.50	0.45
Total vitamin A	0.36	0.44
without supplements	0.26	0.37
Vitamin C	0.38	0.54
without supplements	0.50	0.54
Vitamin B_1	0.32	0.58
without supplements	0.46	0.55
Vitamin B_2	0.33	0.57
without supplements	0.37	0.52
Vitamin B_6	0.50	0.54
without supplements	0.39	0.57
Calcium	0.56	0.56
without supplements	0.46	0.51
Phosphorus (no supplements)	0.32	0.51
Potassium (no supplements)	0.41	0.53
Iron	0.55	0.55
without supplements	0.29	0.28

[a] Diet record data were based on means of four 1-week records. All data were transformed by $\log_e$ to improve normality. Data are based on responses of 150 women.

From Willett et al., 1988.

proach is usually not feasible, as such observations require an artificial environment. Direct observation was used to assess the validity of reported food intake during a specific potluck luncheon, which could be an appropriate reference period for a foodborne outbreak (Decker et al., 1986). During the luncheon, a video recorder and camera were used to record the activities of all 32 attendees under the guise that new equipment was being tested. Two to 3 days later attendees were asked to complete a questionnaire regarding the use or nonuse of all foods that were served, and these responses were compared with the videotaped actual food consumption. Although the associations between reported and recorded intakes were high, only 10 of the 32 subjects made no error. Mullen and colleagues (1984) used direct observation of food consumption by students in a cafeteria on multiple days to compare with their responses to a food-frequency questionnaire. Unfortunately, this carefully collected dataset was analyzed by comparing the frequencies of use (assessed by the two methods) for specific foods *within* each subject, thus providing no information on the capacity of the questionnaire to distinguish among subjects. Baranowski and co-workers (1986) conducted direct observations of school children for two continuous 12-hour days and found over 80% agreement with self-reported food frequency.

Comparison With a Biochemical Indicator of Dietary Intake

Biochemical indicators of dietary intake have great intuitive appeal as the gold standard to assess the validity of a dietary questionnaire. The fundamental advantage of using a biochemical indicator is that measurement errors should be essentially uncorrelated with errors in any dietary questionnaire. Thus, the capacity to demonstrate a correlation between the questionnaire assessment of intake and the biochemical indicator provides almost unquestionable qualitative documentation of validity. Although biochemical markers are undeniably attractive as standards for studies of validity, they have many limitations (see Chapter 9). Biochemical indicators are unlikely to be influenced by dietary intake alone as individuals generally differ to some degree in the absorption and metabolism of most nutrients. These differences cause variability in the biochemical indicator unrelated to intake. Furthermore, other sources of physiologic variation, such as levels of binding proteins or poorly understood fluctuations related to diurnal or

Table 6–11. Correlations between the 1986 questionnaire and nutrients calculated from the 1980 diet records and from 1980 plus 1986 diet records among 92 NHS participants[a]

Nutrients	1986 FFQ[b] vs. 1986 diet records		1986 FFQ vs. 1980 diet records		1986 FFQ vs. 1980 + 1986 diet records	
	r	De-attenuated r	r	De-attenuated r	r	De-attenuated r
Total fat	0.51	0.57	0.49	0.53	0.62	0.67
Saturated fat	0.59	0.68	0.42	0.46	0.64	0.70
Polyunsaturated fat	0.41	0.48	0.45	0.50	0.58	0.64
Monounsaturated fat	0.51	0.58	0.51	0.56	0.63	0.69
Cholesterol	0.62	0.73	0.38	0.42	0.58	0.65
Carbohydrates	0.59	0.64	0.61	0.65	0.69	0.73
Protein	0.42	0.50	0.40	0.44	0.50	0.56
Total vitamin A	0.56	0.79	0.33	0.38	0.57	0.65
Vitamin B_6	0.55	0.64	0.42	0.46	0.60	0.65
Vitamin C	0.63	0.76	0.36	0.38	0.47	0.50
Calcium	0.64	0.75	0.40	0.43	0.49	0.53
Iron	0.47	0.60	0.23	0.25	0.37	0.40

[a] All nutrients adjusted for total energy intakes and do not include supplements.
[b] FFQ, food-frequency questionnaire.

menstrual cycles, may influence the biochemical level.

Variation in dietary intake from day to day will itself cause fluctuation in biochemical indicator levels; the effect of this source of variation differs among indicators depending on their time-integrating capacity. To the extent that the biochemical indicator is serving as a standard for long-term dietary intake, such variation is a source of error. Finally, the technical error associated with laboratory measurement contributes to variation in the biochemical indicator. The net effect of all these sources of variation is to weaken correlations between a dietary questionnaire used to assess long-term intake and the biochemical indicator. For this reason it is likely that the magnitude of such correlations will tend to be rather modest, even when the dietary measurements are highly accurate and precise. Differences in the bioavailability of nutrients from food to food could cause further weakening of these correlations; however, this source of error is probably justifiably attributed to the questionnaire as it is related to a limitation of food composition data.

Several strategies can be employed to account for extraneous variation in the biochemical standard used in a validation study. To the extent that factors causing this variation can be measured, adjustment can be made for them, thus improving observed correlations. For example, vitamin E is nonspecifically carried in lipoprotein particles and is, therefore, strongly correlated with serum cholesterol; adjusting serum vitamin E levels for serum cholesterol thus improves the correlation with both intake (Willett et al., 1983; Stryker et al., 1988) and the availability to functionally relevant tissues (Sokol et al., 1984). Attenuation of correlation coefficients due to true day-to-day variation or random laboratory error can be overcome by either obtaining a large number of replicate samples per subject or by using a smaller number of replicates and correcting statistically for random error (see Chapter 12).

In addition to the limitation that biochemical indicators do not provide a pure reflection of diet, their use is markedly constrained by the lack of any marker for many dietary factors of major interest. For example, biochemical indicators do not exist for intake of total fat, total carbohydrate, sucrose, or fiber. For some other nu-

Table 6–12. Correlation of coefficients for change in energy-adjusted nutrients from 1980 to 1986 assessed by questionnaire and by diet records (n = 92 women)

Nutrient[a]	Crude r	De-attenuated r[b]
Total fat	0.26	0.39
Saturated fat	0.28	0.38
Cholesterol	0.45	0.66
Carbohydrate	0.32	0.44
Vitamin B_6	0.35	0.55
Vitamin A	0.17	0.38
Vitamin C	0.54	0.95

[a] Intakes do not include supplements.

[b] Correlations de-attenuated for week-to-week variation in diet record data. For this adjustment, we calculated two estimates of change from the diet records: one based on two randomly selected 1-week records in 1980 and one 1-week record in 1986 and the other based on the other two 1-week records in 1980 and the other 1-week record in 1986.

trients, biochemical measurements do exist, but homeostatic regulation is so strong (and thus their association with intake so weak) that they are of minimal use as standards in a validation study within the range of typical diets. Such highly regulated nutrients include plasma levels of cholesterol, retinol, and calcium. In spite of these limitations, the use of biochemical markers in a validation study can be helpful when they are available. For example, a null association between a nutrient intake measured by questionnaire and the risk of a disease is more meaningful if the questionnaire measurement has been shown to be correlated with a biochemical indicator.

Examples of questionnaire validations using biochemical measurements are described in Table 6–13. As part of the baseline data in a supplementation trial (Willett et al., 1983), we measured intake of dietary carotene (more specifically, carotenoids with provitamin A activity) and vitamin E, as well as plasma levels of total carotenoids and alpha-tocopherol (the major form of vitamin E). After adjusting nutrient intakes for total caloric intake and plasma nutrients for plasma lipid values, the correlations were 0.35 for carotene and

0.34 for vitamin E. Others have generally observed similar correlations with intakes measured by reasonably complete food-frequency questionnaires.

The ability to demonstrate correlations with biochemical indicators is particularly valuable for nutrients, such as folic acid, for which concern has existed that lability in storage, processing, or preparation might make calculations of intake meaningless. Correlations with blood levels were reported to be 0.63 and 0.56 by Jacques et al. (1993), and Selhub et al. (1993), respectively. For example, as shown in Figure 6–3, folate intake both from foods alone and from food plus supplements was strongly predictive of plasma folate and also plasma homocysteine levels, which are elevated with lower folate intakes (see Chapter 17). Because uncertainty has existed about the ability to calculate intake of variables such as *trans* fatty acids, for which levels in foods are primarily the result of processing practices that change over time, documentation of correlations with objective indicators has also been important (correlations with adipose levels of *trans* fatty acids were reported to be 0.51 and 0.34 by London et al. [1991] and Hunter et al. [1992], respectively). Similar correlations for fatty acids that are not endogenously synthesized have been found in other studies comparing calculated intakes from questionnaires with adipose levels (see Table 6–13). The large study of blood fatty acid levels by Ma and coworkers (1995) included a subset of participants for whom repeated biochemical measurements were made at 2-week intervals. Because appreciable within-person variability existed, the correlation between intakes calculated from the food-frequency questionnaire and blood levels increased from 30% to 80% when corrected for this within-person variability in the biochemical measurement. Because other correlations shown in Table 6–13 have not been corrected in this manner, they are probably substantial underestimates for most nutrients.

Known biochemical responses to a di-

Table 6–13. Correlations between nutrient intakes from food-frequency questionnaires with biochemical indicators of diet[a]

Carotenoids (blood)	0.35[b], 0.25[c], (0.36, 0.42)[e], (0.43, 0.23)[g], 0.51[h], (0.34, 0.30)[i], 0.34[j], 0.51[m], 0.17[p], (alpha 0.26, beta 0.22)[q], (alpha 0.42, beta 0.15)[s], (0.37, −0.25)[t], 0.27[u], (−0.13, 0.18)[v], (0.12, 0.45)[w], (0.25, 0.53)[x], (0.34, 0.27)[y], (0.48, 0.27)[z], (alpha 0.29, beta 0.17, lycopene 0.09, lutein-zeaxanthin 0.03)[aa]
Tocopherols (blood)	0.34[b], (0.53, 0.51)[e], (0.43, 0.23)[g], (0.51, 0.41)[i], 0.19[p], 0.28[u], (0.29, 0.11)[v], (0.31, 0.44)[w], (0.11, 0.12)[x], (0.13, 0.18)[y], (0.19, 0.04)[z]
Ascorbic acid (blood)	0.63[b], 0.21[s], (0.50, 0.04)[t], 0.45[u], (−0.03, 0.65)[w], (0.47, 0.55)[x], 0.29[y], (0.32, 0.15)[z]
Folate (blood)	0.63[l], 0.56[m]
Vitamins B_6, B_{12} (blood)	0.37[d]
trans fatty acid (adipose)	0.51[h]
Marine N-3 fatty acids (blood or adipose)	0.50[f], 0.48[h], 0.49[j], EPA 0.53[n], (DHA 0.21, 0.47)[n], (chol. esters 0.58, phospholipids 0.55)[r]
Linoleic (blood or adipose)	0.35[h], 0.37[j], 0.28[k], 0.42[p], (chol. esters 0.32, phospholipids 0.26[r])
Linolenic acid (blood or adipose)	0.12[h], (chol. esters 0.30, phospholipids 0.26)[r]
Protein (urinary nitrogen)	(0.41,0.30)[t], 0.37[u], (0.40, 0.54)[v], (0.12,0.45)[w], (0.27, 0.07)[x], (0.19,0.31)[y], (0.24,0.36)[z]
Sodium, potassium, calcium, magnesium (urine)	(Sodium 0.66, 0.56)[o], (potassium 0.56, 0.39)[o], (calcium 0.05, 0.18)[o], (magnesium 0.08 / 0.33)[o]

[a] Where reported, correlations are given for both men and women.

[b] Willett et al., 1983 (59 men and women).

[c] Russell-Briefel et al., 1985 (187 men).

[d] Willett, 1985 (94 men and 25 women).

[e] Stryker et al., 1988 (137 men and 193 women).

[f] Silverman et al., 1990 (36 coronary artery disease patients).

[g] Coates et al., 1991 (50 smoking and 41 non-smoking women).

[h] London et al., 1991 (115 women).

[i] Ascherio et al., 1992 (121 men and 186 women).

[j] Hunter et al., 1992 (118 men).

[k] Feunekes et al., 1993 (191 men and women).

[l] Jacques et al., 1993 (57 men and 82 women).

[m] Selhub et al., 1993 (457 men and 703 women).

[n] Tjonneland et al., 1993 (23 men and 63 women).

[o] Joseph, 1994 (127 men and 193 women).

[p] Kardinaal et al., 1995 (82 men and women).

[q] Enger et al., 1995 (215 men and women).

[r] Ma et al., 1995 (2570 men and women).

[s] Bingham et al., 1997 (156 women).

[t] Katsouyanni et al., 1997 (42 men and 38 women).

[u] van Liere et al., 1997 (78–92 women).

[v] Ocke et al., 1997a (68 men and 61 women).

[w] EPIC group of Spain, 1997c (24 men and 29 women).

[x] Riboli et al., 1997 (44 men and 53 women, [13, 12 for protein]).

[y] Pisani et al., 1997 (56 men and 155 women, 12 women for ascorbic acid).

[z] Boeing et al., 1997 (49 men and 55 women).

[aa] Romieu et al., 1997 (110 women).

etary factor can also serve as useful markers in validation studies. For example, in many studies, it has been shown that increases in alcohol consumption produce an elevation in plasma high-density lipoprotein cholesterol (HDL-C) levels. Thus, the demonstration of a correlation between a questionnaire measure of alcohol intake and HDL-C provides qualitative evidence that alcohol intake is being measured with at least some degree of validity. Because other factors affect HDL-C levels, this cannot provide a highly quantitative measure of misclassification. This approach, however, can also be used to estimate the validity of one method relative to an other.

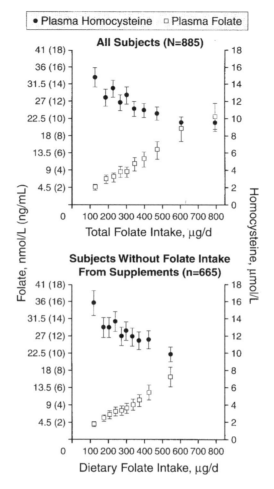

Figure 6–3. Mean plasma folate and homocysteine concentrations (error bars indicate 95% confidence intervals) by deciles of folate intake adjusted for age, sex, and energy intake. (From Tucker et al., 1996; reproduced with permission.)

For example, in the Nurses' Health Study validation substudy (Willett et al., 1987c), we found that the correlation between alcohol intake measured by food-frequency questionnaire and HDL-C was as strong or stronger than the correlation between alcohol intake measured by 28 days of diet record and HDL-C (Fig. 6–4).

Tightly regulated factors such as serum retinol and cholesterol are of limited use in cross-sectional validation analyses because individual metabolic differences may dominate between-person variation; however, studies of *changes* in blood levels within subjects may be more informative. In such studies of change, which are more analogous to controlled metabolic studies of dietary effects within subjects, the variability due to strong individual determinants of blood levels is removed, greatly enhancing the opportunity to see smaller effects of diet. Using this approach in a small dietary intervention study, Sacks and colleagues (1986) observed strong correlations between changes in saturated fat and linoleic acid intake measured by questionnaire before and during intervention and change in serum cholesterol. Similarly, Heller and coworkers (1981) found that change in saturated fat intake measured by a simple

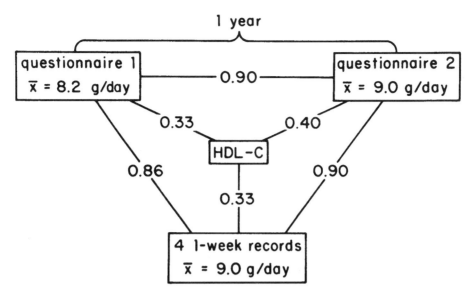

Figure 6–4. Validation of alcohol intake in the Nurses' Health Study. (From Willett et al., 1987a; reproduced with permission.)

eight-item questionnaire was associated with change in serum cholesterol over a period of 4 years among participants in an intervention program. In a variation on this approach, we examined the correlation between baseline total vitamin A intake and the change in serum retinol when all subjects were given a daily supplement of 10,000 IU of preformed vitamin A (Willett et al., 1984). The inverse correlation ($r = -0.50$) indicates the anticipated change: Subjects with low dietary vitamin A intake had the largest increase in serum retinol when given a fixed supplement.

The concept, displayed in Figure 6–5, of using the three-way comparisons between a dietary questionnaire (Q), a more detailed measure of dietary intake such as multiple dietary records (R), and a biochemical measure of intake (B) has been further developed by Kaaks (1997) to estimate the correlations between each method and true intake. This approach addresses the issue that the validity of a questionnaire assessed by the correlation between the questionnaire and records (^rQR) will be underestimated if the record measurement itself is less than perfect or if the

errors in replicate measures of the record used to de-attenuate the obtained correlation are correlated. The method is based on the reasonable assumption that errors in both the questionnaires and records are uncorrelated with errors in the biochemical measure, but also assumes that errors in the questionnaire and record method are uncorrelated, which may not always be true. In the example shown in Figure 6–5, the estimated correlation between the questionnaire and true intake (0.57) is substantially higher than the correlation between the questionnaire and diet record (0.42) or between the questionnaire and biochemical level (0.39). In another example (Ocke and Kaaks, 1997), the correlations for beta-carotene intake from questionnaires were 0.14 with biochemical level and 0.25 with the diet records, but the estimated correlation between the questionnaire and true intake was 0.44. Spiegelman et al. (1997) have further extended the triad approach to quantify any correlated error between the questionnaire and record methods and to estimate the correlation between questionnaire and true intake, allowing for this correlated error.

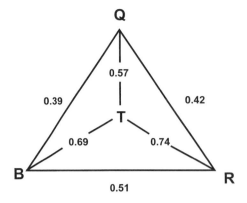

Figure 6–5. Observed correlation for Vitamin C between questionnaire intake (Q), diet record intake (R), and biochemically measured blood level (B). The "method of triads" is used to eliminate the correlation of each method with true intake (T). (Example, based on Ocke and Kaaks, 1997.)

Although the use of biochemical indicators for purposes of questionnaire validation has been limited, this area deserves further pursuit. As discussed in Chapter 5, it is possible that biochemical indicators may be used to identify maximally discriminating questions or to identify food items that fail to be predictive of biochemical levels despite an appreciable content of the nutrient in question. Such failure to predict nutrient levels could result from an unclearly stated questionnaire item, incorrect food composition data, or poor bioavailability of nutrient from that food. Resolution of such a finding could lead to improvement in the questionnaire or its food composition database.

Prediction of a Physiologic Response

The ability of a dietary questionnaire to predict an established relationship between a nutrient intake and a physiologic response may be used as qualitative evidence of validity in a manner analogous to using a biochemical indicator. Unfortunately, relatively few such relationships are well established. Because considerable evidence exists that high potassium intake may lower blood pressure, the demonstration of

an inverse association between potassium intake and incidence of diagnosed hypertension (relative risk = 1.54; 95% confidence interval [1.19–1.96] for less than 2.40 g/day compared with greater than 3.60 g/day [Ascherio et al., 1992a]) supports the validity of the questionnaire's capacity to measure potassium intake. Sandler and colleagues (1985) have demonstrated that bone density among adult women is positively related to the report of milk consumption many years earlier. This observation not only provides qualitative evidence that the questionnaire can measure milk intake but also is one of the few elements of data to suggest that recall of remote dietary intake is feasible.

Prediction of Known Disease Relationships

The use of a questionnaire to demonstrate established relationships between a dietary factor and disease can be interpreted as qualitative support for questionnaire validity. This approach is limited by the small number of relationships between diet and disease that are reasonably well established. For example, because considerable clinical evidence suggests that increased dietary fiber can ameliorate the symptoms of diverticular disease of the colon, the finding of an inverse association between dietary fiber intake and incidence of symptomatic diverticular disease of the colon (relative risk = 0.51, 95% confidence interval [0.37–0.71] for 32 g/day vs. 13 g per day [Aldoori et al., 1994]) supports the validity of the dietary fiber measurement. As data accumulate and the number of established associations increases, it may become more feasible to use the demonstration of such a relationship as a measure of validity; at this time this cannot be a primary approach. In a case–control study such associations could well be due to bias; thus it is probably best that such inferences regarding questionnaire validity be based on prospective studies. In a prospective study, however, failure to find an established association can be due to insufficient sample size or to an inappropriate interval of time between dietary assessment and the diagnosis of disease rather than to low validity of the questionnaire.

DESIGN OF QUESTIONNAIRE VALIDATION STUDIES

Results of studies of diet and disease are often difficult to interpret unless the method used to measure diet has been validated in a population reasonably similar to that being investigated. Without documentation of validity, null associations could simply be due to lack of variation in dietary exposure in the study population or to the inability of the dietary assessment method to detect existing differences in diet. The objectives of a validation study can include

1. Measurement of the true between-subject variation in the dietary factors of interest
2. Qualitative documentation that the dietary assessment method can detect the differences in diet that exist among subjects
3. Calibration of a dietary questionnaire against a true measure of absolute intake, which enhances the capacity to compare findings with other studies
4. Quantitative assessment of exposure measurement error so that measures of association, such as relative risks, can be corrected for measurement error

THE CHOICE OF A POPULATION FOR A VALIDATION STUDY

Ideally, the subjects in a validation study should be a random sample of the study population in which the questionnaire is being used. This is often not practically possible, particularly if the population is widely scattered, as face-to-face contact is usually necessary. For example, the Nurses' Health Study cohort is national, but logistical reasons necessitated a random sample of Boston-area participants for the validation study (Willett et al., 1985). Based on

questionnaires completed by all cohort members, women in the validation study were similar to the other cohort members with respect to intake of most nutrients (unpublished data); however, their use of vitamin supplements was markedly lower than that of women in other parts of the country. To maintain representativeness, maximal efforts to enhance participation are needed once potential validation study subjects are selected, particularly as the time and effort required on their part are substantial. Financial inducements to participation are discouraged by some investigators, but do not seem inappropriate if the time commitment is large and can be useful if they increase the participation rates.

The Choice of a Comparison Method for a Validation Study

As discussed earlier, diet records (particularly when foods are weighed) usually represent an optimal comparison method because sources of error are largely independent of error associated with a dietary questionnaire. Specifically, the diet record method does not depend on memory, is open ended, and allows direct measurement of portion sizes. When cooperation or literacy of study subjects is limited, multiple 24-hour recalls may be the best alternative. Although short-term dietary recalls are less demanding than diet recording and are also less likely to influence the actual diet of subjects, their sources of error tend to be more correlated with error in a dietary questionnaire. For some specific dietary factors (e.g., sodium, potassium, beta-carotene, or certain fatty acids), biochemical indicators, such as urinary excretion, blood levels, or adipose tissue concentrations, may be employed (see Chapter 9).

The Choice of an Appropriate Time Frame

Whatever comparison method(s) are selected, it is critical to consider the conceptually relevant time frame. Because "true" intake is usually the average intake over a long period of time (e.g., 1 or more years) rather than intake over a few days or weeks, it is important that the comparison method reflect this longer time frame. If medium-term variation is likely to exist, such as that due to seasonality, then it is desirable to have multiple measurements during the year, although a few assessments randomly scattered over the time period of interest could be used. Collection of comparison data over a 1-year period is generally appropriate so that seasonal effects and other poorly defined fluctuations in diet are incorporated. Because intake of almost all foods and nutrients varies greatly from day to day (see Chapter 3), collection of data from multiple days per subject is essential to measure the true between-subject variation in dietary factors and the ability of the questionnaire to discriminate among subjects (objectives 1 and 2). However, even a single day of diet record or recall data can be used for calibration or measurement error correction purposes (objectives 3 and 4, see below). Most biochemical markers are also influenced by short-term changes in dietary intake; thus it is also desirable to obtain replicate measures of biochemical markers, at least for a sample of participants.

The Sequence of Data Collection in a Validation Study

In designing a validation study, the sequence of measurements is of concern because it is possible that the process of collecting one measure may affect response to the other method. In particular, the intensive effort involved in daily recording of diet could conceivably sensitize subjects to their food intake and artificially improve their accuracy in completing a questionnaire administered afterward. On the other hand, administering the questionnaire before the detailed assessment of diet results in an artificially low correlation, as the questionnaire relates to diet before the period of detailed assessment. Because questionnaire administration is relatively inex-

pensive, the best solution seems to have subjects complete the questionnaire twice, before and after the period of detailed recording. This provides a conservative estimate of the true correlation between the questionnaire and detailed method (provided by the first questionnaire), as well as an optimistic estimate (provided by the repeat questionnaire). The association with the first questionnaire could also be interpreted as an approximation to the correlation with diet over a period of multiple years.

Because even 1 year may be a short period in relation to the etiologic effect of diet on cancer and heart disease, it may be useful to extend a validation study to a longer interval. Repeated administration of the questionnaire and collection of biochemical specimens after several years will provide useful data on the longer term stability of diet and biochemical indicators. An additional questionnaire focused on the period of detailed diet data collection several years earlier can provide information on the validity of the questionnaire to measure remote diet, which may be particularly relevant for case–control studies.

Number of Subjects and Replicate Measurements for a Validation or Calibration Study

Selecting an appropriate number of subjects for a validation study is less than straightforward as correlations for many nutrients are likely to be examined and the precision required (i.e., the confidence intervals around the coefficients) is somewhat arbitrary. Clearly, we always want to know much more than simply whether a correlation coefficient is different from zero.

A realistic degree of desirable precision might be arrived at by considering that correlations for validity generally tend to be in the range of 0.5 to 0.7. If the observed correlation were 0.6, it would be useful to be reasonably sure that it was actually at least 0.4, as levels of validity lower than this will rather seriously attenuate associations (see Chapter 12). The number of participants required to detect this difference in correlations can be calculated based on the standard one-sample formula for sample size $[n = (Z_\alpha + Z_\beta)^2 \sigma^2/d^2]$ using Fisher's Z transformation of correlation coefficients (Snedecor and Cochran, 1971), where $\sigma^2 = 1$ for the Z-scale. For $\alpha = 0.05$ and $1 - \beta = 0.80$, the number of subjects necessary would be approximately 110. Because one important use of a validation study is to correct observed relative risks for measurement error (see Chapter 12), another approach for choosing an appropriate sample size would be to consider the implications of various sample sizes on the corrected relative risk estimates and their corrected confidence intervals. Rosner and Willett (unpublished data) have examined the influence of validation study sample sizes on these parameters for different degrees of validity and different observed relative risks. In general, fewer subjects are needed for a validation study with higher degrees of validity. Although no sharp cut-off existed to define an optimal sample size, for realistic conditions (correlations between questionnaire and "truth" of 0.5 to 0.7) it was apparent that validation studies larger than 150 to 200 subjects provide little additional precision in corrected confidence intervals. On the other hand, validation studies with as few as 30 subjects lead to a major increase in the width of corrected confidence intervals. A reasonable size for a validation study thus seems to be about 100 to 200 persons. This is adequate for a range of likely degrees of validity and allows the appropriate deletion of some subjects (e.g., those who become seriously ill or pregnant) during the validation study.

The above considerations of sample size assume that a sufficient number of days of dietary information are obtained to reasonably describe an individual's true diet, typically 14 to 28 days, over the reference period. The possibility of using only a small number of replicate measures (e.g., two 24-hour recalls or two 24-hour urines) for the gold standard combined with a statistical adjustment to remove the effects of within-

person variation (Rosner and Willett, 1988) is discussed in Chapter 12. As shown in Chapter 12, similar corrected correlation coefficients were obtained between a food-frequency questionnaire and diet records when either 2 or 4 days of diet recording were used instead of 28 days per subject. In most circumstances, the greatest statistical efficiency (i.e., the lowest variance of the corrected coefficient for a fixed number of measurements) is obtained with only two, and at the most five, replicates per subject. Similar conclusions were reached by Stram and colleagues (1995) and Caroll and colleagues (1997). This approach can have major advantages in terms of cost and feasibility compared with the alternative of obtaining large numbers of replicate measurements per subject. The use of corrected correlation coefficients may also provide more valid conclusions in situations where the burden of obtaining large numbers of replicates would eliminate many subjects (and thus reduce the generalizability of the findings), alter the behavior of the participants (and thus the level of the factor being measured), or potentially affect response to another variable (such as a self-administered questionnaire). The strategy of using a small number of 24-hour recalls per subject (three) was used in a recent questionnaire validation study among adolescents (Rockett et al., 1996). This was done using telephone interviews for the 24-hour recalls with an interactive system for entry and analysis of the dietary data.* This combination provided a highly efficient and relatively low-cost validation process.

If a strategy using a small number of replicates per subject is employed, the number of subjects needs to be increased to maintain the same precision of the corrected correlation coefficient (assessed by standard error or 95% confidence interval). There is not a simple factor by which the

---

*Minnesota Nutrition Data System (NDS), version 2.3, developed by the University of Minnesota Nutrition Coordinating Center.

number of subjects should be increased, because this depends on the intraclass correlation between replicate measures of dietary intake and the underlying true correct correlation as well as the number of replicates per subject. As shown in Figure 6–6, the number of subjects needed to maintain a constant standard error for the corrected correlation is particularly sensitive to the intraclass correlation $(r_I = s_b^2/(s_b^2 + s_w^2)$ or $1/(\lambda + 1)$, where $\lambda = s_w^2/s_b^2)$, which varies greatly among nutrients. As can be seen from Table 3–4, r_I can realistically be as low as 0.2 for some nutrients such as cholesterol or even total fat when expressed as a percentage of total energy. Thus, if a validation study is designed to use 3 days of dietary intake per subject, three times as many persons should ideally be enrolled compared with a study with a large number of replicates per person. This number might be relaxed to about double if somewhat less precision for the more variable nutrients is acceptable. The number rises sharply for nutrients with a low intraclass correlation if only two replicates are used. Overall, it appears that studies using 3 days of dietary information per subject and including 200 to 300 subjects can provide highly informative information on questionnaire validity. As noted by Stram et al. (1995), these days should be randomly dispersed over the time period of interest to include short-and long-term sources of variation, and separate samplings of week versus weekend days is not needed.

An even more extreme approach is to use a single day of dietary information as the gold standard. Such a study design can be used for purposes of calibration and for correction of measurement error, but cannot accomplish the first two aims: the assessment of true between-subject variability or ability of the questionnaire to detect differences among subjects. The simple principle of a calibration study is depicted in Figure 6–7. The conceptual issue is to determine the true intake that corresponds to responses to the questionnaire being evaluated. Counter-intuitively, we do not need a measure of true intake for an individual to accomplish this; the true average for a group of individuals with the same questionnaire response is sufficient (statistically speaking, only an unbiased estimate of true intake). Of course, the precision of the estimate of true intake for a given questionnaire response will be greater if a larger number of days of dietary intake are collected for each person, but the same degree of precision can also be accomplished by increasing the number of subjects with only a single day. As can be appreciated, this is a simple regression analysis problem; the generic principle is that the slope of the regression line is not affected by random error in the dependent (y) variable, but the standard error of the slope is influenced by such random error. This approach to calibration is being employed in the EPIC study, a large multinational cohort study in Europe (Kaaks et al., 1994). Because questionnaires cannot be standard across populations that differ in language and culture, the questionnaire used in each country will be calibrated using an open-ended method (a single 24-hour recall) completed by all participants. This will provide both calibration to a common measure of intake and the data needed to adjust measures of association for error in the food frequency questionnaires (see Chapter 12).

Low-Cost Biochemical Calibration Studies

In some situations, the substantial cost of a validation study is difficult to justify and may preclude the type of questionnaire evaluation described above. For example, if a questionnaire has already been subjected to detailed evaluation, but is to be applied in a new and somewhat different population, a full evaluation may not be warranted. Alternatively, in developing a research proposal, evidence may be needed that a questionnaire can function reasonably, but funds are not available to conduct a full evaluation. In these situations, a low-cost evaluation using biochemical indicators of diet and the calibration principle may be useful. Such an approach would

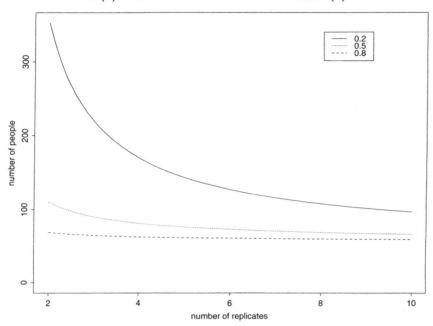

Var(rt) = 0.01 and the corrected correlation (rt) is 0.5

Figure 6–6. Number of subjects needed to maintain a constant precision for the corrected correlation coefficient between a food-frequency questionnaire and intake from the average of multiple replicates of daily intake. Curves are provided for three values of the intraclass correlation (r_I) between repeated replicates, assuming a true correlation of 0.5 with variance = 0.14. (Derivation and figure are courtesy of Bernard Rosner.)

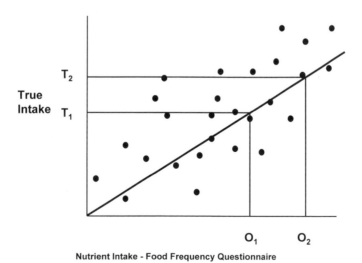

Nutrient Intake - Food Frequency Questionnaire

Figure 6–7. Calibration of food-frequency intake against a measure of true intake. Thus, for observed intakes O_1 and O_2, the true intakes T_1 and T_2 can be estimated.

avoid the expensive repeated contacts necessary for collection of dietary data and the laborsome processing of dietary information. This may be an increasingly useful approach as the basic value of food frequency questionnaires has already been established, and the central question becomes whether the findings of previous validation studies can be extended to other settings.

A central concept of this approach is to select several biochemical measurements that will be sensitive to different aspects of diet; these can act as indicators of questionnaire validity even though they may not include nearly all the aspects of diet that will be assessed. Options are discussed in more detail in Chapter 9, but might include blood levels of specific carotenoids, specific fatty acids in adipose or blood lipid fractions, folic acid, and vitamin D. If there are biochemical indicators related to the hypotheses to be examined, these should certainly be included. The basic design of the study is cross sectional; blood can be collected simultaneously with completion of a single questionnaire. If feasible, collection of blood a few weeks or months before questionnaire completion would in principle be even better as this would avoid artifactual correlation due to proximity in time, although in principle this should be minimal with a questionnaire focused on the past year. A large part of the cost is potentially the biochemical analysis of specimens; if several nutrients are to be analyzed, this can easily cost hundreds of dollars per subject. However, pooling of blood aliquots for individuals with similar nutrient intakes according to the questionnaires *before* biochemical analysis can dramatically reduce the cost. The approach is based on the concept of "actual value for surrogate category," described below. For example, subjects can be grouped into deciles of beta-carotene intake, and aliquots for all persons in each decile are then pooled together and mixed carefully. A single analysis can then be made for each decile pool, dramatically reducing the cost. Obviously, a different set of pooled ali-

quots are needed for each dietary factor as the subjects will not be the same. The values of blood levels across deciles of intake will be informative directly as this will indicate the contrasts that can be presented by the dietary intake data. For example, the demonstration of a twofold difference in blood levels of omega-3 fatty acids from lowest to highest quintiles of intake assessed by questionnaire provided important evidence that informative differences in fish consumption were being measured in one study (Ascherio et al., 1995) (in this study, an analysis of pooled specimens was not used, but the principle applies). Also, a regression line can be fit through the decile values, assigning the median values for intake to each decile; this can be compared with slopes in other populations where this or a similar questionnaire has been used.

The number of subjects to be included in such calibrations depends on an number of factors, including the between- and within-person variations in the biochemical factor, the precision of the laboratory measurement, and the size of contrast across categories that is of interest. Replicate measures for each decile (in a scrambled order with the laboratory blinded to the group) will provide an important estimate of the laboratory precision), and using the average will reduce this source of error. In general, the size of the calibration study should be at least as large as for a full validation study and preferably somewhat larger as a smaller number of laboratory measurements means that this source of error will contribute more importantly to the overall variation.

By using this approach, important information on questionnaire performance can be obtained rapidly and at low cost. Also, the burden on participants is minimal, and thus participation rates are likely to be high. Inevitably, some information is lost, such as the ability to assess the between-person variation and the degree of misclassification, and only a limited number of nutrients can be assessed. However, such information may be sufficient in some situations and will clearly be better than no information on questionnaire performance. This basic approach can also be used to evaluate the capability of a previously validated questionnaire to assess intake of a new dietary factor.

DATA ANALYSIS AND PRESENTATION OF VALIDATION/ CALIBRATION STUDIES

Data obtained in a dietary validation/calibration study are voluminous as they represent multiple measurements of multiple dietary factors using multiple methods. Reducing this information so as to be useful to the investigator interpreting findings from the main epidemiologic study and to be consumable by readers of the literature presents a formidable challenge.

In analyzing data from a validation study, crude nutrient intakes are of interest, but it is also important to adjust nutrient intakes and biochemical factors for variables that are ultimately controlled in an epidemiologic analysis. For example, age and sex are almost always controlled in epidemiologic analyses, so they should also be controlled in the analysis of the validation study. The reason is that the between-person variation in dietary intake due to these covariates tends to increase observed correlations between methods (as by definition $r = s_b^2/(s_b^2 + s_w^2)$. Because this added between-person variation is removed in the epidemiologic analysis adjusting for such covariates, the artifactually increased correlation coefficients are unrealistic. In other words, for typical epidemiologic purposes it is not useful to know that a questionnaire can detect differences in nutrient intake between young men (which will tend to be high) and older women (which will tend to be low) that are simply due to their age and gender. The effect of controlling for age and sex on correlations between a questionnaire and a 1-year diet record are shown in Table 6–14; correlations decreased appreciably after such adjustment. The rationale for adjusting for total energy

intake in epidemiologic analyses is provided in Chapter 11; because it is usually important to adjust for total energy intake in case–control or cohort studies, it is important to adjust for energy intake in validation studies as well.

Many alternatives exist for presenting data on the associations between the questionnaire and comparison methods. Although it is useful to compare means and standard deviations for the two methods, it is most important to provide data on the associations between intakes measured by the two methods. Alternatives include contingency tables (cross classification), correlation coefficients, and regression coefficients. Although contingency tables provide a readily interpretable impression of the agreement between two measures (see Table 6–15 for an example using cholesterol intake), they become cumbersome when many nutrients are being studied. When the relationship between two normally distributed variables is linear (usually reasonably true in the case of validation studies), the correlation coefficient provides, in a single number, essentially the same information as that contained in a contingency table (Walker and Blettner, 1985), thus making this an attractive alternative. Because dietary variables are usually skewed toward higher values, transformations (such as log) to increase normality should be considered before computing correlation coefficients. This has the advantage of reducing the influence of extreme values and of creating a correlation coefficient that can be interpreted in the form of a contingency table. Alternatively, nonparametric correlation coefficients (e.g., Spearman) can be employed when one or both variables are not normally distributed.

A possible disadvantage of the correlation coefficient is that it is a function of true between-person variation in the population being studied as well as of the accuracy of the questionnaire. This limits the generalizability of the correlation coefficient to those populations with similar between-person variation as the test pop-

Table 6–14. Pearson correlation coefficients comparing nutrient intakes from the semiquantitative food-frequency questionnaire with a 1-year diet record[a]

Nutrient	Crude	Calorie-adjusted	Age-, sex-adjusted	Age-, sex-, calorie-adjusted
Total calories	0.67	—	0.37	—
Protein	0.60	0.43	0.46	0.53
Total fat	0.76	0.51	0.57	0.59
Saturated fat	0.74	0.60	0.58	0.62
Linoleic acid	0.74	0.21	0.50	0.28
Total carbohydrate	0.60	0.51	0.37	0.55
Crude fiber	0.44	0.61	0.37	0.65
Cholesterol	0.67	0.38	0.59	0.43
Oleic acid	0.74	0.51	0.55	0.57
Vitamin A	0.63	0.68	0.62	0.70
Niacin	0.48	0.36	0.41	0.37
Vitamin C	0.38	0.46	0.34	0.49
Calcium	0.63	0.55	0.42	0.57
Phosphorus	0.64	0.65	0.52	0.67
Thiamin	0.55	0.41	0.36	0.42
Riboflavin	0.64	0.42	0.55	0.31
Potassium	0.48	0.59	0.33	0.64
Iron	0.47	0.38	0.28	0.40

[a] All variables were transformed by $\log_e$ to improve normality. No supplements are included. Data were provided by 27 men and women aged 20 to 54.

From Willett et al., 1987a.

ulation. Although this dependence on between-person variation has some disadvantages, this can also be viewed as an advantage because the capacity of a questionnaire to discriminate between subjects, and thus the power of a study, is a function of both its accuracy and the be-tween-person variation in exposure within the population.

The relationship between two measures can also be described as a simple regression equation, that is, using the questionnaire (x) to predict true intake (y) (Fig. 6–7). This has direct application in correcting

Table 6–15. Joint classification of calorie-adjusted cholesterol intake assessed by the second semiquantitative food-frequency questionnaire and four 1-week diet records[a]

Questionnaire quintile	Diet record quintile					Total
	1 (low)	2	3	4	5 (high)	
1 (low)	18	9	2	3	2	34
2	8	11	8	4	4	35
3	4	7	9	9	5	34
4	2	8	9	11	6	36
5 (high)	2	0	7	8	17	34
Total	34	35	35	35	34	173

[a] Data based on information provided by 173 registered nurses aged 34–39 years and residing in the Boston area, 1980–1981.

From Willett et al., 1985.

relative risk estimates for measurement error, as described in Chapter 12. Lee and colleagues (1983) have advocated the use of regression coefficients for analyzing data from validation studies and state that "two dietary-intake assessments are interchangeable in comparison studies only if they show a linear regression coefficient that is not statistically different from 1.0." It seems, however, unrealistic to expect that any practical method for assessing diet in an epidemiologic study would be so accurate as to be directly interchangeable with a detailed, open-ended method such as multiple weeks of diet recording. It is also interesting to note that a regression coefficient of 1.0 does imply interchange ability because the method used for true intake (y) only requires an unbiased estimate of true intake, such as a single day of diet record data. Thus, the questionnaire could actually be superior to the method used to estimate truth when the coefficient was 1.0. Moreover, Wahrendorf (1985) has pointed out that the use of a statistical test is not appropriate for the evaluation of validity; the most certain way to ensure that a regression coefficient is not significantly different from 1.0 would be to conduct a very small validation study.

Because the standard deviations are often different for dietary intake assessed by two methods (i.e., their scales may be different even if they nominally use the same units of measurement), it is usually difficult to assess the capacity of a questionnaire to provide a ranking or relative categorization of subjects on the basis of a regression coefficient. For example, it is possible that a questionnaire provides a perfect ranking of subjects but has either an artifactually large standard deviation (resulting in a regression coefficient less than 1.0) or an artifactually small standard deviation (resulting in a regression coefficient greater than 1.0).

The kappa statistic ($P_o - P_e)/(1 - P_e)$; (where P_o is the proportion of subjects observed to be concordant and P_e is the proportion of subjects expected to be concordant on the basis of chance alone) has been increasingly used to compare categories of nutrient intakes measured by two methods. This statistic is an improvement over "percent agreement," as agreement expected on the basis of chance alone is discounted. As pointed out by Maclure and Willett (1987), however, the value of kappa is not readily interpretable, as it will depend on the number of categories into which a continuous variable has been broken. Thus, its use for comparing ordinal variables, such as nutrient intakes, has considerable disadvantages and should be discouraged.

Bland and Altman (1986) have strongly condemned the use of correlation coefficients for comparing two measures and advocated using the mean and standard deviation of the difference between the two. The standard deviation of the difference is not influenced by the between-person variation in exposure; whether this is an advantage or disadvantage is discussed earlier in this chapter. Interpreting this parameter requires considerable knowledge about the usual absolute values and between-person variation, which differ from nutrient to nutrient. Therefore, the mean and standard deviation of the difference between two methods tend to be cumbersome when evaluating many nutrients and interpretable only to the very well informed. A related method is to calculate the standard deviation of the residual from the regression of the true measure on the questionnaire measure, sometimes called the *standard error of the estimate*. This residual represents the variation in true intake that is not accounted for by the surrogate measure.

Another presentation of data from a validation study might be called *actual values for surrogate categories*. In this approach, subjects are first grouped into categories such as quintiles on the basis of the surrogate method, in this case the food-frequency questionnaire. Then, the "true value" for the same subjects based on the more detailed method is assigned to the categories defined by the surrogate method. Such an approach is analogous to the simple regression used for calibration, but is based on categories rather than on a continuous variable. An example of this approach, again based on the validation of the 1980 compressed Nurses' Health Study questionnaire, is shown in Table 6–16. The distinct advantage of this method is that it conveys the actual, quantitative differences in diet that correspond to the relative categories defined by the questionnaire. These values are, of course, a function of both the true variation in diet within the population and the measurement error associated with the questionnaire. In Table 6–16, it can be seen that the variation between subjects in total fat intake as measured by the questionnaire is relatively low and that this variation is further reduced by adjustment for calories, even though adjustment for calories increased the correlation coefficient by reducing correlated error. In contrast, the differences between quintiles were much greater for vitamin A in spite of a lower correlation between methods (see Table 6–7) due to the larger true between-person variation in vitamin A intake. These values, of course, need to be established separately for every study population.

These true values for categories of intake assessed by the questionnaire may be useful in presenting epidemiologic data relating to disease risk as they provide simple and direct presentation of the quantitative relationship between level of a dietary factor and risk of disease. In particular, null findings are more interpretable as it can be readily determined whether the variation in diet and validity of the questionnaire were adequate to evaluate the relationship being considered.

This method of data presentation has another practical advantage in that, like regression analysis, it does not require a large number of days of dietary intake per subject to represent "truth." Because the method merely involves computing means for groups defined by the questionnaire, even a single day of diet recording per subject provides unbiased estimates of the actual values for these categories. This

method may, of course, be extended to analyses based on specific foods.

Because no single method for relating a surrogate measure to a measure of truth conveys all the available information, it is probably best to present the data in several ways. At a minimum, the means and standard deviations of the true and surrogate measures plus their correlations should be provided. This may be supplemented with other data, such as contingency tables and regression coefficients with standard errors (which may be particularly useful for correcting relative risk estimates).

Additional Uses of Validation Studies

In addition to evaluating the overall validity of a food-frequency questionnaire, the validation study can be used to assess the function of specific aspects of the questionnaire; this can provide guidance for using the questionnaire or lead to improvements in the method. The analysis of individual food items described above is one example of this function. As another example, we were able to learn that an ancillary question about the consumption of fat on meat (What do you do with the visible fat on your meat? Eat most of it? Eat some of it? Eat as little as possible?) added to the validity of animal fat intake as measured by diet records (Willett et al., 1988). On the other hand, in a group of Swedish women, additional questions about the use of fat in food preparation did not increase correlation coefficients (Wolk et al., 1997).

We also used a validation study to determine whether a higher number of blank food items was associated with a reduction in questionnaire validity (Rimm et al., 1992). No association was found between number of blank items, up to 70, and the degree of error (assessed as the absolute value of the difference between the questionnaire and the diet record for each person); this information was used to determine exclusion rules for participants in the main cohort study. Similarly, the validation study may be used to identify subgroups among whom the questionnaire performs

Table 6–16. Use of actual values for surrogate categories to compare the 1980 Nurses' Health Study dietary questionnaire with 28 days of diet recording by 173 women

Questionnaire quintile	Mean daily diet record value for women in questionnaire quintile					
	Total fat (g)	Saturated fat (g)	Cholesterol (mg)	Sucrose (g)	Vitamin A[a] (IU)	Vitamin C[a] (mg)
			Crude intake			
1	58	20	252	30	4,684	69
2	64	24	275	35	5,083	117
3	68	23	292	45	6,370	151
4	67	26	320	47	7,356	218
5	79	28	380	60	8,826	436
			Calorie-adjusted			
1	61	21	248	32	4,259	67
2	64	22	281	39	4,761	112
3	67	25	304	42	5,795	124
4	70	26	313	50	7,099	163
5	71	27	374	51	7,593	289

[a] Includes supplements.
From Willett et al., 1985.

poorly and, hence, might be excluded from analyses in the main study.

SUMMARY

The interpretation of any study of diet and disease can be substantially enhanced by quantitative information on the validity of the method used to measure dietary intake. Unless the method employed has been previously studied with respect to validity in a similar population, any major dietary study should include a validation component. Because the degree to which data from one validation study can be generalized to other populations is largely unknown at this time, prudence dictates repeating a validation study if the similarity of populations or circumstances is in doubt.

In general, diet records provide the best available comparison method; biochemical markers are potentially useful but do not exist for many dietary factors. Although multiple weeks of diet recording per subject provide the ideal standard, this process is costly. The use of a small number of replicate measures per subject with statistical correction for within-person variation pro-

vides an alternative approach that should make a validation study feasible in most epidemiologic settings.

REFERENCES

Abramson, J. H., C. Slome, and C. Kosovsky (1963). Food frequency interview as an epidemiological tool. *Am J Public Health 53*, 1093–1101.

Acheson, E. D., and R. Doll (1964). Dietary factors in carcinoma of the stomach: A study of 100 cases and 200 controls. *Gut 5*, 126–131.

Ajani, U. A., W. C. Willett, and J. M. Seddon (1994). Reproducibility of a food frequency questionnaire for use in ocular research. Eye Disease Case–Control Study Group. *Invest Ophthalmol Vis Sci 35*, 2725–2733.

Aldoori, W. H., E. L. Giovannucci, E. B. Rimm, A. L. Wing, D. V. Trichopoulos, and W. C. Willett (1994). A prospective study of diet and the risk of symptomatic diverticular disease in men. *Am J Clin Nutr 60*, 757–764.

Ascherio, A., E. B. Rimm, E. L. Giovannucci, G. A. Colditz, B. Rosner, W. C. Willett, F. Sacks, and M. J. Stampfer (1992a). A prospective study of nutritional factors and hypertension among US men. *Circulation 86*, 1475–1484.

Ascherio, A., E. B. Rimm, M. J. Stampfer, E. Giovannucci, and W. C. Willett (1995). Dietary intake of marine *n*-3 fatty acids, fish intake and the risk of coronary disease among men. *N Engl J Med 332*, 977–982.

Ascherio, A., M. J. Stampfer, G. A. Colditz, E. B. Rimm, L. Litin, and W. C. Willett (1992b). Correlations of vitamin A and E intakes with the plasma concentrations of carotenoids and tocopherols among American men and women. *J Nutr 122*, 1792–1801.

Balogh, M., J. H. Medalie, H. Smith, and J. J. Groen (1968). The development of a dietary questionnaire for an ischemic heart disease survey. *Isr J Med Sci 4*, 195–203.

Baranowski, T., R. Dworkin, J. C. Henske, D. R. Clearman, J. K. Dunn, P. R. Nader, and P. C. Hooks (1986). The accuracy of children's self-reports of diet: Family Health Project. *J Am Diet Assoc 86*, 1381–1385.

Beaton, G. H., J. Milner, V. McGuire, T. E. Feather, and J. A. Little (1983). Source of variance in 24-hour dietary recall data: Implicatons for nutrition study design and interpretation. Carbohydrate sources, vitamins, and minerals. *Am J Clin Nutr 37*, 986–995.

Bingham, S. A., C. Gill, A. Welch, A. Cassidy, S. A. Runswick, S. Oakes, R. Lubin, D. I. Thurnham, T. J. A. Key, L. Roe, K. T. Khaw, and N. E. Day (1997). Validation of dietary assessment methods in the UK arm of EPIC using weighed records, and 24-hour urinary nitrogen and potassium and serum vitamin C and carotenoids as biomarkers. *Int J Epidemiol 26(suppl)*, S137–S151.

Bingham, S. A., C. Gill, A. Welch, K. Day, A. Cassidy, K. T. Khaw, M. J. Sneyd, T. J. A. Key, L. Roe, and N. E. Day (1994). Comparison of dietary assessment methods in nutritional epidemiology: Weighed records v. 24 h recalls, food-frequency questionnaires and estimated-diet records. *Br J Nutr 72*, 619–643.

Bland, J. M., and D. G. Altman (1986). Statistical methods for assessing agreement between two methods of clinical measurement. *Lancet 1*, 307–310.

Block, G., A. M. Hartman, and D. Naughton (1990a). A reduced dietary questionnaire: Development and validation. *Epidemiology 1*, 58–64.

Block, G., F. E. Thompson, A. M. Hartman, F. A. Larkin, and K. E. Guire (1992). Comparison of two dietary questionnaires validated against multiple dietary records collected during a 1-year period. *J Am Diet Assoc 92*, 686–693.

Block, G., M. Woods, A. Potosky, and C. Clifford (1990b). Validation of a self-administered diet history questionnaire using multiple diet records. *J Clin Epidemiol 43*, 1327–1335.

Boeing, H., S. Bohlscheid-Thomas, S. Voss, S. Schneeweiss, and J. Wahrendorf (1997). The relative validity of vitamin intakes derived from a food frequency questionnaire compared to 24-hour recalls, and biological measurements: results from the EPIC pilot study in Germany. European Prospective Investigation into Cancer and Nutrition. *Int J Epidemiol 26(suppl)*, S82–S90.

Bohlscheid-Thomas, S., I. Hoting, H. Boeing, and J. Wahrendorf (1997a). Reproducibility and relative validity of food group intake in a food frequency questionnaire developed for the German part of the EPIC project. European Prospective Investigation into Cancer and Nutrition. *Int J Epidemiol 26(suppl)*, S59–S70.

Bohlscheid-Thomas, S., I. Hoting, H. Boeing, and J. Wahrendorf (1997b). Reproducibilty and relative validity of energy and macronutrient intake of a food frequency questionnaire developed for the German part of the EPIC project. European Prospective Investigation into Cancer and Nutrition. *Int J Epidemiol 26(suppl)*, S71–S81.

Bradburn, N. M., L. J. Rips, and S. K. Shevell (1987). Answering autobiographical questions: The impact of memory and inference on surveys. *Science 236*, 157–161.

Briefel, R. R., M. A. McDowell, K. Alaimo, C. R. Caughman, A. L. Bischof, M. D. Carroll, and C. L. Johnson (1995). Total energy intake of the US population: The third National Health and Nutrition Examination Survey, 1988–1991. *Am J Clin Nutr 62 (suppl)*, 1072S–1080S.

Browe, J. H., R. M. Gofstein, D. M. Morlley, and M. C. McCarthy (1966). Diet and heart disease study in the Cardiovascular Health Center. *J Am Diet Assoc 48*, 95–100.

Byers, T., J. Marshall, E. Anthony, R. Fiedler, and M. Zielezny (1987). The reliability of dietary history from the distant past. *Am J Epidemiol 125*, 999–1011.

Byers, T. E., R. I. Rosenthal, J. R. Marshall T. F. Rzepka, K. M. Cummings, and S. Graham (1983). Dietary history from the distant past: A methodological study. *Nutr Cancer 5*, 69–77.

Callmer, E., E. Riboli, R. Saracci, B. Akesson,

and F. Lindgarde (1993). Dietary assessment methods evaluated in the Malmo food study. *J Intern Med 233*, 53–57.

Carroll, R. J., D. Pee, L. S. Freedman, and C. C. Brown (1997). Statistical design of calibration studies. *Am J Clin Nutr 65 (suppl)*, 1187S–1189S.

Centers for Disease Control and Prevention, National Center for Health Statistics (1994). Daily dietary fat and total food-energy intakes—Third National Health and Nutrition Examination Survey, Phase 1, 1988–91. *MMWR 43(7)*, 116–117.

Chasan-Taber, S., E. B. Rimm, M. J. Stampfer, D. Spiegelman, G. A. Colditz, E. Giovannucci, A. Ascherio, and W. C. Willett (1996). Reproducibility and validity of a self-administered physical activity questionnaire for male health professionals. *Epidemiology 7*, 81–86.

Coates, R. J., J. W. Eley, and G. Block, et al. (1991). An evaluation of a food frequency questionnaire for assessing dietary intake of specific carotenoids and vitamin E among low-income black women. *Am J Epidemiol 134*, 658–671.

Colditz, G. A., W. C. Willett, M. J. Stampfer, L. Sampson, B. Rosner, C. H. Hennekens, and F. E. Speizer (1987). The influence of age, relative weight, smoking, and alcohol intake on the reproducibility of a dietary questionnaire. *Int J Epidemiol 16*, 392–398.

Decker, M. D., A. L. Booth, M. J. Dewey, R. S. Fricker, R. H. Hutcheson Jr, and W. Schaffner (1986). Validity of food consumption histories in a foodborne outbreak investigation. *Am J Epidemiol 124*, 859–863.

Domel, S. B., T. Baranowski, S. B. Leonard, H. Davis, P. Riley, and J. Baranowski (1994). Accuracy of fourth and fifth-grade students' food records compared with school-lunch observations. *Am J Clin Nutr 59*, 218s–220s.

Elmstahl, S., B. Gullberg, E. Riboli, R. Saracci, and F. Lindgarde (1996). The Malmo Food Study: The reproducibility of a novel diet history method and an extensive food frequency questionnaire. *Eur J Clin Nutr 50*, 134–142.

Enger, S. M., M. P. Longnecker, J. M. Shikany, M. E. Swenseid, M. J. Chen, J. M. Harper, and R. W. Haile (1995). Questionnaire assessment of intake of specific carotenoids. *Cancer Epidemiol Biomarkers Prev 4*, 201–205.

Engle, A., L. L. Lynn, K. Koury, and A. P. Boyar (1990). Reproducibility and comparability of a computerized, self-administered food frequency questionnaire. *Nutr Cancer 13*, 281–292.

EPIC Group of Spain (1997a). Relative validity and reproducibility of a diet history questionnaire in Spain. I. Foods. *Int J Epidemiol 26(suppl)*, S91–S99.

EPIC Group of Spain (1997b). Relative validity and reproducibility of a diet history questionnaire in Spain. II. Nutrients. *Int J Epidemiol 26(suppl)*, S100–109.

EPIC Group of Spain (1997c). Relative validity and reproducibility of a diet history questionnaire in Spain. III. Biochemical markers. *Int J Epidemiol 26(suppl)*, S110–S117.

Epstein, L. M., A. Reshef, J. H. Abramson, and O. Bialik (1970). Validity of a short dietary questionnaire. *Isr J Med Sci 6*, 589–597.

Feskanich, D., J. Marshall, E. B. Rimm, L. B. Litin, and W. C. Willett (1994). Simulated validation of a brief food frequency questionnaire. *Ann Epidemiol 4*, 181–187.

Feskanich, D., E. B. Rimm, E. L. Giovannucci, G. A. Colditz, M. J. Stampfer, L. B. Litin, and W. C. Willett (1993). Reproducibility and validity of food intake measurements from a semiquantitative food frequency questionnaire. *J Am Diet Assoc 93*, 790–796.

Feunekes, G. I., W. A. van Staveren, J. H. De Vries, J. Burema, and J. G. Hautvast (1993). Relative and biomarker-based validity of a food-frequency questionnaire estimating intake of fats and cholesterol. *Am J Clin Nutr 58*, 489–496.

Flegal, K. M., and F. A. Larkin (1990). Partitioning macronutrient intake estimates from a food frequency questionnaire. *Am J Epidemiol 131*, 1046–1058.

Goldbohm, R. A., P. A. van den Brandt, H. A. M. Brants, P. van't Veer, M. Al, F. Sturmans, and R. J. J. Hermus (1994). Validation of a dietary questionnaire used in a large-scale prospective cohort study on diet and cancer. *Eur J Clin Nutr 48*, 253–265.

Goldbohm, R. A., P. van't Veer, P. A. van den Brandt, M. A. van't Hof, H. A. M. Brants, F. Sturmans, and R. J. J. Hermus (1995). Reproducibility of a food frequency questionnaire and stability of dietary habits determined from five annually repeated measurements. *Eur J Clin Nutr 49*, 420–429.

Graham, S., A. M. Lilienfeld, and J. E. Tidings (1967). Dietary and purgation factors in the epidemiology of gastric cancer. *Cancer 20*, 2224–2234.

Gray, G. E., A. Paganini-Hill, R. K. Ross, and B. E. Henderson (1984). Assessment of three brief methods of estimation of vitamin A and C intakes for a prospective study of cancer: Comparison with dietary history. *Am J Epidemiol 119*, 581–590.

Hankin, J. H., A. M. Nomura, J. Lee, T. Hirohata, and L. N. Kolonel (1983). Reproducibility of a dietary history questionnaire in a case-control study of breast cancer. *Am J Clin Nutr 37*, 981–985.

Hankin, J. H., G. G. Rhoads, and G. A. Glober (1975). A dietary method for an epidemiologic study of gastrointestinal cancer. *Am J Clin Nutr 28*, 1055–1060.

Heller, R. F., H. D. Pedoe, and G. Rose (1981). A simple method of assessing the effect of dietary advice to reduce plasma cholesterol. *Prev Med 10*, 364–370.

Horwath, C. C. (1993). Validity of a short food frequency questionnaire for estimating nutrient intake in elderly people. *Br J Nutr 70*, 3–14.

Horwath, C. C., and A. Worsley (1990). Assessment of the validity of a food frequency questionnaire as a measure of food use by comparison with direct observation of domestic food stores. *Am J Epidemiol 131*, 1059–1067.

Hunt, I. F., L. S. Luke, N. J. Murphy, V. A. Clark, and A. H. Coulson (1979). Nutrient estimates from computerized questionnaires vs. 24-hr recall interviews. *J Am Diet Assoc 74*, 656–659.

Hunter, D. J., E. B. Rimm, F. M. Sacks, M. J. Stampfer, G. A. Colditz, L. B. Litin, and W. C. Willett (1992). Comparison of measures of fatty acid intake by subcutaneous fat aspirate, food frequency questionnaire, and diet records in a free-living population of US men. *Am J Epidemiol 135*, 418–427.

Jacques, P. F., S. I. Sulsky, J. A. Sadowski, J. C. Phillips, D. Rush, and W. C. Willett (1993). Comparison of micronutrient intake measured by a dietary questionnaire and biochemical indicators of micronutrient status. *Am J Clin Nutr 57*, 182–189.

Jain, M. G., L. Harrison, G. R. Howe, and A. B. Miller (1982). Evaluation of a self-administered questionnaire for use in a cohort study. *Am J Clin Nutr 36*, 931–935.

Jain, M., G. R. Howe, and T. Rohan (1996). Dietary assessment in epidemiology: Comparison of a food frequency and a diet history questionnaire with a 7-day food record. *Am J Epidemiol 143*, 953–960.

Jensen, O. M., J. Wahrendorf, A. Rosenqvist, and A. Geser (1984). The reliability of questionnaire-derived historical dietary information and temporal stability of food habits in individuals. *Am J Epidemiol 120*, 281–290.

Johansson, I., and G. Hallmans (1995). *Impact of Photo Portion Illustrations on Relative Validity of a Food Frequency Questionnaire.* University of Umea, Sweden. Submitted.

Joseph, H. M. (1994). *Assessment of dietary intakes for sodium, potassium, calcium, and magnesium, and factors influencing salt intake.* Thesis. School of Nutrition, Tufts University.

Kaaks, R. (1997). Biochemical markers as an additional measurement in studies of the accuracy of dietary measurements: Conceptual issues. *Am J Clin Nutr 65 (suppl)*, 1232s–1239s.

Kaaks, R., M. Plummer, E. Riboli, J. Esteve, and W. van Staveren (1994). Adjustment for bias due to errors in exposure assessments in multicenter cohort studies on diet and cancer: A calibration approach. *Am J Clin Nutr 59*, 245S–250S.

Kardinaal, A. F., P. van't Veer, H. A. Brants, H. van den Berg, J. van Schoonhoven, and R. J. Hermus (1995). Relations between antioxidant vitamins and adipose tissue, plasma, and diet. *Am J Epidemiol 141*, 440–450.

Katsouyanni, K., E. B. Rimm, C. Gnardellis, D. Trichopoulos, E. Polychronopoulos, and A. Trichopoulou (1997). Reproducibility and relative validity of an extensive semi-quantitative food frequency questionnaire using dietary records and biochemical markers among Greek school teachers. *Int J Epidemiol 26(suppl)*, S118–127.

Larkin, F. A., H. L. Metzner, F. E. Thompson, K. M. Flegal, and K. E. Guire (1989). Comparison of estimated nutrient intakes by food frequency and dietary records in adults. *J Am Diet Assoc 89*, 215–223.

Lee, J., L. N. Kolonel, and J. H. Hankin (1983). On establishing the interchangeability of different dietary-intake assessment methods used in studies of diet and cancer. *Nutr Cancer 5*, 215–218.

London, S. J., F. M. Sacks, J. Caesar, M. J. Stampfer, E. Siguel, and W. C. Willett (1991). Fatty acid composition of subcutaneous adipose tissue and diet in post-menopausal US women. *Am J Clin Nutr 54*, 340–345.

Longnecker, M. P., L. Lissner, J. M. Holden, V. F. Flack, P. R. Taylor, M. J. Stampfer, and W. C. Willett (1993). The reproducibility and validity of a self-administered semi-quantitative food frequency questionnaire in subjects from South Dakota and Wyoming. *Epidemiology 4*, 356–365.

Ma, J., A. R. Folsom, E. Shahar, and J. H. Eckfeldt (1995). Plasma fatty acid composition as an indicator of habitual dietary fat intake in middle-aged adults. The Atherosclerosis Risk in Communities (ARIC) Study. *Am J Clin Nutr 62,* 564–571.

Maclure, M., and W. C. Willett (1987). Misinterpretation and misuse of the kappa statistic. *Am J Epidemiol 126,* 161–169.

Mannisto, S., M. Virtanen, T. Mikkonen, and P. Pietinen (1996). Reproducibility and validity of a food frequency questionnaire in a case–control study on breast cancer. *J Clin Epidemiol 49,* 401–409.

Mullen, B. J., N. J. Krantzler, L. E. Grivetti, H. G. Schutz, and H. L. Meiselman (1984). Validity of a food frequency questionnaire for the determination of individual food intake. *Am J Clin Nutr 39,* 136–143.

Munger, R. G., A. R. Folsom, L. H. Kushi, S. A. Kaye, and T. A. Sellers (1992). Dietary assessment of older Iowa women with a food frequency questionnaire: Nutrient intake, reproducibility, and comparison with 24-hour dietary recall interviews. *Am J Epidemiol 136,* 192–200.

Nomura, A., J. H. Hankin, and G. G. Rhoads (1976). The reproducibility of dietary intake data in a prospective study of gastrointestinal cancer. *Am J Clin Nutr 29,* 1432–1436.

Ocke, M., B. Bueno de Mesquita, E. Feskens, W. van Staveren, and D. Kromhout (1996). Repeated measurements of vegetables, fruits, and antioxidant (pro) vitamins in relation to lung cancer (The Zutphen Study) (thesis). In *Assessment of Vegetable, Fruit, and Antioxidant Vitamin Intake in Cancer Epidemiology.* The Hague, The Netherlands: CIP-Data Koninklijke Bibliotheek.

Ocke, M., H. B. Bueno-de-Mesquita, M. A. Pols, H. A. Smit, W. A. van Staveren, and D. Kromhout (1997a). The Dutch EPIC food frequency questionnaire. II. Relative validity and reproducibility for nutrients. *Int J Epidemiol 26(suppl),* S49–S58.

Ocke, M. C., H. B. Bueno-de-Mesquita, H. E. Goddijn, A. Jansen, M. A. Pols, W. A. van Staveren, and D. Kromhout (1997b). The Dutch EPIC food frequency questionnaire. I. Description of the questionnaire and relative validity and reproducibility for food groups. *Int J Epidemiol 26(suppl),* S37–S48.

Ocke, M. C., and R. J. Kaaks (1997). Biochemical markers as an additional measurement in dietary validity studies: Application of the method of triads with examples from the European Prospective Investigation into Cancer and Nutrition. *Am J Clin Nutr 65 (suppl),* 1240s–1245s.

Pietinen, P., A. M. Hartman, E. Haapa, L. Rasanen, J. Haapakoski, J. Palmgren, D. Albanes, J. Virtamo, and J. K. Huttunen (1988a). Reproducibility and validity of dietary assessment instruments. I. A self-administered food use questionnaire with a portion size picture booklet. *Am J Epidemiol 128,* 655–666.

Pietinen, P., A. M. Hartman, E. Haapa, L. Rasanen, J. Haapakoski, J. Palmgren, D. Albanes, J. Virtamo, and J. K. Huttunen (1988b). Reproducibility and validity of dietary assessment instruments II. A qualitative food-frequency questionnaire. *Am J Epidemiol 128,* 667–676.

Pisani, P., F. Faggiano, V. Krogh, D. Palli, P. Vineis, and F. Berrino (1997). Relative validity and reproducibility of a food frequency dietary questionnaire for use in the Italian EPIC centres. *Int J Epidemiol 26(suppl),* S152–160.

Riboli, E., S. Elmstahl, R. Saracci, B. Gullberg, and F. Lindgarde (1997). The Malmo food study: Validity of two dietary assessment methods for measuring nutrient intake. *Int J Epidemiol 26(suppl),* S161–S173.

Riley, M. D., and L. Blizzard (1995). Comparative validity of a food frequency questionnaire for adults with IDDM. *Diabetes Care 18,* 1249–1254.

Rimm, E. B., E. L. Giovannucci, M. J. Stampfer, G. A. Colditz, L. B. Litin, and W. C. Willett (1992). Reproducibility and validity of a expanded self-administered semiquantitative food frequency questionnaire among male health professionals. *Am J Epidemiol 135,* 1114–1126.

Rockett, H. R., A. M. Wolf, and G. A. Colditz (1995). Development and reproducibility of a food frequency questionnaire to assess diets of older children and adolescents. *J Am Diet Assoc 95,* 336–340.

Rockett, H. R. H., M. Breitenbach, L. Frazier, A. M. Wolf, and G. A. Colditz (1997). Validation of a youth/adolescent food frequency questionnaire. *Prev Med 26,* 808–816.

Rockett, H. R. H., and G. A. Colditz (1997). Assessing diets of children and adolescents. *Am J Clin Nutr, 65 (suppl),* 1116s–1122s.

Rohan, T. E., and J. D. Potter (1984). Retrospective assessment of dietary intake. *Am J Epidemiol 120,* 876–887.

Romieu, I., M. Hernandez, S. Parra, J. Hernandez, H. Madrigal, and W. Willett (1997). Validity and reproducibility of a semiquantitative food frequency questionnaire to assess antioxidants and retinol intake in a Mexican population. Submitted.

Rosner, B., and W. C. Willett (1988). Interval estimates for correlation coefficients corrected for within-person variation: Implications for study design and hypothesis testing. *Am J Epidemiol 127*, 377–386.

Russell-Briefel, R., M. W. Bates, and L. H. Kuller (1985). The relationship of plasma carotenoids to health and biochemical factors in middle-aged men. *Am J Epidemiol 122*, 741–749.

Sacks, F. M., G. H. Handysides, G. E. Marais, B. Rosner, and E. H. Kass (1986). Effects of a low-fat diet on plasma lipoprotein levels. *Arch Intern Med 146*, 1573–1577.

Salvini, S., D. J. Hunter, L. Sampson, M. J. Stampfer, G. A. Colditz, B. Rosner, and W. C. Willett (1989). Food-based validation of a dietary questionnaire: The effects of week-to-week variation in food consumption. *Int J Epidemiol 18*, 858–867.

Sampson, L. (1985). Food frequency questionnaires as a research instrument. *Clin Nutr 4*, 171–178.

Sandler, R. B., C. W. Slemenda, R. E. LaPorte, J. A. Cauley, M. M. Schramm, M. L. Barresi, and A. M. Kriska (1985). Postmenopausal bone density and milk consumption in childhood and adolescence. *Am J Clin Nutr 42*, 270–274.

Selhub, J., P. F. Jacques, P. W. F. Wilson, D. Rush, and I. H. Rosenberg (1993). Vitamin status and intake as primary determinants of homocysteinemia in an elderly population. *J Am Med Assoc 270*, 2693–2698.

Silverman, D. I., G. J. Reis, F. M. Sacks, T. M. Boucher, and R. C. Pasternak (1990). Usefulness of plasma phospholipid *n*-3 fatty acid levels in predicting dietary fish intake in patients with coronary artery disease. *Am J Cardiol 66*, 860–862.

Smith-Warner, S. A., P. J. Elmer, L. Fosdick, T. M. Tharp, and B. Randall (1997). Reliability and comparability of three dietary assessment methods for estimating fruit and vegetable intakes. *Epidemiology 8*, 196–201.

Snedecor, G. W., and W. G. Cochran (1971). *Statistical Methods*. Ames: Iowa State University Press.

Sokol, R. J., J. E. Heubi, S. T. Iannaccone, K. E. Bove, and W. F. Balistreri (1984). Vitamin E deficiency with normal serum vitamin E concentrations in children with chronic cholestasis. *N Engl J Med 310*, 1209–1212.

Spiegelman, D., S. Schneeweiss, and A. McDermott (1997). Measurement error correction for logistic regression models with an "alloyed gold standard." *Am J Epidemiol 145*, 184–196.

Stefanik, P. A., and M. F. Trulson (1962). Determining the frequency of foods in large

group studies. *Am J Clin Nutr 11*, 335–343.

Stein, A. D., S. Shea, C. E. Basch, I. R. Contento, and P. Zybert (1992). Consistency of the Willett semiquantitative food frequency questionnnaire and 24-hour dietary recalls in estimating nutrient intakes of preschool children. *Am J Epidemiol 135*, 667–677.

Stiggelbout, A. M., A. M. van der Giezen, Y. H. Blauw, E. Blok, W. A. van Staveren, and C. E. West (1989). Development and relative validity of a food frequency questionnaire for the estimation of intake of retinol and β-carotene. *Nutr Cancer 12*, 289–299.

Stram, D. O., M. P. Longnecker, L. Shames, L. N. Kolonel, L. R. Wilkens, M. C. Pike, and B. E. Henderson (1995). Cost-efficient design of a diet validation study. *Am J Epidemiol 142*, 353–362.

Stryker, W. S., L. A. Kaplan, E. A. Stein, M. J. Stampfer, A. Sober, and W. C. Willett (1988). The relation of diet, cigarette smoking, and alcohol consumption to plasma beta-carotene and alpha-tocopherol levels. *Am J Epidemiol 127*, 283–296.

Stryker, W. S., L. Sampson, M. J. Stampfer, and G. A. Colditz, et al. (1987). *Contributions of specific foods to nutrient consumption: Absolute intake vs between-person variation*. Doctoral thesis, Boston: Harvard School of Public Health.

Stuff, J. E., C. Garza, E. O. Smith, B. L. Nichols, and C. M. Montandon (1983). A comparison of dietary methods in nutritional studies. *Am J Clin Nutr 37*, 300–306.

Thompson, F. E., D. E. Lamphiear, H. L. Metzner, V. M. Hawthorne, and M. S. Oh (1987). Reproducibility of reports of frequency of food use in the Tecumseh Diet Methodology Study. *Am J Epidemiol 125*, 658–671.

Thompson, F. E., J. E. Moler, L. S. Freedman, C. K. Clifford, G. J. Stables, and W. C. Willett (1997). Register of dietary assessment calibration–validation studies: A status report. *Am J Clin Nutr 65(suppl)*, 1142S–1147S.

Tjonneland, A., K. Overvad, J. Haraldsdottir, S. Bang, M. Ewertz, and O. M. Jensen (1991). Validation of a semiquantitative food frequency questionnaire developed in Denmark. *Int J Epidemiol 20*, 906–912.

Tjonneland, A., K. Overvad, E. Thorling, and M. Ewertz (1993). Adipose tissue fatty acids as biomarkers of dietary exposure in Danish men and women. *Am J Clin Nutr 57*, 629–633.

Treiber, F. A., S. B. Leonard, G. Frank, L. Musante, H. Davis, W. B. Strong, and M. Levy

(1990). Dietary assessment instruments for preschool children: Reliability of parental responses to the 24-hour recall and a food frequency questionnaire. *J Am Diet Assoc 90*, 814–820.

Tsubono, Y., Y. Nishino, A. Fukao, S. Hisamichi, and S. Tsugane (1995). Temporal change in the reproducibility of a self-administered food frequency questionnaire. *Am J Epidemiol 142*, 1231–1235.

Tucker, K. L., B. Mahnken, P. W. F. Wilson, P. Jacques, and J. Selhub (1996). Folic acid fortification of the food supply: Potential benefits and risks for the elderly population. *J Am Med Assoc 276*, 1879–1885.

van Liere, M. J., F. Lucas, F. Clavel, N. Slimani, and S. Villeminot (1997). Relative validity and reproducibility of a French dietary history questionnaire. *Int J Epidemiol 26 (suppl)*, S128–S136.

Wahrendorf, J. (1985). Re: A comparison of frequency and quantitative dietary methods for epidemiologic studies of diet and disease (letter). *Am J Epidemiol 121*, 776.

Walker, A. M., and M. Blettner (1985). Comparing imperfect measures of exposure. *Am J Epidemiol 121*, 783–790.

Willett, W. C. (1985). Does low vitamin B-6 intake increase the risk of coronary heart disease? In Reynolds, R. D., and Leklem, J. E. (eds.): *Vitamin B-6: Its Role in Health and Disease*. New York: Alan R. Liss, pp. 337–346.

Willett, W. C., R. D. Reynolds, S. Cottrell-Hoehner, L. Sampson, and M. L. Browne (1987a). Validation of a semi-quantitative food frequency questionnaire: Comparison with a 1-year diet record. *J Am Diet Assoc 87*, 43–47.

Willett, W. C., L. Sampson, M. L. Browne, M. J. Stampfer, B. Rosner, C. H. Hennekens, and F. E. Speizer (1988). The use of a self-administered questionnaire to assess diet four years in the past. *Am J Epidemiol 127*, 188–199.

Willett, W. C., L. Sampson, M. J. Stampfer, B. Rosner, C. Bain, J. Witschi, C. H. Hennekens, and F. E. Speizer (1985). Reproducibility and validity of a semiquantitative food frequency questionnaire. *Am J Epidemiol 122*, 51–65.

Willett, W. C., M. J. Stampfer, G. A. Colditz, B. A. Rosner, C. H. Hennekens, and F. E. Speizer (1987b). Dietary fat and the risk of breast cancer. *N Engl J Med 316*, 22–28.

Willett, W. C., M. J. Stampfer, G. A. Colditz, B. A. Rosner, C. H. Hennekens, and F. E. Speizer (1987c). Moderate alcohol consumption and the risk of breast cancer. *N Engl J Med 316*, 1174–1180.

Willett, W. C., M. J. Stampfer, B. A. Underwood, L. A. Sampson, C. H. Hennekens, J. C. Wallingford, L. Cooper, C. C. Hsieh, and F. E. Speizer (1984). Vitamin A supplementation and plasma retinol levels: A randomized trial among women. *J Natl Cancer Inst 73*, 1445–1448.

Willett, W. C., M. J. Stampfer, B. A. Underwood, F. E. Speizer, B. Rosner, and C. H. Hennekens (1983). Validation of a dietary questionnaire with plasma carotenoid and alpha-tocopherol levels. *Am J Clin Nutr 38*, 631–639.

Wolf, A., D. Hunter, G. A. Colditz, J. E. Manson, M. J. Stampfer, and K. Corsano, et al. (1994). Reproducibility and validity of a self-administered physical activity questionnaire. *Int J Epidemiol 23*, 991–999.

Wolk, A., H. Ljung, B. Vessby, D. Hunter, W. C. Willett, H.-A. Adami, and the Study Group of MRS SWEA (1998). Effect of additional questions about fat on the validity of fat estimates from a food frequency questionnaire. *Eur J Clin Nutr 52*, 1–7.

7

Recall of Remote Diet

For some diseases, including many cancers, the effect of diet is hypothesized to occur many years before diagnosis; thus, the ability to recall diet in the remote past is of considerable interest. Either relatively unstructured diet histories or food-frequency questionnaires can be used to focus questions on a remote period of time.

The validity of remotely recalled diet can be assessed by resurveying individuals with respect to their past diet who had actually provided detailed dietary information in the past, usually for some other purpose. As discussed in the previous chapter, these dietary assessment methods would ideally be different; the original method should be a very detailed assessment, such as diet recording, and the second method one that could be used epidemiologically, such as a diet history or food-frequency questionnaire. Even the demonstration that the same method used in the past produces similar data when used to recall remote intake, which is evidence more of reproducibility than validity, can be extremely use-

ful. Several studies of recalled remote diet have been published (Table 7–1).

Jensen and colleagues (1984) found fairly low correlations, ranging from 0.13 to 0.42, between intake originally assessed by a detailed household interview and then recalled by a diet history 15 to 25 years later. These correlations were similar in magnitude to those obtained for frequencies of specific food items at a 20-year interval by Byers and coworkers (1983). Stronger correlations, generally in the range of 0.5 to 0.7, were seen in studies in which the interval between dietary assessments ranged from 3 to 10 years (Rohan and Potter, 1984; van Staveren et al., 1986; Byers et al., 1987; Willett et al., 1988).

The interpretation of remotely recalled dietary data is complex, as diet has some consistency over time. Furthermore, it appears that recalled diet is heavily influenced by current diet. For example, in the studies of Jensen and colleagues (1984), Rohan and Potter (1984), and van Staveren and colleagues (1986), the correlations between recalled past diet and current diet were higher than the correlations between actual past diet and recall of past diet. It is, therefore, possible that correlations between actual past diet and recalled diet are simply the result of a tendency for diet to remain consistent over time. Until recently, it has been unclear whether the best assessment of remote diet is actually current diet or recall of past diet. These issues have been addressed in several of the previous studies in which three measurements of diet were made: actual past diet, recall of past diet, and current diet.

In examining the assessment of past diet among Dutch adults, van Staveren and coworkers (1986) found similar correlations between either current or recalled diet and the original measurement of past diet. Similar findings were obtained by Jensen and colleagues (1984) in an investigation among a Danish population. Jensen and colleagues also computed partial correlations between recalled and actual past diet while controlling for current diet; for each nutrient and food examined this partial correlation was positive, although weakly so, indicating that recall of past diet provided some additional information regarding the original diet beyond that obtained by an assessment of current diet. Byers and colleagues (1983, 1987), in substantially larger studies in the United States, found that actual past diet correlated slightly better with recalled diet than with current diet. Byers and coworkers (1987) also explored the possibility that current diet modified by perceived change in diet would correlate better with the actual past diet; however, recall of past diet remained superior. In a study of over 1,000 U.S. men and women who completed food-frequency questionnaires in 1967 and 1982, Thompson and colleagues (1987) found that a retrospective questionnaire completed in 1982 focused on the earlier period provided stronger correlations with the 1967 questionnaire than did an assessment of current diet in 1982. These authors also found that perceived change in the use of food groups

reported in 1982 correlated with change measured by the 1967 and 1982 questionnaires (Metzner et al., 1988); however, like Byers and colleagues, they found that the retrospective questionnaire was superior in describing the earlier diet compared with the combination of current diet in 1982 plus the perception of the change. Bakkum and coworkers (1988), in a study among 40 Dutch men, found that a retrospective diet history correlated more strongly with a similar diet history collected 12 to 14 years earlier than did a diet history focused on current intake (Fig. 7–1). Similar findings were reported by Wu and colleagues (1988) among U.S. men and women, but in a Canadian study (Jain et al., 1989) current and recalled diet were similarly associated with past diet. In an analysis based on foods rather than nutrients, Lindsted and Kuzma (1990) also found that recalled diet was more strongly correlated with past diet than was current diet. Persson and colleagues (1990) also found a strong agreement between recall of past diet and current diet; recall and current diet were similarly associated with actual past diet (Persson et al., 1990). Overall, these studies suggest that, if remote diet is of interest, focusing questions on the period of interest usually provides the most accurate information, although the use of current diet as a surrogate for past diet provides similar information in some instances.

Factors associated with error in recall of diet over a period of 8 years were also examined by Kuzma and Lindsted (1990) among participants in the Adventist Health Study. Greater error (assessed on the absolute difference between original and recall diet) was observed in persons whose diets changed the most over the 8-year period. Greater error in recall was also seen among those with lower education and income, but was not associated with gender or age. The lack of association between error in reporting past diets and age or gender as well as an inverse relation between error and educational level is generally consistent with other observa-

Table 7-1. Studies of recalled remote diet

Source	Subjects	Original method	Recall method	Interval	Range of correlation[a]		
					Original *vs.* recall	Original *vs.* current	Recall *vs.* current
Jensen et al. (1984)	Danish men and women (n=102)	Household survey	Diet history	15–25 yr	r = 0.13 fresh vegetables to 0.42 energy, and whole milk	r = 0.02 fresh fruit to 0.45 fat, and whole milk	r = 0.32 fish 0.63 energy to 0.73 potatoes
van Staveren et al. (1986)	Dutch men and women (n = 102)	Diet history	Diet history	7 yr	r = 0.46 PUFA to 0.75 total carbohydrate	r = 0.32 PUFA to 0.77 total carbohydrate	r = 0.39 PUFA to 0.75 poly-saccharides
Byers et al. (1987)	U.S. men and women (n = 323)	Food-frequency interview	Food-frequency interview	6–10 yr	r = 0.50 fat, 0.61 vitamin A, 0.61 fiber	r = 0.50 fat, 0.49 vitamin A, 0.53 fiber	—
Willett et al. (1988)	U.S. nurses (n = 150)	Four 1-wk frequency records	Food frequency (mailed)	3–4 yr	r = 0.28 iron to 0.61 carbohy-drate	—	—
Byers et al. (1983)	U.S. men and women (n = 175)	Food frequency, 33 items	Food frequency, 33 items	20 yr	r = 0.04 bread to 0.56 coffee	r = 0.00 kale to 0.42 coffee	r = 0.38 bacon, 0.70 bread to 0.99 kale
van Leeuwen et al. (1983)	Dutch men and women (n = 79)	7-day record	Diet history	4 yr	r = 0.47 protein to 0.68 fat and 0.82 alcohol	—	—

Study	Population	Method 1	Method 2	Interval			
Rohan and Potter (1984)	Australian men and women (n = 70)	Food-frequency interview	Food frequency (mailed)	3 yr	$r = 0.25$ protein to 0.78 calcium and 0.87 alcohol	$r = 0.35$ cholesterol to 0.73 vitamin C and 0.91 alcohol	$r = 0.61$ PUFA to 0.91 sugar
Bakkum et al. (1988)	Dutch men (n = 40)[b]	Diet history	Diet history	12–14 yr	$r = 0.68$ carbohydrate to 0.77 energy	$r = 0.48$ fat to 0.58 energy	$r = 0.63$ protein to 0.70 fat
Wu et al. (1988)	U.S. men and women (n = 873)	Food-frequency interview	Food-frequency interview	11 yr	$r = 0.22$ PUFA to 0.39 cholesterol	$r = 0.19$ PUFA to 0.35 kcal	$r = 0.49$ saturated fat to 0.58 PUFA and cholesterol
Jain et al. (1989)	Canadian men and women (n = 94)	Food-frequency interview	Food-frequency interview	7 yr	Mean $r = 0.51$ for 14 nutrients	Mean $r = 0.50$ for 14 nutrients	—
Lindsted and Kuzma (1990)	Adventist men and women (n = 181)	Food-frequency questionnaire	Food-frequency questionnaire	8 yr	Mean $r = 0.47$ for foods	Mean $r = 0.41$ for foods	Mean $r = 0.62$ for foods

[a] PUFA, polyunsaturated fatty acids.

[b] 4 women also studied but not reported separately.

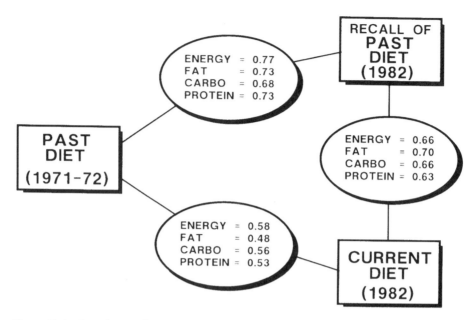

Figure 7–1. Correlations between past diet, recall of past diet, and current diet among 40 Dutch men. (Data from Bakkum et al., 1988.)

tions (for additional references, see Wilkens et al., 1992).

Although most studies of recall of remote diet have focused on diets earlier in adulthood, a few recent analyses have examined the recall of diet during childhood. Hislop and colleagues (1990) examined the reproducibility over a 4- to 6-year interval of recalled diet at four different periods in life: childhood, adolescence, younger adulthood, older adulthood. Among women without a cancer history (which could have perturbed recent diet), reproducibility was similar for these four periods; within each period the weighted kappa values for the 31 foods averaged between 0.42 to 0.46. Frazier et al. (1995) assessed the reproducibility over a 6-year interval of recalled consumption of 24 foods during high school among 275 women currently aged 40 to 75 years. The average Spearman correlation for these foods was 0.66. The average correlation between the first recall and current diet 6 years later was 0.25. Information on the validity, as opposed to reproducibility, of recalled diet during

childhood is limited due to the rarity of childhood intake data from individuals who are now adults and can be traced. In the Harvard Longitudinal Study of Child Health and Development, dietary intake were collected for participants at ages 5 to 7 years, 18 years, and 30 years using a Burke-type diet history. Dwyer and colleagues (1989) recontacted 91 participants (median age 50 years) and used a food-frequency questionnaire to assess retrospectively the diet at the three earlier periods. For foods examined, the median correlations between actual and recalled diets were 0.24 for age 30, 0.12 for age 18, and 0.12 for ages 5 to 7. Correlations of current diet with assessed intakes at these three ages were lower. This level of validity for recalled diet, if correct, is too low to be useful in epidemiologic studies. However, because the validity of the original dietary assessment is also uncertain, the reliability of assessment of recalled diet during childhood and adolescence remains unsettled.

One possible strategy to improve the assessment of past diet is to use current diet with adjustment for reported change in diet. This strategy was assessed in a Japanese population who completed food-frequency questionnaires at baseline and 5 years later; at the repeat administration, subjects were also asked about their changes in consumption of each food between the questionnaires (Tsubono et al., 1995). Reported changes did correspond with differences in consumption frequencies between the two questionnaires, thus providing evidence for the validity of reported change in food consumption. However, adjustment of food frequencies from the second questionnaire for reported changes in food consumption did not appreciably increase the correlation with the first questionnaire. Others have also found that adjusting current diets for reported changes did not substantially improve correlation with earlier diet (Byers et al., 1987; Sobell et al., 1989; Richardson et al., 1993).

POTENTIAL BIAS IN CASE–CONTROL STUDIES

Although remote diet is probably best measured by questions about past diet, the strong influence of current diet on recall raises concerns regarding the possibility of bias when diet has changed after the etiologically relevant period of exposure. This is particularly worrisome in the context of a case–control study when it is possible that the diets of cases, but not controls, may have changed as a result of the diagnosis or the impact of progressive disease and its treatment. This is of increasing concern given the current widespread publicity about diet in relation to cancer and other diseases.

The potential magnitude of recall bias due to the occurrence of disease can be studied by conducting case–control studies within a prospective cohort study of diet and disease. The relationship between dietary factors and disease based on the prospectively collected dietary data would be compared with the same relationship based on dietary data collected after the diagnosis of disease from incident cases and a concurrent sample of subjects without incident disease (the controls).

An assessment of recall bias was conducted by Bloemberg and colleagues (1986) based on a prospective study of diet and coronary heart disease among 615 men in Zutphen, the Netherlands. The original dietary data were collected in 1970 using a diet history interview, and in 1985 the men were again interviewed regarding their diet 15 years earlier. Analyzed prospectively, the men who subsequently became coronary heart disease (CHD) cases consumed 229 kcal/day less than men who remained free of this disease (a consistent finding in studies of CHD). When analyzed using the retrospective data, however, no difference in energy intake was noted between cases and controls. Although this study suggests that serious recall bias may occur in case–control studies of diet, the time between the diagnosis of CHD and the repeat interview may have been many years, which would rarely be the case in the usual incident series case–control study.

Giovannucci et al. (1993) compared retrospectively and prospectively reported diets from breast cancer cases and a sample of noncases in the Nurses' Health Study. Using the prospective data, no association between energy and fat was observed, but in the retrospective assessment, positive associations were seen with both variables. Both biased recall and differences in diets of women who did and did not participate in the retrospective assessment contributed to the distortion in associations (Giovannucci and Willett, 1994). Using a similar design, but one that only assessed recall bias, Friedenreich et al. (1991) found similar results for retrospective and prospectively collected diets. In a multiethnic cohort in Hawaii (Wilkens et al., 1992), retrospectively reported intakes of total and saturated fat were overreported by colon cancer cases compared with controls, but no bias was seen for breast and prostate cancers. This difference for cancers is notable because, for colon cancer in partic- ular, strong positive associations with total energy and saturated fat have been seen with remarkable consistency in case– control studies, whereas in prospective studies associations have tended to be in- verse, sometimes significantly so (see Chap- ter 11 for details). Recall bias was greatest for a greater time interval between the orig- inal and repeat dietary assessment and with more advanced cases of cancer, which may be particularly problematic for cancers that tend to be diagnosed at a late stage. In an- other analysis of recalled past diet nested within a prospective study (Lindsted and Kuzma, 1990), no evidence of biased re- porting for overall frequency of past food consumption was seen, but data were not provided for specific foods and nutrients.

The greatest concern in case–control studies is that cases will systematically over- or underreport past dietary practices com- pared with controls. This would be as- sessed by comparing mean differences be- tween past and recalled diet for cases with the same mean differences for controls. Even if there is no systematic bias, differ- ences in random error, that is, precision in reporting past diet, can distort the shape of dose–response relationships. For example, greater random error for cases than con- trols would create a U-shaped relationship if there was no true overall relationship. Among participants in the Adventist Health Study (Lindsted and Kuzma, 1990), cancer cases reported diets somewhat more precisely than did controls, which appeared to be due to greater changes in diets over time by controls.

SUMMARY

Studies of differential error in reporting of past diets by disease cases and controls in- dicate that biased findings can occur in some circumstances, but not in all studies. Among other factors, the degree of illness of cases and the specific disease being stud- ied appear to influence results, and bias is also likely to be related to specific dietary

factors rather than just overall food intake. Because most of the studies of recall bias in case–control studies have been rather small and have included heterogeneous groups of cancer patients, further evalua- tion of such bias and its determinants are warranted. However, the available data do indicate potential serious pitfalls in case– control studies of dietary factors.

Studies of remote recall have generally used dietary intake data collected in the past for other purposes. There appears to be an unexploited potential for analogous validation studies based on biochemical analyses of specimens collected and pre- served for other reasons. For example, ad- equately stored sera collected in the past could be analyzed for beta-carotene; these levels could then be compared with recalled past intake of carotene-containing foods. Similarly, the demonstration that recalled history of milk intake during early adult- hood (but not recent milk consumption) is correlated with bone density measured many years later provides indirect qualita- tive validity of recalled calcium intake (Sandler et al., 1985).

Overall, studies conducted to date sug- gest that diet may be recalled with accept- able levels of misclassification up to ap- proximately 10 years; beyond this period greater uncertainty exists. Various factors, including educational level, appear to influ- ence the error in reporting past diets. In some circumstances, errors in reporting are associated with disease status, which has important indications for case–control studies. Although studies of recalled diet reported to date have focused on the degree of error, future validation studies should further evaluate factors that influence error and also compare alternative strategies for the collection of recalled dietary data so as to refine and improve existing methods. For example, various types of prompts might be compared as well as different lev- els of detail in the questions about past diet. Further methodologic evaluation and development is required if we are to learn about the long-term health effects of childhood diets by means other than conducting prospective studies that last for many decades.

REFERENCES

Bakkum, A., B. Bloenberg, W. A. van Staveren, M. Verschuren, and C. E. West (1988). The relative validity of a retrospective estimate of food consumption based on a current dietary history and a food frequency list. *Nutr Cancer 11*, 41–53.

Bloemberg, B. P., D. Kromhout, and C. L. Obermann-de Boer (1986). The validity of retrospectively assessed dietary intake data in CHD cases and controls (The Zutphen Study) (abstract). *CVD Epidemiol Newslett 39*, 52.

Byers, T., J. Marshall, E. Anthony, R. Fiedler, and M. Zielezny (1987). The reliability of dietary history from the distant past. *Am J Epidemiol 125*, 999–1011.

Byers, T. E., R. I. Rosenthal, J. R. Marshall, T. F. Rzepka, K. M. Cummings, and S. Graham (1983). Dietary history from the distant past: A methodological study. *Nutr Cancer 5*, 69–77.

Dwyer, J. T., J. Gardner, K. Halvorsen, E. A. Krall, and A. Cohen (1989). Memory of food intake in the distant past. *Am J Epidemiol 130*, 1033–1046.

Frazier, A. L., W. C. Willett, and G. A. Colditz (1995). Reproducibility of recall of adolescent diet: Nurses' Health Study (United States). *Cancer Causes Control 6*, 499–506.

Friedenreich, C. M., G. R. Howe, and A. B. Miller (1991). An investigation of recall bias in the reporting of past food intake among breast cancer cases and controls. *Ann Epidemiol 1*, 439–453.

Giovannucci, E., M. J. Stampfer, G. A. Colditz, J. E. Manson, B. Rosner, M. Longnecker, F. E. Speizer, and W. C. Willett (1993). Recall and selection bias in reporting past alcohol consumption among breast cancer cases. *Cancer Causes Control 4*, 441–448.

Giovannucci, E., and W. C. Willett (1994). Re: A comparison of prospective and retrospective assessments of diet in the study of breast cancer (reply). *Am J Epidemiol 140*, 580–581.

Hislop, T. G., C. W. Lamb, and V. T. Y. Ng (1990). Differential misclassification bias and dietary recall for the distant past using a food frequency questionnaire. *Nutr Cancer 13*, 223–233.

Jain, M., G. R. Howe, L. Harrison, and A. B. Miller (1989). A study of repeatability of dietary data over a seven-year period. *Am J Epidemiol 129*, 422–429.

Jensen, O. M., J. Wahrendorf, A. Rosenqvist, and A. Geser (1984). The reliability of questionnaire-derived historical dietary information and temporal stability of food habits in individuals. *Am J Epidemiol 120*, 281–290.

Kuzma, J. W., and K. D. Lindsted (1990). Determinants of eight-year diet recall ability. *Epidemiology 1*, 386–391.

Lindsted, K. D., and J. W. Kuzma (1990). Reliability of eight-year diet recall in cancer cases and controls. *Epidemiology 1*, 392–401.

Metzner, H. L., F. E. Thompson, D. E. Lamphiear, M. S. Oh, and V. M. Hawthorne (1988). Correspondence between perceptions of change in diet and 15-year change in diet reports in the Tecumseh Diet Methodology Study. *Nutr Cancer 11*, 61–71.

Persson, P. G., A. Ahlbom, and S. E. Norell (1990). Retrospective versus original information on diet: implications for epidemiological studies. *Int J Epidemiol 19*, 343–348.

Richardson, J. L., C. Koprowski, G. T. Mondrus, B. Dietsch, D. Deapen, and T. M. Mack (1993). Perceived change in food frequency among women at elevated risk of breast cancer. *Nutr Cancer 20*, 71–78.

Rohan, T. E., and J. D. Potter (1984). Retrospective assessment of dietary intake. *Am J Epidemiol 120*, 876–887.

Sandler, R. B., C. W. Slemenda, R. E. LaPorte, J. A. Cauley, M. M. Schramm, M. L. Barresi, and A. M. Kriska (1985). Postmenopausal bone density and milk consumption in childhood and adolescence. *Am J Clin Nutr 42*, 270–274.

Sobell, J., G. Block, P. Koslowe, J. Tobin, and R. Andres (1989). Validation of a retrospective questionnaire assessing diet 10–15 years ago. *Am J Epidemiol 130*, 173–187.

Thompson, F. E., D. E. Lamphiear, H. L. Metzner, V. M. Hawthorne, and M. S. Oh (1987). Reproducibility of reports of frequency of food use in the Tecumseh Diet Methodology Study. *Am J Epidemiol 125*, 658–671.

Tsubono, Y., A. Fukao, S. Hisamichi, and S. Tsugane (1995). Perceptions of change in diet have limited utility for improving estimates of past food frequency of individuals. *Nutr Cancer 23*, 299–307.

van Leeuwen, F., H. DeVet, R. Hayes, W. A. van Staveren, C. E. West, and J. G. A. J. Hautvast (1983). An assessment of the relative validity of retrospective interviewing for measuring dietary intake. *Am J Epidemiol 118,* 752–758.

van Staveren, W. A., C. E. West, M. D. Hoffmans, P. Bos, A. F. Kardinaal, G. A. van Poppel, H. J. Schipper, J. G. Hautvast, and R. B. Hayes (1986). Comparison of contemporaneous and retrospective estimates of food consumption made by a dietary history method. *Am J Epidemiol 123,* 884–893.

Wilkens, L. R., J. H. Hankin, C. N. Yoshizawa, L. N. Kolonel, and J. Lee (1992). Comparison of long-term dietary recall between cancer cases and noncases. *Am J Epidemiol 136,* 825–835.

Willett, W. C., L. Sampson, M. L. Browne, M. J. Stampfer, B. Rosner, C. H. Hennekens, and F. E. Speizer (1988). The use of a self-administered questionnaire to assess diet four years in the past. *Am J Epidemiol 127,* 188–199.

Wu, M. L., A. S. Whittemore and D. L. Jung (1988). Errors in reported dietary intakes. II. Long-term recall. *Am J Epidemiol 128,* 1137–1145.

8

Surrogate Sources of Dietary Information

JONATHAN M. SAMET AND ANTHONY J. ALBERG

Many diseases for which dietary hypotheses have been advanced are either immediately or rapidly fatal. For example, median survival after the diagnosis of lung cancer is only 5 months; the prognosis of stomach cancer is equally poor (Axtell et al., 1976). In studying such diseases with a case–control design, surrogate sources of information on diet may be requisite because the index subject is deceased or too ill to provide dietary information. Furthermore, in the setting of severe illness, subjects may alter their dietary pattern so that current consumption, as assessed by a diet record or a recall method, does not reflect the intake relevant to the hypothesis under study. Reporting of past consumption by ill subjects may also be affected by illness-related changes in present consumption (Jain et al., 1980). Such changes may also alter levels of biochemical markers assessed when the subject is ill. Surrogate respondents may also be necessary when the cognitive levels of members of the target population are not sufficient for the collection of dietary data. This situation may arise when the target population encompasses either extreme of the age distribution: the very young, who have yet to attain adequate levels of cognition; and the very old, whose cognition may be impaired (Colsher and Wallace, 1991). Many chronic diseases are associated with cognitive dysfunction (Colsher and Wallace, 1991) and the prevalence of cognitive impairment among the very old is substantial (Kelsey et al., 1989).

Although subjects who cannot provide dietary information directly can be excluded from a study, bias may result if diet affects prognosis. For example, if dietary consumption of beta-carotene were a risk factor for small cell lung cancer but not for other types, exclusion of deceased cases would introduce bias because small cell lung cancer has the poorest prognosis of the various histologic types of lung cancer. Similarly, simply excluding cognitively impaired subjects from a study may be inappropriate because diet is hypothesized to be involved in the etiology of some manifestations of cognitive impairment (Colsher and Wallace, 1991). Exclusion of deceased and ill cases may also lengthen the duration of a study and may be impracticable for some diseases such as fatal myocardial infarction.

Instead of excluding deceased and ill subjects from studies of diet and disease, dietary information may be obtained by interview with a surviving spouse, sibling, child, or other informant. The spouse's diet may also be used as a surrogate measure (Kolonel and Lee, 1981). Complete dietary information, however, may be unavailable from surrogate sources, and measurement error may result from their use. To the extent that spouses share the same dietary pattern, biochemical measurements made on samples from a healthy spouse might be appropriate surrogates for the ill spouse.

In some settings, it is possible that surrogate responses may be less biased than those provided by an index subject. For example, in the context of a case–control study of an illness that alters the diet of the cases, surrogate responses may provide a more accurate assessment of past diet. Although random misclassification might be increased by such use of surrogate respondents, differential misclassification might be reduced. This potential advantage of using surrogate responses has not been evaluated, but merits consideration.

This chapter reviews the literature on surrogate sources of dietary information. The availability of dietary information from surrogates, the validity of such information, and the implications of using surrogates on study design and data analysis are considered.

AVAILABILITY OF INFORMATION FROM SURROGATE RESPONDENTS

Pickle and colleagues (1983) described the availability of information from surrogate respondents in three case–control studies. Although the questionnaires did not include diet, their findings for cigarette smoking have implications for dietary studies. All cigarette smokers were queried about the number of cigarettes smoked daily and the duration of each level of daily smoking. These questions are comparable with those needed to establish temporal variation in consumption of a particular food. This detailed smoking history could be completed by only 56% of spouses, 47% of siblings, and 55% of offspring. The overall pattern of response suggested that siblings were the best source of information about a subject's immediate family or events that occurred during early life, whereas spouses and children were the best information sources for events during adult life.

Nelson and colleagues (1994) reported the degree of nonresponse among 283 surrogate respondents who served as control subjects in a case–control study of subarachnoid hemorrhage. Detailed information concerning cigarette smoking and alcohol drinking were complete for over 90% of the questionnaire items. Spouses provided the most complete data, with more missing data from first-degree relatives and even less complete responses when friends or others served as surrogate respondents. Further analysis showed that the nonresponse did not differ by disease or exposure status (Nelson et al., 1994).

Another study conducted to assess the reliability of surrogate reports for research on Alzheimer's disease assessed cigarette smoking and alcohol drinking as dichotomous exposures. Complete information was provided by all 52 surrogate respondents for these simple measurements (Rocca et al., 1986). Sixty percent of the surrogates were spouses, and the rest were first-degree relatives. In a study of British and Norwegian immigrants to the United States, 83% of the next of kin of those who had died 2 to 6 years earlier were able to provide data about cigarette smoking (Samet et al., 1985).

In a population-based case–control study of lung cancer in New Mexico, interviews were conducted with surrogates for approximately half of the cases (Samet et al.,

1985). Dietary data were collected with a food-frequency approach designed to assess vitamin A consumption, both performed vitamin A and its carotenoid precursors. For each food, the subjects were asked their usual frequency of intake, as measured on a nine-level scale, during a 1-year reference period. For the lung cancer cases with eating habits unaffected by their disease, the reference period was the year ending on the interview date. For cases who changed their eating habits before diagnosis, the reference year ended at the time of the change in diet. The reference year of control subjects was chosen based on the average patient delay interval for lung cancer patients in New Mexico. Usual portion size was determined by reference to pictures of food servings, measuring devices, and convenient units, such as one egg.

Responses for 36 foods were combined to create indices of total vitamin A, preformed vitamin A, and carotene consumption. The extent of missing data for these foods is shown in Table 8–1. Complete information was obtained for nearly all the controls and the self-reported case interviews. In contrast, complete information was obtained for only about 80% of the cases whose data were obtained by surrogate interview. For approximately 10%, indices of vitamin A consumption could not be calculated because of missing data.

Lerchen and Samet (1986) interviewed 80 wives from 1983 through 1984 for the same histories provided earlier by their husbands, who were cases in the lung cancer case–control study in New Mexico described above. The dietary component of the questionnaire was limited; the wives were asked to report their husbands' usual frequency of intake of six foods selected from the original questionnaire: red and green chili pepper sauce, carrots, liver, eggs, and peaches. All of the wives could provide this information for their deceased husbands.

In a similarly designed, but smaller (n = 30 pairs) case–control study of breast can-cer, Hislop and colleagues (1992) found that husbands of deceased breast cancer cases provided more complete dietary information in 1986 to 1987 than their wives did in 1980 to 1982. This surprising finding was of borderline statistical significance ($p = 0.08$). It may be explained by differing modes of data collection. The food-frequency questionnaire was only a small component of a larger questionnaire for the original (self-report) data collection, but was the only data collected in the follow-up (surrogate) interview. Nevertheless, the results of this study suggest that husbands are capable of providing dietary information for their deceased wives.

The results of these studies demonstrate that surrogate respondents can provide dietary information, but that incomplete responses must be anticipated (Table 8–1). The findings of Pickle and coworkers (1983) suggest that the availability of dietary information varies with the relationship of the surrogate respondent to the index subject.

COMPARABILITY OF INFORMATION FROM SURROGATE RESPONDENTS

The comparability of dietary information from a surrogate respondent to that given by an index respondent has been assessed in studies involving simultaneous interviews with spouse pairs. These investigations have not directly addressed the validity of surrogate responses; none has included comparisons of the interview data supplied by the respondents and their surrogates with other measures of intake, such as diet records. The principal studies of spouse pairs are further limited by not replicating the usual interview circumstances with a surviving partner in a case–control or a retrospective cohort study. The findings reviewed in this chapter are predominantly drawn from five studies of the comparability of self-reported and spouse-reported dietary information.

Kolonel and coworkers (1977) interviewed 300 pairs of adults concerning the

Table 8–1. Availability of dietary information from controls, index cases, and case surrogates in a case–control study of lung cancer[a]

| | Controls | | Cases | | | |
| | | | Self-report | | Surrogate-report | |
Missing items	Frequency (%)	Amount (%)	Frequency (%)	Amount (%)	Frequency (%)	Amount (%)
None	97.9	96.1	96.8	94.8	83.1	81.7
1–4	1.8	3.7	1.7	3.5	5.9	7.1
5–9	0.0	0.0	0.0	0.3	0.9	1.5
10–14	0.0	0.3	0.0	0.0	0.0	1.2
≥15	0.3	0.0	1.5	1.4	10.1	8.5

[a]Based on responses to a food-frequency questionnaire. For frequency, 47 items were considered in tabulating the missing data; for amount, 36 items were considered. Amount (usual portion size) considered unavailable if frequency was not reported. Information for all controls was self-reported. The data were obtained from the case–control study reported by Samet et al. (1985).

eating habits of the husband. The subjects were participants in a health survey in Hawaii and were all residents of urban areas on the island of Oahu. Few of the surrogate respondents were elderly; 56% were younger than 45 years of age, and only 5% were 65 years or older. An interview on dietary habits, alcohol consumption, and smoking was administered to both members of the pair. The spouses were interviewed separately and were not permitted to discuss the questions together.

Weekly frequency of consumption was determined for 13 foods and for beverages (Table 8–2) (Kolonel et al., 1977). The mean frequencies of consumption as reported by the index subjects and by their wives were very close. The level of agreement between the two interviews varied with the frequency with which a food was consumed; it tended to be lower for more frequently consumed foods and higher for less frequently consumed foods. The extent of agreement for the foods was comparable with that for age started to smoke and for the number of cigarettes smoked.

A similar study was reported by Marshall and colleagues (1980) (Table 8–3). The index subjects included 67 male cases and 91 male controls in a case–control study in New York state. Within 4 months of the index subject's interview,

the spouse completed the same interviewer-administered questionnaire. Frequency of consumption of an extensive list of foods was determined with an 11-category scale. For assessment of agreement, this scale was reduced to four categories.

The findings (Table 8–3) closely paralleled those reported by Kolonel and colleagues (1977). Mean monthly frequencies were similar as reported by the men and by their wives for them, although the extent of agreement did not vary consistently with the frequency of consumption. The extent of agreement within one unit tended to be extremely high. The limited range of a four-level scale and nonuniform distribution among these categories, however, would ensure a high level of agreement within one unit. The investigators did note, however, that extreme disagreements were infrequent; in less than 2% of the spouse pairs were responses given that placed the frequency in both the maximum and the minimum categories.

In another study, 46 husband–wife pairs were interviewed with a food-frequency questionnaire designed to provide an index of vitamin A consumption (Humble et al., 1984). In 38 pairs, each person answered questions both as a subject and as a surrogate for his or her spouse. In the remaining eight pairs, each individual served

Table 8–2. Comparability of food consumption as reported by male respondents and their spouses for them in a study in Hawaii[a]

	Mean weekly frequency			Agreement (%)	
	Wife	Index subject	Percentage difference[b]	Exact	±1 Unit
Processed meats	2.9	3.0	−3.3	36	63
Beef	3.9	4.3	−9.3	26	56
Pork	1.0	1.0	0.0	50	89
Poultry	1.3	1.5	−13.3	46	85
Eggs	2.7	2.9	−6.9	40	72
Rice	6.9	6.3	9.5	52	65
Pickled vegetables	2.3	2.3	0.0	51	70
Raw vegetables	5.7	5.7	0.0	39	51
Fresh fruit	4.8	5.2	−7.7	40	52
Milk	0.7	0.7	0.0	67	94

[a] The results include other familial relationships but are predominantly (94%) derived from husband–wife pairs.

[b] Percentage difference $= \left(\dfrac{\text{Wife} - \text{Index}}{\text{Index}} \right) \times 100$.

Abstracted from Tables 2 and 3 from Kolonel et al., 1977.

either as a subject or as a surrogate only. A 55-item food-frequency questionnaire, which ascertained frequency of consumption on a nine-level scale, was administered with reference to the year preceding the date of interview. The size of a usual serving was assessed on a six-level scale with food models of standard portions. The past pattern of consumption was categorized as more, the same, or less than the pattern during the reference year.

For individual foods, the findings for frequency of consumption (Tables 8–4 and 8–5) (Humble et al., 1984) were similar to those reported by Kolonel and colleagues (1977) and by Marshall and colleagues (1980). For portion size, the level of agreement varied from 29% to 100% and was 64 % when averaged across all foods. The average agreement for past pattern of consumption was 57%.

Humble and colleagues (1984) used the responses concerning frequency and amount of consumption to calculate two indices of total daily vitamin A intake: one based on frequency alone and the other based on both frequency and amount. For men, similar levels of mean daily consumption were obtained from their own responses

and those of their wives. In contrast, the husbands' responses yielded lower estimates of total daily vitamin A consumption for their wives than were calculated from the wives' own responses. For example, for the index calculated from frequency and portion size, the mean based on the women's responses was 8,602 units, whereas that based on the husbands' responses was 6,518 units ($p < 0.05$).

Agreement of index subject-based and spouse-based indices of total consumption was assessed by Spearman rank order correlation and by comparison of quantile groupings. The extent of agreement tended to be higher for the index based on frequency alone (Spearman $r = 0.49$ for men and $r = 0.52$ for women). Concordance of the quantile rankings ranged from 26% to 52% and varied with the type of index and the choice of quantiles: quintiles, quartiles, and tertiles. For example, with the frequency-based index, the concordance of quintiles was 31% for men and 38% for women.

Using data from the Tecumseh (Michigan) Diet Methodology Study, Metzner and colleagues (1989) compared food-frequency reports from 94 wives as surro-

Table 8–3. Comparability of food consumption as reported by male respondents and their spouses for them in a study in New York state[a]

Food	Mean weekly frequency			Agreement (%)	
	Wife	Index subject	Percentage difference[b]	Exact	±1 Unit
Bacon	5.3	5.6	−5.4	57	90
Hamburger	6.3	6.4	−1.6	75	97
Liver	1.2	1.1	9.1	61	97
Poultry	4.1	3.8	7.9	59	96
Cheese	7.6	7.0	8.6	56	85
Milk	17.3	16.3	6.1	59	83
Broccoli	1.7	1.5	13.3	67	96
Carrots	5.2	4.7	10.6	56	92
Lettuce	12.4	12.1	2.5	62	93
Tomatoes	11.3	10.9	3.7	54	91
Summer squash	1.3	1.2	8.3	63	87
Apples	10.2	9.6	6.3	53	87
Melons	6.0	5.4	11.1	53	84
Peaches	9.2	7.6	21.1	45	85

[a] Ascertained with 11 categories but collapsed to 4 for assessment of agreement.

[b] Percentage difference $= \left(\dfrac{\text{Wife} - \text{Index}}{\text{Index}} \right) \times 100.$

Abstracted from Tables 1 and 2 from Marshall et al., 1980.

Table 8–4. Comparability of food consumption as reported by male respondents and their spouses for them in a study in New Mexico[a]

Food	Mean weekly frequency			Agreement (%)	
	Wife	Index subject	Percentage difference[b]	Exact	±1 Unit
Liver	0.0	0.0	0.0	93	100
Cheese	0.55	0.48	14.6	60	95
Whole milk	0.20	0.21	−4.8	76	95
Eggs	0.37	0.38	−2.6	67	100
Broccoli	0.19	0.19	0.0	57	100
Carrots	0.26	0.27	−3.7	48	100
Lettuce	0.81	0.76	6.6	45	97
Tomatoes	0.60	0.78	−23.1	51	95
Summer squash	0.10	0.13	−23.1	52	93
Cantaloupe	0.20	0.16	25.0	62	100
Peaches	0.25	0.31	19.4	19	90

[a] Ascertained on a nine-level scale.

[b] Percentage difference $= \left(\dfrac{\text{Wife} - \text{Index}}{\text{Index}} \right) \times 100.$

Abstracted from Table 2 from Humble et al., 1984.

Table 8–5. Comparability of food consumption as reported by female respondents and their spouses for them in a study in New Mexico[a]

Food	Mean weekly frequency			Agreement (%)	
	Husband	Index subject	Percentage difference[b]	Exact	±1 Unit
Liver	0.01	0.01	0.0	86	100
Cheese	0.54	0.62	−12.9	43	93
Whole milk	0.26	0.21	23.8	81	88
Eggs	0.34	0.33	3.0	69	100
Broccoli	0.20	0.16	25.0	74	98
Carrots	0.24	0.33	−27.3	40	93
Lettuce	0.92	0.86	7.0	53	97
Tomatoes	0.75	0.80	−6.3	55	93
Summer squash	0.14	0.14	0.0	52	88
Cantaloupe	0.29	0.27	7.4	57	93
Peaches	0.31	0.39	−20.5	43	93

[a] Ascertained on a nine-level scale.

[b] Percentage difference $= \left(\dfrac{\text{Husband} - \text{Index}}{\text{Index}} \right) \times 100$.

Abstracted from Table 3 from Humble et al., 1984.

gates for their husbands and 86 husbands as surrogates for their wives. Portion sizes were not assessed. Indices of vitamins A and C were calculated based solely on how often vitamin-containing foods were consumed. The study subjects were aged 45 to 64 years and long-term participants in a longitudinal study. Their familiarity with the data collection protocols might have improved the quality of reporting.

The results of the Tecumseh study (Table 8–6) (Metzner et al., 1989) reinforce those of the earlier studies. The differences in mean levels between the two sources deviated by up to 20%. Wives were more likely to report that their husbands ate certain foods more frequently than their husbands reported themselves, whereas husbands tended to report that their wives ate certain foods less frequently than their wives reported themselves. These differences were not striking, however. The estimates of exact agreement, based on quintiles derived from an eight-level frequency scale, ranged from 21% to 76% and tended to be similar for both sexes. Allowing for a 1-unit discrepancy improved the agreement to a range of 57% to 94% (Table 8–6).

Herrmann (1985) also reported on the comparability of information from next-of-kin respondents. The subjects were male and female cases and controls in a colon cancer case–control study in Pennsylvania. The index respondents all completed an interviewer-administered food-frequency questionnaire that was referenced to a calendar year several years earlier. The next of kin were assigned at random to complete either the interviewer-administered questionnaire or a self-administered questionnaire. The frequency questions were open ended on the former but were categorized on the latter.

Exact agreement was calculated for cases and controls for the two methods used to collect data from the next of kin (Table 8–7) (Herrmann, 1985). The agreement was lower for the self-completed questionnaire than for the interview. Comparable levels of agreement were observed for cases and controls and for men and women. Herrmann (1985) also noted that agreement tended to be better for the spouse than for other next-of-kin respondents.

Lerchen and Samet (1986) described agreement between the responses of index

Table 8–6. Comparability of food consumption as reported by spouse pairs, Tecumseh Diet Methodology Study[a]

Food	Mean weekly frequency			Agreement (%)	
	Surrogate	Index subject	Percentage difference[b]	Exact	± 1 Unit
Wife Surrogate, Husband Index					
Poultry	0.92	0.93	−1.08	44	89
Meat	6.32	6.46	−2.17	29	63
Dairy	9.57	8.64	10.76	40	78
Citrus	1.35	1.35	0.00	50	83
Vegetables	9.85	8.78	12.19	21	65
Fats and oils	13.54	12.65	7.04	29	65
Sweets	1.96	1.72	13.95	47	81
Alcohol	1.00	1.06	−5.66	76	97
Vitamin A index	6,671.00	5,793.00	15.16	27	64
Vitamin C index	69.10	65.40	5.66	36	78
Husband Surrogate, Wife Index					
Poultry	0.88	1.01	−12.80	46	84
Meat	4.75	4.60	3.26	42	71
Dairy	6.61	7.80	−15.20	35	71
Citrus	2.72	3.40	−20.00	42	72
Vegetables	11.83	12.02	−1.58	30	60
Fats and oils	11.86	12.73	−6.83	22	57
Sweets	1.27	1.40	−9.29	33	74
Alchohol	0.42	0.39	7.69	63	94
Vitamin A index	6,267.00	6,344.00	−1.21	39	68
Vitamin C index	106.80	98.9	7.99	28	71

[a] Ascertained with 8 categories but collapsed to 5 for assessment of agreement.

[b] Percentage difference $= \left(\dfrac{\text{Spouse} - \text{Index}}{\text{Index}} \right) \times 100.$

Abstracted from Tables 2 and 3 from Metzner et al., 1989.

cases and those of their surviving spouses for six foods. As in the other investigations, the means based on the two sets of responses were similar. Exact agreement on a five-level scale was 45% for carrots, 32% for peaches, 51 % for eggs, 52 % for liver, 48% for green chili pepper sauce, and 41% for red chili pepper sauce. Spearman rank order correlation coefficients ranged from 0.38 to 0.56.

The study of Hislop and colleagues (1992), which compared responses from breast cancer cases in 1980 to 1982 who subsequently died, with their husbands' responses 5 years later, was limited by the small number (10–14) of spouse pairs available for analysis. Comparisons by food groups showed that the average re-

ported frequencies of consumption by husbands and wives were fairly similar overall. However, the agreement for specific foods as measured by the weighted kappa statistic ranged widely, with values for foods such as lettuce and certain meats and oils less than would be expected by chance. This high degree of variability may be due to random fluctuation from the small sample size.

All of the studies reviewed thus far were based on food-frequency questionnaires. A small study (data for 12 spouse pairs) is therefore of interest because the wife's report of usual intake during the past year was compared with the husband's 7-day food record (Moore et al., 1970). The Spearman correlation coefficients calcu-

Table 8–7. Comparability of frequency information from cases and controls and from their next of kin in a case–control study of colon cancer in Philadelphia

Food	Exact agreement by interview type	
	Interview (%)	Self-completed (%)
Cases and Next of Kin		
Beverages	77	65
Vegetables	70	49
Fruits	66	49
Meats	71	59
Dairy	67	49
Grains	75	58
Controls and Next of Kin		
Beverages	77	69
Vegetables	66	53
Fruits	63	52
Meats	63	62
Dairy	63	53
Grains	70	63

Abstracted from Table 6 from Herrmann, 1985.

lated from data presented by Moore and colleagues were 0.26 for carbohydrate, 0.53 for fat, 0.60 for cholesterol, and 0.80 for protein. The evidence from this study, albeit limited, is in accord with the findings of studies that relied solely on food-frequency questionnaires.

The results of these studies (see Tables 8–2 through 8–6) demonstrate modest agreement between mean intakes of specific foods reported by interview subjects and their next of kin. The mean intakes are comparable enough that surrogate reports on food consumption may be useful for studies that aim to compare group means, such as cross-cultural or international comparisons.

Surrogate responses may be less useful for case–control and cohort studies. The extent of agreement for individual foods is variable (Tables 8–2 through 8–7) and depends on the frequency with which a food is consumed, the sex of the index subject, the relationship of the surrogate to the index subject, and the method of data col-

lection. The analyses of Humble and colleagues (1984) demonstrate that agreement between subject-based and surrogate-based measures of overall consumption may be less satisfactory than had been suggested by previous studies based on individual foods. As discussed in Chapter 12, even small differences in the quality of reporting, if differential by case–control status, can markedly distort measures of association.

The studies reviewed are limited in the extent to which they replicate the usual circumstances leading to interview with a surrogate respondent. In three of the studies (Kolonel et al., 1977; Humble et al., 1984; Metzner et al., 1989), the study subjects were healthy volunteers, of whom only a small proportion were elderly. Only the small investigations reported by Lerchen and Samet (1986) and Hislop and colleagues (1992) included spouses of deceased index subjects.

USE OF SPOUSE DIET AS A SURROGATE

In several epidemiologic studies of diet and cancer, the diet of one spouse has been used as a surrogate for the diet of the other. For example, Nomura and coworkers (1978) conducted a breast cancer study of wives of men in the Honolulu Heart Study. The diets of the men whose wives had breast cancer were compared with those of the remaining cohort members. In another instance, the dietary habits of surviving spouses of persons who had died from colon or rectal cancer were assessed (Jensen et al., 1980). An implicit assumption underlying such investigations is that married couples share similar diets for a long period of time.

The diets of husbands and wives, however, are not strongly correlated. Kolonel and Lee (1981) described the correlation between the diets of 281 spouse pairs in Hawaii. Average frequency of food consumption tended to be comparable for the men and the women. Exact agreement on frequency was less than 50% for most

foods, and intraclass correlation coefficients ranged from 0.33 to 0.55 for food
items, from 0.15 to 0.32 for nonalcohol-
containing beverages, and from −0.07 to
0.66 for alcoholic beverages. Lee and Kolonel (1982) subsequently reported an expanded investigation that included 1,428
couples. Nutrient indices were derived
from reported intake of 83 food and beverage items. On average, men consumed
more than women, but intake per unit of
body weight was similar. Spearman and intraclass correlation coefficients showed
moderate concordance between the intakes
of the spouses. The Spearman correlation
coefficients for the nutrient indices considered in the report ranged from 0.45 to
0.59; the intraclass coefficients ranged from
0.35 to 0.59.

The findings of these studies suggest that
the diet of a spouse may serve as a surrogate when another source of information is
unavailable. They do not establish, however, that the spouse's diet is a preferable
surrogate to interviewing the surviving case
or control subject. Comparisons of associations estimated from a typical case–control study in which subjects themselves are
interviewed with those from interviews of
spouses of the same cases and controls
would be of considerable methodologic interest.

PARENTS AS SURROGATES
FOR CHILDREN

The nutritional habits of children are of interest because dietary patterns adopted
early in life may influence the risk of
chronic disease in later years. Assessing the
diets of young children is thus important
for evaluating chronic disease risk-
reduction interventions and for research
that seeks to elucidate the determinants of
health behaviors. However, dietary information collected directly from young children may be of uncertain quality. Children
may still be unfamiliar with many foods
and food names and may not be sufficiently

advanced developmentally to have an accurate sense of time and the ability to recall
details from the past (Emmons and Hayes,
1973). Children's short attention spans
may also pose challenges to data collection.
Interest has thus developed in using parents
as surrogate reporters of their children's
diets.

Four relevant studies on 24-hour dietary
recall are summarized in Table 8–8. By
having a trained observer directly record
the child's intake, three of these studies
(Klesges et al., 1987; Eck et al., 1989;
Basch et al., 1990) had independent comparison data to validate surrogate reports
of the children's diet by parents. Comparison of the mean levels of measured foods
and energy sources in two of these studies
shows random but nontrivial differences
between reports of mothers and those of
trained observers (Klesges et al., 1987; Eck
et al., 1989). Both of these studies were
conducted among predominantly middle-
class white populations. In Figure 8–1, results from the Eck et al. study are compared with results from a third study
consisting of a population of Latinos of
lower socioeconomic status residing in
New York City (Basch et al., 1990). In this
study, differences between the two sources
were larger and tended to be in the direction of overreporting by the mother (Fig.
8–1) (Basch et al., 1990).

Together, the three studies show that
mothers can provide dietary information
about their children that agrees to some extent with independent, standardized observations. In the two studies conducted in
white middle-class populations, the correlations between mothers' and objective observers' reports of the index child's diet
were 0.6 or higher for the majority of nutritional categories (Fig. 8–2) (Klesges et
al., 1987; Eck et al., 1989). When compared with results from one of the two
studies described above (Eck et al., 1989),
more variability was observed in the New
York City study, but most of the correlations were still 0.4 or higher; very low cor-

Table 8–8. Summary of designs of studies evaluating parents as surrogate reporters of children's diet

Source	Location	No. of families	Ages of children (yr)	Parent reporting	Recall period	Source of validation
Basch et al. (1990)	New York, NY	46 (Latino)	4–7	Mother	Previous day, 4:00–8:00 p.m.	Observer at home [4:00–8:00 p.m.]
Eck et al. (1989)	Memphis, Tn	33 (caucasian)	4–9	Mother, father	Previous day lunch	Observer in cafeteria, food weighed
Klesges et al. (1987)	Not stated	30 (caucasian)	2–4	Mother (97%)	Same 24 hours, at end of day	Observer at home, food weighed
Emmons and Hayes (1973)	Upstate New York (rural)	431	6–12	Mother	Prior 24 hours	None: parent versus child report

relations were observed for phosphorus, sodium, and calcium (Fig. 8–2) (Basch et al., 1990).

Of further interest is whether the accuracy of surrogate information differs between mothers and fathers. In the study of Eck and colleagues (1989), a family meal outside the home was observed without the family's knowledge. The next day, both parents reported on their child's intake during this meal. The results of this study did not show an appreciable difference between parents (Table 8–9) (Eck et al., 1989). Under usual research circumstances, the surrogate would optimally be the parent/parent figure who had primary responsibility for food preparation.

The fourth study did not include observation, but did provide a comparison of the mother's report with the index child's self-report (Emmons and Hayes, 1973). Over 80% of mothers and children agreed exactly on the child's number of servings for almost one-third of the foods (Table 8–10) (Emmons and Hayes, 1973). However, the foods with low percentage of exact agreement included such childhood staples as milk and bread. The authors concluded that mothers may report what children ate during meals much better than what chil-

dren ate during between-meal snacks. When the mother and child did not agree exactly, mothers were 1.6 times ($p < 0.001$) more likely to report more frequent, rather than less frequent, intake by the child compared with the index child's self-report.

In summary, parents appear to be able to give a moderately valid indication of what their children ate in the previous 24 hours under certain circumstances. Factors that lessen the time parents spend with the index child, such as employment outside of the home and larger family size, could possibly lead to less accurate reporting of the child's diet.

STUDY DESIGN AND DATA ANALYSIS ISSUES

Although the extent and direction of bias from surrogate respondents remain unclear (Gordis, 1982), the possibility of bias must be considered in any data derived from surrogate responses. The potential for bias appears to be greatest when data for one group, such as cases, are obtained from surrogates, whereas data for another, such as controls, are obtained from the index subjects. As discussed by Gordis (1982),

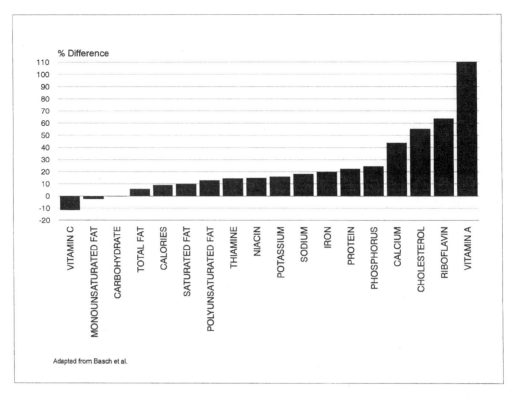

Adapted from Basch et al.

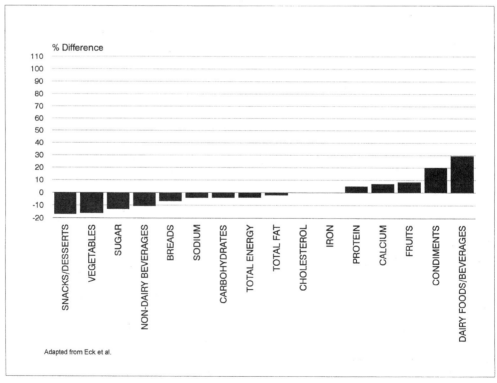

Adapted from Eck et al.

Figure 8–1. Percentage differences in childrens' mean dietary intake between reports of mothers and trained observers, summarized from two studies.

Percentage difference calculated as:

$$\left(\frac{\text{Mother} - \text{Direct Observation}}{\text{Direct Observation}} \right) \times 100$$

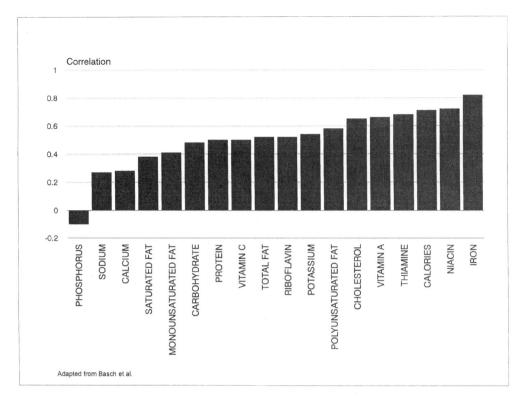

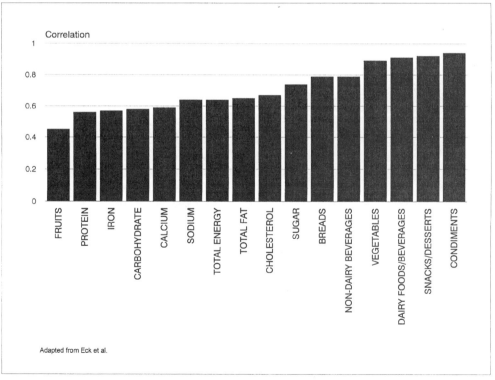

Figure 8–2. Correlations between mothers' and trained observers' reports of child food intake, summarized from two studies.

Table 8–9. Comparison of fathers and mothers as reporters of children's dietary intake

Food group	Percentage difference in mean intake		Correlation with observed intake	
	Mother[a]	Father[b]	Mother	Father
Total energy (kcal)	−3.85	−4.72	0.64	0.83
Energy from protein	4.94	0.00	0.56	0.79
Energy from carbohydrates	−4.00	−2.00	0.58	0.77
Energy from sugar	−12.95	−12.23	0.74	0.88
Energy from total fat	−2.08	−4.17	0.65	0.72
Cholesterol	0.00	−1.33	0.67	0.82
Sodium	−4.10	1.21	0.64	0.70
Iron	0.00	0.00	0.57	0.61
Calcium	6.86	10.78	0.59	0.71
Breads	−6.67	−26.67	0.79	0.54
Nondairy beverages	−10.61	−22.73	0.79	0.54
Dairy foods, beverages	29.41	29.41	0.91	0.72
Vegetables	−16.22	24.32	0.89	0.85
Fruits	8.33	50.00	0.45	0.65
Snacks and desserts	−16.87	−13.25	0.92	0.85
Condiments	20.00	46.67	0.94	0.80

[a]Calculated as $\left(\dfrac{\text{Mother} - \text{Direct observation}}{\text{Direct observation}}\right) \times 100.$

[b]Calculated as $\left(\dfrac{\text{Father} - \text{Direct observation}}{\text{Direct observation}}\right) \times 100.$

Adapted from Table 1 from Eck et al., 1989.

Table 8–10. A comparison of the reliability of parents' and children's reports of children's intake

Percentage exact agreement	Percentage of measured foods	Foods
>90	12	Fish; pasta; soup
81–90	20	Poultry; vegetables—other; cheese; eggs; snack foods
71–80	28	Salad; vegetables—green; vegetables—yellow; ice cream; cereals; legumes; mixed protein
61–70	16	Meat; potatoes and rice; juice; sauces, gravies, and dressings
51–60	8	Fruit; desserts
41–50	4	Milk
31–40	12	Bread, crackers, and pancakes; butter and margarine; sweets

Adapted from Table 1 from Emmons and Hayes, 1973.

the direction of information bias has not been documented and might plausibly be in either a positive or a negative direction.

A study conducted in Hawaii by Wilkens and colleagues (1992) provides reassuring information in this regard. Data on current dietary intake collected at study baseline were compared with dietary intake data referenced to the time of study entry, an average of 7 years earlier. Of the 544 study subjects, 131 went on to develop cancer and 413 did not. Almost one-fifth of the follow-up interviews relied on surrogate respondents; as expected, the proportion of surrogate respondents was greater for the cancer cases than for the noncases. To qualify for the study, a surrogate respondent was required to have lived with the index subject for the 5 years preceding the initial data collection. The authors reported that the ability of cases and noncases to recall past diet was not influenced by respondent type as either a confounder or effect modifier. Under the conditions of this study, differential misclassification appears not to have been a major problem.

As suggested by several of the studies reviewed previously, substantial nondifferential misclassification must be anticipated when surrogate respondents are used. Thus, even if unbiased mean values for cases or controls are provided by surrogate sources, random misclassification in estimates of individual intake may substantially bias measures of association toward null values (Lyon et al., 1992).

Several factors indicate that when planning a study that will include surrogate respondents, sample size estimates need to be inflated (Nelson et al., 1990, 1994). A surrogate who meets the study criteria may be lacking for some index subjects, thereby increasing the number of cases that need to be ascertained. As discussed earlier, more missing data can be expected from surrogate respondents. Finally, the reduced precision in exposure estimates that results from nondifferential misclassification of exposure status diminishes the statistical power of a study.

The value of conducting a substudy to assess the degree of misclassification of dietary exposures that may be introduced by the use of surrogate subjects in a particular study has been recognized (Nelson et al., 1990; Lyon et al., 1992). Such strategies require additional resources that may not always be available, however. Data collection methods aimed at optimizing dietary recall, reviewed elsewhere (Friedenreich et al., 1992), are of even greater importance in studies that rely on surrogate respondents.

In using data from surrogate respondents, certain analytic strategies should be followed. First, the extent of missing data for the various respondent groups should be assessed and a determination made concerning the extent of missing information that is acceptable. For example, in analyzing data from a lung cancer case–control study, Samet and colleagues (1985) excluded subjects with missing data on either frequency or portion size for four or more foods. Second, the responses of the surrogate and index subjects should be compared within homogenous groups for which comparable responses would be anticipated.

Finally, in estimating associations in a case–control or cohort study, it is appropriate to stratify by respondent type to assess its potential role as a confounding or modifying variable. If the exposure–outcome associations are judged not to diverge materially by respondent type, entering indicator variables for respondent type into multiple regression models (e.g., Samet et al., 1985) allows estimation of a summary measure of association that adjusts for respondent type (Walker et al., 1988). Greenland and Robins (1985) have pointed out that this approach may be inappropriate under certain circumstances and therefore emphasized the need to carefully consider data quality issues for a specific study. The demonstration of substantial heterogeneity by respondent type, even without statistically significant interaction, indicates that it would be wise not to pool the study data.

CONCLUSIONS

Reliance on surrogate sources of information may be unavoidable in investigating illnesses that are rapidly fatal or impair cognition significantly. For example, a search of the MEDLINE computerized reference database for articles published from 1991 through 1995 showed that roughly 2% of the abstracts of published case–control studies of diet and cancer referred to the use of surrogate respondents. Despite its acceptance into the epidemiologic repertoire, proxy information concerning diet may introduce measurement error in analytic investigations of dietary hypotheses. The measurement error may be random or may be differential with respect to respondent type. For dietary hypotheses, where the effects of interest are often either unknown or anticipated to be relatively small, misclassification from any source may lead to erroneous conclusions. Use of surrogate sources of dietary information should be minimized in studies of diet and disease.

REFERENCES

Axtell, L. M., A. J. Asire, and M. H. Myers (1976). *Cancer Patient Survival*. No. 5. Bethesda, MD: U.S. Department of Health, Education, and Welfare.

Basch, C. E., S. Shea, R. Arliss, I. R. Contento, J. Rips, B. Gutin, M. Irigoyen, and P. Zybert (1990). Validation of mothers' reports of dietary intake by four to seven year-old children. *Am J Public Health 80*, 1314–1317.

Colsher, P. L., and R. B. Wallace (1991). Epidemiologic considerations in studies of cognitive function in the elderly: Methodology and nondementing acquired dysfunction. *Epidemiol Rev 13*, 1–27.

Eck, L. H., R. C. Klesges, and C. L. Hanson (1989). Recall of a child's intake from one meal: Are parents accurate? *J Am Diet Assoc 89*, 784–789.

Emmons, L., and M. Hayes (1973). Accuracy of 24-hour recalls of young children. *J Am Diet Assoc 62*, 409–415.

Friedenreich, C. M., N. Slimani, and E. Riboli (1992). Measurement of past diet: Review of previous and proposed methods. *Epidemiol Rev 14*, 177–196.

Gordis, L. (1982). Should dead cases be matched to dead controls? *Am J Epidemiol 115*, 1–5.

Greenland, S., and J. M. Robins (1985). Confounding and misclassification. *Am J Epidemiol 122*, 495–506.

Herrmann, N. (1985). Retrospective information from questionnaires. I. Comparability of primary respondents and their next-of-kin. *Am J Epidemiol 121*, 937–947.

Hislop, T. G., A. J. Coldman, Y. Y. Zheng, V. T. Ng, and T. Labo (1992). Reliability of dietary information from surrogate respondents. *Nutr Cancer 18*, 123–129.

Humble, C. G., J. M. Samet, and B. E. Skipper (1984). Comparison of self- and surrogate-reported dietary information. *Am J Epidemiol 119*, 86–98.

Jain, M., G. R. Howe, K. C. Johnson, and A. B. Miller (1980). Evaluation of a diet history questionnaire for epidemiologic studies. *Am J Epidemiol 111*, 212–219.

Jensen, O. M., A. M. Bolander, P. Stigtryggsson, M. Vercelli, X. Nguyen-Dinh, and R. MacLennan (1980). Large bowel cancer in married couples in Sweden. *Lancet 1*, 1161–1163.

Kelsey, J. L., L. A. O'Brien, J. A. Grisso, and S. Hoffman (1989). Issues in carrying out epidemiologic research in the elderly. *Am J Epidemiol 130*, 857–866.

Klesges, R. C., L. M. Klesges, G. Brown, and G. C. Frank (1987). Validation of the 24-hour dietary recall in preschool children. *J Am Diet Assoc 87*, 1383–1385.

Kolonel, L. N., T. Hirohata, and A. M. Nomura (1977). Adequacy of survey data collected from substitute respondents. *Am J Epidemiol 106*, 476–484.

Kolonel, L. N., and J. Lee (1981). Husband-wife correspondence in smoking, drinking, and dietary habits. *Am J Clin Nutr 34*, 99–104.

Lee, J., and L. N. Kolonel (1982). Nutrient intakes of husbands and wives: Implications for epidemiologic research. *Am J Epidemiol 115*, 515–525.

Lerchen, M. L., and J. M. Samet (1986). An assessment of the validity of questionnaire responses provided by a surviving spouse. *Am J Epidemiol 123*, 481–489.

Lyon, J. L., M. J. Egger, L. M. Robison, T. K. French, and R. Gao (1992). Misclassification of exposure in a case–control study: The effects of different types of exposure and different proxy respondents in a study of pancreatic cancer. *Epidemiology 3*, 223–231.

Marshall, J., R. Priore, B. Haughey, T. Rzepka, and S. Graham (1980). Spouse–subject interviews and the reliability of diet studies. *Am J Epidemiol 112*, 675–683.

Metzner, H. L., D. E. Lamphiear, F. E. Thompson, M. S. Oh, and V. M. Hawthorne (1989). Comparison of surrogate and subject reports of dietary practices, smoking habits and weight among married couples in the Tecumseh Diet Methodology Study. *J Clin Epidemiol 42*, 367–375.

Moore, M. C., E. M. Moore, C. D. Beasley, G. J. Hankins, and B. C. Judlin (1970). Dietary-atherosclerosis study on deceased persons. *J Am Diet Assoc 56*, 13–22.

Nelson, L. M., W. T. Longstreth, Jr., T. D. Koepsell, H. Checkoway, and G. van Belle (1994). Completeness and accuracy of interview data from proxy respondents: Demographic, medical, and life-style factors. *Epidemiology 5*, 204–217.

Nelson, L. M., W. T. Longstreth, Jr., T. D. Koepsell, and G. van Belle (1990). Proxy respondents in epidemiologic research. *Epidemiol Rev 12*, 71–86.

Nomura, A., B. E. Henderson, and J. Lee (1978). Breast cancer and diet among the Japanese in Hawaii. *Am J Clin Nutr 31*, 2020–2025.

Pickle, L. W., L. M. Brown, and W. J. Blot (1983). Information available from surrogate respondents in case–control interview studies. *Am J Epidemiol 118*, 99–108.

Rocca, W. A., L. Fratiglioni, L. Bracco, D. Pedone, C. Groppi, and B. S. Schoenberg (1986). The use of surrogate respondents to obtain questionnaire data in case–control studies of neurologic diseases. *J Chronic Dis 39*, 907–912.

Samet, J. M., B. J. Skipper, C. G. Humble, and D. R. Pathak (1985). Lung cancer risk and vitamin A consumption in New Mexico. *Am Rev Respir Dis 131*, 198–202.

Walker, A. M., J. P. Velema, and J. M. Robins (1988). Analysis of case–control data derived in part from proxy respondents. *Am J Epidemiol 127*, 905–914.

Wilkens, L. R., J. H. Hankin, C. N. Yoshizawa, L. N. Kolonel, and J. Lee (1992). Comparison of long-term dietary recall between cancer cases and noncases. *Am J Epidemiol 136*, 825–835.

9

Biochemical Indicators of Dietary Intake

DAVID HUNTER

This chapter considers the utility of biochemical indicators to represent the dietary intakes of specific nutrients in epidemiologic studies. This use of biochemical indicators is different from their common purpose as measures of nutrient status or as predictors of disease risk. Nutritionists and clinicians frequently employ a biochemical indicator as a measure of an individual's current ability to meet physiologic requirements for that nutrient. Nutrient intake is just one determinant of nutrient status, however, because the levels of a nutrient in blood or tissues can be affected by genetic influences, lifestyle factors such as smoking or physical activity, or the intake of other nutrients. A related use of biochemical indicators is to predict disease risk, irrespective of whether the level of the biochemical measure is determined by dietary intake or other factors. For example, serum cholesterol strongly predicts risk of cardiovascular disease, although the association of serum cholesterol with dietary cholesterol is weak due to the influence of nondietary factors such as genetic variation, exercise, and obesity on serum levels (see Chapter 1). Nutritional epidemiologists have a primary interest in the intake of dietary factors as quantifiable determinants of disease, and thus the use of a biochemical indicator is principally as a measure of nutrient intake. The intent of this chapter is to review the relationships between the intake of individual nutrients and their corresponding biochemical indicators rather than to discuss the use of biochemical measurements to predict nutrient status or disease.

First, some general principles of the relationship between nutrient intake and biochemical indicators, which define the utility of these measures for epidemiologic purposes, are discussed. Then some aspects of study design, specimen collection and storage, and measurement, relevant to the validity of biochemical indicators, are reviewed, and the study designs available for validation of biochemical indicators as measures of intake are discussed. To illustrate these principles selenium, a nutrient for which the relationship between dietary intake and levels in various tissues is unusually well characterized, is used as an example. Finally, specific biochemical indicators used to assess intake of selected nutrients of current epidemiologic interest are reviewed.

There are two fundamental uses for biochemical indicators of food and nutrient intake in epidemiologic studies. The most common application is as a surrogate for actual dietary intake in studies of disease occurrence. For nutrients that vary widely in concentration within individual foods and for which food composition tables are inaccurate, a biochemical measure may be the only feasible way to estimate intake. Within-food variation may occur because of differences in food storage, processing, or preparation or may be due to geographic differences in soil nutrient content. For example, Ullrey (1981) demonstrated that the selenium content of corn within the United States can vary by as much as 100-fold and that, in turn, the selenium content of swine muscle varies more than 15-fold. A less common use for biochemical markers, but one that is likely to receive more attention in the future, is to validate other forms of diet assessment. In other words, if a biochemical indicator provides a good index of true intake, then the performance of other assessment techniques can be assessed by comparison with it.

GENERAL PRINCIPLES

Biochemical measures are objective and may, therefore, have a superficial aura of impartiality, especially to the epidemiologist trained to be suspicious of the answers provided by forgetful and potentially biased humans and their interviewers. It is important, however, to be aware that biochemical measures are almost always subject to the same problems of misclassification and bias. The following general principles concern the issues of error in classification with respect to intake and the avoidance or control of sources of bias.

Sensitivity to Intake

The most important requirement of any index of food or nutrient intake is, of course, that it measures what it is supposed to measure. At the extreme, if there is no correlation between blood level of a nutrient and true intake, then the blood levels randomly classify subjects with respect to intake. The magnitude of this correlation depends principally on the degree of homeostatic control of the levels of the nutrient in available biologic samples, on the range of intake in the population to be investigated, and on the existence of determinants other than intake.

Fortunately for humans (if not for nutritional epidemiologists) homeostatic mechanisms control the concentration of many nutrients in body tissues and fluids. These mechanisms may be conceptually simple, such as the saturation of absorption (e.g., iron) or the excretion of excess (e.g., vitamin C), or they may involve complex hormonal pathways (e.g., calcium). These mechanisms mean that the relation between nutrient intake and levels in biologic specimens is rarely linear and may not even be monotonic. For many nutrients, these mechanisms cause the increase in biologic levels with higher nutrient intake to be attenuated or plateau (Fig. 9–1).

The implications of these relationships for biochemical indicators of nutrient intake are several. If the plateau phase of a marker is wide, its concentration may be almost uniform over the range of normal consumption, and thus the indicator is almost useless as a marker of nutrient intake. This is also the case if the range of intake of the study population is relatively narrow and falls in the plateau phase. If the population is more heterogeneous with respect to intake, then the biochemical measure may, at least, be able to discriminate between very low and "average" intakes.

Another relevant consideration in the context of sensitivity to intake is the question of bioavailability. Bioavailability has been defined as "the proportion of a nutrient in food that is absorbed and utilized"

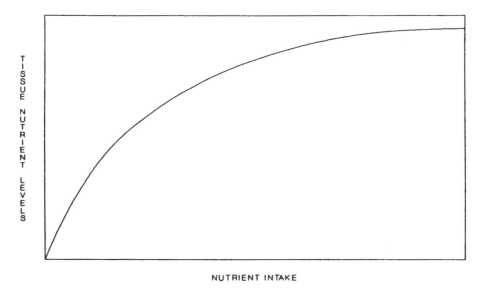

Figure 9–1. Typical relation between nutrient intake and tissue nutrient levels.

(O'Dell, 1984). Some chemical forms of a nutrient may be absorbed far less completely than others. Thus, a biochemical indicator may accurately reflect the intake of a well-absorbed nutrient species, but fail to reflect the intake of a slightly modified compound. This can be a disadvantage if we are interested in absolute dietary intake of the nutrient, such as in hypotheses involving nutrient actions within the intestinal lumen. More often, however, we are concerned with the biologic effects of nutrients after intestinal absorption; in other words, we are interested in the "internal dose" rather than the "external dose." In this regard, biochemical measurements may be more appropriate than estimates of intake based on food composition tables, as these rarely contain information on the relative bioavailability of nutrients in different foods.

Time Integration

Having stressed that the first requirement for a valid biochemical indicator is sensitivity to intake, we must now point out that (in this context) it is possible to have too much of a good thing. Nutrient exposures relevant to disease, like most exposures in chronic disease epidemiology, are usually long term. The induction period of atherosclerotic plaques or the promotion period for cancers may be years or decades. Thus, it is usually desirable that a biochemical indicator reflect the cumulative effect of diet over an extended period of time (Willett, 1987). If the indicator is only sensitive to short-term intake, and if nutrient intake fluctuates from day to day (as it does for most nutrients), then the biochemical indicator reflects nutrient intake for the hours, days, or weeks before sampling, not the months, years, or decades that are truly of interest.

Time integration is largely a function of the nature of the biologic sample being tested. "Longer-lived" specimens are more likely to reflect long-term intake. Nutrients stored in fat tissue, for instance, usually have a slow turnover. For many elements, concentrations of nutrients in erythrocytes are less susceptible to short-term fluctuations in concentration than in plasma or serum. A 24-hour urine collection is more likely to be representative of intake than a random urine sample. Tissue levels, such as liver retinol concentration, may be the best indicators of long-term nutrient status;

however, these are rarely obtainable in epidemiologic studies. Hair and nails are readily available keratinous tissues, which take weeks or months to grow, and thus offer the prospect of measuring long-term intake for certain nutrients.

Information about time integration comes from several sources. Experimental studies, in which nutrient intakes are manipulated, provide good information on the relationship between nutrient intake and the time course of response in different biologic specimens. Less direct but still valuable information can be obtained by simply sampling levels in individuals longitudinally. A high within-person variance in a biochemical measure over time implies a response to short-term fluctuations in intake or to changes in other determinants of its level. In either case, the power of a single measurement to predict long-term average level is low if the within-person variation is large. Sensitivity to recent intake can be overcome to a certain extent by repeated sampling, and Liu and colleagues (1979a) have given a method to calculate the number of replicate measures required to estimate the "true" underlying mean value within a specified range of error (see also Chapter 3). Even if a biochemical measure is a good indicator of dietary intake over the previous months or years, repeated sampling may still be desirable to account for individual change and secular trends in nutrient intake.

Measurement of Nondietary Determinants of Biochemical Indicator Levels

Dietary intake and homeostatic mechanisms are usually not the only determinants of nutrient concentrations in most biologic samples. A wide array of genetic, environmental, and lifestyle factors may also influence nutrient levels. If these factors are not taken into account, then misclassification of subjects with respect to nutrient intake will occur. If such a factor is not associated with disease, then it contributes to random misclassification and attenuates any true association between the biochemical indicator and disease. If the factor is associated with disease, then confounding may occur. For example, vitamin E levels in plasma or serum are related to the concentration of cholesterol in the blood as this lipid-soluble vitamin is transported by the lipoproteins. Among premature infants, low serum vitamin E was not found to be related to clinical vitamin E deficiency unless adjusted for the high lipid levels associated with the liver dysfunction of prematurity (Sokol et al., 1984). The observation that a biochemical indicator of dietary intake is correlated with another factor does not automatically mean that intake levels should be adjusted for this factor; legitimate question may exist as to whether an adjustment should be used. An understanding of the biologic basis for a correlation between the biochemical indicator, such as plasma vitamin E, and the other factor, such as plasma cholesterol, helps resolve this issue. If plasma vitamin E and plasma cholesterol levels were correlated due to an influence of vitamin E intake on serum cholesterol, adjustment would not be appropriate because controlling for an effect of the primary exposure, whether that effect is related to the biologic outcome, would represent "overcontrol." In this example, however, we have information from a randomized trial indicating that vitamin E intake does not affect serum cholesterol levels (Willett et al., 1983c). If, on the other hand, plasma cholesterol levels influence plasma vitamin E levels, as appears to be the case, it may still be unclear whether the variation in plasma vitamin E due to differences in plasma cholesterol is biologically relevant to vitamin concentrations in the tissues of the target organ. The observation among premature infants noted previously, that blood vitamin E levels were not related to clinical vitamin E deficiency unless adjusted for serum cholesterol, provides direct evidence that variation in vitamin E levels due to blood lipids is not biologically relevant and that adjustment is appropriate. Thus, information on whether an association with disease is strengthened by adjustment of the biochemical indicator for another factor can be extremely useful. In addition, information on whether the association between nutrient intake and the biochemical indicator is increased by adjustment for the other factor provides direct guidance as to whether the adjustment is appropriate. Thus, the finding that the correlation between calculated vitamin E intake and plasma vitamin E increased from $r = 0.11$ ($p = 0.19$) to $r = 0.28$ ($p = 0.02$) after adjustment for plasma cholesterol (Willett et al., 1983b) suggests that if blood vitamin E levels are to be used as an indicator of dietary intake they should be adjusted for blood cholesterol and probably other lipid fractions as well.

The same strategies used to control confounding or reduce random error in other contexts are appropriate here. Subjects may be matched on characteristics ascertainable in advance by the investigator, or the study population may be restricted to one in which variability in potential confounding factors is eliminated or reduced. At a minimum, information on potential confounders may be collected to control these in subsequent statistical analyses. Many biochemical measurements vary with age and sex; however, these two variables are almost always routinely controlled for in epidemiologic analyses. As in many other fields of epidemiology, knowledge about other potential confounders is incomplete, and the possibility of uncontrolled confounding must be considered in any assessment of biochemical data.

Genetic Determinants of Biochemical Indicator Level

Inherited factors can influence the relation between nutrient intake and the blood or tissue levels of that nutrient. As detailed later, certain individuals appear to be "hyporesponders" or "hyperresponders" to changes in cholesterol intake, presumably on a genetic basis, partially accounting for the frustrations that some patients and physicians experience when cholesterol reduction may fail to reduce blood choles-

terol levels. Some, but not all, of the between-person differences in responsiveness to dietary cholesterol can be explained by inherited differences in apolipoproteins such as apolipoprotein E (Lehtimaki et al., 1995) and apolipoprotein A-IV (McCombs et al., 1994). Recently, a relatively common mutation was identified in the enzyme that converts 5,10-methylenetetrahydrofolate to 5-methyltetrahydrofolate, the major circulating form of folacin. About 13% of individuals are homozygous for the aberrant enzyme and have lower levels of plasma 5-methyltetrahydrofolate (Ma et al., 1996). Thus, accounting for genotype would improve the predictiveness of plasma folate levels as indicators of folate intake. As our knowledge of these genetic determinants improves, we can expect to improve our ability to interpret biochemical indicators of dietary intake.

Types of Analytic Procedures

There are several broad approaches to biochemical indicator measurement.

Direct Measurement

The most obvious method is direct assay of the concentration of a nutrient, or its metabolic products, in a tissue or a fluid. As new and more refined methods have become available that reduce limits of detection and increase accuracy, direct measurement of more nutrients in a wider variety of specimens has become feasible. As discussed previously, the usefulness of a potential indicator of intake has to be determined individually for each nutrient and for each type of biologic specimen.

Functional Assays

An intuitively appealing alternative to the measurement of nutrient concentrations is the measurement of biochemical functions that depend on specific nutrients. The activities of several nutrient-specific enzymes (e.g., glutathione peroxidase [selenium] and erythrocyte transketolase [thiamine]) have been shown to reflect dietary intake of these nutrients. Care must be taken, however, both that the system used is truly nutrient specific and that its function has not been compromised by some aspect of specimen collection or storage.

In the broadest sense, tests that measure ultimate products of metabolic pathways are tests of the adequacy of intake of participating nutrients (e.g., iron and hemoglobin). Few, if any, however, of these pathways are only influenced by a single nutrient; other nutrients as well as non-nutritional factors may affect the production of the ultimate product. Nonbiochemical tests of physiologic function (e.g., vitamin A and the dark adaptation test) may provide an index of nutrient inadequacy, but rarely provide a measure relevant to the full range of normal intake.

Tolerance Tests

Tolerance tests usually involve taking a blood or urine sample shortly before, and some time after, the administration of a test dose of the relevant nutrient (e.g., vitamin A and the relative dose–response test) (Campos et al., 1987). Poorly nourished individuals frequently retain a larger proportion of the test dose than well-nourished persons, who may simply excrete most of the test dose. The increased logistic demands of these methods limit their use in many epidemiologic studies.

STUDY DESIGN CONSIDERATIONS

Specimen Collection and Storage

Appropriate timing of sampling and proper collection and storage techniques are essential to ensure the validity of biochemical measures. Ideally, all steps involved in the process of delivering biologic specimens to the waiting analyst would be designed such that the concentration of the indicator to be measured is exactly the same as it is in vivo. Biologic reality and the complexities and time course of epidemiologic studies mean that this ideal is rarely attainable. A first requirement of validity, therefore, is that case and control specimens must be

handled in the same way at each step. This must be done to avoid introduction of systematic differences due to study design. A systematic difference, for instance, in the time of storage between the case and the control specimens could bias a study result if the biochemical measure is degraded over time. Substantial degradation in storage of both case and control specimens would, of course, eliminate the ability of finding a difference, even if a difference existed before specimen collection. The storage requirements for different nutrients vary considerably, and, for many, information on stability is sparse.

Seasonal Timing

Nutrient intakes may vary in response to the availability of seasonal foods. For many nutrient markers, therefore, it is important that samples from both cases and controls be collected in the same season, preferably in the same year. If this is not feasible, then adjustment should be made for season of collection in the statistical analysis of the data.

Time of Day

Nutrient markers that are responsive to recent intake may vary substantially over the course of a single day. The collection of early morning fasting blood samples or overnight urine specimens usually minimizes this source of variation. Even measures of long-term intake may be influenced by diurnal variation, and standardization of the time of collection is thus desirable. Again, if this is not possible, time of collection could be controlled for in the analysis.

Options in Study Design

In case–control studies, it may already be too late to collect the relevant samples from cases if the onset, diagnosis, progression, or treatment of the illness affects the levels of the indicator of interest. Results derived from biochemical indices used in case–control studies have not always been confirmed in prospective studies, often because the disease was found to influence nutrient levels (see Chapter 15). One strategy for dealing with this problem is to attempt to enroll cases as soon as possible after the date of diagnosis or even while they are undergoing a diagnostic workup. Many diseases, and especially many cancers, however, have extended preclinical periods, and changes in dietary patterns, or the secretion of tumor products, may affect nutrient levels months before the cases are diagnosed.

Even prospective studies may be prone to this form of bias. For example, low serum cholesterol level was associated with increased cancer risk in the 2 years subsequent to blood collection in the Multiple Risk Factor Intervention Trial (MRFIT) study; however, this effect attenuated over time and may well have been due to preclinical disease (Sherwin et al., 1987). Care should thus be taken in the interpretation of biochemical results in the first years of follow up. In any case, the long induction periods probably associated with many chronic diseases mean that dietary intake years, or decades, before disease onset is the exposure of interest.

The opportunity for efficient and cost-effective assessment of exposures years before disease onset offered by the *nested case–control design* deserves consideration. In a nested case–control study, cases of a disease arising in a cohort are compared with a sample of other cohort members rather than with the entire cohort. If the exposure of interest requires measurement of a biochemical parameter in a stored specimen, this design permits a statistical analysis based on a small fraction of the biochemical analyses that would be required if the relevant biochemical parameter was measured for all members of the cohort. Willett and colleagues (1983a), for example, had available to them frozen sera from 4,480 men and women who had participated in a large clinical trial of treatment for hypertension, as well as information on cancer incidence in the 5 years subsequent to blood collection. Their ex-

posures of interest were retinol, vitamin E, and selenium, and a conventional cohort study approach would have required them to obtain laboratory analyses for measurements on all 4,480 subjects. Using a nested case–control design, however, they matched two control subjects to each of the cancer cases and evaluated the effects of these exposures using data on 333 individuals instead of 4,480. This approach also preserves a high proportion of specimens for subsequent analyses related to other endpoints, leaving the biologic specimen "bank" relatively intact. Nested case–control studies are an efficient method for maximizing the utility of a large cohort study.

A related study design that has been proposed for efficient sampling within a cohort is the case–cohort design (Prentice, 1986). In a case–cohort study a smaller subcohort is selected at the start of the study and biochemical indicator measurements made. The subcohort is then used as the comparison group for cases that arise in the cohort and subsequently have their baseline specimens analyzed. This design has the advantage of spreading the laboratory analysis workload over a longer interval. However, this design is hardly ever desirable in studies using biochemical indicators because any laboratory drift in measurement of the indicator would create a biased comparison, as could even subtle degradation of the case specimens during storage.

Another further design option for maximizing the efficiency of the use of biologic specimens is the possibility of pooling specimens. Aliquots of samples from individuals with a common characteristic (e.g., cases or controls) may be combined and analyzed as a single unit (Peto, 1983). This method provides an obvious economy by replacing many measurements with a single one, an advantage if the analytic test is particularly expensive. In addition, if the test requires a relatively large minimum sample volume relative to the total amount of sample available for each individual, the administrators of the specimens may be very reluctant to lose a large proportion of their samples. Pooling permits a smaller aliquot from each individual to be contributed and thus may be particularly suited for screening hypotheses for more labor-intensive and specimen-intensive investigation. Wahrendorf and colleagues (1986) measured retinol, beta-carotene, and alpha-tocopherol in 610 blood samples and found good relative agreement for retinol and beta-carotene between values measured in pools of 50 specimens and the means of the 50 individual values contributing to each pool. The major disadvantage of the pooling approach is that information is lost on the range of nutrient levels in each comparison group, and the mean levels are susceptible to outlying values about which only individual measurements yield information. In addition, the capacity to address issues of confounding and interaction is reduced. Because only a small number of laboratory measurements are made, the potential influence of technical error becomes large and needs to be carefully considered. Indeed, the expected differences between cases and controls are typically similar to the coefficient of variation for many laboratory measurements.

Contamination

Contamination can occur before, during, or after specimen collection. Precollection contamination is essentially restricted to environmentally exposed biologic specimens such as hair or nails. Hair may be particularly prone to superficial contamination due to its relative porosity and high surface-to-volume ratio. Selenium-containing shampoos, for instance, probably invalidate the use of hair as a substrate for selenium measurement in countries in which their use is widely prevalent (Morris et al., 1983). Attempts to deal with surface contamination by washing must be evaluated on a nutrient-by-nutrient basis, as the possibility of leaching relevant nutrients out of the sample must be considered.

Contamination during or after collection can occur for all types of specimens. The

definition of what constitutes contamination relates to the original concentration of the nutrient in question (Iyengar, 1987). Nutrients such as trace elements, with extremely low concentrations in biologic samples, are more susceptible to a small amount of introduced extraneous material than are nutrients with a greater original concentration. Much of the older published data on levels of many trace elements in biologic samples may be erroneous due to the lack of appreciation of the potential for contamination (Versieck, 1985). All needles, syringes, containers, and solutions that the specimen comes into contact with should be examined for their potential to contaminate the sample. The common anticoagulant EDTA, for instance, contains measurable quantities of iron, zinc, chromium, selenium, and other trace elements (Iyengar, 1987). Standard blood collection tubes and rubber stoppers may be contaminated with zinc; thus, specially prepared tubes should be used for zinc estimation (Smith et al., 1985). Indeed, the declining trends in reported normal values of several trace elements over recent decades may reflect greater control of contamination rather than any underlying secular change in intake (Iyengar, 1987). The articles by Versieck (1985) and Iyengar (1987) provide comprehensive reviews of current knowledge about contamination and trace element analysis.

Stability

Few nutrient measurements relevant to epidemiologic studies can be performed immediately after sampling. Some storage time is thus usual, and specimens may be stored for years or even decades in nested case–control studies. The stability of the relevant nutrients is thus a matter for concern.

If there is any possibility that a nutrient is not completely stable during storage, then identical handling of case and control specimens is again a critical requirement for preventing bias. This may not always be an easy requirement to fulfill. If cases are hospital derived, for instance, and controls are enrolled from the community, then exact matching of the time of day of specimen collection, temperature control, and the length of time between collection and analysis may be difficult to achieve. A log should be kept for each specimen of all events such as sample handling and freezer failure so that the history of the sample storage is known to investigators at the time of analysis. For many nutrients, information is limited on the effects of different methods of long-term storage. This poses a problem for the epidemiologist designing a prospective study or contemplating the analysis of a nutrient in an existing bank of biologic material. In general, simple elements may be less prone to degradation than complex proteins, and samples in which metabolic activity had ceased at the time of sampling, such as hair and nails, may be more stable than those in which enzymatic activities are potentially ongoing. The most common approach to long-term storage of blood components and urine has been freezing in an ordinary freezer ($-20°C$), an ultra-low freezer (approximately $-70°C$) or liquid nitrogen freezer ($-130°C$ or less). Lyophilization (freeze drying) may have advantages for certain samples.

In addition to the influence of duration of storage, the potential impact of multiple freeze–thaw cycles should be considered. At least one freeze–thaw cycle is almost inevitable, unless the entire frozen specimen is given to the laboratory and is thawed immediately prior to analysis. A strategy to minimize the number of freeze–thaw cycles specimens undergo is to pipette multiple aliquots of specimen the first time the original specimen is thawed; these can then be sent to multiple laboratories without further thawing, if, of course, the investigator has guessed correctly about the desirable aliquot sizes! In one of the few tests of multiple freeze–thaw cycles, Hsing et al. (1989) observed remarkably little difference in the mean concentrations of retinol, retinol-binding protein, total carotenoid, beta-carotene, lycopene, and total tocopherol in pooled plasma measured after two, three, and four freeze–thaw cycles. Nevertheless, these investigators recommend storing sera in several small aliquots to avoid unnecessary freeze–thaw cycles.

Specimen Quality Controls

Quality control procedures are as essential in the monitoring of collection and storage procedures as they are in the monitoring of the actual chemical analysis. Quality control, in this context, consists of two activities. Initially, the protocol for collection and storage must be validated with respect to protection from contamination. These procedures should be periodically reviewed. Nutrient stability during storage must also be assessed. This may be accomplished by forming a pool of samples and storing aliquots for periodic analysis. As the aliquots should have the same initial nutrient levels, monitoring these levels over time should provide information about sample stability and "laboratory drift." This procedure also allows calculation of the true between-run coefficient of variation percent ($CV\% = [SD/mean] \times 100\%$) relevant to the time course of an epidemiologic study in which samples may be analyzed over a period of months or years.

ANALYSIS

Practicing epidemiologists rarely have the time, the resources, or the laboratory expertise to actually perform the procedures involved in nutrient analysis. It is important, therefore, to maintain a close liaison with laboratory colleagues and to be aware of potential problems that will affect the interpretation of the exposure measure. Epidemiologists may obtain a rapid initial evaluation of the utility of a laboratory test by sending the laboratory blind specimens that reflect the population range of exposure to the relevant nutrient and splitting each specimen into two or more aliquots.

Calculation of the between-person $CV\%$ gives useful information on the ability of the test to discriminate between individuals, and an analysis of variance comparing different aliquots from the same person provides an assessment of the extent of random laboratory error.

Overview of Analytic Techniques

Much of the stimulus to use biochemical indicators has been derived from the advances that have been made in the measurement of the relevant compounds in biologic tissues. New methods have decreased the random error of measurements so that the small differences in means that are usually relevant to epidemiologic studies (see Chapter 3) may be detectable. Improvements in the lower limit of detection for many nutrients, particularly the trace elements, have meant that new exposure measures are now available.

Minimizing Systematic Error Bias

Reducing random measurement error augments the power of a study to detect between-group differences in that measurement. Reduction of the variance due to random error not only is the domain of the analytic chemist but also depends on the amount of money the epidemiologist (or funding agency) is prepared to spend on expensive analytic methods. Minimization of systematic misclassification or observation bias may be largely achieved by blinding the laboratory to case–control status and by eliminating systematic differences in the way case and control specimens are handled. Laboratory drift, or between-assay variation, occurs in most analytic techniques. It is thus desirable to analyze all specimens in a single run, if possible. Paired cases and controls should be analyzed consecutively (with the within-pair order randomized), and pairs should be randomly ordered with respect to variables of interest so that effects of order (within-run laboratory drift) are not attributed to another variable. If it is not possible to analyze all samples in a single run, then ensuring that cases and their controls are analyzed together in the same batch at least ensures the validity of the paired comparison.

Analytic Quality Control

Quality control is an essential aspect of any program of laboratory analysis. Analytic quality assurance has been called "an attitude of mind" (Parr, 1985), implying that constant awareness of the possibilities of error may be as important as adherence to formal procedures in the pursuit of analytic validity. Regular quantitative estimation of error, both random and systematic, is important. Controlling random error is largely a matter of estimating precision and fine-tuning analytic methods to improve it. The usual measure of precision is the $CV\%$. The within-run $CV\%$ is determined by dividing single samples into two or more aliquots and analyzing them together. To estimate the between-run $CV\%$, aliquots are analyzed in different runs, usually on different days. The larger the $CV\%$ inherent in a measurement technique, the larger will be the sample size necessary to derive stable estimates of the group mean. In general, one expects the within-run $CV\%$ to be less than the between-run $CV\%$, as there is more potential between runs for variation in room temperature, buffer concentrations, personnel, and so on. The between-run $CV\%$ is largely irrelevant if all samples are included in a single run. It is difficult to generalize about acceptable numerical values for the laboratory $CV\%$, as the degree of error acceptable depends on the number of samples available, the mean concentration of the nutrient, between-person variation, and a number of other factors. Reported values of within-run $CV\%$ for modern nutrient analytic procedures are often 5% or less, and this is well within the range of random error tolerable in most epidemiologic studies. It is important to note, however, that published $CV\%$ values may represent the performance of techniques in the hands of highly experienced investigators under optimal conditions and that more error may attend samples run in large batches, in other laboratories, or at later dates.

The other principal component of a quality-assurance program is the use of quality-control standards, either internal standards prepared within the laboratory or certified materials prepared by other laboratories. This not only provides a test of within-laboratory procedures but also allows comparison with other laboratories using the same certified materials, permitting more appropriate interpretation, or even pooling, of the results of different studies. Ideally, reference materials should be used to validate the analytic procedure over the whole relevant working range, not just a single point.

VALIDATION OF BIOCHEMICAL MEASURES AS INDICATORS OF DIETARY INTAKE

Before a biochemical indicator can be used as a measure of nutritional intake, it must be evaluated with respect to its sensitivity to intake of that nutrient. A validation procedure should also assess, if possible, the other important determinants of indicator concentration so that adjustment can be made for these in study design or analysis. Epidemiologists whose principal concern is the relation between diet and disease may be somewhat less interested in exploring the effects of diet on tissue nutrient levels, explorations that seem more appropriate for the metabolic enthusiast. If these indicators are to be used as measures of dietary exposure, however, then the epidemiologist is obviously responsible for ensuring that the exposure measure is a valid representation of long-term intake. In this respect, epidemiologists' requirements of biochemical indicators may be different from those of many nutritionists, who frequently prefer short-term measures of response to therapy. Several strategies are available to

define the relationships between long-term dietary intake and biologic levels.

Animal Studies

The exposure of laboratory animals to nutrients can be tightly controlled, and validation of a biochemical indicator can be attempted by measuring it in animals fed different nutrient intakes. Salbe and Levander (1987), for instance, demonstrated that feeding selenium to rats resulted in increases in hair and nail selenium in a dose–response manner. This approach, however, suffers from the general problem of animal studies, that is, concern about the generalizability of the conclusions to humans.

Geographic Correlation of Intake and Biologic Markers

Specimens from areas of known deficiency of a specific nutrient can be compared with specimens from average and high exposure areas. Thus, Morris and coworkers (1983) correlated geographic differences in selenium intake with group differences in nail selenium concentration. For example, specimens from New Zealand, an area known to have low selenium intake, had uniformly lower selenium levels than those from the United States (Fig. 9–2). With respect to blood measures, studies in New Zealand comparing residents with visitors indicate that plasma selenium concentration is more sensitive to short-term changes than erythrocyte selenium, which provides a selenium index integrated over several months, presumably due to the relatively slow turnover of red blood cells (Rea et al., 1979) (Fig. 9–3). This method has the appeal of using human subjects directly, under natural circumstances, without the potential ethical problems inherent in dietary manipulation. The major problem is that associated with all geographic correlation studies: the difficulty of identifying and controlling confounding factors. International differences in serum cholesterol levels, for instance, may be due to differences in exercise, body composition, or alcohol consumption, as

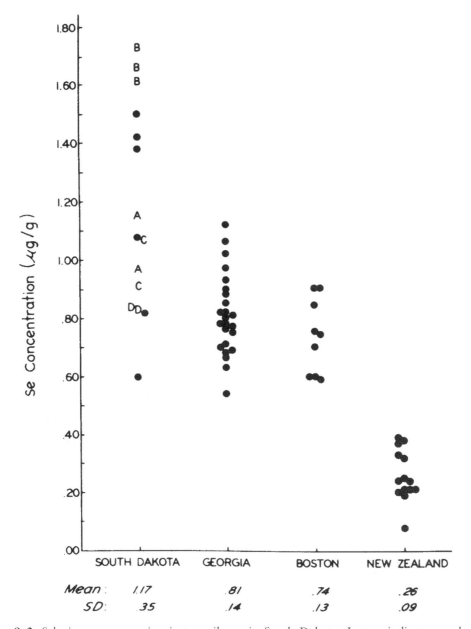

Figure 9–2. Selenium concentration in toenails from four regions. Selenium exposure is known to be unusually low in New Zealand, intermediate in Boston and Georgia, and unusually high in South Dakota. Letters indicate members of the same family; dots indicative unrelated persons. (From Morris et al., 1983; reproduced with permission.)

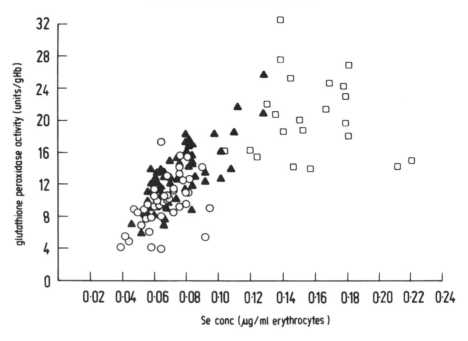

Figure 9–3. Relationship between selenium concentration of erythrocytes and glutathione peroxidase activity of whole blood for Otago patients (O); Otago blood donors (▲); and overseas subjects (□). (From Robinson and Thomson, 1981; reproduced with permission.)

well as differences in cholesterol and fatty acid intake. An important advantage of this approach is that it provides the opportunity for the exposure measure to reflect the long-term intake of settled individuals. Long-term nutrient intake is of greatest interest for most epidemiologic purposes and also the hardest to simulate in dietary manipulation studies.

Correlation With Individual Intake

An observational approach to validation in individuals is to estimate their dietary exposure and determine its relation with biochemical levels. For example, Swanson et al. (1990) calculated selenium intake from analysis of duplicate meals collected from 44 adults in South Dakota; selenium intake correlated well with serum ($r = 0.63$), whole blood ($r = 0.62$), and toenail ($r = 0.59$) selenium measurements. An efficient strategy is to select individuals on the basis of known exposure (e.g., vitamin supplement users). Thus, among U.S. women con-

suming selenium supplements, a linear dose–response relationship was observed between supplement dose and toenail selenium level (Hunter et al., 1987). Another efficient approach if the relevant nutrient has already been measured in a large number of samples is to identify individuals with extreme values and attempt to assess their dietary intake of the nutrient. Dietary intake may be estimated from the analysis of duplicate meals or from diet records, recalls, or food-frequency questionnaires. As long-term intake is usually the exposure of interest, methods with a long reference period are preferable. If the biochemical indicator has been independently validated and is known to reflect intake, then the study design can be reversed, and diet assessment methods can be validated against the biochemical marker.

Dietary Manipulation in Humans

A rigorous test of the relation between nutrient intake and a biochemical indicator may be achieved if a dietary manipulation study is feasible. These trials are usually limited to weeks or months, however, so the measure of dietary intake may be relatively short-term. These studies can take advantage of many of the desirable features of clinical trials, such as randomization, placebo control, or crossover designs. If the intervention involves extensive restructuring of normal diet, however, blinding of the subjects to treatment may not be possible. Studies of vitamin and mineral supplementation, for instance, have been invaluable in delineating the relation between intake and biochemical indicators, allowing, in some instances, complete assessment of the time integration of the dose–response relations. Most studies designed to evaluate indicators for epidemiologic use are performed on free-living subjects. If a more complete understanding of nutrient pathways is desired, then metabolic ward conditions may be necessary. It is desirable to collect information on other determinants of the biochemical measure to control for these in the analysis.

Several experimental studies of selenium intake have provided valuable information on the use of various biologic tissues as indices of selenium exposure. Selenium supplementation increases serum, plasma, and erythrocyte selenium levels (Luoma et al., 1985; C. D. Thomson et al., 1985; Neve et al., 1988; Longnecker et al., 1993). In an experiment to determine the metabolic fate of an oral dose of isotopically labeled selenomethionine, erythrocyte selenium concentration increased and washed out more slowly than plasma selenium, implying a lower sensitivity of erythrocyte selenium to transient changes in exposure (Griffiths et al., 1976). Among 10 Belgian adults supplemented for 60 days with 100 µg Se/day as selenomethionine, plasma selenium level was significantly increased after only 5 days of treatment, whereas erythrocyte selenium level increased only after 45 days (Neve et al., 1988). Similarly, when four New Zealand women consumed 200 µg/

day of selenium in a bread made from selenium-rich wheat, plasma and whole blood selenium levels increased earlier and decreased sooner in the postdosing phase than erythrocyte levels (Thomson C. D. et al., 1985). In an earlier experiment, erythrocyte selenium was still increasing after over 300 days of a selenomethionine supplement (Robinson and Thomson, 1981) (Fig. 9–4). Erythrocyte selenium, therefore, appears to be the preferable blood indicator of long-term exposure status. Whole blood, largely composed of plasma and erythrocytes, has intermediate properties, but suffers from the problem that changes in hematocrit affect selenium concentration. Toenail selenium levels probably provide the most time-integrated measure; Longnecker et al. (1993), using data from an intervention study in which two groups of four men consumed approximately 200 µg and 400 µg of selenium daily, observed that toenail selenium level provided a measure of selenium intake integrated over 26 to 52 weeks.

Repeat Measures

Repeated measures of an indicator over time provide some idea of the within-person variability and thus the likelihood that the indicator is a stable estimate of long-term intake. If repeated measures of a biochemical indicator vary substantially over time in the same individuals, then a single measure does not reflect long-term intake. This lack of consistency may occur because diet has truly changed over the interval between measurements or because the measure is overly sensitive to short-term influences, such as a recent meal. In either event, the single measurements with that indicator do not provide useful tests of hypotheses related to dietary intake over the period represented by the replicate measurements. If variation between repeated measurements is small, then two possibilities exist. The indicator may be a well-integrated measure of long-term intake, or it may be relatively insensitive to

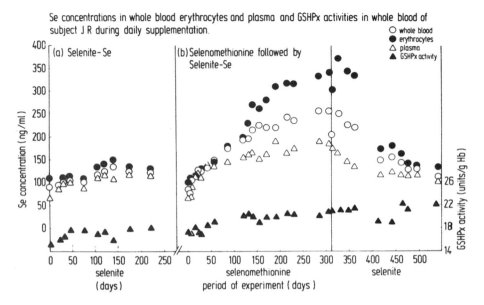

Figure 9–4. Response to daily supplements of 100 μg of selenium during almost 3 years: 31 weeks as selenite; 26 weeks without supplement; 44 weeks as selenomethionine; 26 weeks as selenite. (From Robinson and Thomson, 1981; reproduced with permission.)

both dietary intake and time. To distinguish between these possibilities, information is required from studies in which intake is known. For example, Taylor and colleagues (1987), in a study of the selenium status of 78 adults evaluated at four 3-month intervals, observed intraclass correlation coefficients (representing the average correlation between repeated measurements) of $r = 0.76$ for serum selenium and $r = 0.95$ for whole blood selenium level. This suggests that whole blood selenium level may be less susceptible to temporal variation and thus be a better index of long-term intake than serum selenium. Additional evidence that whole blood selenium level reflects dietary intake was, however, needed before it could be concluded that whole blood selenium level is the superior measure.

The importance of adjusting for relevant covariates in calculating correlation coefficients is demonstrated by the data of Gey and colleagues (personal communication) on vitamin E. The unadjusted correlation coefficient between measures of vitamin E separated by 6 years is $r = 0.65$, implying a satisfactory reproducibility. As previously discussed, however, vitamin E concentration is also strongly related to serum cholesterol level as it is transported in blood lipoproteins. The correlation over 6 years for repeated measures of cholesterol was also $r = 0.65$. This moderate correlation alone generates some correlation of vitamin E levels over time, even if there was no true correlation of serum vitamin E with dietary intake. In fact, adjusting for serum cholesterol reduced the vitamin E correlation to $r = 0.46$, indicating that a substantial proportion of the correlation for unadjusted vitamin E was due to the fact that serum cholesterol was relatively reproducible over the 6 years. Information on the within-person variance in a measure can be used to correct correlation coefficients or relative risks for attenuation due to random within-person variation in the biochemical parameter (see Chapter 12).

USE OF BIOCHEMICAL INDICATORS TO VALIDATE OTHER METHODS OF NUTRIENT INTAKE ASSESSMENT

The relatively few biochemical indicators that provide a sensitive and time-integrated reflection of nutrient intake can be used as reference methods to evaluate other measurements of these nutrients. This approach is less prone to correlated errors that may occur if a subject completes two self-reported forms of dietary assessment (e.g., a subject may distort his or her fat intake on a test method like a food-frequency questionnaire and in a reference method like diet diaries). As an example of this use of a biochemical indicator, Hunter et al. (1992) assessed the polyunsaturated fatty acid (PUFA) intake among 118 Boston-area men by food-frequency questionnaire and 2 weeks of diet records and by analyzing a subcutaneous fat aspirate (FA). The correlation between the food-frequency questionnaire and the diet record measurement of PUFA was $r = 0.60$; the conventional assumption would be that any error (i.e., the reason the correlation was not 1.0) was due to error in the food-frequency questionaire (Fig. 9–5). However, the correlation between the food-frequency questionnaire and FA was $r = 0.50$, equivalent to the correlation between the diet record and FA ($r = 0.49$). This not only tells us that both diet assessment methods measure PUFA intake reasonably well, but it also suggests that the food-frequency questionnaire and diet record may have roughly equivalent validities as a measure of the intake of PUFA over the 1 to 2 years prior to measurement. When using a biochemical indicator as a reference, care must be taken to use an indicator that measures nutrient intake during the period evaluated by the diet assessment instrument being tested. Also, the absence of a correlation between intake assessment and a biochemical indicator should not be automatically interpreted to imply that the intake assessment is invalid. The error may lie with the biochemical indicator if it is not sensitive to intake or is not time integrated. Indeed, because homeostatic and metabolic processes influence biochemical indicator levels, the correlation between an indicator and an assessment of dietary intake can be taken as an estimate of the *lower* limit of the validity of the diet assessment method (Kaaks, 1997).

SPECIFIC BIOCHEMICAL INDICATORS FOR SELECTED NUTRIENTS

The remainder of this chapter is devoted to a review of available biochemical indicators for selected nutrients of current epidemiologic interest. In this rapidly evolving field it is obvious that some of the information will be quickly superseded. Before and during any epidemiologic study employing a biochemical measurement, close collaboration with a biochemically oriented scientist performing the assay or closely familiar with the method, therefore, usually provides optimal results as well as stimulating intellectual exchange. An early review of this subject is that of Sauberlich and colleagues (1974). A report of an ad hoc panel assembled by the Federation of American Societies for Experimental Biology to advise the National Center for

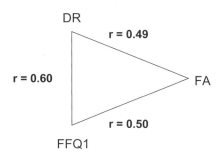

Figure 9–5. Intercorrelations between estimates of polyunsaturated fatty acid intake from a food-frequency questionnaire (FFQ), 2 weeks of diet records (DR), and subcutaneous fat aspirate (FA) among 118 Boston-area men. (From Hunter et al., 1992; reproduced with permission.)

Health Statistics on the conduct of the Health and Nutrition Examination Surveys (HANES) provides much valuable information (Klasing and Pilch, 1985), as does a book by Gibson (1990). A review by Riboli and colleagues (1987) contains much thoughtful detail on methodologic considerations, in addition to specific information on selected indicators of particular interest in cancer research. A review by Winn et al. (1990) contains much information about logistic procedures and policy issues associated with biologic specimen banks.

The overall approach in this section has been to focus on aspects of particular relevance to epidemiologic studies. These include the nature of the indicator itself, its relation to dietary intake and variation within-person over time, the general technical method of measurement and its error, the stability of the compound in storage, and nondietary factors that may influence levels. For many biochemical indicators it is apparent that this basic information is far from complete, and thus the format and detail vary between indicators. A further reason for variation is that we have attempted to make the depth of coverage proportional to the degree of current epidemiologic interest in each nutrient. Most readers will find this section more useful as a reference than as material to be consumed in its entirety.

Vitamin A

Vitamin A may be ingested either as a preformed retinyl ester (which can readily be converted to retinol, the primary form of vitamin A circulating in blood), or as provitamin A carotenoids (of the 600 known carotenoids, only 10% have provitamin A activity and can be converted to retinol in the intestinal epithelium). Preformed vitamin A is naturally found only in food from animal sources, whereas carotenoids are primarily obtained from fruits and vegetables, although a small amount is contained in dairy and seafood products. Postulated associations between vitamin A consumption and endpoints as various as xerophthalmia, childhood survival (Fawzi et al., 1993) and cancer (Sporn and Roberts, 1983) have created considerable interest in the biochemical assessment of vitamin A intake.

Retinol

Retinol can be accurately measured in serum and plasma; however, these measurements have only a limited interpretability as measures of dietary intake in well-nourished populations. In such populations, the liver stores at least 90% of the total body reserve of vitamin A (Olson, 1984) and buffers serum levels over a wide range of dietary vitamin A intake. Thus, serum levels are a poor reflection of vitamin A status unless the liver stores are either very depleted or highly saturated (Russell et al., 1984; Underwood, 1984). Plasma retinol levels are reasonably reproducible; among 265 women the intraclass correlation of four measurements made over 6 months was 0.58 (Liu et al., 1992). However, when 25,000 IU of retinyl palmitate (13,750 retinol equivalents—a dose more than five times a typical dietary intake) was given daily for 8 weeks to 15 healthy, U.S. adults, no appreciable increase in plasma retinol level was observed (Willett et al., 1983c). Wald and colleagues (1985), using supplements of between 10,000 and 36,000 IU of retinyl palmitate daily, demonstrated a small (2%) increase in serum retinol concentrations after 3 months of supplementation. A supplement of 10,000 IU of vitamin A daily for 4 weeks also resulted in a small, statistically significant mean increase in plasma retinol level (9% over baseline values) in a group of apparently healthy U.S. women previously identified as having relatively low plasma retinol levels (Willett et al., 1984b). The correlation between preformed vitamin A intake (estimated from a self-administered seimiquantitative food-frequency questionnaire) and plasma retinol was weak ($r = 0.17$ adjusted for age, gender, total caloric intake, and plasma lipids) and not statistically significant ($p = 0.12$). Among 1,182 participants in an intervention study, baseline serum retinol level was only weakly correlated with a food-frequency questionnaire estimate ($r = 0.10$) (Goodman et al., 1996). Thus, blood retinol measurements may be used in well-nourished populations to identify the rare persons with unusually low intakes, but are likely to misclassify individuals over a wide range of typical intakes. Blood retinol level may be a more sensitive indicator of vitamin A status in undernourished populations in which prolonged low intake of vitamin A is common. Patwardhan (1969) demonstrated a strong correlation between mean vitamin A intake and mean serum retinol levels using survey data from developing countries. The mean serum vitamin A levels in Indonesian children with night blindness or Bitot's spots, or both (signs of vitamin A deficiency), were less than two-thirds those of normal control children (Sommer et al., 1980). Plasma retinol concentrations of <10 mg/dl are usually associated with clinical signs of vitamin A deficiency (International Vitamin Consultative Group, 1993).

Retinyl Esters

Under normal conditions of vitamin A nutriture the concentration of retinyl esters is low (less than 5% of total serum vitamin A) (Smith and Goodman, 1976). When vitamin A intake is excessive, serum retinol level may be only slightly elevated, but serum retinyl esters are markedly increased. If hypervitaminosis A is an exposure of interest in an epidemiologic study, then a fasting retinyl ester level is probably the most discriminating test available.

Relative Dose–Response Test

The relative dose–response (RDR) test is based on the observation that in vitamin A–deficient individuals, retinol-binding protein (RBP) accumulates in the liver (Loerch et al., 1979; Campos et al., 1987). When a small vitamin A challenge is given, RBP-bound vitamin A is rapidly released into the blood. The method involves taking a blood sample immediately before and 5 hours after a small oral dose (e.g., 1,500 IU) of vitamin A. The RDR% is calculated as

$$\frac{\begin{array}{c}(\text{Plasma retinol at 5 hours})\\ -\ (\text{Plasma retinol at 0 hours})\end{array}}{(\text{Plasma retinol at 5 hours})} \times 100\%$$

Thus, higher values of RDR% are associated with decreased liver retinol stores. In a study of 12 children with liver disease, for instance, Amedee-Manesme and co-workers (1987b) report that five out of five children with RDR% values of >20% had total liver vitamin A concentrations of less than 20 µg/g, whereas six out of seven children with an RDR% of <10% had liver vitamin A values of more than 20 µg/g.

Like serum retinol, however, the RDR test is quite insensitive in well-nourished populations, and its utility in undernourished populations remains to be fully defined (Russell et al., 1984). Conditions that affect protein metabolism (malabsorption, liver disease, severe protein malnutrition) may influence RBP availability and thus confound the test (Russell et al., 1983). The necessity to obtain two blood samples 5 hours apart imposes substantial logistical constraints and limits compliance.

The Modified Relative Dose–Response Test

In the modified RDR assay, a single dose of a retinol analogue, 3,4-didehydroretinol (100 µg/kg body weight), is given orally and the ratio of 3,4-didehydroretinol/retinol is measured in serum 4 to 6 hours later (Tanumihardjo, 1993). In vitamin A deficiency a higher proportion of the test dose is released into the serum bound to RBP; ratios ≥0.06 are evidence of marginal vitamin A status. Reproducibility is high in healthy individuals (Tanumihardjo and Olson, 1991), and only one blood sample is required. Vitamin A deficiency as indicated by the modified RDR fell from 73% to 13% among Indonesian pregnant women given 35 daily doses of 8,000 IU of vitamin A (Tanumihardjo et al., 1996).

Serum Retinol-Binding Protein

Determinations of serum RBP levels have also been used to assess vitamin A status. Because RBP and vitamin A circulate as a trimolecular complex with transthyretin, little unbound RBP is present in blood. Measurement of RBP on a molar basis should be closely related to blood retinol. Indeed, serum retinol levels are highly correlated to RBP (Vahlquist et al., 1978; Willett et al., 1984a). Because RBP is also sensitive to the disease processes listed previously, it may not be a good indicator of vitamin A status when these conditions exist. Due to the dependence of retinol on RBP for transport to tissues, however, this may be a measure of the physiologically available form (Underwood, 1984).

Retinal Rod Function

Tests of night blindness are relatively sensitive measures of vitamin A deficiency (Russell et al., 1984). Classic testing of dark adaptation requires an expensive and delicate dark adaptometer and is thus unsuitable for large epidemiologic studies. The rapid dark adaptation test (Thornton, 1977) requires only simple equipment, takes 5 to 15 minutes to perform, and is practical for field studies (Solomons et al., 1982). False-positive results may occur due to congenital night blindness and other nutritional deficiencies that affect dark adaptation (e.g., zinc and protein deficiency). Substantial interobserver variation (Russell et al., 1984) and its inappropriateness for young children limit the use of this functional test in epidemiologic studies.

Impression Cytology

A relatively simple test for detection of severe vitamin A deficiency is the determi-

nation that ocular goblet cells are absent from the epithelium of the bulbar conjunctiva (Wittpenn et al., 1986; Amedee-Manesme et al., 1987a). In the simplest version of this test, a strip of filter paper is applied to the bulbar conjunctiva of the eye, the cells transferred to a glass slide, and the cells fixed, stained, and examined. This test, yet to be extensively evaluated in large populations, offers substantial logistic advantages relative to the collection, storage, and analysis of blood and may prove to be a useful clinical and research tool in developing countries. The test may be better suited for assessing the community prevalence of vitamin A deficiency than for individual assessment (Keenum, 1993).

Laboratory Techniques

High-performance liquid chromatography (HPLC), with either ultraviolet or fluorometric detection, is the preferred method for serum retinol determination in microsamples (Bieri et al., 1979; Kalman et al., 1987). W. J. Driskell and colleagues (1985) note that application of this technique to long-term frozen sera may result in substantial degradation of vitamin A during the procedure unless a modification of the technique is employed. Although older calorimetric techniques are reasonably comparable to HPLC for the measurement of total vitamin A (Pilch, 1985), HPLC has the advantage that it separates retinol from its esters (Bankson et al., 1986). The between-run CV% for serum retinol determined by HPLC by Biesalski and coworkers (1986) were 3.5% to 3.9%. Speek and colleagues (1986) have used an HPLC method to measure retinol in 5-μl aliquots of plasma collected from over 2,000 Thai children and report a within-assay CV% of 3.9% and a between-assay CV% of 5.0%.

RBP may be measured in serum obtained by finger prick using a radial immunodiffusion assay technique (Arroyave et al., 1982), which has the advantage that diffusion plates can be taken into the field for use.

Stability

HPLC recovery of retinol from heparinized plasma is equivalent to that from serum. Oxalate or citrate as anticoagulants, however, reduce retinol concentrations, and it is possible that EDTA also causes a slight reduction (Nierenberg, 1984; Peng et al., 1987). Retinol is sensitive to ultraviolet light; thus samples must be protected from any unnecessary sunlight exposure. Retinol and RBP concentrations in samples maintained at 26° to 28°C for 24 hours were 11.9% and 8.4% less, respectively, than in samples kept at 4°C (Mejia and Arroyave, 1983); in another experiment no difference was noted between retinol levels in plasma frozen immediately after separation and kept at room temperature for 24 hours (Craft et al., 1988). No statistically significant loss of blood retinol occurred in samples stored on ice and kept in the dark for 24 hours before centrifuging (Peng et al., 1987); however, only three samples from each of two subjects were tested. Serum retinol appears to be quite stable when frozen at -80°C for periods up to 7 years (Willett et al., 1984b; Comstock et al., 1995). No loss of retinol occurred in plasma stored at -20°C for 12 months (Peng et al., 1987). RBP is more stable than retinol during extended storage and may be a better indicator of initial vitamin A status, especially if storage conditions have been less than optimal (Olson, 1984).

Other Determinants of Serum Retinol

In addition to a variety of clinical conditions that alter serum retinol levels (Klasing and Pilch, 1985), serum retinol increases with age (Russell et al., 1983). Serum retinol levels also tend to be higher among men, among users of oral contraceptives (Bamji and Ahmed, 1978; Stryker et al., 1988), and users of postmenopausal estrogens (Nierenberg et al., 1989). Comstock and colleagues (1988) observed slightly lower serum retinol levels among male smokers and slightly higher levels among female smokers; Nierenberg et al. (1989) observed slightly lower plasma retinol lev-

els among smokers of both genders. In a study of 201 subjects, plasma retinol level was increased among subjects drinking more than 44 g of alcohol per day (Herbeth et al., 1988). Plasma retinol is positively correlated with plasma cholesterol (Russell-Briefel et al., 1985) for reasons that are not clear, as it is not transported in the lipoprotein particles.

Carotenoids

Carotenoids are red and yellow fat-soluble pigments synthesized in nature exclusively by photosynthetic microorganisms and plants. The basic structure of eight isoprenoid units can be modified by a variety of chemical reactions, producing a group of compounds with a heterogeneous biologic activity. The major carotenoids with vitamin A activity in common food sources are beta-carotene, alpha-carotene, gamma-carotene, and cryptoxanthin. Some carotenoid pigments have no detectable vitamin A activity (e.g., lycopene) (Underwood, 1984). Carotenoids have been suggested to play a role in protection from cancer, cardiovascular disease, and a variety of other diseases such as macular degeneration.

Plasma and Serum

Blood carotenoid levels are very sensitive to dietary intake as they are not closely regulated by homeostatic mechanisms. A daily beta-carotene supplement of 30 mg (5,000 retinol equivalents) approximately tripled plasma total carotenoid levels after 8 weeks (Willett et al., 1983c). In a similar study using 30 mg beta-carotene daily over 6 weeks, total plasma carotenoid levels increased by more than fourfold, but plasma beta-carotene level increased more than 25-fold (Micozzi et al., 1992). When a similar dose was fed as carrots, plasma carotenoid levels increased by twofold, while plasma beta-carotene level increased over fivefold. This suggests that blood levels are much more responsive to supplemental beta-carotene than to beta-carotene from food sources. In a study of 98 nonsmoking premenopausal women, the correlation between plasma beta-carotene level (averaged from two samples taken 1 week apart) and a 7-day diet record estimate of beta-carotene intake was $r = 0.51$ (Yong et al., 1994). Among 99 men and women in Minnesota, a food-frequency questionnaire estimate of intake of beta-carotene–rich foods was positively correlated with plasma levels ($r = 0.41$) (Campbell et al., 1994). Among 1,182 participants in the CARET randomized trial, the correlation between a food-frequency questionnaire estimate of beta-carotene intake and baseline plasma levels was $r = 0.24$ (Goodman et al., 1996). Among 24 male subjects who provided four consecutive weekly blood specimens, the within-to-between-person variance ratio for plasma beta-carotene level was 0.62 (intraclass $r = 0.79$) (Tangney et al., 1987). In the Basel Family Study the correlation for carotene (80% beta-carotene, 20% alpha-carotene) between two measurements taken 6 years apart was $r = 0.45$ (Stahelin et al., 1991). This sensitivity to intake and the capacity to integrate over a period of several weeks makes even a single measurement of blood beta-carotene a potentially good index of dietary intake.

Plasma levels of several other carotenoids are also reasonably correlated with intake estimates. In an intervention study, plasma alpha-carotene levels increased more than 12-fold in response to 272 g of carrots daily, and plasma lutein increased 2.5-fold in response to daily consumption of 300 g of broccoli (Micozzi et al., 1992). In the study of 98 women referred to above, correlations between average plasma measures (from two samples taken 1 week apart) and diet record estimates of intake were alpha-carotene, $r = 0.58$; beta-cryptoxanthin, $r = 0.49$; lutein plus zeaxanthin, $r = 0.31$; and lycopene, $r = 0.50$. Less is known about the within-person variability of plasma levels of these carotenoids, although the correlations over 1 week were all $r \geq 0.80$ (Yong et al., 1994).

Concern has been expressed that high doses of beta-carotene supplements may reduce blood levels of other carotenoids and/ or vitamin E, perhaps leading to deleterious effects of beta-carotene supplementation. Xu et al. (1992), for instance, observed a 40% reduction in plasma alpha-tocopherol after 9 months of supplementation with up to 60 mg/day of beta-carotene. However, no other studies have observed such changes (Bendich, 1992). Fotouhi et al. (1996) studied 29 men who had been taking 50 mg beta-carotene every other day for 12 years and compared their carotenoid and tocopherol levels with those of 30 men who had been taking a placebo. Beta-carotene plasma levels were 3.2 times higher in the supplemented group; no difference was seen in levels of alpha-carotene, lutein, cryptoxanthin, lycopene, or alpha-or gamma-tocopherol.

Adipose Carotenoid Concentration

Relatively few studies have assessed the relations of dietary intake of individual carotenoids and their levels in adipose tissue. Six months of supplementation with 30 mg/day of beta-carotene increased adipose tissue (obtained by subcutaneous FA) beta-carotene concentrations by sixfold among 25 subjects in the Netherlands (Kardinaal et al., 1995). The correlation between adipose and plasma beta-carotene levels among 77 subjects in this study was $r = 0.56$. However, the correlation between adipose beta-carotene measurements taken 4 months apart was only $r = 0.50$, and the correlation with diet assessed by a food-frequency questionnaire was $r = 0.20$ (n = 74, not statistically significant). The correlation over 4 months is substantially lower than is observed for repeated measures of adipose fatty acids, suggesting that relatively high turnover in adipose beta-carotene may be responsible for the weak association with dietary intake. Among 11 subjects who consumed a single 120-mg dose of beta-carotene, adipose beta-carotene levels were significantly increased by 50% after only 5 days, consistent with a shorter half-life for beta-carotene in adipose than that associated with fatty acids (Johnson et al., 1995). A similar weakness of correlations between adipose and dietary measures of alpha-carotene, beta-carotene, beta-cryptoxanthin, lutein, and lycopene has also been observed in a small study of Boston area women (Zhang et al., 1997). More data are needed to assess the utility of adipose carotenoid levels as indicators of intake of individual carotenoids.

Laboratory Techniques
Total carotenoid levels may be measured spectrophotometrically and by HPLC (Bieri et al., 1985; Motchnik et al., 1994). The HPLC method differentiates alpha-carotene, beta-carotene, cryptoxanthin, and lycopene from other carotenoids, the sum of these peaks accounting for more than 90% of the total carotenoids in a total lipid extract. The between-assay CV% for beta-carotene measured by HPLC on consecutive days by Vuilleumier and colleagues (1983) was 3%.

Storage
Beta-carotene, like retinol, is sensitive to light and heat. Beta-carotene levels declined by 6.7% per day in blood samples stored in ambient light at room temperature for 3 days (Hankinson et al., 1989). Samples stored at −20°C for 15 months deteriorated by approximately 24% for lutein/zeaxanthin, 51% for lycopene, 10% for alpha-carotene, and 26% for beta-carotene (Craft et al., 1988); thus storage at lower temperatures is necessary. Degradation of beta-carotene is detectable in samples stored at −40°C to −50°C (Comstock et al., 1993); however, no degradation was observed in levels of alpha-carotene, beta-carotene, cryptoxanthin, lutein, and lycopene after 4 years of storage at −70°C (Comstock et al., 1995).

Other Determinants of Carotenoids
The mean level of beta-carotene was approximately 20% higher among women in Washington County, MD, than the level observed among men, and there was a small increase with age (Comstock et al.,

1988). In a study of 1,750 participants in a clinical trial, plasma beta-carotene was 27% higher among women, and no association with age was observed (Nierenberg et al., 1989). Smoking is associated with reduced serum beta-carotene levels in both sexes (Stryker et al., 1988; Goodman et al., 1996), and these effects do not appear to be explained entirely by differences in dietary carotene intake. In multiple regression analyses controlling for dietary carotene, smoking, and alcohol consumption, the investigators observed a significantly positive association of carotene with plasma cholesterol and a significantly inverse relationship with plasma triglycerides. In a crossover study of the effect of daily ingestion of 30 g of alcohol among premenopausal women, alcohol increased plasma alpha-carotene and beta-carotene levels and decreased plasma lutein/zeaxanthin levels (Forman et al., 1995). In the Basel cohort, plasma beta-carotene levels tended to be higher from August to November and lower from January to May, presumably reflecting seasonal changes in diet (Gey et al., personal communication). More extreme seasonal variations may be seen in developing countries (see Chapter 3).

Vitamin E
Vitamin E is a powerful intracellular antioxidant that reduces lipid peroxidation and lowers transformation frequencies in in vitro carcinogenesis assays. In humans, clinical vitamin E deficiency has been reported only in premature infants, newborns, and persons with fat absorption disorders. The two principal forms of vitamin E in the diet are alpha-tocopherol and gamma-tocopherol, of which the former has the greater biologic activity. In a cross-sectional study, serum alpha-tocopherol concentrations were between 5.6 and 8.3 times higher than gamma-tocopherol concentrations (Behrens and Madere, 1986). Alpha-tocopherol is transported in blood as part of a lipoprotein complex, mainly in association with low-density lipoprotein cholesterol (LDL-C). Unlike vitamin A,

there is no principal storage organ for vitamin E.

Plasma and Serum

The most common tests of vitamin E nutriture have been measurements of either alpha-tocopherol or total vitamin E in blood. The major problem with interpretation of these results is confounding by blood lipid concentration due to the strong positive correlation between vitamin E levels and serum cholesterol and total lipid concentrations. Willett and colleagues (1983b) calculated correlations between plasma alpha-tocopherol and total cholesterol ($r = 0.59$), high-density lipoprotein (HDL) ($r = -0.02$), and LDL ($r = 0.56$, $p \leq 0.001$). A concurrent measurement of either serum cholesterol or LDL permits adjustment of the alpha-tocopherol measurement; without this, considerable misclassification results. Jordan et al. (1995) recommend a regression-based adjustment for both cholesterol and triglycerides simultaneously.

Plasma levels are moderately responsive to alpha-tocopherol intake. A daily alpha-tocopherol supplement of 800 IU (approximately 100 times usual dietary intake) approximately doubled plasma alpha-tocopherol levels in well-nourished adults after 16 weeks (Willett et al., 1983c). The simple correlation between vitamin E intake estimated from a self-administered semi-quantitative food-frequency questionnaire and plasma alpha-tocopherol level was $r = 0.12$ ($p = 0.19$). Adjustment for total plasma cholesterol level increased the correlation to $r = 0.28$ ($p = 0.02$), and adjustment for age, sex, total caloric intake, and plasma triglycerides further increased the partial correlation to 0.34 ($p = 0.006$). Jacques et al. (1994), among 139 Boston-area subjects, observed correlations of $r = 0.53$ for lipid-adjusted alpha-tocopherol measurements and estimated intake, including supplement, and $r = 0.35$ after excluding supplement users. Knekt and colleagues (1988) observed a correlation of $r = 0.65$ between measures of vitamin E obtained 4 years apart from 105 adults in Finland. Over a 6-year period, Gey and coworkers (personal communication) also found a correlation of $r = 0.65$ for repeated measures. Lipid adjustment, however, reduced this correlation to $r = 0.46$, implying that part of the original correlation was determined by the fact that cholesterol measurements were also highly correlated over the 6-year period, which exaggerated the correlation for total vitamin E. Nevertheless, it does appear that a single measurement of plasma alpha-tocopherol, adjusted for blood lipids, can represent long-term vitamin E intake to a modest degree, reflecting both a capacity to integrate intake over a few weeks and an element of long-term stability of diet among persons.

Erythrocyte Tocopherol

Alpha-tocopherol and its beta, delta, and gamma analogues can be measured in red blood cells by HPLC. The alpha-tocopherol content of both red blood cells and platelets increased in a dose–response manner among 20 subjects consuming 41 IU per day, and then 136 IU per day, for two 6-week periods (Lehmann et al., 1988).

Among 261 healthy Japanese children, red cell alpha-tocopherol level was highly correlated with plasma alpha-tocopherol level ($r = 0.59$, $p < 0.001$). It has been suggested that red blood cell alpha-tocopherol level may be a more appropriate measure of bioavailable vitamin E than plasma alpha-tocopherol level, particularly if lipid adjustment is not possible (Mino and Nagamatu, 1986). The exact relationships between vitamin E intake, plasma and red blood cell tocopherol, and plasma lipids, however, remain to be determined.

Adipose Tissue Tocopherol

As much as 90% of body tocopherol is contained in adipose tissue, and large oral doses of vitamin E increase tocopherol levels in adipose tissue obtained from patients with abetalipoproteinemia, whose initial levels are low (Traber and Kayden, 1987). Adipose alpha-tocopherol levels were only weakly correlated with vitamin E intake among 74 men and women in the Netherlands ($r = 0.24$); the correlation between specimens taken 4 months apart was $r = 0.78$ (Kardinaal et al., 1995). In a small sample of Boston-area women, vitamin E supplementation was associated with significantly higher adipose alpha-tocopherol levels, but the association with vitamin E intake from foods was weak (Zhang et al., 1997). A report of substantial variability in alpha-tocopherol/cholesterol ratios between needle FA from different anatomic sites suggests that standardization of needle aspirate site may be advisable (Handelman et al., 1988).

Erythrocyte Hemolysis Test

The ability of erythrocytes to resist hemolysis when stressed with hydrogen peroxide is a test of the antioxidant protection provided by vitamin E to the membrane (Russell et al., 1984). The rate of hemolysis is inversely correlated with serum tocopherol levels; however, deficiencies of other nutrients that play a role in cellular antioxidant function, such as selenium, may also influence the hemolysis rate (Klasing and Pilch, 1985). The requirement for fresh erythrocyte samples also limits the applicability of this test in many epidemiologic studies.

Pentane-Ethane Breath Test

The concentrations of pentane and ethane (products of the peroxidation of linolenic and linoleic acids) may be measured in exhaled breath by gas chromatography, and high levels may indicate vitamin E deficiency (Russell et al., 1984). Among 10 adult subjects, pentane output was negatively correlated with plasma vitamin E levels ($r = -0.66$, $p < 0.01$), and breath pentane was significantly reduced in 5 subjects supplemented with 1,000 IU of alpha-tocopherol for 10 days (Lemoyne et al., 1987). Application of this test in large epidemiologic studies is obviously problematic.

Laboratory Techniques

Although vitamin E may be measured by colorimetric or spectrofluorometric techniques, HPLC is probably the method of choice. HPLC allows the differentiation of alpha-tocopherol and gamma-tocopherol (Behrens and Madere, 1986) and the simultaneous determination of serum retinol (Bieri et al., 1979). Biesalski and colleagues (1986) report CV% between assays of 4% to 4.5%.

Storage and Stability

In a study of 12 adult subjects, alpha-tocopherol decreased by 1.6% per day, and gamma-tocopherol increased by 4.9% per day, in blood stored at room temperature in the dark for 3 days (Hankinson et al., 1989). Alpha-tocopherol was stable during 28 months of storage at both −20°C and −70°C (Craft et al., 1988), and both alpha-tocopherol and gamma-tocopherol were stable during 4 years of storage at −70°C (Comstock et al., 1995).

Measurement of Other Determinants

When assessing serum or plasma vitamin E levels, it is desirable to obtain concurrent measurements of serum cholesterol or total lipids. In multiple regression analyses controlling for plasma cholesterol, neither age nor sex was a significant predictor of plasma alpha-tocopherol (Willett et al., 1983b). Cigarette use and alcohol consumption also do not appear to be important determinants of plasma alpha-tocopherol levels (Comstock et al., 1988; Stryker et al., 1988). Jacques et al. (1995), among 665 elderly individuals, observed positive associations between intake of vitamin C and plasma alpha-tocopherol level and between carotenoid intake and plasma alpha-tocopherol level after adjusting for vitamin E intake, but the reasons for these associations are not clear.

Vitamin D

Epidemiologic studies of vitamin D status in children have traditionally been concerned with rickets, now relatively rare in developed countries subsequent to the for-tification of milk. Recent interest in vitamin D nutrition in adults centers on osteoporosis, hypertension (Sowers et al., 1985), and colorectal cancer (Garland et al., 1985).

Vitamin D may be absorbed from the diet or synthesized in the sun-exposed skin. The relative contributions of these two sources varies. Clinical vitamin D deficiency is unlikely, however, unless the supply from both sources is reduced (Parfitt et al., 1982). Vitamin D is synthesized in the skin by the ultraviolet catalyzed conversion of 7-dehydrocholesterol to vitamin D_3 (cholecalciferol), which is slowly released into the bloodstream bound to an alpha-globulin (transcalciferin). Elderly subjects exposed to a standard dose of simulated solar radiation achieve only 25% of the increase in circulating vitamin D that occurs in young adults, presumably due to the fact that skin thickness declines with age and thus 7-dehydrocholesterol levels are much lower in the elderly (Holick, 1995). Natural sources of dietary vitamin D are few; however, many countries fortify margarine or dairy products either with vitamin D_2 (ergocalciferol) or vitamin D_3. Plasma derivatives of vitamin D_2 are thus of exogenous origin only, whereas derivatives of vitamin D_3 may arise from either diet or skin (Parfitt et al., 1982). The metabolic fate of both of these compounds is the same.

Vitamin D must be metabolically activated before functioning biochemically, initially by 25-hydroxylation in the liver to form 25-hydroxyvitamin D (25[OH]D), the major circulating metabolite, and then by 1-alpha-hydroxylation in the kidney to produce 1,25-dihydroxyvitamin D (1,25 $[OH]_2$D), which is the active metabolite. This last step is the principal site of regulation of vitamin D metabolism. Formation of 1,25$(OH)_2$D is increased by low serum phosphate levels and by low serum calcium mediated by parathyroid hormone. Correction of these deficits reduces the stimulus

for 1-alpha-hydroxylation, thus closing the feedback loop (Haussler and McCain, 1977; DeLuca, 1979). Cellular receptors for 1,25$(OH)_2$D have been found not only in the intestine and bone but also in many other tissues, suggesting that 1,25$(OH)_2$D is fundamental to the metabolism of many cell types, probably because of its role in intracellular calcium regulation (Dickson, 1987).

D25(OH)D

The most useful measure of vitamin D status is the plasma level of the major circulating metabolite 25(OH)D (Parfitt et al., 1982; Russell et al., 1984). In six normal subjects, more than 80% of the total 25(OH)D existed in the form 25(OH)D_3 (Haddad and Hahn, 1973). Substantial seasonal variation exists, especially in elderly populations, with plasma 25(OH)D levels reaching a nadir in winter and rising during the summer, presumably reflecting seasonal ultraviolet-sunlight exposure (Holick, 1995). Values are higher in men than women and higher in vitamin D supplement users than nonusers (Omdahl et al., 1982). In an international correlation study, serum 25(OH)D level was inversely related to latitude and positively correlated with mean vitamin D intake (McKenna et al., 1985). In countries with vitamin D fortification of foods, the population most likely to be both deprived of sunlight and inadequate consumers of dietary vitamin D is the elderly. Significantly lower plasma 25(OH)D concentrations in elderly subjects than in younger controls have been demonstrated in several studies (Omdahl et al., 1982; Parfitt et al., 1982). Vitamin D insufficiency in the elderly can be prevented by increasing sunlight exposure and/or consumption of 100 µg (400 IU) of vitamin D daily (Holick, 1995).

In a study of 373 healthy, noninstitutionalized women, Sowers and colleagues (1986) observed a weak ($r = 0.11$) positive correlation between estimated vitamin D intake from food (based on a 24-hour recall) and serum 25(OH)D level. This correlation improved to $r = 0.24$ when vitamin D from supplements was included in the diet score. The correlation between estimated sunlight exposure and serum 25(OH)D was $r = 0.26$. In a study of 139 subjects, a food-frequency questionnaire estimate of vitamin D intake including supplements was more strongly correlated with plasma 25(OH)D level ($r = 0.35$) than when supplement users were excluded ($r = 0.25$) (Jacques et al., 1993). Newton and colleagues (1985) investigated the relationship between vitamin D intake and plasma 25(OH)D among 57 institutionalized elderly women (whose sunlight exposure was minimal). Both vitamin D_2 and vitamin D_3 intakes were strongly correlated with plasma 25(OH)D_2 and 25(OH)D_3 levels, respectively, as were total vitamin D intake and total plasma 25(OH)D level ($r = 0.55$). In a study of 125 patients with hip fractures (Lips et al., 1987), a significant correlation was observed between vitamin D intake and serum 25(OH)D level only among patients with low sunshine exposure ($r = 0.54$). These data suggest that sunshine exposure is the most important determinant of total 25(OH)D level and that total 25(OH)D level is a better marker of dietary intake in subjects with low sun exposure.

In patients with hypervitaminosis D, plasma 25(OH)D levels were approximately 15 times higher than those of normal controls (Hughes et al., 1976). As this was exogenous vitamin D, most of the plasma metabolites were of the 25(OH)D_2 form. Hypercalcemia frequently coexists with high levels of 25(OH)D and is a useful marker of hypervitaminosis D (Klasing and Pilch, 1985).

1,25(OH)₂D
Although measurement of 1,25(OH)₂D is a direct measurement of vitamin D hormone activity, it is not a good reflection of vitamin D nutritional status because of the influences of calcium and phosphate levels and parathyroid hormone, described previously.

Serum Alkaline Phosphatase Activity
Alkaline phosphatase activity was used as an indirect measure of vitamin D status before the availability of direct measurements of vitamin D metabolites. Alkaline phosphatase activity increases in proportion to vitamin D deficiency; however, it is susceptible to other disease processes such as Paget's disease, hyperparathyroidism (increased), and protein-energy malnutrition (decreased), which may confound the relation with vitamin D (Sauberlich et al., 1974).

Methods
Until recently, a competitive protein-binding assay was widely used to measure 25(OH)D (Belsey et al., 1974). Measurement of 1,25(OH)₂D, and distinction between 25(OH)D_2 and 25(OH)D_3, can be achieved chromatographically (Omdahl, 1978). HPLC for measurement of vitamin D metabolites is now the method of choice (Klasing and Pilch, 1985).

Storage
25(OH)D concentrations were significantly reduced by 9.3% in plasma stored for 11 months at $-18°C$, suggesting that long-term storage may not be feasible if vitamin D analyses are desired (Norris et al., 1986) or that colder temperatures are needed.

Vitamin K

Vitamin K is essential for the activation of four proteins in the clotting cascade prothrombin, factor VII, factor IX, and factor X; deficiency results in a hemorrhagic tendency. Vitamin K occurs in two forms, phylloquinone, found in foods, and the menaquinones, produced by bacteria (Suttie, 1992). About half of the human vitamin K requirement is derived from green leafy vegetables, meat, and dairy products and the remainder from biosynthesis by the intestinal flora (Olson, 1980). As vitamin K is widely distributed in food sources, and endogenously synthesized in the gut, vitamin K deficiency is unusual in healthy adults, and vitamin K status is a weak indicator of vitamin K intake. Newborn infants born without intestinal flora and adults with fat malabsorption syndromes, liver disease, or inflammatory bowel disease or taking gut-sterilizing antibiotics may be prone to vitamin K deficiency.

Vitamin K status has traditionally been determined by functional methods that measure prothrombin activity. Recent development of immunochemical assays has made direct measurement of phylloquinone in plasma feasible. The concentrations of undercarboxylated prothrombin and osteocalcin are also used because the carboxylase enzyme is vitamin K dependent.

Functional Assays
Of the many tests for bleeding abnormalities, the most specific for vitamin K deficiency is the prothrombin time, which tests the time plasma takes to clot when excess calcium and thromboplastin are added. The prothrombin time does not become prolonged until circulating prothrombin is less than 40% of normal. Thus, it is not a good test for mild vitamin K deficiency (Russell et al., 1984).

Direct Assays
Recently, HPLC has been used to measure vitamin K in human plasma (Shearer et al., 1982). Immunoassays for the direct measurement of both normal prothrombin and the undercarboxylated forms that appear during vitamin K deficiency (Blanchard et al., 1981) are much more sensitive indicators of mild vitamin K deficiency than the prothrombin time. The undercarboxylation of serum osteocalcin is reduced by phylloquinone supplementation in postmenopausal women (Knapen et al., 1989) and newborn babies and their mothers (Jie et al., 1992) and is inversely correlated with plasma phylloquinone concentrations ($r = 0.35$, $p < 0.001$) (Sokoll and Sadowski, 1996).

Measurement of Other Determinants
Information about disorders interfering with endogenous synthesis (e.g., bowel disease) or requiring chronic antibiotic treatment is useful in the interpretation of vitamin K status (Olson, 1987). Undercarboxylated prothrombin and osteocalcin, and plasma phylloquinone, have variable relations with age, gender, and menopause (Sokoll and Sadowski, 1996); thus, these need to be carefully controlled for in epidemiologic analyses.

Vitamin C

Vitamin C occupies a special place in the history of nutritional epidemiology because the discovery that scurvy was preventable by dietary manipulation remains a classic demonstration of the relationship between a specific dietary deficiency and a specific disease. Indeed, James Lind's study (1753) of the treatment of scurvy was one of the first intervention studies performed (MacMahon and Pugh, 1970), although the sample size he used (two patients for each treatment) was small by modern standards! Enthusiasm for high-dose administration of vitamin C as a treatment for cancer (Cameron and Pauling, 1978) and the suggestion that low vitamin C intake may predispose to cancer (Cameron et al., 1979) have led to renewed epidemiologic interest in this vitamin.

The pharmacokinetics of vitamin C are well described. Over the range of usual dietary intake, vitamin C is readily absorbed from the small intestine, the absorption efficiency being 90% or more (Olson and Hodges, 1987). The unadjusted correlation coefficients between questionnaire-derived dietary ascorbic acid intake and plasma and leukocyte ascorbic acid concentrations in a heterogenous population were $r = 0.43$ and $r = 0.31$, respectively (Loh, 1972). Among 196 Scottish men, the partial correlations (adjusted for total energy intake, body mass index, and serum cholesterol level) between a food-frequency questionnaire estimate of vitamin C intake and serum vitamin C values were $r = 0.55$

(for smokers) and $r = 0.58$ (for nonsmokers) (Bolton-Smith et al., 1991). Vitamin C is not protein bound and thus circulates freely between plasma and tissues, with concentrations in certain tissues being 3 to 10 times higher (Olson and Hodges, 1987). As ascorbic acid intake increases, plasma, serum, buffy coat (platelets and leukocytes), and leukocyte levels increase monotonically, although the rate of increase levels off as intake approaches the upper end of the normal range (Basu and Schorah, 1982; Jacob et al., 1987). Saturation of plasma is achieved at 1,000 mg/day (Levine et al., 1996). When dietary vitamin C is completely eliminated, ascorbic acid becomes undetectable in plasma after 35 to 40 days, in whole blood after 80 to 90 days, and in leukocytes after 100 to 120 days (Baker et al., 1980). This suggests that leukocyte vitamin C level would be a preferable measure of long-term intake, whereas plasma and serum levels reflect more recent intake (Jacob et al., 1987). This sensitivity to short-term intake was reflected in the Basel study in which the correlation between plasma vitamin C values in men obtained 6 years apart ($r = 0.28$) was much lower than the correlations obtained for vitamin E and beta-carotene (Gey, personal communication). This suggests that a single plasma vitamin C determination will misclassify many individuals with respect to their actual long-term intake. The fact that leukocytes become saturated at the low daily intake of 100 mg (Levine et al., 1996) means that plasma or whole blood is the most appropriate measure despite their higher within-person variability. The best method for measuring vitamin C nutritional status is total body pool estimation using isotope dilution or excretion techniques. Although inapplicable to large studies, they remain the standard for evaluating other methods.

Urinary ascorbate is a less sensitive measure than plasma over the normal range of vitamin C intake, but as renal clearance increases at high intakes (when the plasma values plateau), urinary measures may identify megadose vitamin C supplement users.

Methods

The classic method for blood and serum vitamin C measurement has been derivatization with 2,4-dinitrophenylhydrazine with calorimetric analysis. HPLC methods are available and are associated with recoveries of almost 100% and high precision (Margolis and Davis, 1988).

Stability

Without special preservation, vitamin C deteriorates rapidly during frozen storage (Basu and Schorah, 1982). Plasma samples should be acid stabilized (e.g., with trichloroacetic or metaphosphoric acid) and frozen at $-70°C$. Vitamin C in samples stabilized with metaphosphoric acid were stable at $-70°C$ after 3.5 years of storage.

Measurement of Other Determinants

Ascorbic acid levels are higher in the plasma and leukocytes of vitamin C supplement users. Several studies have demonstrated lower plasma and leukocyte vitamin C levels among cigarette smokers (Brook and Grimshaw, 1968). Gey and colleagues (personal communication) identified seasonal variations in plasma vitamin C similar to, but weaker than, those observed for beta-carotene. Acute and chronic infections also lower plasma vitamin C levels (Irwin and Hutchins, 1976).

Vitamin B_1 (Thiamine)

Vitamin B deficiency is the cause of beriberi, which principally occurs in regions where polished rice is the staple food. In developed countries, improved nutrition and thiamine fortification of flour has made clinical vitamin B_1 deficiency rare, except among patients with chronic gastrointestinal syndromes and chronic alcoholics, in whom thiamine deficiency may cause Wernicke's encephalopathy. Iber and colleagues (1982) have estimated that 5% of U.S. adults over 60 years old have impaired thiamine status and that the prevalence is higher among the poor, the chronically ill, and the institutionalized. The principal dietary thiamine sources are cereals, legumes, other fresh vegetables, pork, and beef

The best method for assessing thiamine nutriture in the general population is the measurement of the stimulation of erythrocyte transketolase by thiamine pyrophosphate (TPP) (Sauberlich et al., 1974). Transketolase is an enzyme in the pentose phosphate pathway and requires TPP. The assay measures transketolase activity before and after the addition of TPP, and a large enhancement of enzyme activity by TPP implies a relative deficiency of endogenous thiamine (Sauberlich et al., 1974). Recent improvements in the precision of this test, and the development of automated procedures, make this method more applicable to large studies (Sauberlich, 1984). Basu and colleagues (1974) have developed a calorimetric method to measure transketolase activity in as little as 50 µl of whole blood. However, Jacques et al. (1993) obtained a correlation of $r = 0.02$ between this measure and thiamine intake measured by a food-frequency questionnaire among 139 subjects.

Although HPLC is a precise technique for measuring vitamin B_1 in plasma and whole blood (Bettendorff et al., 1986), this is not a useful measure of thiamine status because even in deficiency the reduction in blood thiamine level is small. Similarly, urinary thiamine level is not a good index of thiamine nutriture over the normal range of intake, although it may be useful to confirm clinically suspected thiamine deficiency (Sauberlich, 1984). The recent development of HPLC methods to measure thiamine in erythrocytes and whole blood (Herve et al., 1994) suggests that direct measurement may become the method of choice; however, the relation of these measurements with thiamine intake remains to be determined.

Methods
Automated methods of measuring erythrocyte transketolase stimulation provide reproducible and sensitive results that correlate well with manual methods (Waring et al., 1982). The coefficient of variation between repeated determinations using an automated method was 2.7% (within-run) and 4.1% (between-run) (Doolman et al., 1995).

Storage and Stability
Long-term stability of erythrocyte transketolase is uncertain.

Measurement of Other Determinants
Subjects with diabetes mellitus and polyneuritis have low erythrocyte transketolase activity independent of thiamine intake, whereas activity is increased in patients with pernicious anemia (Kjosen and Seim, 1977). Heavy alcohol intake not only inhibits thiamine absorption but affects its metabolism (Iber et al., 1982).

Vitamin B_2 (Riboflavin)
Clinical riboflavin deficiency is rare in developed countries. The principal dietary sources are dairy foods, meat, and riboflavin-enriched flour.

The best indicator of riboflavin nutritional status is the erythrocyte glutathione reductase (EGR) assay. This measures the increase in activity of the enzyme glutathione reductase after the in vitro addition of flavin adenine dinucleotide (FAD). This is expressed as the erythrocyte glutathione reductase assay coefficient (EGRAC), which is the ratio of enzyme activity with and without added FAD (Tillotson and Baker, 1972). In normal subjects little increase occurs, whereas in those with an inadequate intake of riboflavin the increase is marked, and guidelines for the interpretation of EGRAC have been given (McCormick, 1985). Jacques et al. (1993) observed a correlation of $r = -0.13$ between this test and estimated riboflavin intake, consistent with the suggestion that the assay only reflects riboflavin intake at very low intake levels.

In a study of the behavioral effects of riboflavin restriction (Sterner and Price, 1973), the EGRAC rose monotonically with increasing length of riboflavin depletion and then returned to baseline during the repletion period. EGRAC was a more stable index of riboflavin status than urinary riboflavin, which displayed more within-person variation. Confirming a high EGRAC value with a low urinary riboflavin value has been recommended for the accurate diagnosis of riboflavin deficiency (Horwitt, 1987). Direct measurement of riboflavin in plasma is possible using HPLC. Oral doses of riboflavin result in a rapid transient increase in plasma riboflavin levels with a half-life of less than 5 hours (Zempleni et al., 1996). This sensitivity to short-term intake suggests that blood riboflavin levels may not be good indicators of long-term intake.

Methods
For the EGR assay, erythrocytes are separated soon after blood collection and then may be frozen. Only a small sample is required, and automated calorimetric methods are available (Sauberlich, 1984).

Measurement of Other Determinants
The EGR assay is not a good measure of riboflavin nutriture in persons with glucose-6-phosphate dehydrogenase deficiency (Thurnham, 1972) and certain endocrine disorders. A modest circadian variation in plasma and urinary riboflavin levels, with lower concentrations in the afternoon, has been described (Zempleni et al., 1996).

Vitamin B_6

The term *vitamin B_6* embraces a family of compounds with a structural relationship to pyridoxal 5'-phosphate (PLP). Vitamin B_6 occurs naturally in three forms, pyridoxal, pyridoxamine, and pyridoxine, which are converted in the liver to PLP (Leklem, 1996). This enzyme has a function in over 100 different enzyme systems, most of which are involved in amino acid and protein metabolism (Sauberlich et al., 1974). Frank clinical vitamin B_6 deficiency is uncommon, although among at-risk groups such as the elderly (Driskell, 1978) and adolescent girls (J. A. Driskell et al., 1985) inadequate vitamin B_6 status, measured biochemically, may be more prevalent. Low vitamin B_6 intake has been implicated in the etiology of cancer (Thanassi et al., 1985) and coronary heart disease (Willett, 1985).

Measures
Several different approaches to vitamin B_6 status assessment exist, and the most physiologically appropriate measure has yet to be determined (Reynolds and Leklem, 1985). The most common procedure is the direct measurement of plasma PLP. PLP is the major circulating and coenzymatic form of vitamin B_6, comprising over half the total body pool (Lumeng et al., 1985). In an experiment in which subjects ingested constant diets that were normal, restricted, or supplemented with vitamin B_6, plasma PLP level discriminated well between the different dietary regimens, and there was low within-person fluctuation of plasma PLP level. A dose–response relation exists between increasing vitamin B_6 supplement dose and plasma PLP level (Schultz and Leklem, 1985). Response to oral vitamin B_6 supplementation in previously unsupplemented subjects, however, is rapid (Thakker et al., 1987), with a half-life of less than 48 hours after supplementation (Mascher, 1993), suggesting that PLP is a better measure of short-term than long-term intake. In a study of 19 adults, Schuster et al. (1984) observed a correlation of $r = 0.61$ between plasma PLP level and vitamin B_6 intake on the previous day. This may be the reason that only modest correlations were found by Willett (1985) between a food-frequency questionnaire estimate of vitamin B_6 intake over 1 year and a single fasting plasma PLP level among 280 healthy men and women ($r = 0.37$ for men and $r = 0.39$ for women).

Vitamin B_6 measurements in random morning urine samples have been found to correlate reasonably well with 24-hour excretion (Sauberlich et al., 1974). Urinary vitamin B_6 may be even more responsive to recent dietary intake than plasma PLP level, however, and thus a poorer indicator of long-term intake. The measurement of the principal metabolic endproduct of vitamin B_6, 4-pyridoxic acid (4PA), has also been found to reflect vitamin B_6 intake when measured in 24-hour urine collections (Schultz and Leklem, 1985). 4PA measured in random urine samples is correlated ($r = 0.72$) with 4PA in 24-hour urine samples (Schuster et al., 1984).

Measurements of erythrocyte transaminase enzymes, such as glutamate oxaloacetate transaminase and aspartate aminotransferase, provide a limited indication of vitamin B_6 status (Sauberlich et al., 1974). Liu et al. (1992) measured AST activity among 265 women and obtained an intraclass correlation of 0.65 for four measurements over 6 months; however, correlations with calculated vitamin B_6 intake were negative. Jacques et al. (1993) observed similar inverse correlations, suggesting that the enzyme response is saturated at normal levels of intake. A stimulation test measuring the in vitro effect of adding PLP also lacks sensitivity and specificity (Sauberlich, 1984). Another functional test, the tryptophan load test, measures the excretion of tryptophan metabolites in the urine after a tryptophan load, testing the integrity of the tryptophan metabolic pathway, which requires PLP as a coenzyme for several reactions. Many factors other than vitamin B_6 intake affect tryptophan metabolism, and the necessity for a 24-hour urine collection makes this test unwieldy for large field studies.

Methods
Several well-validated chemical and enzymatic assays for measuring PLP in plasma exist (Sauberlich, 1984). HPLC procedures have the advantage that they can be used to separate and quantitate the different vitamin B_6 compounds. Vitamin B_6 measurements in finger prick blood samples correlated well with measurements using venous blood (Andon and Reynolds, 1987).

Storage
Howard and colleagues (1984) found PLP levels to be highly stable in plasma frozen at $-20°C$ over a 700-day period. Based on 113 determinations of aliquots from a stored pool over this interval, the rate of decline was only 2.2% per year. Camp and coworkers (1983) found PLP to be stable in plasma stored at $-80°C$ for at least 10 days.

Measurement of Other Determinants
Willett (1985) observed little relationship between plasma PLP and age, gender, or obesity. In a study of 10 men aged 20 to 30 and 10 aged 60 to 70 years, no differences in baseline plasma PLP levels or in the bioavailability of radiolabeled pyridoxine were observed (Ferroli and Trumbo, 1994). A transient increase in plasma PLP level and urinary vitamin B_6 occurs after strenuous physical activity (Leklem, 1985; Manore et al., 1987), and women using oral contraceptives or postmenopausal estrogens may be at higher risk of developing vitamin B_6 deficiency (Miller, 1985). Certain drugs and ethanol also lower plasma PLP levels (Bhagavan, 1985), as can increased protein intake and smoking (Leklem, 1990).

Folacin and Folic Acid
Folacin is a generic term for compounds with chemical structures and nutritional functions similar to folic acid (also called *pteroylglutamic acid*). The principal dietary sources of folacin are leafy vegetables, fruits, fortified cereals, and tea. Between one-half and two-thirds of ingested folacin is absorbed (Herbert, 1987). Folacin analogues function as coenzymes in the metabolism of single-carbon compounds, in particular, nucleic acid synthesis and amino acid metabolism. N-5-methyltetrahydrofolate is the methyl donor in the conversion of homocysteine to methionine;

thus, folate levels are inversely associated with plasma homocysteine (Selhub et al., 1993).

The principal manifestation of folate deficiency is megaloblastic anemia. Inadequate folate intake in the periconceptional period is a major cause of neural tube defects in infants (see Chapter 18). In the second National Health and Nutritional Examination survey, 1976–1980 (NHANES II), the greatest prevalence of low folate status was among women of childbearing age. Folate deficiency and megaloblastic anemia are more common in developing countries. Low folate intake may also be related to heart disease and colorectal cancer (Selhub and Rosenberg, 1996).

Measures

The most commonly employed assays of folacin nutriture are serum and red blood cell folate levels. Serum levels of folate decline 3 weeks after the initiation of a low folate diet; however, red blood cell folate level remains in the normal range for approximately 17 weeks (Herbert, 1987). The decrease in red blood cell folate level coincides closely with the depletion of liver folate stores (liver is the major storage organ for folate) and the onset of morphologic abnormalities in erythrocytes. Red blood cell folate correlates well with dietary folate intake (Bates et al., 1982) ($r = 0.51, p = 0.02$, among 19 elderly subjects). Serum folate level also correlates well with folate intake ($r = 0.56$ among 385 members of the Framingham Heart Study) (Selhub et al., 1993), as does plasma folate level ($r = 0.63$ among 139 Boston-area subjects) (Jacques et al., 1993).

An alternative approach to folacin status assessment is the measurement of polymorphonuclear leukocyte lobe counts. Hypersegmented neutrophils appear in the bone marrow after about 5 weeks of folate deficiency and in the blood after about 7 weeks (Herbert, 1987). Hypersegmentation is commonly assessed as the percentage of

polymorphonuclear leukocytes in peripheral blood smears with five or more lobes or for a more rapid assessment, the presence or absence of a single six-lobed cell. Polymorphonuclear leukocyte hypersegmentation may also be due to vitamin B_{12} deficiency and is an unreliable indicator of folacin deficiency during pregnancy (Sauberlich, 1984).

Methods

The two principal approaches to folacin measurement in serum and red blood cells have been microbiologic and radiodilution assays. The microbiologic assay, using the growth dependency of *Lactobacillus casei* on folacin, is regarded as the standard procedure for folacin measurement in biologic specimens. A variety of radiodilutables exist in commercial kit form, although there is some concern over their validity (Sauberlich, 1984). Both methods were used in NHANES II, and both were subject to relatively high within-run CV%s (on the order of 10% to 20%) (Senti and Pilch, 1984). Independent quality control and validation are, therefore, desirable for investigators using either method. In the Framingham Heart Study, Selhub et al. (1993) used both measures on a subset of 385 men and women. The correlation between folate intake measured by a semiquantitative food frequency questionnaire and plasma folate measured by the microbiological assay was stronger ($r = 0.56$) than for the radioassay ($r = 0.43$).

Storage

The effect of storage on measures of folacin status is uncertain.

Measurement of Other Determinants

Serum and red blood cell folate levels are reduced in smokers and in many pregnant or highly parous women (three live births) and are increased in multivitamin supplement users (Senti and Pilch, 1984). Alcohol and prescription drugs (e.g., folate antagonists, phenytoin, and oral contraceptives) may antagonize folacin absorption. Red blood cell folate level may also be reduced in patients with a primary vitamin B_{12} deficiency (pernicious anemia) (Sauberlich et al., 1974).

Selenium

Selenium has attracted much scientific attention due principally to its possible role as a cancer-preventive agent (Schrauzer et al., 1977; Clark, 1985; Willett, 1986; Clark et al., 1996). Low selenium intake has been linked with a regional cardiomyopathy in China (Keshan Disease Research Group of the Chinese Academy of Medical Sciences, 1979).

Measures

As previously described, several lines of evidence indicate that selenium may be meaningfully measured in blood components and that erythrocyte selenium level is probably superior to serum selenium level as a measure of long-term intake. The antioxidant function of the selenium-dependent enzyme glutathione peroxidase, measured in plasma, serum, erythrocytes, platelets, or whole blood, may be a useful functional test of selenium status. Glutathione peroxidase activity is reduced among subjects with low serum selenium level (Thomson et al., 1977) and increases with selenium supplementation if a deficiency exists (C. D. Thomson et al., 1985). Enzyme activity, however, plateaus in selenium-replete individuals and hence is a poor measure of selenium intake among persons with moderate and high exposure. Thus, in Finland, which had low levels of dietary selenium, the addition of selenium to fertilizers substantially blunted the increase in platelet glutathione peroxidase activity obtained after consumption of 200 µg of selenium/day (Alfthan et al., 1991). These authors calculated that daily intake of about 100 µg of selenium was almost enough to saturate glutathione peroxidase in platelets and sufficient to saturate plasma and erythrocyte glutathione peroxidase. Similarly, a linear relationship exists between erythrocyte selenium and glutathione peroxidase activity among New Zealand residents, but the two are essentially uncorrelated among short-term visitors to the country (Rea et al., 1979) (Fig. 9–3).

Hair selenium level is well correlated with blood selenium level in China (Chen et al., 1980). Selenium-containing shampoos, however, represent a major source of environmental contamination in developed countries. Toenail clippings are less exposed to environmental contamination (at least in countries where wearing shoes is the norm) and present major logistic advantages in ease of specimen collection, transport, and storage compared with blood or urine samples. Toenail selenium levels appear to reflect selenium intake. In a study of South Dakotans with high dietary selenium intake, a good correlation was observed between serum and toenail selenium levels ($r = 0.66$) (Longnecker et al., 1987). As toenails grow slowly and are different lengths, if toenails are clipped from all toes simultaneously, these specimens provide a time-integrated measure of intake. Longnecker et al. (1993) calculated, from an intervention study, that toenail selenium levels provided a measure of intake over 26 to 52 weeks. Garland et al. (1993) observed a correlation of $r = 0.48$ for selenium levels in toenails collected 6 years apart from 127 U.S. women. The feasibility of collecting toenails from large numbers of subjects has been demonstrated in the Nurses' Health Study, in which two-thirds (more than 68,000 women) of the cohort responded to a mailed request to return a set of toenail clippings. Good correlations have been observed between dietary selenium intake and 24-hour urinary excretion; however, recent dietary intake greatly affects random urine samples (Robinson et al., 1985).

Methods

Several accurate technical methods exist for the measurement of selenium in biologic tissues, including fluorometric analysis, atomic absorption spectrophotometry, and neutron activation analysis. This last technique has the advantage that it does not destroy the specimen, which can be reused for other analyses. The coefficient of variation for duplicate selenium neutron activation analysis in serum is 7.5%, and for nails approximately 4% (J. S. Morris, personal communication). Automated methods are available for the assay of glutathione peroxidase (McAdam et al., 1984).

Storage

As an inorganic element, selenium is not prone to degradation in storage. Levander (1985) states that glutathione peroxidase, however, loses activity in stored samples, although no quantitative results are described.

Measurement of Other Determinants

Lloyd and coworkers (1983) reported that plasma, whole blood, and erythrocyte selenium, but not whole blood glutathione peroxidase, levels were reduced in older persons. Hunter and colleagues (1987) similarly observed an inverse relationship between age and toenail selenium level. Smoking is associated with reduced selenium status. Among men older than 30 years, plasma, whole blood, and erythrocyte selenium levels and glutathione peroxidase activity were all significantly reduced among smokers compared with nonsmokers (Lloyd et al., 1983). Toenail selenium level was significantly lower among female smokers than nonsmokers, and an inverse dose–response relation was observed between increasing daily cigarette consumption and decreasing toenail selenium levels (Hunter et al., 1987). Swanson et al. (1990) also observed lower toenail selenium levels among smokers in South Dakota; at least part of this association was probably due to lower intake of selenium among smokers. Serum selenium level is reduced among alcoholics (Korpela et al., 1985), perhaps because alcoholic beverages are low in selenium, and thus dietary selenium is reduced in those who consume a high proportion of total calories from alcohol. The effect of moderate alcohol consumption on selenium status is minimal (Hunter et al., 1987).

The relationship of selenium with disease may be modified by other antioxidants. Willett and colleagues (1983a) observed, for instance, that the relative risk of cancer among subjects with low serum selenium level was increased among those who also had a low serum vitamin E level. Thus, information on vitamin E, and possibly vitamin C, status may be useful for the interpretation of epidemiologic studies involving selenium.

Iron

Iron deficiency may be the most common deficiency of a single nutrient in both the developing and the developed world. Iron is essential for the formation of hemoglobin and many intracellular heme enzymes. Dietary iron requirements are determined by blood loss (including menstrual blood loss), as well as by the needs of growth in children, adolescents, and pregnant women.

Intestinal iron absorption is closely regulated and inversely related to body iron stores. Reduced body iron stores may be caused by inadequate dietary iron, excessive blood loss, or both. Thus, information on the extent and source of blood loss is essential to the interpretation of biochemical measures of iron status as markers of dietary intake. In many developing countries, blood loss due to hookworm infestation or to the demands of repeated cycles of pregnancy and lactation combine with poor nutritional intake to produce biochemical and clinical evidence of iron deficiency. In addition, it is important to recognize that the bioavailability of iron from different foods varies considerably. Nonheme iron (mainly from vegetables) and heme iron (from meat and fish) have independent absorption pathways in the intestinal mucosa, the absorption of heme iron being much less efficiently regulated (Ascherio et al., 1994). Absorption of nonheme iron is influenced by other dietary factors. In a study of 49 subjects (Hallberg and Rossander, 1984), consumption of 65 g of ascorbic acid in cauliflower more than tripled nonheme iron absorption, whereas 1 g of citric acid reduced it by two-thirds. Biochemical data may be used to identify groups whose iron requirements are not being met, but are a poor indication of dietary intake for individuals without substantial additional information about other dietary components, growth requirements, and blood loss.

Serum Ferritin

Ferritin is the principal iron storage protein, and serum ferritin level provides the best single indicator of iron stores (Cook and Skikne, 1982). Ferritin is decreased in proportion to the frequency of phlebotomy and increased in proportion to supplementation. Serum ferritin is increased in iron overload (Cavill et al., 1986). The average within-subject CV% for serum ferritin drawn from 13 adults over 15 days was 14.5% (for a technique with a within-assay CV% of 4.3%) (Pilon et al., 1981). In a study of healthy childbearing women, Soustre and coworkers (1986) did not observe a significant correlation between total daily iron intake and serum ferritin level. Meat intake, however, was a significant predictor of serum ferritin level, suggesting that serum ferritin level does provide a measure of heme iron. Similarly, in a study of 123 men, Ascherio et al. (1994) observed Spearman correlations of $r = 0.16$ ($p = 0.07$) of plasma ferritin level with heme iron intake, $r = 0.22$ ($p = 0.03$) with red meat intake, and $r = -0.15$ ($p = 0.08$) with total iron intake.

Serum Iron

Serum iron level is highly variable, and changes of more than 20% have been observed within 10 minutes among healthy subjects (Cavill et al., 1986). This short-term variability makes serum iron an unreliable long-term measure.

Transferrin Saturation and Total Iron-Binding Capacity

Transferrin is the plasma iron-transport protein. Transferrin saturation is measured as the ratio of serum iron and total iron-binding capacity. As the total iron-binding capacity of the transferrin pool is relatively stable, transferrin saturation is determined principally by changes in the serum iron concentration and is, thus, equally subject to short-term variation.

Erythrocyte Protoporphyrin

A deficiency of iron results in impaired heme synthesis and the accumulation of protoporphyrin, a heme precursor, in erythrocytes. Measurement of erythrocyte protoporphyrin (EP) level is a sensitive indicator of iron deficiency, but provides no information about iron overload. Among 4,160 children in Minneapolis (Yip et al., 1983), an EP value <35 mg/dl was associated with 88% sensitivity and 90% specificity when compared with iron deficiency diagnosed based on a serum ferritin level of ≤15 mg/L; over all subjects the correlation of EP with serum ferritin level was −0.66. Cavill and colleagues (1986) have emphasized the advantages of this test for large-scale surveys: the small sample size (about 20 μl of blood) required and the relative simplicity and reproducibility of the measurement.

Mean Corpuscular Volume

Microcytosis of erythrocytes is a morphologic indicator of iron deficiency, but can also be caused by thalassemia and inflammation.

Hemoglobin or Hematocrit

More severe and long-standing iron deficiency results in reduced hemoglobin level. Over hydration, the hemoglobinopathies, vitamin B_{12} deficiency, and a wide variety of chronic disease conditions also cause lowered hemoglobin level.

Hair and Nails

The biologic significance of iron in hair and nails remains to be determined. Hunter et al. (personal communication) observed that toenail iron levels were higher among patients with hemochromatosis than among controls; however, this observation gives little information about levels over the normal range of iron intake.

Other Determinants

The major determinant of iron stores, other than dietary intake, is blood loss. A history of blood donations and a menstrual history in women are valuable in the interpretation of iron measurements. Serum ferritin is significantly increased among oral contraceptive users, possibly due to reduced menstrual blood loss (Frassinelli-Gunderson et al., 1985).

Summary

Pilch and Senti (1984a) have emphasized that the use of several biochemical indicators of iron status provides a more sensitive and specific assessment than any single indicator alone. If the aim is to categorize subjects according to diagnostic groups, then the choice of appropriate cut-off values is a source of continuing controversy. Extensive additional information about the other determinants of iron stores is necessary to interpret biochemical measures of iron status in individuals.

Sodium

On the basis of geographic correlation studies, it has been suggested that salt intake is positively correlated with blood pressure; results from experimental studies have confirmed a modest relationship. Consumption of salt-cured foods has been hypothesized to increase the risk of stomach cancer (Committee on Diet Nutrition and Cancer, Assembly of Life Sciences, National Research Council, 1982). A continuing problem in studies of sodium intake has been its measurement, because day-to-day variation in sodium intake is high (Caggiula et al., 1985).

Measures

Measurement of sodium in the blood provides almost no information about sodium intake due to tight homeostatic control mechanisms that minimize variation in blood sodium level. Urinary sodium level, in contrast, is a good measure of short-term sodium intake. In a study of free-living subjects, average absorption of sodium from food was 98%, and average urinary excretion was 86% (Holbrook et al., 1984). A measurement of average urinary output is thus a good indicator of dietary intake. The problem is that sodium excretion is determined by recent intake and is thus almost as variable as intake itself. Liu and coworkers (1979a) estimated the ratio of day-to-day within-person to between-person variation in 24-hour sodium excretion to be greater than 3. Thus, a single 24-hour urine collection is a poor guide to true long-term intake. Nevertheless, Caggiula and colleagues (1985) observed a high correlation ($r = 0.61$) between sodium estimated from a 6-day food record and a single 24-hour urine measurement among 50 adult subjects. Similarly, Holbrook and colleagues (1984) reported a correlation of $r = 0.76$ between sodium intake calculated from analysis of four 7-day duplicate meal collections and four 24-hour urine sodium measurements among 28 individuals. Although these correlations are impressive, it is important to note that the dietary reference periods were relatively short and that correlations with long-term intake would be substantially lower. In a study of 160 women who kept 16 days of weighed food records and collected an average of six 24-hour urine samples in the course of 1 year, Bingham et al. (1995) observed a correlation of $r = 0.30$ between dietary intake of sodium and the average of the 24-hour urine sodium levels. Joseph (1994) compared sodium intakes estimated from two 7-day diet records and the average of two 24-hour urine samples and observed correlations of $r = 0.33$ among 127 men and $r = 0.41$ among 193 women.

Given the logistic difficulties that attend

24-hour urine collection in large studies, the alternative of using overnight specimens has been considered. Liu and colleagues (1979b) estimated a correlation coefficient of 0.73 between mean 24-hour and overnight urine sodium excretion measurements in children. Watson and Langford (1970) observed a correlation of $r = 0.76$ between overnight and 24-hour sodium excretion measurements among adults. Given the relative ease of obtaining overnight urine specimens, it appears that for many epidemiologic studies, collection of a greater number of overnight urine samples per subject may be preferable to a smaller number of 24-hour collections. If an absolute, rather than a relative, estimate of 24-hour sodium excretion is required, then a 24-hour sample is necessary due to the diurnal variation in sodium excretion. Of interest is the report by Farleigh and coworkers (1985), who observed a statistically significant correlation ($r = 0.28$) between the sodium concentration in saliva and the preceding (but not the same) day 24-hour urine sodium excretion.

Storage
As long as the total original volume is noted, preservation of an aliquot of urine results in substantial saving of freezer space.

Stability
Sodium is stable in frozen urine.

Measurement
Sodium can be accurately measured in urine by flame atomic absorption spectrophotometry or ion-selective electrode potentiometry.

Measurement of Other Determinants
Holbrook and colleagues (1984) observed a small, but significant, decrease in the percentage of dietary sodium excreted in summer compared with winter, possibly due to increased excretion in sweat.

Potassium

The principal epidemiologic interest in potassium relates to the putative association of low potassium intake with the development of hypertension (McCarron et al., 1984) and, possibly, strokes (Khaw and Barrett-Connor, 1987).

Blood potassium level is under tight homeostatic control and does not reflect potassium intake over its normal range. The proportion of ingested potassium excreted in urine, 77% in the study of Holbrook and colleagues (1984), is less than that for sodium, as relatively more potassium is excreted in stool. Nonetheless, the correlation between potassium intake and four 24-hour urinary excretion was $r = 0.82$, and the correlation of a single 24-hour urine and 6 days of food records was $r = 0.62$ (Caggiula et al., 1985). In the study of Bingham et al. (1995), the correlation between potassium intake estimated from 16 days of food records and urine potassium level in an average of six 24-hour urine samples was $r = 0.73$. Joseph (1994) observed correlations of $r = 0.64$ and $r = 0.53$ among 127 men and 193 women, respectively, who completed two 7-day diet records and two 24-hour urine collections.

Measurement of Other Determinants
Potassium-wasting diuretics or potassium supplements may affect potassium excretion.

Calcium

It has been suggested that dietary calcium protects against hypertension (McCarron et al., 1984) and colorectal cancer (Garland et al., 1985). In addition, the relationship between dietary calcium, osteoporosis, and fractures is a subject of much activity and considerable controversy.

Blood calcium level is under tight homeostatic control and thus not a useful indicator of intake. Few data are available on the relation between calcium intake and urinary calcium level. Twenty-four–hour calcium excretion was lower in subjects consuming a low-calcium diet whose calcium intake was estimated to be approximately 75% of those consuming a high-calcium diet (Castenmiller et al., 1985). Interestingly, in this study, sodium supplementation appeared to increase calcium excretion, independent of calcium intake. Among 22 omnivorous, healthy male subjects, a calcium supplement of 1. 12 g daily (a mean increase of 92% above normal dietary intake) resulted in a 20% increase in mean urinary calcium excretion (Aalberts et al., 1988). However, Joseph (1994) observed correlations of $r = 0.05$ and $r = 0.16$ among 127 men and 193 women, respectively, who kept two 7-day diet records and collected two 24-hour urine samples. This suggests that urine calcium is not a good indicator of calcium intake in the normal range.

Magnesium

Relative deficiency of dietary magnesium has been associated with hypertension and coronary heart disease in some studies (Luoma et al., 1983; Joffres et al., 1987).

Although serum is homeostatically controlled, among 139 men and women Jacques et al. (1993) observed weak positive correlations between estimated intake and serum magnesium level ($r = 0.27$ including supplement users, $r = 0.15$ after excluding them). One mechanism of magnesium regulation is urinary excretion, and a reduction in magnesium intake reduces urinary excretion (Wacker, 1980). In the study described above, Joseph (1994) observed correlations of $r = 0.27$ for 127 men and $r = 0.34$ for 193 women, suggesting that multiple 24-hour urine collections would be required to indicate magnesium intake. A loading test that measures the amount of magnesium excreted in urine after a slow intravenous infusion of magnesium has been proposed as a measure of magnesium deficiency (Ryzen et al., 1985); the lack of utility to large epidemiologic studies is obvious, although the method has

been used to assess the prevalence of magnesium deficiency in ischemic heart disease patients (Rasmussen et al., 1988).

Copper

Although copper-dependent enzymes and copper-containing proteins are numerous, clinical diagnosis of copper deficiency appears to be rare, presumably due to the wide distribution of copper in foods and cooking utensils. Concern has been expressed, however, that per capita copper intakes in the United States may be substantially lower than the recommended dietary allowance of 2 to 3 mg/day suggested by the Food and Nutrition Board of the National Research Council (Klevay et al., 1980). Reduced copper status has been associated with ischemic heart disease (Klevay, 1983) and cardiac arrhythmias (Reiser et al., 1985).

Serum and Plasma

Few data are available on the relation between dietary copper intake and serum or plasma levels. Plasma levels in patients on total parenteral nutrition solutions deficient in copper were observed to fall steadily until copper repletion restored normal levels (Solomons et al., 1976). No increase in serum copper level was observed, however, among seven subjects who consumed 10 mg of copper per day for 12 weeks (Pratt et al., 1985). A further reason that circulating copper levels are a poor guide to copper status is the large number of lifestyle factors (e.g., oral contraceptive use, smoking) and pathologic conditions (e.g., infections and inflammation) that profoundly alter blood copper concentration (Solomons, 1985).

Ceruloplasmin

Delves (1976) found 94% of circulating copper bound to the cuproprotein ceruloplasmin, and it has been suggested that this would be a more reliable measure of copper status. Ceruloplasmin production is also, however, influenced by many factors other than dietary intake (Solomons, 1985).

Erythrocyte Superoxidase Dismutase

Measurement of the function of the copper-and zinc-dependent enzyme superoxide dismutase (SoD) may be a better index of copper status. Among four men fed a copper-deficient diet for 4 months, erythrocyte SoD activity declined markedly in all four, whereas plasma copper level declined in only one, and copper repletion restored normal SoD values (Milne et al., 1982). In a similar experiment on nine men consuming a low-copper diet containing 20% fructose, erythrocyte SoD activity, but not plasma copper or ceruloplasmin level, reflected both copper depletion and repletion (Reiser et al., 1985). Cytochrome *c* activity in leukocytes and platelets is reduced in copper deficiency before SoD activity is reduced and may be a useful marker of early copper deficiency (Olivares and Uauy, 1996).

Hair

Copper level can be measured in hair, but it is not elevated in Wilson's disease (Martin, 1964). Hambidge (1973) demonstrated a progressive increase in mean copper concentration in hair with increasing distance from the scalp, data highly suggestive of external contamination.

Nails

Copper concentration was moderately elevated in the fingernails of two out of three patients with Wilson's disease (Martin, 1964). It remains to be determined, however, whether nail levels reflect differences in normal dietary intake.

Urine

The major excretory route for copper is bile, and only small amounts are lost in urine (Cousins, 1985). In a study of 12 subjects who collected 24-hour urine specimens for 5 days, the between-day $CV\%$ was 53%, suggesting that large day-to-day fluctuations in urinary copper excretion

make this an unreliable indicator of long-term copper status (Yang et al., 1986).

Methods

Atomic absorption spectrophotometry (AAS) is the most common analytic technique with which to determine copper level in serum or plasma. There are several methods available for measurement of ceruloplasmin and SoD activity; however, these are all quite labor intensive (Klasing and Pilch, 1985). Hair and nail copper levels can be measured using neutron activation analysis or AAS.

Storage

Copper is stable in blood. The stability of ceruloplasmin and SoD is uncertain.

Measurement of Other Determinants

Blood levels of copper are sensitive to a number of nondietary determinants. An example of the extent of this problem is the fact that the reference range for serum copper among oral contraceptive users is higher than, and does not even overlap, the range for nonusers (Alpers et al., 1983). Several other dietary components appear to influence copper absorption; amino acids appear to increase absorption, whereas ascorbic acid, fiber, and zinc have been observed to decrease copper absorption (Cousins, 1985). Collection of information about all of these factors, and in particular the use of vitamin C and zinc supplements, should theoretically aid in the interpretation of measures of copper status.

Zinc

Marginal zinc nutriture has been linked to a variety of clinical conditions and to suboptimal physiologic performance (Pilch and Senti, 1984b). No single measure of zinc status is a reliable measure of intake. Although zinc supplementation increases plasma zinc levels (Fischer et al., 1984), dietary zinc deprivation may not result in lowered plasma zinc level (Prasad et al., 1978). Thus, zinc deficiency may coexist with a normal plasma zinc level (Sandstead et al., 1982). In a study of 24 elderly sub-jects, zinc intake was not significantly cor-related with zinc concentrations in plasma, whole blood, or leukocytes (Bunker et al., 1984). Furthermore, blood zinc level is sen-sitive to a wide range of nondietary factors (Solomons, 1985). Measurements of zinc in erythrocytes and hair have not been widely accepted as indices of dietary intake (Klas-ing and Pilch, 1985). No increase in hair zinc levels was observed among 52 preg-nant women whose mean dietary zinc in-take was estimated to be about 50% of the recommended daily allowance and who consumed 20 mg of zinc daily for a mean of 4.5 months (Hunt et al., 1983). Among 13 men consuming a zinc supplement of 40 mg/day (almost four times their estimated dietary intake) for 12 weeks, a transient rise in serum zinc level was observed, but levels declined to baseline after 4 weeks (Black et al., 1988). Among seven subjects on a zinc-deficient diet for 8 days, plasma zinc level fell 7%, while erythrocyte meta-llothionein (a zinc-binding protein) levels fell 59% (Grider et al., 1990). Supplemen-tation with zinc rapidly increased meta-llothionein levels, suggesting that they may be a useful marker of short-term intake. Suggested functional tests, such as taste and smell acuity and neuropsychologic function, are clearly not specific for zinc de-ficiency.

Lipids

The relationship between diet and coro-nary heart disease has been of major inter-est over the last three decades, and the lipid composition of diet has been identified as a predictor of this disease (Shekelle et al., 1981; Kushi et al., 1985). The general ac-ceptance of this association has been de-layed by the controversy over the re-lationship between the lipid composition of diet and the levels of cholesterol and lipo-proteins in blood, cells, and fat. In recent years these relationships have become bet-ter understood, principally because many sources of variance in both dietary fats and biochemical parameters have been deter-

mined (see Chapter 17). These develop-ments allow a better evaluation of lipid bi-ochemical indicators as measures of lipid intake.

Given the epidemiologic interest in the relation of total fat intake to the occurrence of both cardiovascular disease and cancer, it is unfortunate that there is no biochem-ical measure of total dietary fat. This also leads to problems in the interpretation of the measurement of specific lipids. A find-ing, for instance, that the concentration of a specific fatty acid is equal in the adipose tissue of cases of a disease and of controls could have two interpretations. The abso-lute intake of the fatty acid might be equal in both groups in the context of equal total fat intake. On the other hand, the absolute intakes may differ, but differences in the same direction in total intake may mean that consumption of the fatty acid as a per-cent of total fat is equal and there is no relative difference. These alternatives would lead to different causal interpreta-tions and dietary recommendations, but without a measure of total fat intake it is not possible to distinguish between them.

Lipid Physiology: A Simple Overview
Dietary fats are largely consumed as tri-glycerides (molecules of glycerol and fatty acids). Cholesterol, derived solely from an-imal sources, is emulsified with bile acids and absorbed into the portal circulation. Triglycerides, available from both plant and animal sources, are hydrolyzed into monoglycerides and diglycerides by pancre-atic lipase before absorption through the intestinal mucosa, re-formation into tri-glycerides, and transport via blood and lymph in chylomicrons (Linscheer and Ver-groesen, 1988). Dietary cholesterol is trans-ported to the liver, which also synthesizes cholesterol de novo. Endogenous choles-terol synthesis in the liver is more than twice the typical American dietary choles-terol consumption, and feedback mecha-nisms cause changes in endogenous syn-thesis to partially counteract changes in dietary intake (Samuel et al., 1983). Cho-

lesterol and triglycerides are synthesized in the hepatocytes, combined with proteins and phospholipids to form lipoproteins, and then secreted into the blood. There are four basic types of lipoproteins, chylomicrons, very low-density lipoproteins (VLDL), LDL, and HDL, listed in order of decreasing size and increasing density. The protein moieties of these transport particles are called *apolipoproteins*, some of which function as activators of the enzymes of cholesterol and triglyceride metabolism and as ligands for cell surface receptors. VLDL and chylomicrons are the primary transport particles for triglycerides to cells, whereas LDL is the major vehicle for cholesterol transport. HDL scavenges excess cholesterol from cells, returning it to other lipoproteins, to the liver, and to extrahepatic cells that require cholesterol for steroid hormone production and membrane biosynthesis.

There are large differences in plasma total cholesterol and LDL-C levels between populations, and the diversity within most populations is also large. Population differences in average levels of LDL-C are determined by differential rates of LDL production and catabolism. It is not known, however, if these rates are controlled by dietary intakes or other environmental factors (International Collaborative Study Group, 1986). Within populations, large interindividual differences exist in the ability of subjects to suppress endogenous cholesterol synthesis when challenged with increased dietary cholesterol (McNamara et al., 1987). Large differences have also been observed in individual responses of plasma concentrations of total cholesterol and LDL-C to the substitution of saturated fatty acids for unsaturated fatty acids (Grundy and Vega, 1988). These differences, presumably genetic in origin, may be the most important determinants of individual cholesterol levels (Tikkanen et al., 1990).

Recently, some of this inherited component in the between-person variability in response to changes in intake of cholesterol and fatty acids has been elucidated. Apolipoprotein E (ApoE) mediates the uptake of VLDL and chylomicron remnants by the liver. Three alleles (E2, E3, and E4) exist; the E2 allele is associated with lower serum LDL-C and total cholesterol levels, and the E4 is associated with higher levels (Lehtimaki et al., 1995). In an observational study of Finnish youths, Lehtimaki et al. (1995) showed that the ApoE–serum cholesterol association was substantially stronger among subjects with high dietary cholesterol and saturated fat intakes, suggesting that the genotype is less influential when the "environmental" or dietary exposure is low. Some (e.g., Manttari et al., 1991), but not all (e.g., Boerwinkle 1991), studies have shown that the ApoE genotype modulates the individual serum lipid response to changes in dietary cholesterol and saturated fatty acid intake. The apolipoprotein A-IV plays a role in HDL metabolism, and a common polymorphism (ApoA-IV-2) is present in approximately 8% of whites (McCombs et al., 1994). Carriers of the ApoA-IV-2 allele had attenuated serum cholesterol response to short-term ingestion of four eggs per day (McCombs et al., 1994). At the present, these and other genotypes explain only some of the heterogeneity in response to changes in cholesterol and lipid intake. Ultimately, these and other genotypes should improve our ability to infer lipid intake on the basis of serum lipid levels.

Serum Total, LDL-C, and HDL-C Levels

Both serum total cholesterol and LDL-C levels have a positive relationship with coronary heart disease incidence, whereas HDL-C is inversely related (Gordon et al., 1977; Wallace and Anderson, 1987). There has been much discussion about the extent and shape of the relationship between dietary and total serum cholesterol. Based on metabolic ward studies, both Keys and colleagues (1965) and Hegsted and colleagues (1965) proposed equations that predict serum cholesterol from dietary intake of cholesterol and saturated and polyunsaturated fatty acids. The Keys equation* proposes that plasma cholesterol level increases in proportion to the square root of dietary cholesterol intake (in mg/1,000 kcal per day). It thus predicts that plasma cholesterol level will increase more for a given increase in cholesterol consumption if this increase occurs from a low, rather than a high, baseline. The Hegsted equation† proposed a linear relationship. Both equations appear to perform reasonably well over the usual range of dietary cholesterol in developed countries. In the low and high range of cholesterol intake, however, the nonlinear Keys equation appears to be superior (Keys, 1984). The fact that dietary intake of saturated and polyunsaturated fatty acids is a predictor of serum cholesterol level indicates that dietary cholesterol is not the only dietary determinant of serum levels. The performance of plasma cholesterol as an indicator of dietary intake can be partially deduced from the shape of the Keys relation. Plasma cholesterol level rises less steeply as dietary cholesterol intake increases. Thus, it will probably be a better index of cholesterol consumption in the low than in the moderate and high range. The increases predicted by these equations are small in comparison with the known variance of serum cholesterol in the population. This suggests that, although they may predict changes in serum cholesterol in response to dietary change for groups, the use of serum cholesterol to calculate the dietary cholesterol intake of individuals results in severe misclassification (see Chapter 1).

Data from the many intervention studies and the few observational studies that have been conducted to study this issue support this deduction. Subjects in the Leiden Intervention Study (Arntzenius et al., 1985), whose diets were already low in cholesterol and whose dietary cholesterol was reduced from a daily mean of 89.6 to 29.5 mg/1,000 kcal, were observed to have a reduction of serum cholesterol level from 6.9 to 6.2 mmol/L. Thus, a dietary intervention that effectively reduced dietary cholesterol by two-thirds resulted in a 10% reduction in serum cholesterol level. In the National Diet Heart Study, among subjects whose dietary cholesterol intake was representative of normal U.S. intake (approximately 200 mg/1,000 kcal per day) and who consumed a diet that reduced cholesterol alone, a reduction of approximately 100 mg/1,000 kcal per day (approximately a 50% decrease in cholesterol intake) was associated with a less than 3% reduction in serum cholesterol level (National Diet Heart Study Research Group, 1968). In an intervention study in the Netherlands (Katan et al., 1986), 94 healthy men and women had their cholesterol intake increased from a daily average of 49 to 234 mg/1,000 kcal; serum cholesterol levels increased an average of 5.25 mmol/L and by an average of 0.50 mmol/L after 13 days. In this study, two groups of 15 "hyporesponders" and 17 "hyperresponders" were identified, and the hyporesponders had a significantly lower increase in serum cholesterol level than the hyperresponders when challenged with a larger increase in dietary cholesterol (349 mg/1,000 kcal/day), indicating that variability of response to dietary cholesterol exists within populations, possibly due to genetic influences, as previously discussed. In cross-sectional observational studies, correlations between dietary cholesterol intake and serum cholesterol values depend on the range of cholesterol intake in the population being examined. In a macrobiotic vegetarian population with a mean dietary cholesterol intake of 42.3 mg/1,000 kcal per day, the unadjusted correlation coefficient between dietary cholesterol consumption and serum

---

*The Keys equation is $\Delta y = 1.35 (2\Delta S - \Delta P) + 1.5\Delta Z$, where Δy = change in serum cholesterol (mg/dl); ΔS and ΔP = change in dietary intake of saturated and polyunsaturated fatty acids expressed as percentage of calories; and $\Delta Z = (x_1^{0.5} - x_2^{0.5})$, where x_1 and x_2 are the dietary cholesterols of the two diets being compared in mg/1,000 kcal.

†The Hegsted equation is $\Delta y = 2.16\Delta S - 1.65\Delta P + 0.176\Delta C$, where ΔC is change in cholesterol intake in mg/1,000 kcal.

cholesterol level was $r = 0.46$ (Kushi et al., 1988). Shekelle and coworkers (1981), however, observed an unadjusted correlation of $r = 0.08$ between the calculated Keys score (which includes cholesterol and saturated and polyunsaturated fatty acid intake) and serum cholesterol levels among 1,900 middle-aged men whose mean dietary cholesterol intake was 240.5 mg/1,000 kcal per day. It is thus apparent that, although serum cholesterol level reflects dietary intake at low intake levels, it is a poor measure of differences in cholesterol intake between individuals consuming typical Western diets.

About two-thirds of total serum cholesterol is contained in LDLs, and the relationship between cholesterol intake and level of LDL is very similar to the relationship with total cholesterol. In a large dietary intervention study among hypercholesterolemic men (Glueck et al., 1986), a decrease in cholesterol intake was associated with reductions in both total plasma cholesterol and LDL-C. Dietary saturated fat (a positive relation) and dietary polyunsaturated fat (a negative relation), however, were stronger determinants of total cholesterol and HDL-C. Numerous studies have demonstrated that replacement of dietary saturated fatty acids with polyunsaturated fatty acids lowers LDL-C and total cholesterol, although the mechanism is still unclear (Beynen and Katan, 1985b). Not all dietary saturated fatty acids, however, have the same metabolic effects. A diet high in stearic acid (18:0) did not raise total cholesterol or LDL-C levels among men, in contrast with increases seen with a diet high in palmitic acid (16:0) (Bonanome and Grundy, 1988). Lauric acid (12:0) raises serum cholesterol levels more than palmitic acid (Temme et al., 1996). While replacement of saturated fats with polyunsaturated fats reduces serum cholesterol level, monounsaturated fats have almost the same effect (Grundy, 1996). In summary, lipoproteins may be useful in intervention studies as markers of average response for groups. In observational studies, however, lipoprotein levels, like serum total cholesterol levels, are poor indicators of individual dietary cholesterol or fatty acid intake, at least in developed countries.

Laboratory Techniques

A variety of reliable, automated chemical and enzymatic methods are available for the measurement of total cholesterol in serum. Lipoproteins may be measured by ultracentrifugation, which is the generally accepted reference method, or by column chromatography, electrophoresis, or precipitation reactions (Naito and David, 1984). Use of certified reference materials, such as those available from the Centers for Disease Control and Prevention, is essential to ensure the validity of total cholesterol and HDL-C measurements (Hainline et al., 1978).

Measurements of cholesterol and the lipoproteins exhibit an appreciable degree of within-person day-to-day variation. Coefficients of variation between the initial and second visit for 7,055 white participants in the Lipid Research Clinics Prevalence Study were 8% for fasting plasma cholesterol level and 25% for fasting plasma triglyceride level (Jacobs and Barrett-Connor, 1982). Mjos and coworkers (1979) observed within-person coefficients of variation of approximately 8% for total cholesterol, 9% for HDL-C, 11% for LDL-C, and 26% for triglycerides. Even under metabolic ward conditions with constant dietary intake, coefficients of variation of 3.1% to 9.0% for serum cholesterol levels have been observed (Hegsted and Nicolosi, 1987). This degree of variability, the cause of which is poorly understood, means that a single, or even several, measurements of serum cholesterol, lipoproteins, and triglycerides, will misclassify many subjects with respect to their long-term average levels. This further reduces our ability to observe any underlying association with dietary intake.

Increases of approximately 10% in the levels of total cholesterol, HDL-C, LDL-C,

VLDL-C, and triglycerides were observed when blood was taken after 30 minutes of standing relative to 30 minutes in the supine position (Kjeldsen et al., 1983). These changes, attributable to an orthostatic decrease in plasma volume, emphasize the necessity for strict standardization of procedures for blood drawing and subject posture in the measurement of all biochemical parameters in blood.

Stability

Total cholesterol is stable in frozen serum (Wood et al., 1980). Repeated freezing and thawing degrades lipoproteins, with HDL being particularly susceptible. HDL-C values were more stable when stored at $-60°C$ than at $-20°C$ over 10 months (Cooper, 1979). Thus, storage at the lower temperature seems advisable; the validity of measurements made in serum or plasma stored for more than 1 year needs to be determined.

Measurements of Other Determinants

A further reason that cholesterol and lipoproteins are poor indicators of dietary intake is the influence of nondietary factors. Levels of LDL-C are positively correlated with Quetelet's index and smoking (Glueck et al., 1986). HDL-C is increased by exercise and alcohol consumption and has an inverse relationship with smoking and body mass index (Hulley et al., 1977). Even after adjusting for these factors, the correlation of lipoproteins with dietary cholesterol remains poor.

Fatty Acids

Specific fatty acid levels in blood, cell membranes, and subcutaneous fats are more promising indicators of dietary fat intake than cholesterol or lipoprotein measurements. Although this field is not new, recent improvements in gas chromatography and HPLC methods have made the measurement of many individual fatty acids and their isomers more feasible in large studies.

Fatty acids are numbered by their carbon chain length. Saturated fatty acids have no double bonds between carbon atoms, monounsaturated fatty acids have one, and polyunsaturated fatty acids have two or more double bonds. The standard numbering system for fatty acids gives the number of carbon atoms, the number of double bonds (after a colon), and the position of the first double bond (after the Greek letter ω) counting from the end of the carbon chain opposite the carboxyl group. Thus, oleic acid (18:1ω-9) is a monounsaturated fatty acid with its single double bond nine carbon atoms from the C18 end of the chain. In *trans* isomers of fatty acids, the two hydrogen atoms attached to the carbon atoms linked by a double bond are on opposite sides of the molecule. These hydrogen atoms are in the *cis* configuration, on the same side of the molecule, in most dietary unsaturated fatty acids.

It seems reasonable to expect that the best markers of dietary intake would be the fatty acids that cannot be endogenously synthesized from carbohydrates. These are largely the omega-3 fatty acids (long chain lengths derived from some plants, and extra long chain lengths from sea animals), the omega-6 family (mostly from vegetable oils,) *trans*-fatty acids (primarily from partially hydrogenated fats and ruminants), and odd-numbered and branched chain fatty acids (from dairy products). Linoleic acid (18:2ω-6) is the principal dietary essential fatty acid, and it is capable of being metabolized to longer-chain, more highly unsaturated, omega-6 fatty acids, including arachidonic acid (20:4ω-6). Similarly, linolenic acid (18:3ω-3) gives rise to a sequence of longer chain omega-3 fatty acids. Oleic acid (18:1ω-9) may be endogenously synthesized and is the starting point for synthesis of omega-9 fatty acids. The relationship between dietary intake of these three principal precursors (18:3ω-3, 18:2ω-6, and 18:1ω-9) and the levels of their metabolites in human tissues is complex, largely because intake of one inhibits the elongation and unsaturation of the others (Holman, 1986). The majority of studies comparing fatty acid intake with fatty acid levels have concentrated on linoleic acid and oleic acid. More recently, limited information on the interpretation of other fatty acid peaks has become available.

Caution is appropriate in the interpretation of markers of fatty acid intake. Results are usually expressed as relative percentages of total fatty acid. Thus, an increase in dietary intake of one fatty acid, if incorporated into the substrate for analysis, results in a decrease in the relative amounts of all other fatty acids. This decrease should not necessarily be taken as evidence for a metabolic interaction. Such interactions may exist, however (e.g., the inhibition of metabolism of omega-3 fatty acids by dietary intake of omega-6 fatty acids described by Holman [1986]), and further complicate the interpretation of relative differences with respect to dietary intake. Metabolic inhibition of one fatty acid by another leads to the possibility that the between-person intake of a particular fatty acid may be confounded by differences in the between-person intake of an interacting fatty acid. Much work needs to be done to define the nature of these relationships. In general, however, biochemical fatty acid profiles may be interpreted as indicating relative patterns of fatty acid intake rather than absolute amounts.

Plasma Fractions, Cell Membranes, and Adipose Tissue

The measurement of individual fatty acids is further complicated by the fact that they may be measured in erythrocytes, platelets, and adipose tissue, as well as in several lipid subfractions found in plasma. Data are sparse on the relationships of fatty acid intake and their levels in these substrates, and interpretation of the existing data is frequently difficult because otherwise comparable studies have often measured fatty acid levels in different fractions.

Individual fatty acids may be measured in the cholesterol ester, phospholipid, and triglyceride fractions of serum or plasma or as free fatty acids. These fractions are usu-

ally separated by thin layer chromatography before proceeding with isolation and identification of individual fatty acids. Cross-sectional studies reveal major differences in the relative contribution of individual fatty acids to different fractions among subjects eating a Western diet. Linoleic acid concentration is typically approximately two to three times higher than oleic acid in the cholesterol ester fraction of plasma. This predominance is reduced to a factor of between one and a half to two in plasma phospholipids. The ratio is reversed in triglycerides, where oleic acid predominates. Oleic acid is also the major free fatty acid found in plasma and is three to four times more common than linoleic acid in both platelet phospholipids and adipose tissue. Although palmitic acid levels are higher than stearic acid levels in almost all these substrates, the ratio of palmitic acid to stearic acid varies from about 2 in plasma phospholipids to more than 10 in plasma cholesterol esters. Arachidonic acid ($20:4\omega\text{-}6$) constitutes 2.3% of total fatty acids in plasma triglycerides, 11.5% in plasma phospholipids, less than 1% in adipose tissue, but 27% in platelet phospholipids (Hirsch et al., 1960; Dayton et al., 1966; Phillips and Dodge, 1967; Manku et al., 1983; Sacks et al., 1987; Wood et al., 1987). In a study of 84 subjects, dietary polyunsaturated and saturated fat intakes were equivalently correlated with their serum levels measured in the cholesteryl ester and triglyceride fractions; correlations between intake and phospholipid fraction levels were lower (Nikkari et al., 1995).

The distribution of fatty acids in the phospholipid fraction of plasma is closely related to their distribution in the phospholipids of erythrocyte membranes. In a study of 10 healthy subjects, Phillips and Dodge (1967) observed correlations between fatty acids in plasma and erythrocyte phospholipids of $r = 0.42$ (stearic acid), $r = 0.80$ (palmitic acid), $r = 0.51$ (oleic acid), and $r = 0.73$ (linoleic acid). Changes in the oleic and linoleic acid contents of diet are reflected in erythrocyte phospholipids within weeks of dietary change, suggesting that membrane fatty acids have a dynamic relationship with plasma levels and are not fixed at the time of erythropoiesis (Farquhar and Ahrens, 1963). In a study of 67 healthy men, Boberg and colleagues (1985) observed a correlation of $r = 0.78$ between the proportions of linoleic acid in platelet phospholipids and in plasma phospholipids.

These differences in fatty acid composition of various tissues or plasma lipid fractions are due to the endogenous production of some fatty acids, the different roles of these fractions as vehicles for fatty acid transport, and the physiologic functions of individual fatty acids. In some tissues, the fatty acid levels may largely passively reflect diet, whereas in others these levels may be actively regulated, which is likely to be true when they are playing an important structural or functional role. The situation is further complicated if we examine the relationship of dietary change and fatty acid levels, as factors such as the half-lives of cholesteryl ester fractions or red cell membranes are additional influences on the rate of incorporation of individual fatty acids. For use as an epidemiologic marker of fatty acid intake, the choice of a specific lipid fraction or substrate for measurement depends largely on two characteristics: the responsiveness or sensitivity of the substrate to changes in dietary fatty acids and the degree to which fatty acid levels in the substrate integrate intake over time. For example, in the study of Sacks and colleagues (1987), the largest responses to changes in intake of both linoleic and oleic acid were measured in the triglyceride fraction of plasma. Although this responsiveness is an advantage, the triglyceride fraction could be less useful as a measure of long-term intake if the day-to-day variation in fatty acid content was greater than for the other lipid fractions. In a study of fasting samples collected from 50 subjects 3 years apart, correlations for the major fatty acids measured in cholesterol esters (stearic, palmitic, oleic, and linoleic acids) were >0.65; these correlations in the phospholipid fraction were slightly lower (Ma et al., 1995a). In a follow-up study of 759 Finnish youths, with measurement of cholesterol ester fatty acids at baseline and after 6 years, correlations were palmitic acid $r = 0.34$; oleic acid, $r = 0.45$; linoleic acid, $r = 0.50$; eicosopentaenoic acid, $r = 0.38$; and docosohexaenoic acid, $r = 0.38$ (Moilanen et al., 1992). These suggest that plasma fatty acid measures may represent a time-integrated reflection of intake of these fatty acids. If a generalization can be made at this stage, it is that the long half-life associated with fatty acid turnover in adipose tissue probably means that this tissue provides the best measure of long-term intake of the dietary fatty acids that are incorporated into fat. In studies seeking to monitor short-term dietary change, plasma lipid fractions and erythrocyte or platelet membrane phospholipids may provide a more rapidly responding measure. More data are needed before definite recommendations can be made on which fatty acid measurements reflect dietary intake and, for each fatty acid, which plasma fraction or tissue is most suitable for measurement.

Linoleic, Linolenic, and Oleic Acid

Cross-sectional studies of fatty acid intake and fatty acid profiles measured in plasma have generally failed to demonstrate strong positive relations. In a geographic correlation study, where large dietary differences were involved, mean intakes of linoleic acid among subjects in Italy, Finland, and the United States correlated with the mean levels of linoleic acid in plasma (Dougherty et al., 1987). The daily estimated consumption of linoleic acid (as a percentage of energy intake in kcal) was 2.2% in the Italian center, 3.5% in the Finnish center, and 4.9% in the U.S. center. The corresponding percent contributions of linoleic acid to major fatty acids measured in the cholesteryl ester fraction of plasma were 33.4%, 41.2%, and 57.4%. In a small group of 29 healthy free-living volunteers whose normal diet was unusually well characterized, no consistent correlation between dietary linoleic acid intake and plasma linoleic acid concentration was observed (Reeves et al., 1984), possibly because the between-person variation in intake appears to have been small. In a cross-sectional study of 3,570 middle-aged adults, Ma et al. (1995b) compared dietary linoleic acid intake measured by a 66-item food-frequency questionnaire with levels in plasma. The correlations were $r = 0.28$ for linoleic acid measured in the cholesterol ester fraction and $r = 0.22$ in the phospholipid fraction. In an intervention study in which 17 healthy adults increased their linoleic acid consumption from 5% to 15% of calories over 4 weeks, the linoleic acid content of plasma rose 33% in the triglyceride fraction, 7% in the cholesteryl ester fraction, and 8% among phospholipids (Sacks et al., 1987). Dayton and colleagues (1966) reported on 393 institutionalized men whose diet was altered to increase the linoleic acid content from 11% to almost 40% of total fatty acid while oleic acid intake was held constant. Linoleic acid measured in the cholesteryl ester, phospholipid, and triglyceride fractions of serum increased substantially, the largest change being seen in the serum triglyceride fraction (Fig. 9–6). This situation is analogous to that for cholesterol, as plasma linoleic acid can discriminate between groups with relatively large differences in intake, but performs less well on an individual basis.

For most purposes, the best readily available tissue for fatty acid measurement is adipose tissue. Hirsch and colleagues (1960) demonstrated that subcutaneous fat aspiration with a needle and syringe was a simple, virtually painless method of obtaining a fat sample. The fatty acid composition of subcutaneous fat is very similar to omental fat (Gurr et al., 1982). Several well-conducted studies have defined the kinetics of linoleic acid in adipose tissue. In the study of Dayton and coworkers (1966) (Fig. 9–7), the linoleic acid content of total fatty acid in subcutaneous fat increased

from 11% to 32% after 5 years among elderly, institutionalized men whose diet was altered to increase the linoleic acid content from 11% to almost 40% of total fatty acid while oleic acid was held constant. Repeated sampling from these subjects allowed the half-life of adipose tissue linoleic acid to be estimated at about 680 days. Thus, the fatty acid content of subcutaneous fat provides a qualitative measure of fatty acid intake over the previous 2 or more years. Based on pooled data from seven studies, Beynen and coworkers (1980) observed a correlation of $r = 0.80$ between the percentage of polyunsaturated fatty acids relative to total fatty acid intake and the relative percentage of adipose tissue polyunsaturated fatty acids. These relations, observed in intervention and geographic correlation studies, have also been observed in cross-sectional studies conducted within single populations. In a study of 164 Scottish men, M. Thomson and colleagues (1985) observed a correlation of $r = 0.57$ between dietary linoleic acid intake determined from 7-day weighed diet records and the relative proportion of linoleic acid in adipose tissue. In a study of 59 Dutch women, van Staveren and colleagues (1986) also observed a high correlation ($r = 0.70$) between the dietary linoleic acid content of diet and subcutaneous fat. Hunter et al. (1992), in a study of 118 Boston-area men, observed a correlation of $r = 0.48$ between linoleic acid measured in adipose and calculated from a food frequency questionnaire. Among 140 women, Garland et al. (1997) observed a correlation of $r = 0.37$ for linoleic acid and $r = 0.34$ for linolenic acid, comparing adipose tissue and the average of two food-frequency questionnaire estimates of intake. Part of the reason for a stronger correlation between diet and adipose as compared with plasma levels may be that fatty acid concentrations are more regulated in the cholesteryl ester and plasma phospholipid fractions and thus respond less to alteration in intake. (Compare the response to an increase in dietary linoleic

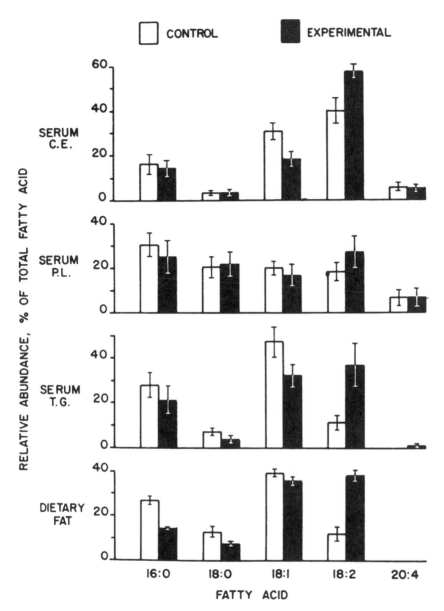

Figure 9–6. Fatty acids in the major serum lipid fractions (C.E., cholesteryl ester; P.L., phospholipids; T.G., triglycerides) compared with dietary fat. Subjects were elderly, institutionalized men whose diet was unaltered (control) or whose diet was altered (experimental) to increase the linoleic acid content from 11% to almost 40% of total fatty acid while oleic acid was held constant. Data are presented for 10 subjects in each group after 3 years. Subjects were selected for adherence to dietary protocol of 88.6% or better. Values are shown as mean ± SD. Note the larger change in linoleic (18:2) acid and oleic (18:1) acid response in the triglyceride fraction relative to the cholesteryl ester and phospholipid fractions. (From Dayton et al., 1966; reproduced with permission.)

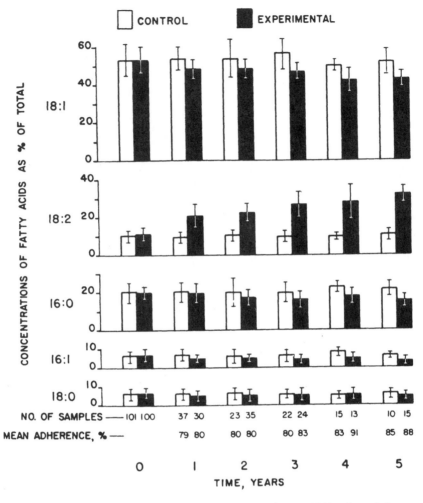

Figure 9–7. Fatty acids of aspirated adipose tissue in control and experimental subjects. Subjects were elderly, institutionalized men, and men in the experimental group had their diet altered to increase the linoleic acid content from 11% to almost 40% of total fatty acid while oleic acid was held constant. Time intervals shown are ± 30 days. Values are shown as mean ± SD. (From Dayton et al., 1966; reproduced with permission.)

acid measured in serum cholesterol ester, phospholipids, and adipose tissue in Figs. 9–6 and 9–7.)

Marine Omega-3 Fatty Acids

A substantial literature supports the idea that long chain omega-3 marine fatty acids measured in human tissues do reflect dietary intake. Levels of eicosapentaenoic acid ($20:5\omega$-3) and docosahexaenoic acid ($22:6\omega$-3) measured in serum phospholipids were much higher in residents of a Japa-

nese seaside fishing village than among inland Americans (3.7 times higher for $20:5\omega$-3; 9.9 times higher for $22:6\omega$-3) (Yamori et al., 1985). Similar differences were noted in plasma and platelet eicosapentaenoic acid concentrations when Greenland Eskimos, having very high marine oil consumption, were compared with Danish controls (Dyerberg et al., 1975; Dyerberg and Bang, 1979). High fish oil consumption in the Japanese subjects was also reflected in a higher percentage of 20:

5ω-3 and $22:6\omega$-3 in adipose tissue. It should be noted that the dietary differences involved here are large. After one subject consumed an "Eskimo diet" (seal, fish, and other marine animals) containing 14 g of eicosapentaenoic acid daily for 74 days, adipose tissue eicosapentaenoic acid concentration rose from 0% to only 0.5%. Eicosapentaenoic acid concentration in the phospholipids of erythrocytes, however, rose from 2.3% to 12.8%. After 36 months of consuming 1.8 g of eicosapentaenoic acid daily as fish oil, mean eicosapentaenoic acid concentration in adipose tissue among 28 subjects was 0.51%, whereas levels were not detectable among 28 controls (Sinclair and Gale, 1987). In a cross-sectional study, 15 subjects with a daily dietary omega-3 fatty acid intake of less than 0.10 g/day were observed to have 3.8% of omega-3 fatty acids in plasma phospholipids compared with subjects consuming greater than 0.20 g/day whose mean plasma omega-3 fatty acid proportion was 5.2% ($p < 0.05$) (Silverman et al., 1988). In their study of 3,570 adults, Ma et al. (1995b) observed correlations of $r = 0.23$ (cholesterol ester fraction) and $r = 0.20$ (phospholipid fraction) for eicosapentaenoic acid intake and $r = 0.42$ (cholesterol ester) and $r = 0.42$ (phospholipid) for docosahexaenoic acid intake. In an intervention study among 20 healthy men, supplementation with 4 g/day of eicosapentaenoic acid quadrupled its levels in erythrocyte phospholipids, but levels returned to baseline after 3 months, indicating that this was a medium-term marker (Prisco et al., 1996). Marckmann et al. (1995) measured the reproducibility of these fatty acids over 8 months in 27 men and women aged 20 to 29 years. The correlation over 8 months was $r = 0.68$ for eicosapentaenoic acid and $r = 0.93$ for docosahexaenoic acid. The average adipose levels were moderately correlated with intakes estimated from three 7-day weighted food records ($r = 0.40$ for eicosapentaenoic acid, $r = 0.66$ for docosahexaenoic acid), suggesting that the latter may be a more reliable marker of fish intake. London et al. (1991) observed a correlation of $r = 0.48$ for the sum of these two marine fatty acids compared with adipose levels. These data suggest that eicosapentaenoic acid in adipose tissue, plasma, and erythrocytes discriminates between long-term fish eaters and nonfish eaters; however, the dose–response relation remains to be determined.

Oleic Acid

Oleic acid is the principal monounsaturated fatty acid in the diet. Although most studies have demonstrated a positive relation between oleic acid intake and oleic acid measured in blood and adipose tissue, the relation is not as strong as that observed for linoleic acid, possibly because oleic acid can be synthesized endogenously from carbohydrate and because the range of intake is less. In the study of Dougherty and coworkers (1987) referred to previously, the oleic acid contribution to major fatty acids in the cholesterol ester fraction of plasma was 37.8% among Italian subjects and 18.6% among U.S. subjects, although the calculated oleic acid composition of the diets in the two centers was equivalent. The difference may be due to the fact that most of the oleic acid in the Italian diets is probably the *cis* isomer derived from olive oil, whereas much of that in the U.S. diet is probably the *trans* isomer derived from partial hydrogenation of vegetable oils in margarine. In the intervention study referred to earlier, an increase of oleic acid intake from 11% to 20% of calories had a variable effect on plasma oleic acid, increasing it by 14% among triglycerides, 0% in cholesteryl esters, and 9% in phospholipids (Sacks et al., 1987). Similarly, Ma et al. (1995b) observed only weak correlations between oleic acid intake and oleic acid levels in plasma cholesterol esters ($r = 0.03$) and phospholipids ($r = 0.08$). Hunter et al. (1992) observed an only slightly stronger correlation ($r = 0.13$) for oleic acid in adipose compared with a food-frequency questionnaire estimate in

118 men; and Garland et al. (1997) reported $r = 0.12$ in 140 women. In the study of Beynen and coworkers (1980), pooling seven datasets, the correlation between relative percentages of monounsaturated fats in diet and adipose tissue was $r = 0.46$. In a study in Crete, high levels of oleic acid in adipose tissue were attributed to the diet high in olive oil (Fordyce et al., 1983). Thus, plasma levels are poor predictors of oleic acid intake, but adipose tissue may weakly reflect oleic acid intake.

Saturated Fatty Acids

The principal saturated fatty acids in both diet and tissues are palmitic acid (16:0), the most abundant, and stearic acid (18:0). Levels of these fatty acids in plasma do not provide a simple index of intake. In the study of Dougherty and coworkers (1987), for instance, although calculated intake of saturated fatty acids in the U.S. subjects (17.4% of calories) was double that of the Italian subjects (8.7% of calories), levels of saturated fatty acids in the cholesteryl ester fraction of plasma were actually lower in the U.S. subjects. It is possible that consumption of linoleic acid (higher in the U.S. subjects) and other polyunsaturated fatty acids reduces saturated fatty acid levels in plasma.

Interestingly, Ma et al. (1995b) in their study of 3,570 adults, observed similar strengths of correlations between plasma cholesterol ester saturated fatty acid levels and saturated fat intake ($r = 0.23$) and polyunsaturated fat intake ($r = 0.24$). Among 20 healthy subjects, correlations between normal intake of total saturated fatty acids and fatty acid composition of triglycerides in adipose tissue were $r = 0.57$ for palmitic acid and $r = 0.56$ for stearic acid (Field et al., 1985). Hunter et al. (1992) observed a lower correlation for palmitic acid ($r = 0.27$), comparing an adipose tissue measurement with a food-frequency questionnaire estimate among 118 men; and Garland et al. (1997) reported a correlation of $r = 0.14$ among 140 women. In the intervention study of Dayton and coworkers

(1966), in which dietary intake of saturated fat (initially about 40% of total fatty acid) was approximately halved, differences in serum palmitic and stearic acid compositions were slight after 3 years of the intervention, whether measured in the cholesteryl ester, phospholipid, or triglyceride fraction. Substantial reductions in palmitic and stearic acid levels in adipose tissue were observed, however, suggesting that long-term saturated fatty acid intake may be reflected in adipose tissue levels.

A novel approach was taken by McMurchie and colleagues (1984b), who compared fatty acid levels in human cheek epithelial cell phospholipids collected from vegetarians and a group of nonvegetarians. Cheek cells are collected in a noninvasive manner by asking subjects to rinse their mouths with distilled water and centrifuging the expectorated fluid. Saturated fat as a percentage of total fat intake (21% among vegetarians, 27% among nonvegetarians) was closely reflected in the saturated fatty acid composition of the cheek cell phospholipids (21% among vegetarians, 34% among nonvegetarians). Little difference in polyunsaturated fatty acid intake was present, and the monounsaturated fatty acid composition of phospholipids was actually higher among the vegetarians despite a substantially lower dietary intake. In an intervention study (McMurchie et al., 1984a) 16 subjects had their dietary polyunsaturated to saturated fat ratio increased from a mean of 0.27 to 1.06, principally by the replacement of saturated and monounsaturated fatty acids with linoleic acid. After 6 weeks, the mean plasma linoleic acid level had increased by 9.0% of total plasma fatty acid, whereas linoleic acid in cheek cells had increased by 36.4% of total cheek cell fatty acids; however, there was no significant change among saturated fatty acids. These results are intriguing, but partially paradoxical, and more data are needed to define the utility of cheek cell fatty acid levels as measures of dietary intake.

Trans-Fatty Acids

Concern has been expressed about the health effects of *trans*-fatty acids in the modern diet. The only natural sources of *trans*-fatty acids are foods containing ruminant fats (e.g., dairy products, beef fat) and breast milk, and levels in these sources are relatively low. Industrial hydrogenation of vegetable oils (e.g., margarine) alters fatty acids from the *cis* isomer to the *trans* geometry (Ohlrogge et al., 1981).

The average *trans*-fatty acid content of the U.S. food supply is approximately 5% to 6% of total fat intake, which is similar to the *trans*-fatty acid content of human adipose tissue (Senti, 1985). Similar agreement has been found in the United Kingdom, where the average *trans*-fat intake of 5.4% of fat estimated in the average diet was similar to the average of 5.2% of adipose fat obtained from 95 subjects (Thomas et al., 1981). Among 118 Boston-area men, Hunter et al. (1992) observed a modest ($r = 0.29$) correlation between *trans* fatty acid measured in adipose and by food-frequency questionnaire. Among 140 Boston-area women, Garland et al. (1997) found a stronger correlation of $r = 0.40$ between adipose *trans* and intake estimated from the average of two food-frequency questionnaires; the correlation with animal *trans* sources was much weaker than the correlation with vegetable *trans*. In a previous validation study among 115 Boston-area women, London et al. (1991) observed a correlation of $r = 0.51$ between *trans* intake estimated from a single food-frequency questionnaire and an FA measure. The variability in these estimates derived from Boston-area studies using similar diet assessment methods may be due to chance or to small differences in study procedures; alternatively, temporal changes in the *trans* contents of manufactured products such as oils and margarines may cause misclassification in intake estimates derived by using nutrient composition databases that do not reflect these changes.

Laboratory Techniques

If cholesteryl esters or phospholipids are used for fatty acid analysis, it is probably not necessary to collect fasting blood samples. Subjects, however, should be fasting if the triglyceride fraction or free plasma levels are to be analyzed. Zambon et al. (1993) observed that in subjects with high triglyceride levels, free fatty acids were artificially elevated due to the postvenisection lipolytic activity of lipoprotein lipase. This elevation could be eliminated by immediate freezing of the plasma at $-70°C$ or the use of paraoxon (which blocks lipoprotein lipase activity) in the vacutainer tubes.

The techniques of subcutaneous fat aspiration are well described by Hirsch and colleagues (1960). Subsequent modifications of this technique eliminating the use of saline injection, and possibly local anesthetic, have made it even more applicable to large epidemiologic studies (Beynen and Katan, 1985a; Handelman et al., 1988). Use of glass apparatus and rigorous cleaning with organic solvents is most important. Separation of the triglyceride, cholesteryl esters, phospholipid, and free fatty acid fractions requires preparative thin layer chromatography. Gas–liquid chromatography or HPLC methods may be used to separate and measure the fatty acids within each fraction. Fatty acids are identified by their known chromatographic characteristics and by comparison with known standards, and they are quantitated by calculating the area under each peak. The sum of these individual fatty acids accounts for as much as 98% of the total peak area of fatty acids on the chromatogram. A typical high resolution chromatogram is displayed in Figure 9–8.

Stability

Beynen and Katan (1985a) observed no significant alterations in the fatty acid compositions of abdominal adipose tissue stored at 4°C, $-20°C$, and $-80°C$ for up to 18 months.

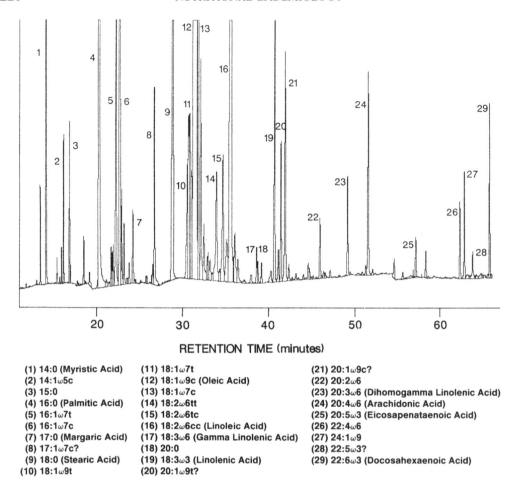

RETENTION TIME (minutes)

(1) 14:0 (Myristic Acid)	(11) 18:1ω7t	(21) 20:1ω9c?
(2) 14:1ω5c	(12) 18:1ω9c (Oleic Acid)	(22) 20:2ω6
(3) 15:0	(13) 18:1ω7c	(23) 20:3ω6 (Dihomogamma Linolenic Acid)
(4) 16:0 (Palmitic Acid)	(14) 18:2ω6tt	(24) 20:4ω6 (Arachidonic Acid)
(5) 16:1ω7t	(15) 18:2ω6tc	(25) 20:5ω3 (Eicosapenataenoic Acid)
(6) 16:1ω7c	(16) 18:2ω6cc (Linoleic Acid)	(26) 22:4ω6
(7) 17:0 (Margaric Acid)	(17) 18:3ω6 (Gamma Linolenic Acid)	(27) 24:1ω9
(8) 17:1ω7c?	(18) 20:0	(28) 22:5ω3?
(9) 18:0 (Stearic Acid)	(19) 18:3ω3 (Linolenic Acid)	(29) 22:6ω3 (Docosahexaenoic Acid)
(10) 18:1ω9t	(20) 20:1ω9t?	

Figure 9–8. A high resolution gas-liquid chromatography chromatogram of a fatty acid profile.

Other Determinants

Ma et al. (1995b) observed that plasma saturated fatty acid levels tended to be higher, and/or linoleic acid levels were lower, in overweight subjects, alcohol drinkers, and smokers, even after standardizing for reported dietary intake. These observations could reflect differential validity of reporting of dietary intake in these groups or true modification of the relations of intake with plasma fat levels.

Protein

No single biochemical measure is adequate for the assessment of protein intake. In NHANES I, protein intake was a signifi-

cant predictor of both serum total protein and serum albumin in multiple regression analyses. Even after adjustment for constitutional and sociodemographic factors, however, protein intake explained less than 10% of the variance in these biochemical measures (Kerr et al., 1982). In populations where protein intake is low or marginal, serum levels may be more useful. The other common measure of protein intake is urinary nitrogen excretion. Most of the nitrogen derived from amino acids produced by protein catabolism is excreted in urine. When dietary protein is reduced, these amino acids are used more efficiently, and thus less nitrogen is excreted (Young and

Pellett, 1987). Excess ingested protein increases nitrogen excretion. In a study of eight healthy subjects, Bingham and Cummings (1985) measured daily protein intake and urinary nitrogen excretion for 28 consecutive days. The mean within-person CV% in protein intake was 21%, whereas the mean within-person CV% in urinary nitrogen was substantially less at 13%. The high day-to-day variation in protein intake, reflected in the smaller, but still substantial variation in 24-hour urinary nitrogen level, means that a single 24-hour urinary nitrogen level will be a poor marker of long-term intake. In a subsequent study of 160 women who kept 16 days of weighed food records and collected an average of six 24-hour urine samples in the course of 1 year, Bingham and Cummings (1985) observed a correlation of $r = 0.69$ between nitrogen intake estimated from the diet records and the average of the 24-hour urine nitrogen levels; thus, several 24-hour urine samples are needed to provide a stable estimate of nitrogen intake. Nitrogen excretion increases with body size and exercise, and decreased caloric intake results in a less efficient utilization of amino acids and higher urinary nitrogen excretion (Alpers et al., 1983). These nondietary influences should be considered in the interpretability of urinary nitrogen as a measure of dietary protein.

Urinary measurement of 3-methylhistidine has been proposed as a specific indicator of meat consumption. The correlation between 24-hour urinary 3-methylhistidine and a food-frequency questionnaire meat score among 24 Canadian men was remarkably high ($r = 0.77$) (McKeown-Eyssen et al., 1986); this relationship needs to be examined further. The requirement for a 24-hour urine sample limits the usefulness of these markers for large epidemiologic studies.

Fiber

Low fiber intake has been hypothesized to increase a wide range of chronic diseases, but few studies have been conducted be-cause of difficulties in collection of stool specimens. Dietary fiber can be classified as soluble or insoluble. Neutral detergent fiber (NDF) includes insoluble hemicellulose, cellulose, and lignin. Daily fecal weight, but not stool frequency, increases with increasing NDF consumption in isocaloric diets (Tucker et al., 1981; Kelsay and Clark, 1984). Dietary fiber intake was positively correlated with daily stool weight ($r = 0.84$) in a meta-analysis including 206 individual subjects (Cummings et al., 1992). In a study in which total fiber intake was estimated from 2-day food records, significant correlations were found between fiber intake and fecal hemicellulose ($r = 0.54$) and percentage of water ($r = 0.37$), and a nonsignificant positive correlation was observed with total fecal fiber ($r = 0.27$) (McKeown-Eyssen et al., 1986). Similar correlations were found with fiber intake estimated from a food-frequency questionnaire 1 year before the stool specimens were collected. These data suggest that total fiber, and its insoluble components measured in stool, may be good indices of fiber intake. The difficulty of obtaining stool specimens from subjects in large epidemiologic studies severely limits the utility of this form of biochemical assessment.

SUMMARY

Biochemical measurements of nutrient levels in blood or other tissues can provide a useful assessment of the intake of certain nutrients. This approach is especially important for nutrients that are measured poorly by other methods due to large within-food variation in nutrient content. The principal biochemical indicators that are used in epidemiologic studies are listed in Table 9–1, along with representative values from the literature of their reproducibility and validity.

The selection of a method for estimating intake of a particular nutrient must be made on a nutrient-by-nutrient basis. For several important nutrients, no feasible biochemical indicator of intake is available.

Table 9–1. Principal biochemical indicators of nutrient intake used in epidemiologic studies for which information on validity exists

Nutrient	Analytic procedure[a]	Biologic tissue	Reproducibility (Time)[a]	Validity[b,c]
Retinol	HPLC	Plasma	0.58 (6 mo)	0.17
Beta-carotene	HPLC	Plasma	0.45 (6 yr)	0.51
		Adipose	0.50 (4 mo)	0.20
Alpha-carotene	HPLC	Plasma	—	0.58
Beta-cryptoxanthin	HPLC	Plasma	—	0.49
Lutein/zeaxanthin	HPLC	Plasma	—	0.31
Lycopene	HPLC	Plasma	—	0.50
Vitamin E	HPLC	Plasma	0.65 (6 yr)	0.35 (diet)
		Plasma	—	0.53 (+ suppl)
		Adipose	0.78 (4 mo)	0.24
Vitamin D	HPLC	Plasma	—	0.25 (diet)
		Plasma	—	0.35 (+ suppl)
Vitamin C	HPLC	Plasma	0.28 (6 yr)	0.38 (diet)
		Plasma	—	0.43 (+ suppl)
Vitamin B_6	PLP assay	Plasma	—	0.37
Folacin	Microbiologic assays	Serum	—	0.56
		Erythrocyte	—	0.51
Selenium	Neutron activation AAS	Serum	0.76 (1 yr)	0.63
		Toenails	0.48 (6 yr)	0.59
	Glutathione perox- idase activity	Blood	—	Plateaus at 100 μg/day intake
Iron	Ferritin	Serum	—	0.16
Sodium	AAS	Urine (24-hr)	—	0.41
Calcium	AAS	Urine (24-hr)	—	0.16
Potassium	AAS	Urine (24-hr)	—	0.53
Magnesium	AAS	Urine (24-hr)	—	0.34
Cholesterol	Ultracentrifugation	Blood	0.60 (1 yr)	0.46 (low intake)
				0.08 (high intake)
Palmitic acid	HPLC	Plasma	>0.65 (1 yr)	0.23
		Adipose	—	0.27
Oleic acid	HPLC	Plasma	>0.65 (1 yr)	0.03
		Adipose	—	0.13
Linoleic acid	HPLC	Plasma	>0.65 (1 yr)	0.28
		Adipose	—	0.48
Trans fatty acids	HPLC	Adipose	—	0.40
Eicosapentaenoic acid	HPLC	Adipose	0.68 (8 mo)	0.40
Docosahexaenoic acid	HPLC	Adipose	0.93 (8 mo)	0.66
Nitrogen	Kjeldahl	Six 24-hr urines	—	0.69
Sodium	Flame photometry	Six 24-hr urines	—	0.30
Potassium	Flame photometry	Six 24-hr urines	—	0.73
Magnesium	Flame photometry	Two 24-hr urines	—	0.34
Fiber	Hemicellulose	Stool	—	0.54

[a] AAS, atomic absorption spectrophotometry; HPLC, high-performance liquid chromatography; PLP, pyridoxol 5'-phosphate.

[b] Representative values from the literature; for specific references see text for each nutrient.

[c] Correlations of biochemical indicator values with an appropriate dietary assessment method; for details see text for each nutrient. These are generally underestimates of true validity due to misclassification in measuring dietary intake.

For others, within-person variation in level of the indicator or the existence of other strong determinants make correlations with long-term intake weak. For some nutrients, a biochemical indicator of intake exists that is sufficiently valid to be the method of choice. Careful attention to specimen collection, storage, and analysis is vital to avoid misclassification or bias. As analytic methods improve and more biochemical indicators are validated as measures of dietary intake, their use in nutritional epidemiology is likely to expand.

REFERENCES

Aalberts, J. S., P. L. Weegels, L. van der Heijden, M. H. Borst, J. Burema, J. G. Hautvast, and T. Kouwenhoven (1988). Calcium supplementation: Effect on blood pressure and urinary mineral excretion in normotensive male lactoovovegetarians and omnivores. *Am J Clin Nutr* 48, 131–138.

Alfthan, G., A. Aro, H. Arvilommi, and J. K. Huttunen (1991). Selenium metabolism and platelet glutathione peroxidase activity in healthy Finnish men: Effects of selenium yeast, selenite, and selenate. *Am J Clin Nutr* 53, 120–125.

Alpers, D. H., R. E. Clouse, and W. F. Stenson (1983). *Manual of Nutritional Therapeutics*. Boston, MA: Little, Brown and Co.

Amedee-Manesme, O., R. Luzeau, C. Carlier, and A. Ellrodt (1987a). Simple impression cytology method for detecting vitamin A deficiency (letter). *Lancet 1*, 1263.

Amedee-Manesme, O., M. S. Mourey, A. Hanck, and J. Therasse (1987b). Vitamin A relative dose response test: Validation by intravenous injection in children with liver disease. *Am J Clin Nutr* 46, 286–289.

Andon, M. B., and R. D. Reynolds (1987). A comparison of plasma pyridoxal 5'-phosphate concentrations in capillary (finger prick) and venous blood. *Am J Clin Nutr* 45, 1461–1465.

Arntzenius, A. C., D. Kromhout, J. D. Barth, J. H. Reiber, A. V. Bruschke, B. Buis, C. M. van Gent, N. Kempen-Voogd, S. Strikwerda, and E. A. van der Velde (1985). Diet, lipoproteins, and the progression of coronary atherosclerosis. The Leiden Intervention Trial. *N Engl J Med 312*, 805–811.

Arroyave, G., C. O. Chichester, H. Flores, J. Glover, L. A. Mejia, J. A. Olson, K. L. Simpson, and B. A. Underwood (1982). *Biochemical Methodology for the Assessment of Vitamin A Status*. Report of IVACG. Washington, DC: Nutrition Foundation.

Ascherio, A., W. C. Willett, E. B. Rimm, E. L. Giovannucci, and M. J. Stampfer (1994). Dietary iron intake and risk of coronary disease among men. *Circulation 89*, 969–974.

Baker, H., O. Frank, and S. H. Hutner (1980). Vitamin analyses in medicine. In: Goodhart, R. S., and Shils, M. E. (eds.): *Modern Nutrition in Health and Disease*. Philadelphia: Lea and Febiger, pp. 631–632.

Bamji, M. S., and F. Ahmed (1978). Effect of oral contraceptive steroids on vitamin status of women and female rats. *World Rev Nutr Diet 31*, 135–140.

Bankson, D. D., R. M. Russell, and J. A. Sadowski (1986). Determination of retinyl esters and retinol in serum or plasma by normal-phase liquid chromatography: Method and applications. *Clin Chem 32 (pt 1)*, 35–40.

Basu, T. K., D. R. Patel, and D. C. Williams (1974). A simplified microassay of transketolase in human blood. *Int J Vitam Nutr Res 44*, 319–326.

Basu, T. K., and C. J. Schorah (1982). Vitamin C reserves and requirements in health and disease. In Basu, T. K., and Schorah, C. S. (eds.): *Vitamin C in Health and Disease*. Westport, CT: AVI Publishing, pp. 61–92.

Bates, C. J., A. E. Black, D. R. Phillips, A. J. Wright, and D. A. Southgate (1982). The discrepancy between normal folate intakes and the folate RDA. *Hum Nutr Appl Nutr 36*, 422–429.

Behrens, W. A., and R. Madere (1986). Alpha- and gamma-tocopherol concentrations in human serum. *J Am Coll Nutr 5*, 91–96.

Belsey, R. E., H. F. DeLuca, and J. T. Potts Jr. (1974). A rapid assay for 25-OH-vitamin D_3 without preparative chromatography. *J Clin Endocrinol Metab 38*, 1046–1051.

Bendich, A. (1992). Safety issues regarding the use of vitamin supplements. *Ann NY Acad Sci 669*, 300–312.

Bettendorff, L., C. Grandfils, C. De Rycker, and E. Schoffeniels (1986). Determination of thiamine and its phosphate esters in human blood serum at femtomole levels. *J Chromatog 382*, 297–302.

Beynen, A. C., R. J. Hermus, and J. G. Hautvast (1980). A mathematical relationship between the fatty acid composition of the diet and that of the adipose tissue in man. *Am J Clin Nutr 33*, 81–85.

Beynen, A. C., and M. B. Katan (1985a). Rapid sampling and long-term storage of subcutaneous adipose-tissue biopsies for determination of fatty acid composition. *Am J Clin Nutr 42*, 317–322.

Beynen, A. C., and M. B. Katan (1985b). Why do polyunsaturated fatty acids lower serum cholesterol? *Am J Clin Nutr 42*, 560–563.

Bhagavan, H. N. (1985). Interaction between vitamin B-6 and drugs. In Reynolds, R. D., and Leklem, J. E. (eds.): *Vitamin B₆: Its Role in Health and Disease*. New York: Alan R. Liss, pp. 401–415.

Bieri, J. G., E. D. Brown, and J. C. Smith, Jr. (1985). Determination of individual carotenoids in human plasma by high performance liquid chromatography. *J Liquid Chromatogr 8*, 473–84.

Bieri, J. G., T. J. Tolliver, and G. L. Catignani (1979). Simultaneous determination of alpha-tocopherol and retinol in plasma or red cells by high pressure liquid chromatography. *Am J Clin Nutr 32*, 2143–2149.

Biesalski, H., H. Greiff, K. Brodda, G. Hafner, and K. H. Bassler (1986). Rapid determination of vitamin A (retinol) and vitamin E (alpha-tocopherol) in human serum by isocratic adsorption HPLC. *Int J Vitam Nutr Res 56*, 319–327.

Bingham, S. A., A. Cassidy, T. J. Cole, A. Welch, S. A. Runswick, A. E. Black, D. Thurnham, C. Bates, K. T. Khaw, T. J. A. Key, and N. E. Day (1995). Validation of weighed records and other methods of dietary assessment using the 24 h urine nitrogen technique and other biological markers. *Br J Nutr 73*, 531–550.

Bingham, S. A., and J. H. Cummings (1985). Urine nitrogen as an independent validatory measure of dietary intake: A study of nitrogen balance in individuals consuming their normal diet. *Am J Clin Nutr 42*, 1276–1289.

Black, M. R., D. M. Medeiros, E. Brunett, and R. Welke (1988). Zinc supplements and serum lipids in young adult white males. *Am J Clin Nutr 47*, 970–975.

Blanchard, R. A., B. C. Furie, M. Jorgensen, S. F. Kruger, and B. Furie (1981). Acquired vitamin K–dependent carboxylation deficiency in liver disease. *N Engl J Med 305*, 242–248.

Boberg, M., L. B. Croon, I. B. Gustafsson, and B. Vessby (1985). Platelet fatty acid composition in relation to fatty acid composition in plasma and to serum lipoprotein lipids in healthy subjects with special reference to the linoleic acid pathway. *Clin Sci 68*, 581–587.

Boerwinkle, E., S. A. Brown, K. Rohrbach, A. M. Gotto, Jr., and W. Patsch (1991). Role of apolipoprotein E and B gene vari-

ation in determining response of lipid, lipoprotein, and apolipoprotein levels to increased dietary cholesterol. *Am J Hum Genet 49*, 1145–1154.

Bolton-Smith, C., C. E. Casey, K. F. Gey, W. C. Smith, and H. Tunstall-Pedoe (1991). Antioxidant vitamin intakes assessed using a food-frequency questionnaire: Correlation with biochemical status in smokers and non-smokers. *Br J Nutr 65*, 337–346.

Bonanome, A., and S. M. Grundy (1988). Effect of dietary stearic acid on plasma cholesterol and lipoprotein levels. *N Engl J Med 318*, 1244–1248.

Brook, M., and J. J. Grimshaw (1968). Vitamin C concentration of plasma and leukocytes as related to smoking habit, age, and sex of humans. *Am J Clin Nutr 21*, 1254–1258.

Bunker, V. W., L. J. Hinks, M. S. Lawson, and B. E. Clayton (1984). Assessment of zinc and copper status of healthy elderly people using metabolic balance studies and measurement of leukocyte concentrations. *Am J Clin Nutr 40*, 1096–1102.

Caggiula, A. W., R. R. Wing, M. P. Nowalk, N. C. Milas, S. Lee, and H. Langford (1985). The measurement of sodium and potassium intake. *Am J Clin Nut 42*, 391–398.

Cameron, E., and L. Pauling (1978). Supplemental ascorbate in the supportive treatment of cancer: Reevaluation of prolongation of survival times in terminal human cancer. *Proc Natl Acad Sci USA 75*, 4538–4542.

Cameron, E., L. Pauling, and B. Leibovitz (1979). Ascorbic acid and cancer: A review. *Cancer Res 39*, 663–681.

Camp, V. M., J. Chipponi, and B. A. Faraj (1983). Radioenzymatic assay for direct measurement of plasma pyridoxal 5'-phosphate. *Clin Chem 29*, 642–644.

Campbell, D. R., M. D. Gross, M. C. Martini, G. A. Grandits, J. L. Slavin, and J. D. Potter (1994). Plasma carotenoids as biomarkers of vegetable and fruit intake. *Cancer Epidemiol Biomark Prev 3*, 493–500.

Campos, F. A., H. Flores, and B. A. Underwood (1987). Effect of an infection on vitamin A status of children as measured by the relative dose response (RDR). *Am J Clin Nutr 46*, 91–94.

Castenmiller, J. J., R. P. Mensink, L. van der Heijden, T. Kouwenhoven, J. G. Hautvast, P. W. de Leeuw, and G. Schaafsma (1985). The effect of dietary sodium on urinary calcium and potassium excretion in normotensive men with different calcium intakes. *Am J Clin Nutr 41*, 52–60.

Cavill, I., A. Jacobs, and M. Worwood (1986). Diagnostic methods for iron status. *Ann Clin Biochem 23*, 168–171.

Chen, X., G. Q. Yang, J. Chen, X. Chen, Z. Wen, and K. Ge (1980). Studies on the relations of selenium and Keshan disease. *Biol Trace Element Res 2*, 91–107.

Clark, L. C. (1985). The epidemiology of selenium and cancer. *Fed Proc 44*, 2584–2589.

Clark, L. C., G. F. Combs Jr., B. W. Turnbull, E. H. Slate, D. K. Chalker, J. Chow, L. S. Davis, R. A. Glover, G. F. Graham, E. G. Gross, A. Krongrad, J. L. Lesher, Jr., H. K. Park, B. B. Sanders, Jr., C. L. Smith, and J. R. Taylor (1996). Effects of selenium supplementation for cancer prevention in patients with carcinoma of the skin. A randomized controlled trial. Nutritional Prevention of Cancer Study Group. *JAMA 276*, 1957–1963.

Committee on Diet Nutrition and Cancer, Assembly of Life Sciences, National Research Council (1982). *Diet, Nutrition, and Cancer*. Washington, DC: National Academy Press.

Comstock, G. W., A. J. Alberg, and K. J. Helzlsouer (1993). Reported effects of long-term freezer storage on concentrations of retinol, β-carotene, and α-tocopherol in serum or plasma summarized. *Clin Chem 39*, 1075–1078.

Comstock, G. W., M. S. Menkes, S. E. Schober, J. P. Vuilleumier, and K. J. Helsing (1988). Serum levels of retinol, beta-carotene, and alpha-tocopherol in older adults. *Am J Epidemiol 127*, 114–123.

Comstock, G. W., E. P. Norkus, S. C. Hoffman, M. W. Xu, and K. J. Helzlsouer (1995). Stability of ascorbic acids, carotenoids, retinol, and tocopherols in plasma stored at −70 degrees C for 4 years. *Cancer Epidemiol Biomark Prev 4*, 505–507.

Cook, J. D., and B. S. Skikne (1982). Serum ferritin: A possible model for the assessment of nutrient stores. *Am J Clin Nutr 35*, 1180–1185.

Cooper, G. R. (1979). High density lipoprotein reference materials. In Lippel, K. (ed.): *Report of the High Density Lipoprotein Methodology Workshop*. Bethesda, MD: U.S. Government Printing Office, DHEW Publ. No. 79–1661, pp. 178–188.

Cousins, R. J. (1985). Absorption, transport, and hepatic metabolism of copper and zinc: Special reference to metallothionein and ceruloplasmin. *Physiol Rev 65*, 238–309.

Craft, N. E., E. D. Brown, and J. C. Smith Jr. (1988). Effects of storage and handling conditions on concentrations of individual carotenoids, retinol, tocopherol in plasma. *Clin Chem 34*, 44–48.

Cummings, J. H., S. A. Bingham, K. W. Heaton, and M. A. Eastwood (1992). Fecal weight, colon cancer risk, and dietary intake of nonstarch polysaccharides (dietary fiber). *Gastroenterology 103*, 1783–1789.

Dayton, S., S. Hashimoto, W. Dixon, and M. L. Pearce (1966). Composition of lipids in human serum and adipose tissue during prolonged feeding of a diet high in unsaturated fat. *J Lipid Res 7*, 103–111.

DeLuca, H. F. (1979). The vitamin D system in the regulation of calcium and phosphorus metabolism. *Nutr Rev 37*, 161–193.

Delves, H. T. (1976). The microdetermination of copper in plasma protein fractions. *Clin Chim Acta 71*, 495–500.

Dickson, I. (1987). New approaches to vitamin D. *Nature 325*, 18.

Doolman, R., A. Dinbar, and B. A. Sela (1995). Improved measurement of transketolase activity in the assessment of "TPP effect." *Eur J Clin Chem Clin Biochem 33*, 445–446.

Dougherty, R. M., C. Galli, A. Ferro-Luzzi, and J. M. Iacono (1987). Lipid and phospholipid fatty acid composition of plasma, red blood cells, and platelets and how they are affected by dietary lipids: A study of normal subjects from Italy, Finland, and the USA. *Am J Clin Nutr 45*, 443–455.

Driskell, J. A. (1978). Vitamin B-6 status of the elderly. In *Human Vitamin B-6 Requirements*. National Research Council, Food and Nutrition Board. Washington, DC: National Academy of Sciences, pp. 252–256.

Driskell, J. A., A. J. Clark, T. L. Bazzarre, L. F. Chopin, H. McCoy, M. A. Kenney, and S. W. Moak (1985). Vitamin B-6 status of Southern adolescent girls. *J Am Diet Assoc 85*, 46–49.

Driskell, W. J., M. M. Bashor, and J. W. Neese (1985). Loss of vitamin A in long-term stored, frozen sera. *Clin Chim Acta 147*, 25–30.

Dyerberg, J., and H. O. Bang (1979). Haemostatic function and platelet polyunsaturated fatty acids in Eskimos. *Lancet 2*, 433–435.

Dyerberg, J., H. O. Bang, and N. Hjorne (1975). Fatty acid composition of the plasma lipids in Greenland Eskimos. *Am J Clin Nutr 28*, 958–966.

Farleigh, C. A., R. Shepherd, and D. G. Land (1985). Measurement of sodium intake and its relationship to blood pressure and salivary sodium concentration. *Nutr Res 5*, 815–816.

Farquhar, J. W., and E. H. Ahrens, Jr. (1963).

Effects of dietary fats on human erythro-cyte fatty acid patterns. *J Clin Invest 42*, 675–685.

Fawzi, W. W., T. C. Chalmers, M. G. Herrera, and F. Mosteller (1993). Vitamin A supplementation and child mortality: A meta-analysis. *JAMA 269*, 898–903.

Ferroli, C. E., and P. R. Trumbo (1994). Bioavailability of vitamin B-6 in young and older men. *Am J Clin Nutr 60*, 68–71.

Field, C. J., A. Angel, and M. T. Clandinin (1985). Relationship of diet to the fatty acid composition of human adipose tissue structural and stored lipids. *Am J Clin Nutr 42*, 1206–1220.

Fischer, P. W., A. Giroux, and M. R. L'Abbe (1984). Effect of zinc supplementation on copper status in adult men. *Am J Clin Nutr 40*, 743–746.

Fordyce, M. K., G. Christakis, A. Kafatos, R. Duncan, and J. Cassady (1983). Adipose tissue fatty acid composition of adolescents in a US–Greece cross-cultural study of coronary heart disease risk factors. *J Chronic Dis 36*, 481–486.

Forman, M. R., G. R. Beecher, E. Lanza, M. E. Reichman, B. I. Graubard, W. S. Campbell, T. Marr, L. C. Yong, J. T. Judd, and P. R. Taylor (1995). Effect of alcohol consumption on plasma carotenoid concentrations in premenopausal women: A controlled dietary study. *Am J Clin Nutr 62*, 131–135.

Fotouhi, N., M. Meydani, M. S. Santos, S. N. Meydani, C. H. Hennekens, and J. M. Gaziano (1996). Carotenoid and tocopherol concentrations in plasma, peripheral blood mononuclear cells, and red blood cells after long-term β-carotene supplementation in men. *Am J Clin Nutr 63*, 553–558.

Frassinelli-Gunderson, E. P., S. Margen, and J. R. Brown (1985). Iron stores in users of oral contraceptive agents. *Am J Clin Nutr 41*, 703–712.

Garland, C., R. B. Shekelle, E. Barrett-Conner, M. H. Criqui, A. H. Rossof, and O. Paul (1985). Dietary vitamin D and calcium and risk of colorectal cancer: A 19-year prospective study in men. *Lancet 1*, 307–309.

Garland, M., J. S. Morris, B. A. Rosner, M. J. Stampfer, V. L. Spate, C. J. Baskett, W. C. Willett, and D. J. Hunter (1993). Toenail trace element levels as biomarkers: Reproducibility over a 6-year period. *Cancer Epidemiol Biomark Prev 2*, 493–497.

Garland, M., F. M. Sacks, G. A. Colditz, E. B. Rimm, L. A. Sampson, W. C. Willett, and D. J. Hunter (1997). The relationship between fatty acid intake as assessed by food frequency questionnaires, diet records, and

adipose tissue fatty acid composition among a population of U.S. women. *AJCN* (in press).

Gibson, R. S. (1990). *Principles of Nutritional Assessment*. New York: Oxford University Press.

Glueck, C. J., D. J. Gordon, J. J. Nelson, C. E. Davis, and H. A. Tyroler (1986). Dietary and other correlates of changes in total and low density lipoprotein cholesterol in hypercholesterolemic men. The lipid research clinics coronary primary prevention trial. *Am J Clin Nutr 44*, 489–500.

Goodman, E. G., M. Thornquist, M. Kestin, B. Metch, G. Anderson, and G. S. Omenn (1996). The association between participant characteristics and serum concentrations of β-carotene, retinol, retinyl palmitate, and α-tocopherol among participants in the Carotene and Retinol Efficacy Trial (CARET) for prevention of lung cancer. *Cancer Epidemiol Biomark Prev 5*, 815–821.

Gordon, T., W. P. Castelli, M. C. Hjortland, W. B. Kannel, and T. R. Dawber (1977). High density lipoprotein as a protective factor against coronary heart disease. The Framingham Study. *Am J Med 62*, 707–714.

Grider, A., L. B. Bailey, and R. J. Cousins (1990). Erythrocyte metallothionein as an index of zinc status in humans. *Proc Natl Acad Sci USA 87*, 1259–1262.

Griffiths, N. M., R. D. Stewart, and M. F. Robinson (1976). The metabolism of [75Se] selenomethionine in four women. *Br J Nutr 35*, 373–382.

Grundy, S. M. (1996). Dietary fat. In Ziegler, E. E., and Filer, Jr., J. J. (eds.): *Present Knowledge in Nutrition*. 7th ed. Washington, DC: ILSI Press, pp. 44–57.

Grundy, S. M., and G. L. Vega (1988). Plasma cholesterol responsiveness to saturated fatty acids. *Am J Clin Nutr 47*, 822–824.

Gurr, M. I., R. T. Jung, M. P. Robinson, and W. P. James (1982). Adipose tissue cellularity in man: The relationship between fat cell size and number, the mass and distribution of body fat and the history of weight gain and loss. *Int J Obesity 6*, 419–436.

Haddad, J. G., Jr., and T. J. Hahn (1973). Natural and synthetic sources of circulating 25-hydroxyvitamin D in man. *Nature 244*, 515–517.

Hainline, A., Jr., C. L. Winn, G. R. Cooper, D. T. Miller, and D. D. Bayse (1978). The CDC cooperative cholesterol and triglyceride standardization program—Twenty years experience. *Clin Chem 24*, 1020.

Hallberg, L., and L. Rossander (1984). Improvement of iron nutrition in developing countries: Comparison of adding meat, soy protein, ascorbic acid, citric acid, and ferrous sulphate on iron absorption from a simple Latin American–type of meal. *Am J Clin Nutr 39*, 577–583.

Hambidge, K. M. (1973). Increase in hair copper concentration with increasing distance from the scalp. *Am J Clin Nutr 26*, 1212–1215.

Handelman, G. J., W. L. Epstein, L. J. Machlin, F. J. van Kuijk, and E. A. Dratz (1988). Biopsy method for human adipose with vitamin E and lipid measurements. *Lipids 23*, 598–604.

Hankinson, S. E., S. J. London, C. G. Chute, R. L. Barbieri, L. Jones, L. A. Kaplan, F. M. Sacks, and M. J. Stampfer (1989). Effect of transport conditions on the stability of biochemical markers in blood. *Clin Chem 35*, 2313–2316.

Haussler, M. R., and T. A. McCain (1977). Basic and clinical concepts related to vitamin D metabolism and action. *N Engl J Med 297*, 974–983.

Hegsted, D. M., R. B. McGandy, M. L. Myers, and F. J. Stare (1965). Quantitative effects of dietary fat on serum cholesterol in man. *Am J Clin Nutr 17*, 281–295.

Hegsted, D. M., and R. J. Nicolosi (1987). Individual variation in serum cholesterol levels. *Proc Natl Acad Sci USA 84*, 6259–6261.

Herbert, V. (1987). Recommended dietary intakes (RDI) of folate in humans. *Am J Clin Nutr 45*, 661–670.

Herbeth, B., L. Didelot-Barthelemy, A. Lemoine, and C. Le Devehat (1988). Plasma fat-soluble vitamins and alcohol consumption (letter). *Am J Clin Nutr 47*, 343–344.

Herve, C., P. Beyne, and E. Delacoux (1994). Determination of thiamine and its phosphate esters in human erythrocytes by high-performance liquid chromatography with isocratic elution. *J Chromatogr B Biomed Appl 653*, 217–220.

Hirsch, J., J. W. Farquhar, E. H. Ahrens, Jr., M. L. Peterson, and W. Stoffel (1960). Studies of adipose tissue in man; A microtechnic for sampling and analysis. *Am J Clin Nutr 8*, 499–511.

Holbrook, J. T., K. Y. Patterson, J. E. Bodner, L. W. Douglas, C. Veillon, J. L. Kelsay, W. Mertz, and J. C. Smith, Jr. (1984). Sodium and potassium intake and balance in adults consuming self-selected diets. *Am J Clin Nutr 40*, 786–793.

Holick, M. F. (1995). Environmental factors that influence the cutaneous production of vitamin D. *Am J Clin Nutr 61 (suppl)*, 638S–645S.

Holman, R. T. (1986). Control of polyunsaturated acids in tissue lipids. *J Am Coll Nutr 5*, 183–211.

Horwitt, M. K. (1987). Human requirements for riboflavin: Reply to letter by Bates. *Am J Clin Nutr 46*, 123.

Howard, M. P., M. A. Andon, and R. D. Reynolds (1984). Long-term stability of pyridoxal phosphate in frozen human plasma. *Fed Proc 43*, 486.

Hsing, A. W., G. W. Comstock, and B. F. Polk (1989). Effect of repeated freezing and thawing on vitamins and hormones in serum. *Clin Chem 35*, 2145.

Hughes, M. R., D. J. Baylink, P. G. Jones, and M. R. Haussler (1976). Radioligand receptor assay for 25-hydroxyvitamin D-2/D-3 and 1 alpha, 25-dihydroxyvitamin D-2/D-3. *J Clin Invest 58*, 61–70.

Hulley, S. B., R. Cohen, and G. Widdowson (1977). Plasma high-density lipoprotein cholesterol level: Influence of risk factor intervention. *JAMA 238*, 2269–2271.

Hunt, I. F., N. J. Murphy, A. E. Cleaver, B. Faraji, M. E. Swendseid, A. H. Coulson, V. A. Clark, N. Laine, C. A. Davis, and J. C. Smith, Jr. (1983). Zinc supplementation during pregnancy: Zinc concentration of serum and hair from low-income women of Mexican descent. *Am J Clin Nutr 37*, 572–582.

Hunter, D. J., C. G. Chute, E. Kushner, G. A. Colditz, M. J. Stampfer, F. E. Speizer, J. S. Morris, and W. C. Willett (1987). Predictors of selenium concentration in nail tissue. *Am J Epidemiol 126*, 743.

Hunter, D. J., E. B. Rimm, F. M. Sacks, M. J. Stampfer, G. A. Colditz, L. B. Litin, and W. C. Willett (1992). Comparison of measures of fatty acid intake by subcutaneous fat aspirate, food frequency questionnaire, and diet records in a free-living population of US men. *Am J Epidemiol 135*, 418–427.

Iber, F. L., J. P. Blass, M. Brin, and C. M. Leevy (1982). Thiamin in the elderly—relation to alcoholism and to neurological degenerative disease. *Am J Clin Nutr 36(suppl)*, 1067–1082.

International Collaborative Study Group (1986). Metabolic epidemiology of plasma cholesterol: Mechanisms of variation of plasma cholesterol within populations and between populations. *Lancet 2*, 991–996.

International Vitamin Consultative Group (IVACG) (1993). *A Brief Guide to Current Methods of Assessing Vitamin A status.* Washington, DC: The Nutrition Foundation, Inc.

Irwin, M. I., and B. K. Hutchins (1976). A conspectus of research on vitamin C requirements of man. *J Nutr* 106, 821–879.

Iyengar, V. (1987). Dietary intake studies of nutrients and selected toxic elements in human studies: Analytical approaches. *Clin Nutr* 6, 105–117.

Jacob, R. A., J. H. Skala, and S. J. Omaye (1987). Biochemical indices of human vitamin C status. *Am J Clin Nutr* 46, 818–826.

Jacobs, D. R., Jr., and E. Barrett-Connor (1982). Retest reliability of plasma cholesterol and triglyceride. The Lipid Research Clinics Prevalence Study. *Am J Epidemiol* 116, 878–885.

Jacques, P. F., A. D. Halpner, and J. B. Blumberg (1995). Influence of combined antioxidant nutrient intakes on their plasma concentrations in an elderly population. *Am J Clin Nutr* 62, 1228–1233.

Jacques, P. F., S. I. Sulsky, G. A. Perrone, and E. J. Schaefer (1994). Ascorbic acid and plasma lipids. *Epidemiology* 5, 19–26.

Jacques, P. F., S. I. Sulsky, J. A. Sadowski, J. C. Phillips, D. Rush, and W. C. Willett (1993). Comparison of micronutrient intake measured by a dietary questionnaire and biochemical indicators of micronutrient status. *Am J Clin Nutr* 57, 182–189.

Jie, K. S., K. Hamulyak, B. L. Gisjsbers, F. J. Roumen, and C. Vermeer (1992). Serum osteocalcin as a marker for vitamin K-status in pregnant women and their newborn babies. *Thromb Haemost* 68, 388–391.

Joffres, M. R., D. M. Reed, and K. Yano (1987). Relationship of magnesium intake and other dietary factors to blood pressure: The Honolulu Heart Study. *Am J Clin Nutr* 45, 469–475.

Johnson, E. J., P. M. Suter, N. Sahyoun, J. D. Ribaya-Mercado, and R. M. Russell (1995). Relation between β-carotene intake and plasma and adipose tissue concentrations of carotenoids and retinoids. *Am J Clin Nutr* 62, 598–603.

Jordan, P., D. Brubacher, U. Moser, H. B. Stahelin, and K. F. Gey (1995). Vitamin E and vitamin A concentrations in plasma adjusted for cholesterol and triglycerides by multiple regression. *Clin Chem* 41, 924–927.

Joseph, H. M. (1994). *Assessment of Dietary Intakes for Sodium, Potassium, Calcium, and Magnesium, and Factors Influencing Salt Intake.* Thesis, School of Nutrition, Tufts University.

Kaaks, R. (1997). Validation and calibration of dietary intake measurements in the EPIC project methodologic considerations *International J Epidemiol* 26(suppl 1) 515–525.

Kalman, D. A., G. E. Goodman, G. S. Omenn, G. Bellamy, and B. Rollins (1987). Micronutrient assay for cancer prevention clinical trials: Serum retinol, retinyl palmitate, alpha-carotene, and beta-carotene with the use of high-performance liquid chromatography. *J Natl Cancer Inst* 79, 975–982.

Kardinaal, A. F., P. van't Veer, H. A. Brants, H. van den Berg, J. van Schoonhoven, and R. J. Hermus (1995). Relations between antioxidant vitamins and adipose tissue, plasma, and diet. *Am J Epidemiol* 141, 440–450.

Katan, M. B., A. C. Beynen, J. H. de Vries, and A. Nobels (1986). Existence of consistent hypo-and hyperresponders to dietary cholesterol in man. *Am J Epidemiol* 123, 221–234.

Keenum, D. (1993). Conjunctival impression cytology. In Underwood, B. A., and Olson, J. A., (eds.): *IVACG—A Brief Guide to Current Methods of Assessing Vitamin A Status.* Washington, DC: The Nutrition Foundation, Inc., pp. 19–21.

Kelsay, J. L., and W. M. Clark (1984). Fiber intakes, stool frequency, and stool weights of subjects consuming self-selected diets. *Am J Clin Nutr* 40, 1357–1360.

Kerr, G. R., E. S. Lee, M. K. Lam, R. J. Lorimor, E. Randall, R. N. Forthofer, M. A. Davis, and S. M. Magnetti (1982). Relationship between dietary and biochemical measures of nutritional status in HANES I data. *Am J Clin Nutr* 35, 294–307.

Keshan Disease Research Group of the Chinese Academy of Medical Sciences (1979). Epidemiologic studies on the etiologic relationship of selenium and Keshan disease. *Chin Med J* 92, 477–482.

Keys, A. (1984). Serum-cholesterol response to dietary cholesterol. *Am J Clin Nutr* 40, 351–359.

Keys, A., J. T. Anderson, and F. Grande (1965). Serum cholesterol response to changes in the diet. I. Iodine value of dietary fat versus 2S-P. *Metabolism* 14, 747–758.

Khaw, K. T., and E. Barrett-Connor (1987). Dietary potassium and stroke-associated mortality. A 12-year prospective population study. *N Engl J Med* 316, 235–240.

Kjeldsen, S. E., I. Eide, P. Leren, and O. P. Foss (1983). Effects of posture on serum cholesterol fractions, cholesterol ratio and triglycerides. *Scand J Clin Lab Invest* 43, 119–121.

Kjosen, B., and S. H. Seim (1977). The transketolase assay of thiamine in some diseases. *Am J Clin Nutr* 30, 1591–1596.

Klasing, S. A., and S. M. Pilch (eds.) (1985). *Suggested Measures of Nutritional Status and Health Conditions for the Third National Health and Nutrition Examination Survey.* Bethesda, MD: Federation of American Societies for Experimental Biology.

Klevay, L. M. (1983). Copper and ischemic heart disease. *Biol Trace Element Res 5,* 245–255.

Klevay, L. M., S. J. Reck, R. A. Jacob, G. M. Logan, Jr., J. M. Munoz, and H. H. Sandstead (1980). The human requirement for copper. I. Healthy men fed conventional, American diets. *Am J Clin Nutr 33,* 45–50.

Knapen, M. H. J., K. Hamulyak, and C. Vermeer (1989). The effect of vitamin K supplementation on circulating osteocalcin (bone gla protein) and urinary calcium excretion. *Ann Intern Med 111,* 1001–1005.

Knekt, P., A. Aromaa, J. Maatela, R. K. Aaran, T. Nikkari, M. Hakama, T. Hakulinen, R. Peto, E. Saxen, and T. L. (1988). Serum vitamin E and risk of cancer among Finnish men during a 10-year follow-up. *Am J Epidemiol 127,* 28–41.

Korpela, H., J. Kumpulainen, P. V. Luoma, A. J. Arranto, and E. A. Sotaniemi (1985). Decreased serum selenium in alcoholics as related to liver structure and function. *Am J Clin Nutr 42,* 147–151.

Kushi, L. H., R. A. Lew, F. J. Stare, C. R. Ellison, M. el Lozy, G. Bourke, L. Daly, I. Graham, N. Hickey, R. Mulcahy, and J. Kevancy (1985). Diet and 20-year mortality from coronary heart disease: The Ireland–Boston Diet-Heart study. *N Engl J Med 312,* 811–818.

Kushi, L. H., K. W. Samonds, J. M. Lacey, P. T. Brown, J. G. Bergan, and F. M. Sacks (1988). The association of dietary fat with serum cholesterol in vegetarians: The effect of dietary assessment on the correlation coefficient. *Am J Epidemiol 128,* 1054–1064.

Lehmann, J., D. D. Rao, J. J. Canary, and J. T. Judd (1988). Vitamin E and relationships among tocopherols in human plasma, platelets, lymphocytes, and red blood cells. *Am J Clin Nutr 47,* 470–474.

Lehtimaki, T., T. Moilanen, K. Porkka, H. K. Akerblom, T. Ronnemaa, L. Rasanen, J. Viikari, C. Ehnholm, and T. Nikkari (1995). Association between serum lipids and apolipoprotein E phenotype is influenced by diet in a population-based sample of free-living children and young adults: The Cardiovascular Risk in Young Finns Study. *J Lipid Res 36,* 653–661.

Leklem, J. E. (1985). Physical activity and vitamin B-6 metabolism in men and women: Interrelationship with fuel needs. In Reynolds, R. D., and Leklem, J. E. (eds.): *Vitamin B-$_6$: Its Role in Health and Disease.* New York: Alan R. Liss, pp. 221–241.

Leklem, J. E. (1990). Vitamin B-6: A status report. *J Nutr 120(suppl),* 1503–1507.

Leklem, J. E. (1996). Vitamin B-6. In In Ziegler, E. E., and Filer, L. J., Jr., (eds.): *Present Knowledge in Nutrition,* 7th ed. Washington, DC: ILSI Press, pp. 174–183.

Lemoyne, M., A. Van Gossum, R. Kurian, M. Ostro, J. Axler, and K. N. Jeejeebhoy (1987). Breath pentane analysis as an index of lipid peroxidation: A functional test of vitamin E status. *Am J Clin Nutr 46,* 267–272.

Levander, O. A. (1985). Considerations on the assessment of selenium status. *Fed Proc 44,* 2579–2583.

Levine, M., C. Conry-Cantilena, Y. Wang, R. W. Welch, P. W. Washko, K. R. Dhariwal, J. B. Park, A. Lazarev, J. F. Graumlich, J. King, and L. R. Cantilena (1996). Vitamin C pharmacokinetics in healthy volunteers: Evidence for a recommended dietary allowance. *Proc Natl Acad Sci USA 93,* 3704–3709.

Lind, J. (1753). *A Treatise on the Scurvy.* Republished, Edinburgh: Edinburgh University Press, 1953.

Linscheer, W. G., and A. J. Vergroesen (1988). Lipids. In Shils, M. E., and Young, V. R. (eds.): *Modern Nutrition in Health and Disease.* Philadelphia: Lea and Febiger, pp. 72–107.

Lips, P., F. C. van Ginkel, M. J. Jongen, F. Rubertus, W. J. van der Vijgh, and J. C. Netelenbos (1987). Determinants of vitamin D status in patients with hip fracture and in elderly control subjects. *Am J Clin Nutr 46,* 1005–1010.

Liu, K., R. Cooper, J. McKeever, P. McKeever, R. Byington, I. Soltero, R. Stamler, F. Gosch, E. Stevens, and J. Stamler (1979a). Assessment of the association between habitual salt intake and high blood pressure: Methodological problems. *Am J Epidemiol 110,* 219–226.

Liu, K., R. Cooper, I. Soltero, and J. Stamler (1979b). Variability in 24-hour urine sodium excretion in children. *Hypertension 1,* 631–636.

Liu, T., N. P. Wilson, C. B. Craig, T. Tamura, S. Soong, H. E. Sauberlich, P. Cole, and C. E. Butterworth Jr. (1992). Evaluation of three nutritional assessment methods in a group of women. *Epidemiology 3,* 496–502.

Lloyd, B., R. S. Lloyd, and B. E. Clayton (1983). Effect of smoking, alcohol and other factors on the selenium status of a healthy population. *J Epidemiol Commun Health 37*, 213–217.

Loerch, J. D., B. A. Underwood, and K. C. Lewis (1979). Response of plasma levels of vitamin A to a dose of vitamin A as an indicator of hepatic vitamin A reserves in rats. *J Nutr 109*, 778–786.

Loh, H. S. (1972). The relationship between dietary ascorbic acid intake and buffy coat and plasma ascorbic acid concentrations at different ages. *Int J Vitam Nutr Res 42*, 80–85.

London, S. J., F. M. Sacks, J. Caesar, M. J. Stampfer, E. Siguel, and W. C. Willett (1991). Fatty acid composition of subcutaneous adipose tissue and diet in postmenopausal US women. *Am J Clin Nutr 54*, 340–345.

Longnecker, M. P., M. J. Stampfer, J. S. Morris, V. Spate, C. Baskett, M. Mason, and W. C. Willett (1993). A 1-y trial of the effect of high-selenium bread on selenium concentrations in blood and toenails. *Am J Clin Nutr 57*, 408–413.

Longnecker, M. P., P. R. Taylor, O. A. Levander, M. Howe, C. Veillon, P. A. McAdam, K. Y. Patterson, J. M. Holden, M. J. Stampfer, J. S. Morris, and W. C. Willett (1987). Tissue selenium (Se) levels and indices of Se exposure in a seleniferous area. *Fed Proc 46*, 587.

Lumeng, L., T. K. Li, and A. Lui (1985). The interorgan transport and metabolism of vitamin B-6. In Reynolds, R. D., and Leklem, J. F. (eds.): *Vitamin B-₆: Its Role in Health and Disease.* New York: Alan R Liss, pp. 35–54.

Luoma, H., A. Aromaa, S. Helminen, H. Murtomaa, L. Kiviluoto, S. Punsar, and P. Knekt (1983). Risk of myocardial infarction in Finnish men in relation to fluoride, magnesium and calcium concentration in drinking water. *Acta Med Scand 213*, 171–176.

Luoma, P. V., H. Korpela, E. A. Sotaniemi, and J. Kumpulainen (1985). Serum selenium, glutathione peroxidase, lipids, and human liver microsomal enzyme activity. *Biol Trace Element Res 8*, 113–121.

Ma, J., A. R. Folsom, J. H. Eckfeldt, L. Lewis, and L. E. Chambless (1995a). Short-and long-term repeatability of fatty acid composition of human plasma phospholipids and cholesterol esters. The Atherosclerosis Risk in Communities (ARIC) Study Investigators. *Am J Clin Nutr 62*, 572–578.

Ma, J., A. R. Folsom, E. Shahar, and J. H. Eckfeldt (1995b). Plasma fatty acid composition as an indicator of habitual dietary fat intake in middle-aged adults. The Atherosclerosis Risk in Communities (ARIC) Study. *Am J Clin Nutr 62*, 564–571.

Ma, J., M. J. Stampfer, C. H. Hennekens, P. Frosst, J. Selhub, J. Horsford, M. R. Malinow, W. C. Willett, and R. Rozen (1996). Methylenetetrahydrofolate reductase polymorphism, plasma folate, homocysteine, and risk of myocardial infarction in U.S. physicians. *Circulation 94*, 2410–2416.

MacMahon, B., and T. F. Pugh (1970). *Epidemiology: Principles and Methods.* Boston, MA: Little, Brown and Company.

Manku, M. S., D. F. Horrobin, Y. S. Huang, and N. Morse (1983). Fatty acids in plasma and red cell membranes in normal humans. *Lipids 18*, 906–908.

Manore, M. N., J. E. Leklem, and M. C. Walter (1987). Vitamin B-6 metabolism as affected by exercise in trained and untrained women fed diets differing in carbohydrate and vitamin B-6 content. *Am J Clin Nutr 46*, 995–1004.

Manttari, M., P. Koskinen, C. Ehnholm, J. K. Huttunen, and V. Manninen (1991). Apolipoprotein E polymorphism influences the serum cholesterol response to dietary intervention. *Metabolism 40*, 217–221.

Marckmann, P., A. Lassen, J. Haraldsdottir, and B. Sandstrom (1995). Biomarkers of habitual fish intake in adipose tissue. *Am J Clin Nutr 62*, 956–959.

Margolis, S. A., and T. P. Davis (1988). Stabilization of ascorbic acid in human plasma, and its liquid-chromatographic measurement. *Clin Chem 34*, 2217–2223.

Martin, G. M. (1964). Copper content of hair and nails of normal individuals and of patients with hepatolenticular degeneration. *Nature 202*, 903–904.

Mascher, H. (1993). Determination of total pyridoxal in human plasma following oral administration of vitamin B₆ by high-performance liquid chromatography with post-column derivatization. *J Pharmaceut Sci 82*, 972–974.

McAdam, P. A., V. C. Morris, and O. A. Levander (1984). Automated determination of glutathione peroxidase (GSU-Px) activity in tissue from rats of different selenium (Se) status (abstract). *Fed Proc 43*, 867.

McCarron, D. A., C. D. Morris, H. J. Henry, and J. L. Stanton (1984). Blood pressure and nutrient intake in the United States. *Science 224*, 1392–1398.

McCombs, R. J., D. E. Marcadis, J. Ellis, and R. B. Weinberg (1994). Attenuated hypercholesterolemic response to a high-cholesterol diet in subjects heterozygous for the apolipoprotein A-IV-2 allele. *N Engl J Med 331*, 706–710.

McCormick, D. B. (1985). Vitamins. In Tietz, N. W. (ed.): *Textbook of Clinical Chemistry*. Philadelphia; W. B. Saunders.

McKenna, M. J., R. Freaney, A. Meade, and F. P. Muldowney (1985). Hypovitaminosis D and elevated serum alkaline phosphatase in elderly Irish people. *Am J Clin Nutr 41*, 101–109.

McKeown-Eyssen, G. E., K. S. Yeung, and E. Bright-See (1986). Assessment of past diet in epidemiologic studies. *Am J Epidemiol 124*, 94–103.

McMurchie, E. J., B. M. Margetts, L. J. Beilin, K. D. Croft, R. Vandongen, and B. K. Armstrong (1984a). Dietary-induced changes in the fatty acid composition of human cheek cell phospholipids: Correlation with changes in the dietary polyunsaturated/saturated fat ratio. *Am J Clin Nutr 39*, 975–980.

McMurchie, E. J., J. D. Potter, T. E. Rohan, and B. S. Hetzel (1984b). Human cheek cells; a non-invasive method for determining tissue lipid profiles in dietary and nutritional studies. *Nutr Rep Int 29*, 519–526.

McNamara, D. J., R. Kolb, T. S. Parker, H. Batwin, P. Samuel, C. D. Brown, and E. H. Ahrens, Jr. (1987). Heterogeneity of cholesterol homeostasis in men. Response to changes in dietary fat quality and cholesterol quantity. *J Clin Invest 79*, 1729–1739.

Mejia, L. A., and G. Arroyave (1983). Determination of vitamin A in blood. Some practical considerations on the time of collection of the specimens and the stability of the vitamin. *Am J Clin Nutr 37*, 147–151.

Micozzi, M. S., E. D. Brown, B. K. Edwards, J. G. Bieri, P. R. Taylor, F. Khachik, G. R. Beecher, and J. C. Smith, Jr. (1992). Plasma carotenoid response to chronic intake of selected foods and beta-carotene supplements in men. *Am J Clin Nutr 55*, 1120–1125.

Miller, L. T. (1985). Oral contraceptives and vitamin B-6 metabolism. In Reynolds, R. D., and Leklem, J. E. (eds.): *Vitamin B-6: Its Role in Health and Disease*. New York: Alan R Liss, pp. 243–255.

Milne, D. B., S. Gallagher, C. Stjern, L. M. Klevay, and H. H. Sandstead (1982). Superoxide dismutase activity as an index of copper nutriture in man (abstract). *Fed Proc 41*, 785.

Mino, M., and M. Nagamatu (1986). An evaluation of nutritional status of vitamin E in pregnant women with respect to red blood cell tocopherol level. *Int J Vitam Nutr Res 56*, 149–153.

Mjos, O. D., S. N. Rao, L. Bjoru, T. Henden, D. S. Thelle, O. H. Forde, and N. E. Miller (1979). A longitudinal study of the biological variability of plasma lipoproteins in healthy young adults. *Atherosclerosis 34*, 75–81.

Moilanen, T., L. Rasanen, J. Viikari, H. K. Akerblom, and T. Nikkan (1992). Tracking of serum fatty acid composition: A 6-year follow-up study of Finnish youths. *Am J Epidemiol 136*, 1487–1492.

Morris, J. S., M. J. Stampfer, and W. C. Willett (1983). Dietary selenium in humans: Toenails as an indicator. *Biol Trace Element Res 5*, 529–537.

Motchnik, P. A., B. Frei, and B. N. Ames (1994). Measurement of antioxidants in human blood plasma. *Methods Enzymol 234*, 269–279.

Naito, H. K., and J. A. David (1984). Laboratory considerations: Determination of cholesterol, triglyceride, phospholipid, and other lipids in blood and tissues. *Lab Res Methods Biol Med 10*, 1–76.

National Diet Heart Study Research Group (1968). *The National Diet Heart Study Final Report. Chapter XII. Serum Cholesterol Response. I:181–223*. No. Monograph No. 18. New York: American Heart Association.

Neve, J., F. Vertongen, and P. Capel (1988). Selenium supplementation in healthy Belgian adults: Response in platelet glutathione peroxidase activity and other blood indices. *Am J Clin Nutr 48*, 139–143.

Newton, H. M., M. Sheltawy, A. W. Hay, and B. Morgan (1985). The relations between vitamin D_2 and D_3 in the diet and plasma 250HD$_2$ and 250HD$_3$ in elderly women in Great Britain. *Am J Clin Nutr 41*, 760–764.

Nierenberg, D. W. (1984). Determination of serum and plasma concentrations of retinol using high-performance liquid chromatography. *J Chromatogr Biomed Appl 311*, 239–248.

Nierenberg, D. W., T. A. Stukel, J. A. Baron, B. J. Dain, E. R. Greenberg, and The Skin Cancer Prevention Study Group (1989). Determinants of plasma levels of beta-carotene and retinol. *Am J Epidemiol 130*, 511–521.

Nikkari, T., P. Luukkainen, P. Pietinen, and P. Puska (1995). Fatty acid composition of serum lipid fractions in relation to gender and quality of dietary fat. *Ann Med 27*, 491–498.

Norris, R. L., M. J. Thomas, and P. W. Craswell (1986). Assessment of a two-step high-performance liquid chromatographic assay using dual-wavelength ultraviolet monitoring for 25-hydroxyergocalciferol and 25-hydroxycholecalciferol in human serum or plasma. *J Chromatogr 381*, 53–61.

O'Dell, B. L. (1984). Bioavailability of trace elements. *Nutr Rev 42*, 301–308.

Ohlrogge, J. B., E. A. Emken, and R. M. Gulley (1981). Human tissue lipids: Occurrence of fatty acid isomers from dietary hydrogenated oils. *J Lipid Res 22*, 955–960.

Olivares, M., and R. Uauy (1996). Copper as an essential nutrient. *Am J Clin Nutr 63 (suppl)*, 791S–796S.

Olson, J. A. (1984). Serum levels of vitamin A and carotenoids as reflectors of nutritional status. *JNCI 73*, 1439–1444.

Olson, J. A. (1987). Recommended dietary intakes (RDI) of vitamin K in humans. *Am J Clin Nutr 45*, 687–692.

Olson, J. A., and R. E. Hodges (1987). Recommended dietary intakes (RDI) of vitamin C in humans. *Am J Clin Nutr 45*, 693–703.

Olson, R. E. (1980). Vitamin K. In Goodhart, R. S., and Shils, M. G. (eds.). *Modern Nutrition in Health and Disease*. Philadelphia: Lea and Febiger, pp. 170–180.

Omdahl, J. L. (1978). Interaction of the parathyroid and 1,25-dihydroxyvitamin D_3 in the control of renal 25-hydroxyvitamin D_3 metabolism. *J Clin Biol Chem 253*, 8474–8478.

Omdahl, J. L., P. J. Garry, L. A. Hunsaker, W. C. Hunt, and J. S. Goodwin (1982). Nutritional status in a healthy elderly population: Vitamin D. *Am J Clin Nutr 36*, 1225–1233.

Parfitt, A. M., J. C. Gallagher, R. P. Heaney, C. C. Johnston, R. Neer, and G. D. Whedon (1982). Vitamin D and bone health in the elderly. *Am J Clin Nutr 36(suppl)*, 1014–1031.

Parr, R. M. (1985). Quality assurance of trace element analyses. *Nutr Res (suppl (1)*, 5–11.

Patwardhan, V. N. (1969). Hypovitaminosis A and epidemiology of xerophthalmia. *Am J Clinc Nutr 22*, 1106–1118.

Peng, Y. M., M. J. Xu, and D. S. Alberts (1987). Analysis and stability of retinol in plasma. *JNCI 78*, 95–99.

Peto, R. (1983). The marked differences between carotenoids and retinoids: Methodological implications for biochemical epidemiology. *Cancer Surv 2*, 327–40.

Phillips, G. B., and J. T. Dodge (1967). Composition of phospholipids and phospholipid fatty acids of human plasma. *J Lipid Res 8*, 676–681.

Pilch, S. M. (ed.) (1985). *Assessment of the Vitamin A Nutritional Status of the U.S. Population Based on Data Collected in the Health and Nutrition Examination Surveys*. Bethesda, MD: Life Sciences Research Office, Federation of American Societies for Experimental Biology.

Pilch, S. M., and F. R. Senti (1984a). *Assessment of the Iron Nutritional Status of the U.S. Population Based on Data Collected in the Second National Health and Nutrition Examination Survey, 1976–1980*. Bethesda, MD: Life Sciences Research Office, FASEB.

Pilch, S. M., and F. R. Senti (eds.): (1984b). Assessment of the zinc nutritional status of the U.S. population based on data collected in the second national health and nutrition examination survey, 1976–1980. Bethesda, MD: Life Sciences Research Office, FASEB.

Pilon, V. A., P. J. Howanitz, J. H. Howanitz, and N. Domres (1981). Day-to-day variation in serum ferritin concentration in healthy subjects. *Clin Chem 27*, 78–82.

Prasad, A. S., P. Rabbani, A. Abbasii, E. Bowersox, and M. R. Fox (1978). Experimental zinc deficiency in humans. *Ann Intern Med 89*, 483–490.

Pratt, W. B., J. L. Omdahl, and J. R. Sorenson (1985). Lack of effects of copper gluconate supplementation. *Am J Clin Nutr 42*, 681–682.

Prentice, R. L. (1986). A case–cohort design for epidemiologic cohort studies and disease prevention trials. *Biometrika 73*, 1–12.

Prisco, D., M. Filippini, I. Francalanci, R. Paniccia, G. F. Gensini, R. Abbate, and G. G. N. Serneri (1996). Effect of n-3 polyunsaturated fatty acid intake on phospholipid fatty acid composition in plasma and erythrocytes. *Am J Clin Nutr 63*, 925–932.

Rasmussen, H. S., P. McNair, L. Goransson, S. Balslov, O. G. Larsen, and P. Aurup (1988). Magnesium deficiency in patients with ischemic heart disease with and without acute myocardial infarction uncovered by an Intravenous Loading Test. *Arch Intern Med 148*, 329–332.

Rea, H. M., C. D. Thomson, D. R. Campbell, and M. F. Robinson (1979). Relation between erythrocyte selenium concentrations and glutathione peroxidase (EC I, II,1,9) activities of New Zealand residents and visitors to New Zealand. *Br J Nutr 42*, 201–208.

Reeves, V. B., E. J. Matusik, Jr., and J. L. Kelsay (1984). Variations in plasma fatty acid concentrations during a one-year self-selected dietary intake study. *Am J Clin Nutr 40(suppl)*, 1345–1351.

Reiser, S., J. C. Smith Jr., W. Mertz, J. T. Holbrook, D. J. Scholfield, A. S. Powell, W. K. Canfield, and J. J. Canary (1985). Indices of copper status in humans consuming a typical American diet containing either fructose or starch. *Am J Clin Nutr 42*, 242–251.

Reynolds, R. D., and J. E. Leklem (1985). Implications on the role of vitamin B$_6$ in health and disease—A summary. In Reynolds, R. D., and Leklem, J. F. (eds.). *Vitamin B$_6$: Its Role in Health and Disease.* New York: Alan R Liss, pp. 481–489.

Riboli, E., H. Ronnholm, and R. Saracci (1987). Biologic markers of diet. *Cancer Surv 6*, 685–718.

Robinson, J. R., M. F. Robinson, O. A. Levander, and C. D. Thomson (1985). Urinary excretion of selenium by New Zealand and North American human subjects on differing intakes. *Am J Clin Nutr 41*, 1023–1031.

Robinson, M. F., and C. D. Thomson (1981). Selenium levels in humans vs. environmental sources. In Spallholz, J. E., et al, (eds.): *Selenium in Biology and Medicine.* Westport, CT: AVI Publishing Company, pp. 283–302.

Russell, R. M., F. L. Iber, S. D. Krasinski, and P. Miller (1983). Protein-energy malnutrition and liver dysfunction limit the usefulness of the relative dose response (RDR) test for predicting vitamin A deficiency. *Hum Nutr Clin Nutr 37*, 361–71.

Russell, R. M., S. D. Krasinski, and B. Dawson-Hughes (1984). Indices of fat-soluble vitamin states. *Clin Nutr 3*, 161–168.

Russell-Briefel, R., M. W. Bates, and L. H. Kuller (1985). The relationship of plasma carotenoids to health and biochemical factors in middle-aged men. *Am J Epidemiol 122*, 741–749.

Ryzen, E., N. Elbaum, F. R. Singer, and R. K. Rude (1985). Parenteral magnesium tolerance testing in the evaluation of magnesium deficiency. *Magnesium 4*, 137–147.

Sacks, F. M., M. J. Stampfer, A. Munoz, K. McManus, M. Canessa, and E. H. Kass (1987). Effect of linoleic and oleic acids on blood pressure, blood viscosity, and erythrocyte cation transport. *J Am Coll Nutr 6*, 179–185.

Salbe, A. O., and O. A. Levander (1987). Hair and nails as indicators of selenium (Se) status in rats fed elevated dietary levels of Se as L-selenomethionine (Se Met) or sodium selenate (Na2Se04). *Fed Proc 46*, 1153.

Samuel, P., D. J. McNamara, and J. Shapiro (1983). The role of diet in the etiology and treatment of atherosclerosis. *Annu Rev Med 34*, 179–194.

Sandstead, H. H., L. K. Henriksen, J. L. Greger, A. S. Prasad, and R. A. Good (1982). Zinc nutriture in the elderly in relation to taste acuity, immune response, and wound healing. *Am J Clin Nutr 36*, 1046–1059.

Sauberlich, H. E. (1984). Newer laboratory methods for assessing nutriture of selected B-complex vitamins. *Annu Rev Nutr 4*, 377–407.

Sauberlich, H. G., J. H. Skala, and R. P. Dowdy (1974). *Laboratory Tests for the Assessment of Nutritional Status.* Cleveland, OH: CRC Press Inc.

Schrauzer, G. N., D. A. White, and C. J. Schneider (1977). Cancer mortality correlation studies—III: Statistical associations with dietary selenium intakes. *Bioinorg Chem 7*, 23–31.

Schultz, T. D., and J. E. Leklem (1985). Supplementation and vitamin B$_6$ metabolism. In Reynolds, R. D., and Leklem, J. E. (eds.): *Vitamin B$_6$: Its Role in Health and Disease.* New York: Alan R. Liss, pp. 419–427.

Schuster, K., L. B. Bailey, J. J. Cerda, and J. F. Gregory (1984). Urinary 4-pyridoxic acid excretion in 24-hour versus random urine samples as a measurement of vitamin B$_6$ status in humans. *Am J Clin Nutr 39*, 466–470.

Selhub, J., P. F. Jacques, P. W. F. Wilson, D. Rush, and I. H. Rosenberg (1993). Vitamin status and intake as primary determinants of homocysteinemia in an elderly population. *JAMA 270*, 2693–2698.

Selhub, J., and I. H. Rosenberg (1996). Folic acid. In Ziegler, E. E., and Filer, Jr., J. J. (eds.): *Present Knowledge in Nutrition*, 7th ed. Washington, DC: ILSI Press, pp. 206–219.

Senti, F. R. (ed.) (1985). *Health Aspects of Dietary Trans Fatty Acids. Report Prepared for Center for Food Safety and Applied Nutrition. Food and Drug Administration, Department of Health and Human Services.* Bethesda, MD: Life Sciences Research Office, Federation of the American Societies for Experimental Biology.

Senti, F. R., and S. M. Pilch (1984). *Assessment of the Folate Nutritional Status of the U.S. Population Based on Data Collected in the Second National Health and Nutrition Examination Survey, 1976–1980.* Bethesda, MD: Life Sciences Research Office, Federation of American Societies for Experimental Biology.

Shearer, M. J., J. Oyeyi, S. Rahim, Y. Haroon,

and P. Barkhan (1982). Endogenous vitamin K1 in human plasma measured by high-performance liquid chromatography. *J Br Soc Haematol 50,* 690.

Shekelle, R. B., A. M. Shryock, O. Paul, M. Lepper, J. Stamler, S. Liu, and W. J. Raynor, Jr. (1981). Diet, serum cholesterol, and death from coronary heart disease: The Western Electric Study. *N Engl J Med 304,* 65–70.

Sherwin, R. W., D. N. Wentworth, J. A. Cutler, S. B. Hulley, L. H. Kuller, and J. Stamler (1987). Serum cholesterol levels and cancer mortality in 361, 662 men screened for the Multiple Risk Factor Intervention Trial. *JAMA 257,* 943–948.

Silverman, D. I., G. J. Reis, F. M. Sacks, T. M. Boucher, M. E. Slipperly, and R. C. Pasternak (1988). Plasma phospholipid FPA levels: A new measure of dietary fish consumption. *Circulation 78(suppl),* 227.

Sinclair, H., and M. Gale (1987). Eicosopentaenoic acid in fat. *Lancet 1,* 1202.

Smith, F. R., and D. S. Goodman (1976). Vitamin A transport in human vitamin A toxicity. *N Engl J Med 294,* 805–808.

Smith, J. C., J. T. Holbrook, and D. E. Danford (1985). Analysis and evaluation of zinc and copper in human plasma and serum. *J Am Coll Nutr 4,* 627–638.

Sokol, R. J., J. E. Heubi, S. T. Iannaccone, K. E. Bove, and W. F. Balistreri (1984). Vitamin E deficiency with normal serum vitamin E concentrations in children with chronic cholestasis. *N Engl J Med 310,* 1209–1212.

Sokoll, L. J., and J. A. Sadowski (1996). Comparison of biochemical indexes for assessing vitamin K nutritional status in a healthy adult population. *Am J Clin Nutr 63,* 566–573.

Solomons, N. W. (1985). Biochemical, metabolic, and clinical role of copper in human nutrition. *J Am Coll Nutr 4,* 83–105.

Solomons, N. W., T. J. Layden I. H. Rosenberg, K. Vo-Khactu, and H. H. Sandstead (1976). Plasma trace metals during total parenteral alimentation. *Gastroenterology 70,* 1022–1025.

Solomons, N. W., R. M. Russell, E. Vinton, A. M. Guerrero, and L. Mejia (1982). Application of a rapid dark adaptation test in children. *J Pediatr Gastroenterol Nutr 1,* 571–574.

Sommer, A., G. Hussaini, Muhilal, I. Tarwotjo, D. Susanto, and J. S. Saroso (1980). History of night blindness: A simple tool for xerophthalmia screening. *Am J Clin Nutr 33,* 887–891.

Soustre, Y., M. C. Dop, P. Galan, and S. Herc-
berg (1986). Dietary determinants of the iron status in menstruating women. *Int J Vitam Nutr Res 56,* 281–286.

Sowers, M. R., R. B. Wallace, B. W. Hollis, and J. H. Lemke (1986). Parameters related to 25-OH-D levels in a population-based study of women. *Am J Clin Nutr 43,* 621–628.

Sowers, M. R., R. B. Wallace, and J. H. Lemke (1985). The association of intakes of vitamin D and calcium with blood pressure among women. *Am J Clin Nutr 42,* 135–142.

Speek, A. J., C. Wongkham, N. Limratana, S. Saowakontha, and W. H. Schreurs (1986). Microdetermination of vitamin A in human plasma using high-performance liquid chromatography with fluorescence detection. *J Chromatogr 382,* 284–289.

Sporn, M. B., and A. B. Roberts (1983). Role of retinoids in differentiation and carcinogenesis. *Cancer Res 43,* 3034–3040.

Stahelin, H. B., K. F. Gey, M. Eichholzer, and E. Ludin (1991). Beta-carotene and cancer prevention: The Basel Study. *Am J Clin Nutr 53 (suppl),* 265S–269S.

Sterner, R. T., and W. R. Price (1973). Restricted riboflavin: Within-subject behavioral effects in humans. *Am J Clin Nutr 26,* 150–160.

Stryker, W. S., L. A. Kaplan, E. A. Stein, M. J. Stampfer, A. Sober, and W. C. Willett (1988). The relation of diet, cigarette smoking, and alcohol consumption to plasma beta-carotene and alpha-tocopherol levels. *Am J Epidemiol 127,* 283–296.

Suttie, J. W. (1992). Vitamin K and human nutrition. *J Am Diet Assoc 92,* 585–590.

Swanson, C. A., M. P. Longnecker, C. Veillon, M. Howe, O. A. Levander, P. R. Taylor, P. A. McAdam, C. C. Brown, M. J. Stampfer, and W. C. Willett (1990). Selenium intake, age, gender, and smoking in relation to indices of selenium status of adults residing in a seleniferous area. *Am J Clin Nutr 52,* 858–862.

Tangney, C. C., R. B. Shekelle, W. Raynor, M. Gale, and E. P. Betz (1987). Intra-and interindividual variation in measurements of beta-carotene, retinol, and tocopherols in diet and plasma. *Am J Clin Nutr 45,* 764–769.

Tanumihardjo, S. A. (1993). The modified relative dose-response assay. In Underwood, B. A., and Olson, J. A., (eds.): *IVACG—A Brief Guide to Current Methods of Assessing Vitamin A Status.* Washington, DC: The Nutrition Foundation, Inc., pp. 14–15.

Tanumihardjo, S. A., Muherdiyantiningsih, D.

Permaesih, Komala, Muhilal, D. Karyadi, and J. A. Olson (1996). Daily supplements of vitamin A (8.4 μmol, 8,000 IU) improve the vitamin A status of lactating Indonesian women. *Am J Clin Nutr 63*, 32–35.

Tanumihardjo, S. A., and J. A. Olson (1991). The reproducibility of the modified relative dose response (MRDR) assay in healthy individuals over time and its comparison with conjunctival impression cytology (CIC). *Eur J Clin Nutr 45*, 407–411.

Taylor, P. R., M. P. Longnecker, O. A. Levander, S. M. Howe, W. C. Willett, C. Veillon, P. A. McAdam, K. Y. Patterson, J. M. Holden, and M. J. Stampfer (1987). Seasonal variation in selenium (Se) status among free-living persons in South Dakota. *Fed Proc 46*, 882.

Temme, E. H. M., R. P. Mensink, and G. Hornstra (1996). Comparison of the effects of diets enriched in lauric, palmitic, or oleic acids on serum lipids and lipoproteins in healthy women and men. *Am J Clin Nutr 63*, 897–903.

Thakker, K. M., H. S. Sitren, J. F. Gregory 3rd., G. L. Schmidt, and T. G. Baumgartner (1987). Dosage form and formulation effects on the bioavailability of vitamin E, riboflavin, and vitamin B-6 from multivitamin preparations. *Am J Clin Nutr 45*, 1472–1479.

Thanassi, J. W., N. T. Meisler and J. M. Kittler (1985). Vitamin B₆ metabolism and cancer. In Reynolds, R. D., and Leklem, J. E. (eds.): *Vitamin B₆: Its Role in Health and Disease*. New York: Alan R Liss, pp. 319–336.

Thomas, L. H., P. R. Jones, J. A. Winter, and H. Smith (1981). Hydrogenated oils and fats: The presence of chemically-modified fatty acids in human adipose tissue. *Am J Clin Nutr 34*, 877–886.

Thomson, C. D., L. K. Ong, and M. F. Robinson (1985). Effects of supplementation with high-selenium wheat bread on selenium, glutathione peroxidase and related enzymes in blood components of New Zealand residents. *Am J Clin Nutr 41*, 1015–1022.

Thomson, C. D., H. M. Rea, V. M. Doesburg, and M. F. Robinson (1977). Selenium concentrations and glutathione peroxidase activities in whole blood of New Zealand residents. *Br J Nutr 37*, 457–460.

Thomson, M., M. Fulton, D. A. Wood, S. Brown, R. A. Elton, A. Birtwhistle, and M. F. Oliver (1985). A comparison of the nutrient intake of some Scotsmen with dietary recommendations. *Hum Nutr Appl Nutr 39*, 443–455.

Thornton, S. P. (1977). A rapid test for dark adaptation. *Ann Ophthalmol 9*, 731–734.

Thurnham, D. I. (1972). Influence of glucose-6-phosphate dehydrogenase deficiency on the glutathione reductase test for ariboflavinosis. *Ann Trop Med Parasitol 66*, 505–508.

Tikkanen, M. J., J. K. Huttunen, C. Ehnholm, and P. Pietinen (1990). Apolipoprotein E₄ homozygosity predisposes to serum cholesterol elevation during high fat diet. *Arteriosclerosis 10*, 285–288.

Tillotson, J. A., and E. M. Baker (1972). An enzymatic measurement of the riboflavin status in man. *Am J Clin Nutr 25*, 425–431.

Traber, M. G., and H. J. Kayden (1987). Tocopherol distribution and intracellular localization in human adipose tissue. *Am J Clin Nutr 46*, 488–495.

Tucker, D. M., H. H. Sandstead, G. M. Logan, Jr., L. M. Klevay, J. Mahalko, L. K. Johnson, L. Inman, and G. E. Inglett (1981). Dietary fiber and personality factors as determinants of stool output. *Gastroenterology 81*, 879–883.

Ullrey, D. E. (1981). Selenium in the soil-plant-food chain. In Spallhotz, J. E., et al. (eds.): *Selenium in Biology and Medicine*. Westport, CT: AVI Publishing, pp. 176–191.

Underwood, B. A. (1984). Vitamin A in animal and human nutrition. In Sporn, M. B., Roberts, A. B., and Goodman, D. S., (eds): *The Retinoids*, vol. 1. Orlando, FL: Academic Press, pp. 281–392.

Vahlquist, A., G. Michaelsson, and L. Juhlin (1978). Acne treatment with oral zinc and vitamin A: Effects on the serum levels of zinc and retinol binding protein. *Acta Dermatol Venereol 58*, 437–442.

van Staveren, W. A., P. Deurenberg, M. B. Katan, J. Burema, L. C. de Groot, and M. D. Hoffmans (1986). Validity of the fatty acid composition of subcutaneous fat tissue microbiopsies as an estimate of the long-term average fatty acid composition of the diet of separate individuals. *Am J Epidemiol 123*, 455–463.

Versieck, J. (1985). Trace elements in human body fluids and tissues. *Crit Rev Clin Lab Sci 22*, 97–184.

Vuilleumier, J. P., H. E. Keller, D. Gysel, and F. Hunziker (1983). Clinical chemical methods for the routine assessment of the vitamin status in human populations. Part I: The fat-soluble vitamins A and E, and beta-carotene. *Int J Vitam Nutr Res 53*, 265–272.

Wacker, W. E. (1980). *Magnesium and Man*. Cambridge, MA: Harvard University Press.

Wahrendorf, J., A. B. Hanck, N. Munoz, J. P. Vuilleumier, and A. M. Walker (1986). Vitamin measurements in pooled blood samples. *Am J Epidemiol 123*, 544–550.

Wald, N. J., H. S. Cuckle, R. D. Barlow, P. Thompson, K. Nanchahal, R. J. Blow, I. Brown, C. C. Harling, W. J. McCulloch, J. Morgan, and A. A. Reid (1985). The effect of vitamin A supplementation on serum retinol and retinol binding protein levels. *Cancer Lett 29*, 203–213.

Wallace, R. B., and R. A. Anderson (1987). Blood lipids, lipid-related measures, and the risk of atherosclerotic cardiovascular disease. *Epidemiol Rev 9*, 95–119.

Waring, P. P., D. Fisher, J. McDonnell, E. L. McGown, and H. E. Sauberlich (1982). A continuous-flow (Auto Analyzer II) procedure for measuring erythrocyte transketolase activity. *Clin Chem 28*, 2206–2213.

Watson, R. L., and H. G. Langford (1970). Usefulness of overnight urines in population groups. Pilot studies of sodium, potassium, and calcium excretion. *Am J Clin Nutr 23*, 290–304.

Willett, W. (1987). Nutritional epidemiology: Issues and challenges. *Int J Epidemiol 16*, 312–317.

Willett, W. C. (1985). Does low vitamin B_6 intake increase the risk of coronary heart disease? In Reynolds, R. D., and Leklem, J. E. (eds.): *Vitamin B_6: It's Role in Health and Disease*. New York: Alan R. Liss, pp. 337–346.

Willett, W. C. (1986). Vitamin A and selenium intake in relation to human cancer risk. In Hayashi, Y. (ed.): *Diet, Nutrition and Cancer*. Utrecht: VNU Science Press, pp. 237–245.

Willett, W. C., B. F. Polk, J. S. Morris, M. J. Stampfer, S. Pressel, B. Rosner, J. O. Taylor, K. Schneider, and C. G. Hames (1983a). Prediagnostic serum selenium and risk of cancer. *Lancet 2*, 130–134.

Willett, W. C., B. F. Polk, B. A. Underwood, and C. G. Hames (1984a). Hypertension detection and follow-up program study of serum retinol, retinol-binding protein, total carotenoids, and cancer risk: A summary. *JNCI 73*, 1459–1462.

Willett, W. C., M. J. Stampfer, B. A. Underwood, L. A. Sampson, C. H. Hennekens, J. C. Wallingford, L. Cooper, C. C. Hsieh, and F. E. Speizer (1984b). Vitamin A supplementation and plasma retinol levels: A randomized trial among women. *JNCI 73*, 1445–1448.

Willett, W. C., M. J. Stampfer, B. A. Underwood, F. E. Speizer, B. Rosner, and C. H. Hennekens (1983b). Validation of a dietary

questionnaire with plasma carotenoid and alpha-tocopherol levels. *Am J Clin Nutr 38*, 631–639.

Willett, W. C., M. J. Stampfer, B. A. Underwood, J. O. Taylor, and C. H. Hennekens (1983c). Vitamins A, E, and carotene: Effects of supplementation on their plasma levels. *Am J Clin Nutr 38*, 559–566.

Winn, D. M., M. E. Reichman, and E. Gunter (1990). Epidemiologic issues in the design and use of biologic specimen banks. *Epidemiol Rev 12*, 56–70.

Wittpenn, J., S. C. Tseng, and A. Sommer (1986). Detection of early xerophthalmia by impression cytology. *Arch Ophthalmol 104*, 237–239.

Wood, D. A., R. A. Riemersma, S. Butler, M. Thomson, C. Macintyre, R. A. Elton, and M. F. Oliver (1987). Linoleic and eicosapentaenoic acids in adipose tissue and platelets and risk of coronary heart disease. *Lancet 1*, 177–183.

Wood, P. D., P. S. Bachorik, J. J. Albers, C. C. Stewart, C. Winn, and K. Lippel (1980). Effects of sample aging on total cholesterol values determined by the automated ferric chloride-sulfuric acid and Liebermann-Burchard procedures. *Clin Chem 26*, 592–597.

Xu, M. J., P. M. Plezia, D. S. Alberts, S. S. Emerson, Y. M. Peng, S. M. Sayers, Y. Liu, C. Ritenbaugh, and H. L. Gensler (1992). Reduction in plasma or skin alpha-tocopherol concentration with long-term oral administration of beta-carotene in humans and mice. *JNCI 84*, 1559–1565.

Yamori, Y., Y. Nara, N. Iritani, R. J. Workman, and T. Inagami (1985). Comparison of serum phospholipid fatty acids among fishing and farming Japanese populations and American inlanders. *J Nutr Sci Vitaminol 31*, 417–422.

Yang, X. Y., H. K. Naito, and R. S. Galen (1986). Urinary calcium, phosphorus, magnesium and copper in 24-hour and random samples from normal subjects. *Trace Element Med 3*, 81–86.

Yip, R., S. Schwartz, and A. S. Deinard (1983). Screening for iron deficiency with the erythrocyte protoporphyrin test. *Pediatrics 72*, 214–219.

Yong, L. C., M. R. Forman, G. R. Beecher, B. I. Graubard, W. S. Campbell, M. E. Reichman, P. R. Taylor, E. Lanza, J. M. Holden, and J. T. Judd (1994). Relationship between dietary intake and plasma concentrations of carotenoids in premenopausal women: Application of the USDA-NCI carotenoid food-composition database. *Am J Clin Nutr 60*, 223–230.

Young, V. R., and P. L. Pellett (1987). Protein intake and requirements with reference to diet and health. *Am J Clin Nutr 45(suppl)*, 1323–1343.

Zambon, A., S. I. Hashimoto, and J. D. Brunzell (1993). Analysis of techniques to obtain plasma for measurement of levels of free fatty acids. *J Lipid Res 34*, 1021–1028.

Zempleni, J., J. R. Galloway, and D. B. McCormick (1996). Pharmacokinetics of orally and intravenously administered riboflavin in healthy humans. *Am J Clin Nutr 63*, 54–66.

Zhang, S., G. Tang, R. M. Russell, K. A. Mayzel, M. J. Stampfer, W. C. Willett, and D. J. Hunter (1997). Measurement of retinoids and carotenoids in breast adipose tissue and a comparison of concentrations in breast cancer cases and control subjects. *Am J Clin Nutr, 66*: 626–632.

10

Anthropometric Measures and Body Composition

Anthropometric variables, particularly weight and height, are the most commonly employed measures of nutritional status in epidemiologic studies because of their simplicity and ease of collection. In adults, measures of body dimensions and mass are used to represent nutritional status directly, to compute the absolute size of the major body compartments, such as lean body mass and adipose mass, to estimate relative body composition, such as fatness, and to describe body fat distribution.

This chapter begins with an overview of weight and height, including their relationships to nutritional status, their use in epidemiologic studies, and the reproducibility and validity of these measurements. Next, the concept of major body compartments is discussed, and methods of measuring them are considered. The major part of the chapter addresses the assessment of relative body composition, specifically fatness, using densitometry, combinations of weight and height, skinfold thicknesses, and the newer methods of bioelectric resistance and dual energy x-ray absorptiometry. Finally, the evaluation of body fat distribution is reviewed, and the use of such measurements in epidemiologic analyses is examined.

Throughout, an emphasis is given to methods that are likely to be used by epidemiologists themselves. Methods more suitable for laboratory application are described briefly, as they can provide standards against which field methods can be compared. For each method, attention is given to measurement error. Other reviews of methods for assessing human body composition that may be helpful have been published by Lukaski (1987), Roche and colleagues (1987, 1996), and the World Health Organization (1995). A video has also been prepared by the Centers for Disease Control and Prevention that provides instruction for standardized anthropometric measurements that were used in the Third National Health and Nutrition Examination Survey.*

*Available by calling the Government Printing Office (202-512-1800) and requesting the NHANES III An-

244

WEIGHT AND HEIGHT

Relationship to Nutritional Status

The voluminous literature regarding the use of weight and height to represent childhood nutritional status is largely related to the assessment of protein-energy deficiency and is outside the scope of this book. Excellent reviews are available elsewhere (Garn, 1979; Zerfar, 1979; World Health Organization, 1983). In adults, weight and height are sometimes used directly to represent nutritional status. In populations where food is widely available, such as the United States and most other industrialized countries, height is predominantly determined by genetic factors. However, adult height clearly does reflect nutritional factors in many cultures. For example, Japanese-Americans have attained substantially greater height during successive generations (Insull et al., 1968), and major secular increases in height have been observed within Japan (Hirayama, 1978).

The effect of nutrition on height is complex, as early unconstrained intake will not only accelerate growth, but will also cause early maturity (Frisch and McArthur, 1974) and closure of the epiphyses, resulting in cessation of long bone growth. Because growth of the trunk can continue, sitting height may provide a more sensitive indicator of energy availability before age 20, particularly during adolescence. Biacromial (between the tips of the clavicles) and biiliac diameters also reflect growth during development and thus, potentially, early nutritional factors.

Use of Height and Weight in Epidemiologic Studies

Height and other measures of frame size may be particularly useful in epidemiologic studies because they may reflect an influence of diet in the remote past that may be difficult to measure in any other way. Furthermore, in case–control studies, these measurements are generally not affected by disease or its treatment (except, perhaps, in the case of spinal metastases). For example, Brinkley and coworkers (1971) have used measurements of height and other body dimensions in a case–control study of breast cancer; the positive associations they observed with biacromial and biiliac diameters support the hypothesis that early nutritional status is associated with breast cancer risk. Unfortunately, their data on sitting height (which was inversely related to breast cancer risk) are difficult to interpret because this decreases at older ages due to compression of the vertebrae, and they did not account for the older age of the breast cancer cases in their analysis.

Micozzi (1985) has used height as a measure to address the hypothesis proposed by de Waard (1975) that early energy availability might explain some of the international differences in breast cancer risk. In an ecologic study he observed a strong correlation ($r = 0.68$) between average height at age 18 and national age-specific breast cancer incidence.

Limitations of height as a measure of early nutritional status are apparent: Some of these measurements may be difficult to obtain in many studies, and in older adults vertebral collapse causes a reduction in height. Because genetic factors strongly influence these dimensions, failure to find associations in epidemiologic studies may simply reflect a lack of variation in energy availability during growth within the study population. In addition to energy intake, the composition of childhood diet, such as its animal protein and zinc content, may contribute to adult height.

Weight itself is rarely used alone in studies among adults as it is related to both height and body composition. *Change* in weight over time, however, in effect controls for overall body size and is thus frequently used as a measure of change in body composition.

thropometric Procedure Video, Stock Number 017-022-01335-5. The cost is $19.00.

Reproducibility and Validity of Weight and Height Measurements

Details of methods to ensure optimal precision and accuracy in the collection of weight, height, and other anthropometric variables are discussed elsewhere (Rose and Blackburn, 1982; Lohman et al., 1988; Roche et al., 1996) and are mentioned only briefly here. The manuals by Lohman and colleagues (1988) and Roche and colleagues (1996) contain detailed instructions with photographs and provide the standard for these measurements. Weight is optimally measured on a platform (beam balance) scale with the subject nude or lightly clad and not wearing shoes. Unfortunately, platform scales are often not sufficiently portable for many epidemiologic applications, such as in-home interviews. In this case, it may be necessary to use spring (e.g., bathroom-type) scales. Particular care must be taken to calibrate thesescales regularly using standard weights. When direct measurement of standing height is possible, it should be made without shoes, the back square against a metal wall tape, and with eyes looking straight ahead. A set square should rest on the scalp and against the wall tape to read the height, which is recorded to the nearest 0.5 cm (Rose and Blackburn, 1982).

In general, body weight is among the most precise biologic measurements, even with simple and imperfect conditions. For repeated measurements of weight within the hour among children, a standard deviation of ± 0.02 kg has been reported by Habicht and colleagues (1979). If a single measurement is used to represent weight over a longer period, such as months, factors such as changes in hydration, recency of food intake, and intended weight change will increase error substantially more than that due to the technical aspect of weighing. The net effect of both biologic and technical sources of variation can be evaluated by repeated measurements over a period of months. For example, we found a correlation of 0.96 for repeated assess-

ments of weight at an interval of approximately 1 year among adult women, even though the first value was based on self-report and the other on measurement using a bathroom-type scale. This degree of reproducibility is far greater than for most biochemical or physiologic measurements and indicates that, with reasonable care, imprecision in measurement of weight is not likely to be a serious issue in most epidemiologic studies. In studies that involve *change* in weight over months or a few years, precision in measurement is much more critical as measurement errors contribute twice (at the beginning and the end) and the magnitude of weight changes is usually small compared with differences in attained weight between persons.

Self-Reported Weight and Height

In many epidemiologic studies weight and height are necessarily based on self-reports. The validity of these self-reports has been addressed by several investigators (Stunkard and Albaum, 1981; Palta et al., 1982; Stewart, 1982; Stewart et al., 1987). Stunkard and Albaum (1981) found that reported weight averaged slightly lower (2 to 6 lb) than directly measured weight, but the correlation between them was 0.99 among U.S. men and women. These authors, however, found that self-report among Danish men and women was less valid ($r = 0.91$ to 0.97 for groups defined by age and sex). Stewart (1982) observed correlations of 0.98 or more among both U.S. men and women when reported and measured weights were compared. Palta and coworkers (1982) also found that errors were small among a large group of U.S. adults for self-reported weight and height when the report was compared with direct measurements. Weight was understated by 1.6% among men and by 3.1% among women, whereas height was overstated by 1.3% by men and 0.6% by women. Stewart and colleagues (1987) observed similar small systematic tendencies to underreport weight and over report height among 1,598 subjects in New Zealand; the correlation between reported and direct measures was 0.96 for height, 0.98 for weight, and 0.94 for relative weight. These authors point out that, due to the small tendencies to underreport weight and overreport height, relative weight based on these measures will be biased downward. This causes a small degree of systematic error when comparing data on an absolute scale, such as weight/height^2 (often called body mass index [BMI] or Quetelet's index). Epidemiologic measures of association, such as relative risks, however, will not be appreciably affected by this degree of measurement error (see Chapter 12).

Even recalled weight from many years earlier appears to be highly valid, although the error is greater than for self-report of current weight. In a study among 1,805 Japanese men living in Honolulu, Rhoads and Kagan (1983) compared the report of weight at age 25 recalled 20 to 30 years later with actual weights at age 25 recorded at the time of draft registration. Recalled weight averaged 2.2% higher than that recorded at registration, and the correlation between estimates was 0.80. Similarly, Stevens et al. (1990) found a correlation of 0.82 between actual weight and its recall 28 years later. Subjects who were older or less educated or who performed less well on a test of cognitive function reported their earlier weight less accurately. Troy and colleagues (1995) compared weight at age 18 years reported by female nurses currently 25 to 42 years of age with their medical records at admission to nursing school. Nurses underreported by an average of only 1.4 kg, and the correlation was 0.87. Using self-reported weight and height to calculate BMI at age 18, the correlation with body mass index calculated from the records was 0.84. Must and colleagues (1993) used data on weight and height obtained in the Harvard Longitudinal Study at ages 13 to 18 to assess the validity of self-reported values at ages 71 to 76. The correlations between self-reported and measured values at age 18 for weight, height, and BMI were 0.64, 0.91, and 0.91 for men and 0.84, 0.92 and 0.92 for women. Recall of earlier weights is likely to be poor and, even if valid, would not be interpretable without information on height at the same age. However, in the same study useful information was obtained by asking the elderly participants to describe their body profile at ages 5, 10, 15, and 20 using a series of pictograms developed by Sorensen et al. (1983) that ranged from very lean to massively obese. Correlations (male/female) between BMI calculated from actual measurements and the pictogram level were 0.53, 0.66 at age 20, 0.60, 0.75 at age 15, and 0.66, 0.65 at age 10.

Probing even earlier in life, self-report of birth weight also appears to be reasonably valid, at least in some populations. Among women in the Nurses' Health study, self-reported birth weight (as multiple-choice categories) was correlated with both actual birth records ($r = 0.74$) and with maternal report ($r = 0.75$) (Troy et al., 1996). Among male health professionals, the correlation between self-reported birth weight and maternal report was 0.72 (unpublished data). Sorensen et al. (1983) have also documented that adults can reasonably describe their parent's level of adiposity 15 years earlier, either by reporting their weight and height from which BMI can be calculated or with the use of multiple-choice pictograms noted earlier.

In summary, even self-reported weight and height appear to be sufficiently accurate and precise in most circumstances so that their errors have minimal effect on epidemiologic measures of association. A more serious degree of error arises when combinations of weight and height are used to represent body fat composition (discussed later).

MEASUREMENT OF MAJOR BODY COMPARTMENTS

The human body has frequently been considered as two major compartments: adipose (storage fat) and lean tissue. Conceptually, lean mass is involved in highly active metabolic processes, so that nutritional requirements are primarily related to the size of this compartment. Adipose, in contrast, has traditionally been regarded as metabolically inactive, and its main energy requirement is for transportation, as cargo, from place to place. This concept, although serving as a useful first approximation in many instances, is quite incomplete. A somewhat more detailed scheme is described later.

Body compartments are most often of interest as determinants of disease when considered in relation to overall body size. For example, it is likely that a large absolute fat mass will have more adverse metabolic effects in a person whose other body compartments are small than in a person who is large in all respects. Similarly, a small absolute bone mass will be more likely to fracture in a large person than in a small person. For some methods of determining relative body composition, such as percent body fat, it is first necessary to measure absolute compartments. The absolute size of compartments may also be inherently interesting. In particular, effects of absolute intakes of specific nutritional factors are probably important in relation to the absolute size of body compartments rather than to their relative size.

Adipose is tissue primarily composed of storage fat, mainly in the form of triglyceride. Although certainly less metabolically active in terms of energy and nutrient requirements, adipose tissue does play an important role in hormone metabolism, such as in the synthesis of estrogen in postmenopausal women (Grodin et al., 1973). The major fat stores are under the skin and in the abdomen, although considerable amounts can also be located within muscles and around other organs such as the heart and kidneys.

Lean body mass is considered to be the body component that is not adipose and is, therefore, more metabolically active. Lean body mass is, of course, extremely heterogeneous as it includes bone, muscle, extracellular water, nervous tissue, various or-

gans, and all cells other than adipocytes (Fig. 10–1). If the lean body mass (weight) is known, the adipose component can be calculated as the difference between the lean and total body masses.

The division of the body into adipose and lean body mass provides a useful anatomic distinction. Adipose tissue, however, does not include all fat in the body, such as the lipid contained within other cells, hepatocytes, or important structural lipids in cell membranes or the nervous system. Thus, it is sometimes convenient to partition the body on the basis of chemical composition, rather than anatomy, between fat mass and fat-free mass components. These compartments correspond closely, but not exactly, to adipose and lean body mass for the reasons noted previously. The distinction, however, does not appear to be of major practical importance as lipid comprises only about 2% of the lean body mass (Sheng and Huggins, 1979). At present, few practical methods exist to measure the adipose or total fat mass components directly (for review, see Jebb and Elia, 1993). Indirect methods are discussed later.

The traditional measurement of lean body mass usually involves two basic assumptions: that water is distributed only to

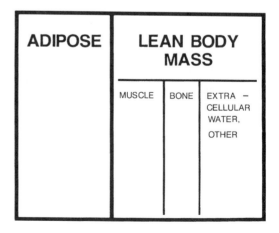

Figure 10–1. Components of total body mass.

this component (as the water content of adipose tissue is very low) and that the concentration of water in the lean body mass is constant among persons. Based primarily on data from animals, it has been estimated that the fraction of water in the lean body mass is 0.732. Thus, lean body mass = total body water/0.732. The limitations of using total body water to estimate lean body mass (and indirectly body fat composition) have been reviewed by Sheng and Huggins (1979). They note that the assumption of a constant proportion of water in the fat-free mass cannot be perfectly correct, as this varies depending on the state of hydration and the relative subcomponents of this mass. For example, bone mass, which contains relatively little water but is quite dense, can vary considerably among postmenopausal women.

Measurement of total body water is usually accomplished by dilution; a known amount of a substance that is distributed to the total body water is administered and, after sufficient time for "mixing," the concentration of this substance in the body water is measured (Schoeller, 1996). The total amount administered is then divided by the concentration, providing a measure of total body water. Deuterium oxide (heavy water, derived from a stable isotope of hydrogen) is commonly employed for this determination (Lukaski and Johnson, 1985); tritium oxide has also been used. Dilution methods are sufficiently simple and inexpensive to be practical in many epidemiologic settings: An oral dose is administered, and urine or saliva samples are collected over the next 2 to 4 hours. To minimize error, subjects should be fully hydrated but not edematous; this is usually not problematic in healthy adult populations.

Total body water (and thus lean body mass) has been extensively studied in relation to anthropometric measurements. Although the human body is three-dimensional, lean body mass appears to have a direct linear relationship with height among adults rather than an exponential

relationship; presumably the adult body is closer to a straight line than a sphere (Fig. 10–2). Thus, height can be used as a first approximation to represent lean body mass in epidemiologic analyses. Lean body mass, however, is correlated with weight even among people of the same height both because lean mass itself has weight and because adiposity is positively correlated with lean body mass (Roche, 1984). Thus, improved estimates of lean body mass can be calculated using measures of both height and weight. Such equations have been provided by Watson and colleagues (1980), who have also summarized equations derived from other populations. These authors found that calculations of total body water based on age, height, and weight were highly correlated with measurements by dilution ($r = 0.84$ for men and 0.86 for women); using exponential terms of weight and height did not improve these correlations. The equations predicting total body water (liters) from age (years), height (cm), and weight (kg) were

Men:

$$\text{Total body water} = 2.447 - 0.09516 \text{ age} + 0.1074 \text{ height} + 0.3362 \text{ weight}$$

Women:

$$\text{Total body water} = -2.097 + 0.1069 \text{ height} + 0.2466 \text{ weight}$$

As noted, age appeared to be an important variable for men, but not for women. The development and use of prediction equations are also discussed in detail by Roche et al. (1996).

Body cell mass represents the part of lean body mass composed of cells, which is mainly muscle, and excludes extracellular water and bone minerals (Moore et al., 1963). Although less frequently used because it is difficult to measure, this is the component of lean body mass that is most active with respect to energy utilization.

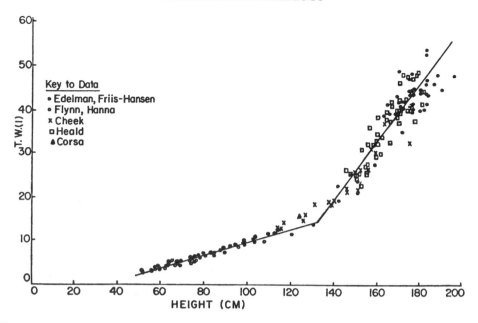

Figure 10–2. Total body water in relation to height. (From Mellits and Cheek, 1970; reproduced with permission).

Measurement of active cell mass is usually based on the determination of total body potassium, using the fact that body potassium is largely intracellular. This measurement is best accomplished by counting the gamma-ray emissions of potassium-40, a naturally occurring radioisotope. Because this method measures a natural isotope (which occurs as a known proportion of all potassium isotopes), no administration of a tracer is required; however, the method requires a special, generally unavailable, counting chamber (Lukaski, 1987; Jebb and Elia, 1993).

Bone mass is the other major component of lean body mass. Bone mass measurement can enhance the accuracy of other body components that are measured indirectly and is of inherent interest in the study of fractures. Photon absorptiometry is most commonly used to measure bone mass and is based on the principle that the mineral content of the bone being studied is directly proportional to the absorbed energy from a photon beam emitted by a radionuclide. Lukaski (1987) provides a detailed review of this technology and its accuracy. Single photon absorptiometry uses a simple and relatively inexpensive device to measure bone mass or density in the arm or legs; a site over the distal radius is the most commonly used. Although highly reproducible, even multiple measurements do not provide an accurate assessment of total bone mass, in part because much of the bone mass is contained in the axial skeleton and the densities at various sites are only moderately correlated. Dual photon absorptiometry uses the differential absorption of photon beams with two distinct energy levels to differentiate between bone mineral and soft tissue mass. Coupled with a body scanning device, this provides an accurate measurement of total body bone mass. A similar method, dual-energy x-ray absorptiometry (DEXA), in which an x-ray generator replaces the photon source, has more recently been used to measure bone mass as well as lean and fat mass (see below).

MEASUREMENT OF RELATIVE BODY COMPOSITION

Because of widespread interest in the health effects of obesity, the most frequent use of anthropometry in epidemiologic studies is to estimate adiposity. In general, adiposity has been expressed as percent body fat (fat mass/total mass $\times$ 100%), although there may be reason to question whether this is truly the most biologically relevant measure of adiposity (see below). In epidemiologic studies, the most commonly used methods to estimate relative body composition are combinations of weight and height, skinfold thickness, and body circumferences. Newer methods based on electrical resistance and impedance, DEXA, magnetic resonance imaging, and computer-assisted tomography have become available. Because these methods measure adiposity indirectly, it is crucial to consider the degree of error associated with their use, as well as their feasibility. Because densitometry has been the generally accepted standard for measuring the percentage of body weight that is fat, this method is described first, even though it is impractical for most epidemiologic applications.

Densitometry

Densitometry (also called hydrostatic weighing) is based on the principle that fat tissue is lighter than fat-free tissue. The ratio of weights measured in air and under water, therefore, provides an estimate of the proportion of total body mass that is composed of fat. In the most widely used technique, subjects wearing a swimming suit are submerged seated on a scale in a tank of water (with a known weight strapped to their body so that they do not float). Because the air in the lungs influences weight under water, residual lung volume is measured by having subjects breath through a snorkel into a special device (for a detailed description of densitometry, see Going, 1996). Formulas for the calculation of percentage of body fat from these data have been developed by Siri (1961) and Brozek and colleagues (1963). Both biologic variation in the density of fat and lean body mass and technical variation in the measurement of density contribute to error in estimating body fat composition by densitometry. Of these factors, variation in the water content of the lean body mass, in bone size, and the density of bone appear to be the primary sources of error and may lead to errors of 3% to 4% in predicting body fatness (Lohman, 1981; Lukaski, 1987). Within a population of similar age, sex, and race, however, the biologic sources of error should be considerably less important than in the heterogeneous groups in which sources of error have been evaluated. For demographically homogeneous groups, the magnitude of error associated with densitometry is not well defined.

Combinations of Weight and Height

Weight and height are the most commonly available anthropometric measurements in epidemiologic settings; the literature regarding methods of combining them to best represent adiposity is enormous. The criteria usually employed are (1) that the index should be highly correlated with percent body fat and (2) that the index be uncorrelated with height. The first criterion is obviously most important, but also the most difficult to evaluate because a perfect standard for adiposity is not available and the best methods, such as densitometry, are difficult for practical reasons. More attention has been focused on the second criterion, probably because it is far easier to evaluate. This criterion, however, has become less important with the advent of computers because many multivariate procedures are widely available that can easily provide a statistical adjustment for height (discussed later). If height is not associated with the disease being investigated, the second criterion is largely irrelevant in that setting. Moreover, the second criterion makes the implicit assumption that adiposity is unrelated to height. This appears to be generally true for adults, but is not for children; before puberty, obese children tend to be taller than lean children (discussed later and by Roche, 1984). The two most commonly employed measures of obesity are relative weight (a standardized ratio) and indices of weight and height that are not related to a standard.

Relative weight is the ratio of a subject's observed weight to a standard or expected weight; this may also be expressed as a percentage above or below the standard. The standard weights are frequently derived from a large group of persons of the same height, sex, and (sometimes) age. These may be obtained from an external population, such as the widely used Metropolitan Life Insurance "desirable weights" (Metropolitan Life Insurance Co, 1959); these are based on associations with minimal mortality among insurees and are revised periodically. In some large investigations, such as the American Cancer Society cohort of 750,000 men and women (Lew and Garfinkel, 1979), the average weights for study participants of the same height, sex, and age are used as standards.

The use of relative weight provides a readily interpretable measure; to say that a group of subjects was 140% to 150% of the average weight for their age, sex, and height conveys a meaningful image to almost any reader. The distinct disadvantage of this approach is that findings from different studies are difficult to compare as a wide variety of standards may have been employed. It is not often appreciated, for example, that the Metropolitan Life standards are substantially below the standards based on average weights in other U.S.

studies (Manson et al., 1987). Differences in standards are likely to be even greater internationally.

Obesity indices are combinations of weight and height that are not related to a standard. More than 100 years ago, Quetelet (1869) pointed out that weight/height^2 (also called the body mass index or BMI) was minimally correlated with height. Other investigators have advocated the use of weight/height, weight/height$^{1.5}$, and weight/height^3. Collectively, these have been called power indices. Benn (1971) has advocated the use of an empirically fit value for the exponent of height (p) based on the specific population being studied so that, by definition, the index (weight/height^p) is uncorrelated with height. He has further shown that such an index is perfectly correlated with relative weight based on a standard from within the same population. The use of these obesity indices, with the exception of the Benn index, has the considerable advantage that they provide measurement scales that do not vary from study to study, thus facilitating the comparison of findings. The relative merits of the different indices should be considered on the basis of their relationships with true adiposity and, to a much lesser degree, on being uncorrelated with height.

Multivariate adjustment for height provides a simple alternative to the use of relative weight or obesity indices. Weight and height can both be entered as independent variables in a multiple regression model predicting the outcome of interest; this provides a measure of the effect of weight independent of height, thus by definition weight uncorrelated with height. Conceptually, this can be thought of as the effect of weight among individuals of identical height.

Although the meaning of weight in this multivariate model containing weight and height is relatively clear, the converse is not; the interpretation of height adjusted for weight is conceptually unclear and of little interest as it is strongly related to body composition. (This was appreciated by the wit of yore who commented that he was not fat, just short for his weight.) If both height and weight-adjusted-for-height (an estimate of obesity) are of interest, a two-step procedure analogous to that suggested for adjusting nutrient intake for total caloric intake can be employed (see Chapter 11). First, a simple regression model is used with height as the independent variable (x) and weight as the dependent variable (y). The resulting residual of weight on height provides, by definition, a measure of weight uncorrelated with height. (This measure thus has all the advantages of the Benn index, with the added feature of having the usual scale of weight, i.e., kilograms or pounds.) In the second step, height and the residual of weight on height can both be entered in the multivariate model. This simultaneously provides the full effect of height as well as a measure of weight independent of height.

The assumption that true adiposity is unrelated to height is central to the interpretation of relative weight and obesity indices. This relationship has been addressed by examining the correlations between height and adiposity measured by skin folds or by densitometry (Table 10–1). In adults, it does appear that the correlation between height and adiposity is minimal; in only the data of Womersley and Durnin (1977) does there appear to be a slight inverse relationship.

Among the obesity indices shown in Table 10–1, the correlation with height has generally been lowest for BMI (weight/height^2). The Benn index, using an empirically fit exponent for weight (Benn, 1971; Lee et al., 1981), does not seem to provide any clear advantage as the correlation between height and weight/height^2 is typically already small (Garn and Pesick, 1982; Colliver et al., 1983). Others have found that the exponent of 1.5 produces a slightly lower correlation with height among women (Micozzi et al., 1986).

Relationships of height and weight

among children are considerably more complex, probably because this is a period of active growth; an exhaustive review is beyond the scope of this book. At some ages, however, height is positively associated with adiposity to a degree such that an assumption of independence is materially violated (Killeen et al., 1978). In this situation one could use the combination of weight and height most strongly correlated with obesity and adjust for height, if it is related to the outcome being studied, with multivariate analysis. Alternatively, the use of a more direct measure, such as skinfolds, may be preferable.

The validity of combinations of weight and height as measures of adiposity has frequently been assessed by correlating these with skinfold thickness (Table 10–2). Because skinfold thicknesses themselves are imperfect indicators of adiposity, the absolute value of these correlations should not be interpreted as a direct measure of validity. Comparing the correlations of skinfolds with different combinations of weight and height, however, may be useful to assess their relative degrees of validity. As shown in Table 10–2, the correlations with skinfolds are quite similar whether one uses weight/height or weight/height^2, and the correlations with weight/height^3 are only slightly reduced. Indeed, the use of weight alone is nearly as good as any weight index. This result is not surprising as it can be readily appreciated that most variation in weight between individuals is independent of height because adult heights do not vary dramatically; within one age and sex group the range from the tallest to the shortest is typically only about 20%.

The Influence of Frame Size

It is commonly assumed that weight should be evaluated in relation to frame size and that an accurate measurement of skeletal dimensions may improve the validity of obesity indices that are based simply on weight and height. Indeed, height itself is

Table 10–1. Correlation coefficients between height and selected indices of obesity (Pearson r)

Source	Subjects	Wt	Wt/Ht	Wt/Ht^2	Wt/Ht^3	Wt/$\overline{\text{W}}$t	Log skinfold	Body fat (densitometry)
Allen et al. (1956)[a]	55 men	—	0.41	0.16	−0.16	—	—	0.03
	26 women	—	0.27	0.03	−0.24	—	—	0.05
Khosla and Lowe (1967)	5,000 men (15–64 yr)	0.43/0.59	0.19/0.37	−0.10/0.08	−0.36/−0.24	—	—	—
Evans and Prior (1969)	432 men	0.44	0.25	0.02	−0.21	—	−0.13[b]/0.15[b]	—
	378 women	0.55	0.33	0.05	−0.18	—	−0.06[b]/0.19[b]	—
Florey (1970)	1,723 men	0.48	—	—			0.12 (trcps) 0.04 (infscp) 0.02 (trcps) 0.02 (infscp) −0.08 (infscp) −0.08 (infscp)	— — — — — —
Keys et al. (1972)	2,202 women	0.25	—	—	—	—	—	—
	180 students	0.46	0.25	0.02	−0.24[c]	0.04	0.04	—
	249 executives	0.40	0.18	0.06	−0.30[c]	0.01	0.02	—
Goldbourt and Medalie (1974)	9,475 men	0.52	0.28	−0.03	−0.31[c]	—	0.09 (trcps) 0.05 (infscp)	—
Womersley and Durnin (1977)	245 men	—	0.01	−0.22	−0.43[c]	−0.08	−0.13	−0.22
	324 women	—	0.06	−0.10	−0.26[c]	−0.04	−0.06	−0.13
Revicki and Israel (1986)	474 men	0.19	−0.03	−0.24	—	0.01	0.02	—
Killeen et al. (1978)	13,867 children 6–17 yr (by race and sex)	0.21/0.71	−0.01/0.38[d]	−0.36/0.18	—	—	0.02 0.34 (infscp)	—
Michielutte et al. (1984)	832 boys	—	0.76	0.44	−0.27	—	—	—
	836 girls aged 5–12 yr	—	0.78	0.50	−0.18	—	—	—
Micozzi et al. (1986)	5,808 men (25–74 yr)	0.42	0.08/0.24	~0.00/−0.08	−0.22/−0.33	—	—	—
	8,592 women (25–74 yr)	0.21	~0.00/0.08	~0.00/−0.13	−0.25/−0.31	—	—	—

[a] Calculations from Womersley and Durnin (1977).

[b] Sum of triceps (trcps) and infrascapular (infscp).

[c] Correlations are for cube root of weight divided by height (ponderal index).

[d] Strongest positive correlations for youngest children.

Table 10–2. Correlation of skinfold measures with anthropometric indices of obesity (Pearson r)

Source	Subjects	Skinfold	Ht	Wt	Wt/Ht	Wt/Ht²	Wt/Ht³
Flory (1970)	1,723 men	Triceps	0.12	0.44	0.45	0.42	0.36[a]
	1,723 men	Infrascapular	0.04	0.59	0.64	0.64	0.59[a]
	2,202 women	Triceps	0.02	0.47	0.47	0.46	0.44[a]
	2,202 women	Infrascapular	0.08	0.61	0.65	0.66	0.64[a]
Keys et al. (1972)	180 students 18–24 yr	Sum of triceps + infrascapular	0.06	0.78	0.83	0.85	0.81[a]
	249 executives		0.00	0.72	0.77	0.78	0.74[a]
Goldbourt and Medalie (1974)	9,475 Israeli men	Triceps	0.09	0.39	0.42	0.40	0.36[a]
		Infrascapular	0.05	0.54	0.60	0.60	0.56[a]
Killen et al. (1978)	13,687 children 6–17 yr by age and sex	Infrascapular	—	—	0.55–0.81	0.61–0.83[b]	0.47–0.81
Michielutte et al. (1984)	832 boys 5–12 yr	Triceps	—	—	0.73	0.81[b]	0.69
	835 girls 5–12 yr	Triceps	—	—	0.73	0.81[b]	0.64
Revicki and Israel (1986)	474 men	7 skinfolds (computed % fat)	0.01	0.71 0.70[c]	0.75 0.74[c]	0.76 0.72[c]	0.73 0.72[c]
Micozzi et al. (1986)	5,808 men	Infrascapular	~0.00	0.69	0.75	0.77	0.74
	8,592 women	Infrascapular	−0.09	0.76	0.79	0.80	0.79

[a] Correlations for cube root of weight divided by height (ponderal index).

[b] Correlations lowest for younger children.

[c] Age-adjusted.

basically a one-dimensional measure of frame size that is easily available in most studies. Widely used "ideal weights," such as those published by Metropolitan Life, are often provided for small, medium, and large frame sizes. These categories of frame size, however, have no quantitative definition and are left to individual judgment.

In addition to height, other measures of skeletal dimensions include biacromial diameter, knee and elbow width (Frisancho, 1984), biiliac diameter, and chest depth (Garn et al., 1986); such measurements have sometimes been combined into indices of frame size (Katch and Freedson, 1982). Katch and colleagues (1982) have demonstrated that frame sizes based on self-report or on a subjective rating by an expert correspond poorly with a standardized measurement of frame size. Roche (1984) has reviewed studies that address

the issue of whether measures of frame size improve the prediction of body fat composition above and beyond that provided by simple weight and height. Overall, there appears to be no consistent evidence that frame size measurements in addition to height provide any important refinement in the estimation of obesity. This is probably expected because, as demonstrated by the data in Tables 10–2 and 10–3, even height provides only a modest incremental improvement in prediction of body fat composition; further refinements in frame size estimation are likely to produce smaller marginal gains. Although additional work is warranted to identify simple measures of frame size that may improve the interpretation of weight, the cost and difficulty involved in obtaining such measurements are unlikely to be justified in epidemiologic studies of obesity.

Table 10–3. Correlation coefficients between densitometry estimates of body fat composition and anthropometric indices of obesity (Pearson r)

Source	Subjects	Wt	Wt/Ht	Wt/Ht^2	Wt/Ht^3	Skinfold
Allen et at.	55 men	—	0.70	0.72	0.68	—
(1956)[a]	26 women	—	0.74	0.80	0.77	—
Parizkova	62 normal adolescents	—	—	—	—	0.74 (triceps)
(1961)						0.80 (infrascapular)
Seltzer et al.	32 obese adolescent	—	—	—	—	0.69 (triceps)
(1965)	girls					0.59 (infrascapular)
Keys et al.	180 students	—	0.83	0.85	0.79[b]	0.85[c]
(1972)	249 executives	—	0.66	0.67	0.66[b]	0.82[c]
Womersley and	245 men	—	0.68	0.71	0.72[b]	0.84
Durnin	324 women	—	0.81	0.82	0.84[b]	0.86
(1977)						
Harsha et al.	242 black and white	0.32	—	—	—	0.81 (triceps)
	children					0.76 (infrascapular)
Roche et al.	68 boys (6–12 yr)	0.33	0.73	0.68	0.74	0.84 (triceps)
(1981)						0.74 (infrascapular)
	49 girls (6–12 yr)	0.23	0.69	0.55	0.62	0.83 (triceps)
						0.68 (infrascapular)
	63 boys (13–17 yr)	0.30	0.71	0.61	0.71	0.78 (infrascapular)
						0.72 (infrascapular)
	81 girls (13–17 yr)	0.72	0.77	0.77	0.74	0.83 (triceps)
						0.81 (infrascapular)
	141 men (18–49 yr)	0.67	0.64	0.77	0.75	0.70 (triceps)
						0.75 (infrascapular)
	135 women	0.70	0.69	0.76	0.75	0.77 (triceps)
	(18–49 yr)					0.71 (infrascapular)
Revicki and	474 men	0.66	0.70	0.71	0.69	0.84 (7 measures)
Israel (1986)		—	0.52[d]	0.58[d]	0.58[d]	

[a] Calculations from Womersley and Durnin (1977).

[b] Correlations are for cube root of weight divided by height (ponderal index).

[c] Sum of triceps and infrascapular.

[d] Age-adjusted.

Skinfold Measurements

Next to combinations of height and weight, skinfolds are probably the most widely used method to measure body composition in epidemiologic studies. This method has conceptual appeal because it provides a direct measure of body fat; its major limitations are that not all fat is accessible to the calipers (such as intraabdominal and intramuscular fat) and that the distribution of subcutaneous fat can vary considerably over the body. This variability in distribution of subcutaneous fat creates difficulties when measurements at one or only a few sites are used to represent overall body fat composition; however,

these distributions may be of interest in their own right (discussed later).

The technical aspects of skinfold measurements and considerations for selecting specific sites are discussed in detail elsewhere (Habicht et al., 1979; Lohman, 1981; Mueller and Stallones, 1981; Rose and Blackburn, 1982; Roche, 1984; Roche et al., 1996). In general, skinfold measurements are substantially less reproducible than most other anthropometric measures, such as weight, height, and limb and girth circumferences (Bray et al., 1978; Habicht et al., 1979; Lukaski, 1987).

Ruiz and colleagues (1971) formally investigated sources of variation in skinfold thickness measurements. They found that a small difference (2.5 cm) in the site of measuring the triceps skinfold, for example, resulted in a difference as large as 50% in the average skinfold. Other factors, such as the manner in which the skinfold was picked up and the depth of caliper bite, contributed less to variation. Jointly, these factors contribute to the substantial inter-observer variation that has typically been reported for such measurements. Because of this relatively high degree of error variance, skinfold thickness measurements are of limited use in following changes in obesity over time (Bray et al., 1978).

The validity of skinfold thickness assessed by calipers as a measure of true subcutaneous adipose thickness (as opposed to being a measure of body fat composition, which is discussed next) has been assessed by comparing data obtained by calipers and by computed tomography or ultrasound (Roche, 1996). Fanelli and Kuczmarski (1984) and Kuczmarski and colleagues (1987) found that subcutaneous fat measurements by ultrasound were not superior to skinfold measurements by caliper in predicting body fat composition determined by densitometry among relatively lean individuals. Among obese adults, however, the ultrasonic measurements proved to be superior. Among the obese group, correlations between skinfold thickness and ultrasonic measurements at the same site ranged from 0.30 (waist) to 0.72 (thigh and biceps). Abe and colleagues (1994), however, found that subcutaneous adipose estimated by ultrasound was overall more predictive of body fat measured by densitometry than when measured by calipers. Seidell and colleagues (1987) compared the sum of paraumbilical and suprailiac skinfolds with the cross-sectional area of subcutaneous fat measured by computed tomography. They observed high correlations for both men (0.83) and women (0.88).

It is possible that ultrasound measurements may become commonly used in epidemiologic studies, as the method is simple and safe. It should be noted that many of

the same limitations of the traditional skinfold technique (sensitivity to the exact placement of the device and the general variation of subcutaneous fat over the body) also applies to the ultrasound method.

Another method to measure thickness of subcutaneous adipose that uses a beam of near-infrared radiation is also commercially available (Jebb and Elia, 1993). However, this approach appears to have limitations similar to traditional skinfold measurements plus relatively low validity.

Validity of Relative Weights, Obesity Indices, and Skinfold Thicknesses as Measures of Body Fat Composition

The validity of epidemiologic measures of body composition can be assessed by comparison with more accurate and precise methods. Because even the best methods are indirect, the choice of an optimal "gold standard," as for dietary intake, is not completely clear. In addition to being highly accurate, it would be desirable that any error associated with the gold standard be independent of error in the method being evaluated so that correlation does not occur simply on the basis of errors that are common to both approaches. Until the present, most studies of validity have employed densitometry (underwater weighing) as the standard method. Although this method is not perfect due, for example, to variation in the bone density of subjects, it is a reasonable choice as any errors should be independent, and it has been in widespread use for decades. It would be reassuring if several of the more sophisticated approaches for measuring obesity (e.g., densitometry, deuterium dilution, electrical conductance, and x-ray absorptiometry) were compared with each other; if very high correlations were observed between them, say on the order of 0.95, this would provide reassurance that they were all providing similarly precise information and could equally serve as standards. A number of studies in which obesity indices and skinfold thicknesses have been compared with densitometry measurements are summarized in Table 10–3. Correlations with obesity indices have ranged from approximately 0.60 to 0.85. Although the correlations with weight/height, weight/height^2, and weight/height^3 are similar, BMI (weight/height^2) tends to be slightly more strongly correlated. The Benn index (weight/height^p) had no higher correlation with densitometry than weight/height^2 in a large study among men (Revicki and Israel, 1986). The correlations of skinfold thicknesses with densitometry have a similar range of coefficients and are not clearly higher than for the obesity indices; it is possible that the use of multiple skinfolds may improve the correlation with densitometry.

Using another approach to evaluate the relative validity of different epidemiologic measures of obesity, Criqui and coworkers (1982) compared various indices with blood triglyceride level, total cholesterol level, blood pressure, and fasting glucose level (which are all known to be related to obesity) among a large population of men and women (Table 10–4). For each outcome, weight/height^2 and relative weight exhibited the strongest correlations, providing evidence that these are the most biologically relevant measures of obesity.

Although the correlations with densitometry seen in Table 10–3 are reasonably high, there are several reasons to believe that they overrepresent the validity of obesity indices and skinfolds in the context of most epidemiologic studies. Because the magnitude of a correlation coefficient is directly related to the degree of variation in the parameter being studied, in this case the between-person variation in obesity, the observed correlation coefficient is applicable only to study populations with a similar variation in obesity. In the published studies, it is often unclear how subjects were selected; however, it seems that they were frequently enriched with an atypically high representation of obese subjects. This would tend to lead to higher correlations than would be observed, given the same de-

gree of accuracy, in a general population. Furthermore, correlations have not been adjusted for age in most published reports. This also overstates the relevant variation in obesity because obesity tends to be strongly correlated with age, and virtually all epidemiologic analyses adjust for age. Not only does BMI increase with age in Western populations, for the same BMI, older persons (and women) tend to have a higher body fat composition (Gallagher et al., 1996). In a study that examined the association of weight-for-height indices with obesity measured by densitometry, Womersley and Durnin (1977) found a correlation of 0.71 for weight/height^2 among men when all ages were combined, but correlations ranging from 0.49 to 0.62 within specific 10-year age groups. Correlations with weight/height^2 were somewhat higher among women, being 0.81 overall, and ranging from 0.64 to 0.91 within specific age groups. Similarly, in a study among 474 men (with unclear basis for selection), Revicki and Israel (1986) found that the correlation between weight/height^2 decreased from 0.71 to 0.58 with adjustment for age. For these reasons, it is difficult to determine the true degree of validity for measures such as BMI in the context of epidemiologic studies on the basis of published data. It seems likely, however, that the correlation with true percent body fat composition in general populations is likely to be on the order of 0.5 or 0.6 for men and perhaps slightly higher for women.

Although use of population samples with atypically large variations in adiposity and the failure to control for basic demographic characteristics may tend to exaggerate correlations between anthropometric indices and percent body fat assessed by densitometry, the validity of these indices may also have been underestimated if percent body fat is not truly the biologically relevant measure of adiposity. Although BMI is typically thought of as an estimate of percent body fat, it is actually more a measure of absolute mass adjusted for height, which is conceptually similar to the residual of weight adjusted for height described above. Thus, comparisons of BMI with percent body fat do not really compare like with like. Data on percent body fat from densitometry in combination with weight can be used to calculate absolute fat mass, and this can be adjusted for height in regression analysis to create a variable that is conceptually analogous with BMI. Using a large dataset to make such calculations, Spiegelman and colleagues (1992) found remarkably high correlations between BMI and absolute fat mass adjusted for height, even after accounting for age and gender (correlations were between 0.82 and 0.91). Thus, BMI appears to be an excellent measure of fat mass adjusted for height, with somewhat less validity as a measure of percent body fat (the correlations ranged from 0.60 to 0.71).

Using the same dataset, Spiegelman and colleagues (1992) examined the degree to which percent body fat and absolute fat mass adjusted for height, both measured by densitometry, predicted blood pressure and fasting blood glucose level. In both men and women, absolute fat mass adjusted for height appeared to be the better predictor. A variety of other combinations of weight and height as well as measures of body fat distribution were not found to be superior to BMI. These findings suggest that an increase in lean body mass, which would reduce percent body fat, does not offset the adverse effect of excess fat mass. Furthermore, these findings may explain why BMI has been such a strong predictor of health outcomes in a vast epidemiologic literature: It is both a biologically relevant expression of adiposity (apparently better than percent body fat), and it is an excellent measure of adiposity, at least in the young adult and middle-aged population studied by Spiegelman and coworkers.

Despite the excellent performance of BMI as noted above, there are reasons to suspect that this index performs less well in older adults. The basic reason for a high degree of validity is that the vast majority of variation in weight among middle-aged adults of the same gender that is not accounted for by height is fat (muscle builders may be exceptions, but they are rare). However, in the elderly many, but not all, individuals lose substantial amounts of lean body mass (Gallagher et al., 1996), often because of greatly reduced activity. Therefore, variation in lean body mass can contribute to a much greater degree to differences in weight and changes in weight, thus reducing the validity of BMI as a measure of adiposity. Even individuals who maintain the same weight can have substantial changes in adiposity. The observation that men on average do not gain weight appreciably after about age 50, but do greatly expand their abdominal circumference, attests to this redistribution. Indeed, Micozzi and Harris (1990) found that the correlation between BMI and arm fat area tended to decrease with age, and the correlation between BMI and arm muscle area tended to increase with age. Thus, for men over age 65, BMI was similarly correlated with fatness and muscularity, and for women, the correlation with fat area was only modestly greater. It may be that other measures of adiposity will be more appropriate for the elderly. For example, changes in abdominal circumference unequivocally reflect adipose rather than muscle and may thus be a better indicator of overall adiposity than weight or weight indices in some groups.

In summary, on the basis of the previous data, one or two skinfold measurements or any of the obesity indices provide approximately similar estimates of relative body fat composition. Among the obesity indices, weight/height^2 appears at least as good as the others as a measure of relative adiposity and is usually optimal with respect to lack of correlation with height. Although the use of other exponents for height may slightly reduce the correlation with height in a particular population, this rarely outweighs the substantial advantages in comparability among studies that use weight/height^2. Keys and colleagues (1972) have concluded similarly that weight/

Table 10–4. Correlations of height (Ht), weight (Wt), and obesity indices with risk factors in men

	Men aged 20–79 yr (n = 2,266)						
	Wt	Ht	Wt/Ht	Wt/Ht²	$\sqrt[3]{\text{Wt}}/\text{Ht}$	$-\text{Ht}/\sqrt[3]{\text{Wt}}$	Relative weight
Age	−0.16	−0.29	−0.09	0.00	−0.14	−0.14	−0.01
Cholesterol	0.01	−0.08	0.04	0.07	0.02	0.03	0.07
Log triglyceride	0.21	0.01	0.23	0.24	0.22	0.22	0.25
Systolic blood pressure	0.01	−0.17	0.07	0.12	0.03	0.02	0.12
Diastolic blood pressure	0.14	−0.04	0.17	0.19	0.15	0.15	0.19
Fasting plasma glucose	0.08	−0.03	0.10	0.12	0.09	0.09	0.12

[a]All correlations of absolute magnitude, 0.07 in women and 0.08 in men, or greater, are significant at $p < 0.001$.
From Criqui et al., 1982.

height² is the preferable measure of relative weight in epidemiologic studies. Nevertheless, if height is strongly associated with disease in a particular study, it is important to be certain that the obesity index used is not associated with height. If so, any of a variety of multivariate methods can be used to control for confounding due to height.

The validity of BMI and other obesity indices as measures of relative body composition, represented by the correlations in Table 10–3, is clearly less than perfect. As noted before, part of the reason correlations are not higher is that these represent conceptually different variables. Also, as discussed earlier, only moderate correlation is not the result of error in measuring weight or height; the primary source of error is that these indices reflect the weight of both lean body mass and fat tissue. Bone mass and muscle mass both contribute to the correlation of lean body mass with obesity indices based on weight and height. It is, therefore, important to consider that associations between obesity indices and other variables can be due to differences in lean body mass as well as adiposity. This potential for confounding, however, is due not only to the technical imperfection of the obesity indices as measures of adiposity, but also to the biologic correlation of lean body mass and percent body fat. Thus, the possibility must be considered that an observed association between any measure of obesity and disease is due to an associ-ation with lean body mass rather than adiposity.

Dual Energy X-Ray Absorptiometry (DEXA)

In the mid-1980s, DEXA, which uses an x-ray beam with high- and low-energy peaks combined with a whole body scanner, was developed to measure bone mass and has subsequently been used to measure soft tissue composition as well (for further details, see Roubenoff et al., 1993; Lohman, 1996). The method is able to distinguish fat mass, fat-free mass, and bone mineral mass, both for the total body and for specific regions, by the differential absorption of the high- and low-energy x-rays by these tissues. Because the total radiation dose is extremely low, the method can be used for research across all age groups, except pregnant women. It is far easier for participants than underwater weighing. The x-ray and scanning unit is expensive and must be accompanied by software used to estimate body components.

For measurements both within the same day and over months, DEXA provides quite reproducible measurements of body components. For percent body fat, the standard deviation is about 1%, the coefficient of variation (SD/mean × 100%) has been 4% to 7%, depending on the mean body fat in the sample (Lohman, 1996).

The validity of DEXA as assessed by comparison with densitometry appears to and women aged 20–79 years, Rancho Bernardo, California, 1972–1974[a]

	Women aged 20–79 yr (n = 2,690)						
	Wt	Ht	Wt/Ht	Wt/Ht^2	$\sqrt[3]{Wt}/Ht$	$-Ht/\sqrt[3]{Wt}$	Relative weight
Age	0.04	−0.29	0.11	0.19	0.06	0.07	0.17
Cholesterol	0.06	−0.17	0.10	0.15	0.07	0.09	0.14
Log triglyceride	0.19	−0.10	0.23	0.25	0.21	0.20	0.25
Systolic blood pressure	0.14	−0.20	0.20	0.25	0.16	0.15	0.25
Diastolic blood pressure	0.19	−0.09	0.22	0.24	0.20	0.19	0.25
Fasting plasma glucose	0.10	−0.06	0.12	0.13	0.10	0.10	0.13

be quite high in most populations, but substantial systematic errors have been seen in older and younger individuals (Lohman, 1996). Clark et al. (1993) reported a high correlation (r=0.91) between percent body fat and body density among young white men. In this study, the standard error of the estimate was 3.0% body fat ($s.e.e. = \sqrt{\Sigma(Y_o - Y_e)^2/(N-2)}$, where Y_o is the observed conductivity measurement and Y_e is the conductivity measurement predicted by densitometry; this has been referred to elsewhere as the standard deviation of the residual, see Chapter 6). Hansen et al. (1993) found a similar correlation (0.92) between percent body fat estimated by DEXA and by densitometry among 100 premenopausal women; the standard error of the estimate was 2.4% body fat.

The DEXA method has already found widespread use in clinical studies and may become a standard for other measures of body composition. Whether it or densitometry is a more valid measure of body fat composition is difficult to determine at this point; simultaneous comparisons of both methods with other indicators of body fat would be particularly useful to assess their relative validity.

Bioelectrical Impedance Analysis

In recent years great interest has developed in the use of bioelectrical impedance (or resistance) and conductance measurements to estimate lean body mass and body fat composition (i.e., percent body fat). These measurements are based on the principle that the lean body mass, which consists largely of ions in a water solution, conducts electricity far better than does fat tissue (Van Itallie et al., 1986; Anonymous, 1996; Baumgartner, 1996). Therefore, the resistance (technically impedance in the case of an alternating current) of the body to an electrical current is inversely related to the lean body mass. Such measurements should, therefore, provide the same information as obtained with deuterium oxide or other dilution methods. If the total body mass is known, the fat mass and percent body fat can easily be calculated. Electrical resistance is affected also by body shape, so that correcting measurements for height using empirically derived regression formulas or the ratio height^2/resistance can improve the prediction of body composition. Prediction of lean mass can be further improved by accounting for gender as well as height and weight.*

The bioelectrical impedance method is extremely simple in practice. Electrodes (either two or four) are attached to a person's extremities while recumbent but clothed. A weak radio frequency signal is applied to the electrodes, and the impedance is measured. Usually several measurements are

*A widely accepted prediction equation (Lukaski et al., 1986) is: Fat-free mass (kg) = $-4.03 + 0.734 \cdot (Ht^2/R) + 0.116 \cdot (\text{weight}) + 0.096\ (Xc) + 0.984 \cdot$ Sex, where Ht is in cm, weight is in kg, Xc is impedance in ohms, and sex = 0 for F and 1 for M.

made, but the whole procedure takes less than 1 minute. The signal generator and recording device (which costs a few thousand dollars) is the size of an attache case and is thus fully portable.

Another method, the "total body electrical conductivity" technique (Segal et al., 1985; Van Itallie et al., 1986), is also based on the differential electrical properties of lean and fat mass. The measuring device consists of a large coil into which a radio frequency current is injected. When a conducting material, such as a body, is passed though the coil, the impedance to the radio frequency current is decreased in relation to the mass of conducting material. Because a person is simply passed through a large coil, no electrodes are required and the procedure is very rapid. The device is, however, expensive and not portable. Largely for these reasons, these instruments are no longer manufactured and thus are not discussed further here.

Because the impedance measurements are extremely simple, rapid, safe, and portable, they are potentially useful in epidemiologic settings. Their reproducibility and validity, therefore, deserve considerable attention. As discussed for combinations of weight and height, validity in the epidemiologic context is most realistically evaluated by examining the association of the new method with a gold standard after controlling for age and sex (as these are controlled for in any epidemiologic analysis) and in a population with a typical distribution of body fat composition (as opposed to a population with artificially inflated heterogeneity in body composition). Validation studies have generally used densitometry as the standard method, although dilution methods have also been employed. Studies of *relative* validity in which a new measure as well as other standard measures (such as BMI or skinfolds) are all compared with a gold standard (or a biologic indicator such as blood pressure or blood glucose) are particularly useful. As discussed in Chapter 6, three-way comparisons (the method triangles) can be used

to estimate the correlation between each of the individual methods and truth, assuming the errors in methods are not correlated, which is probably a reasonable assumption when the technologies used to measure body fat are different. This approach does not appear to have been applied in the field of body composition.

Measurements of bioelectrical impedance appear to be highly reproducible (Baumgartner, 1996). Among a population of overweight men and women, Helenius and colleagues (1987) observed an extremely high correlation ($r = 0.99$) for repeated measurements made on the same day. Even in a more homogenous group of 37 healthy young men measured at an interval of 5 days, Lukaski and colleagues (1985) also observed a correlation of 0.99 for replicate measures. Although impedance measurements appear to be remarkably reproducible, their validity as a measure of absolute and relative body components is a more complex issue.

Among 37 healthy young men, Lukaski and colleagues (1985) found impedance measurements (expressed as height^2/resistance) to be highly correlated with total body water ($r = 0.95$). Kushner and Schoeller (1986) found similarly high correlations between height^2/resistance and total body water measured with deuterium ($r = 0.96$ for men and $r = 0.85$ for women). Lukaski and coworkers (1986) compared measurements of both lean body mass and percent body fat based on impedance with the same parameters based on densitometry. Among 84 men, the correlation was 0.98 for fat-free mass and 0.93 for percent body fat. Among 67 women the correlation was 0.95 for fat-free mass and 0.88 for percent body fat. In this study, the estimation of percent body fat among men based on impedance ($r = 0.93$) was only slightly better than that based on four skinfolds (0.88), although this difference was statistically significant. Segal and colleagues (1985) reported correlations between height^2/resistance and densitometrically determined lean body mass of 0.82 for men and 0.92 for women. Based on a much larger sample, Hodgdon and Fitzgerald (1987) observed correlations between percent body fat based on impedance and densitometry measurements of 0.79 among 403 men and 0.82 among 135 women.

The validity of the body fat assessment by impedance methods has also been expressed as the standard error of the estimate, which has ranged from 3.5 to 5.0 percent body fat (Baumgartner, 1996). Although these errors are appreciable, they may be an underestimate because the prediction equations on which they are based have not been independently validated. However, because the standard error of the densitometry method compared with theoretical truth has been estimated to be on the order of 2.5 percent body fat (Lohman, 1981), Segal and coworkers (1985) have pointed out that an appreciable part of the apparent error of other methods assessed by comparison with densitometry may be due to error in the gold standard. Among 100 premenopausal women, Hansen et al. (1993) evaluated percent body fat assessed by electrical impedance as well as BMI, DEXA, and the sum of four skinfolds in relation to percent body fat measured by densitometry, thus providing an assessment of the relative validity of the three methods. The standard errors of the estimates of percent body fat were 2.92 for the resistance method, 3.25 for BMI ($r = 0.83$), 3.00 for sum of skinfolds ($r = 0.84$), and 2.40 for DEXA ($r = 0.92$). In this population, DEXA appears to provide the best measure of percent body fat, and the other methods were only modestly less valid.

At this time, few of the validation studies of impedance measurements have been analyzed in a manner that makes their epidemiologic relevance directly interpretable. In general, correlations with lean body mass have tended to be relatively strong and higher than for percent body fat, presumably because lean body mass has varied more between subjects in these studies than has percent body fat. The correlations observed in a large study (Hodgdon and Fitzgerald, 1987) were similar to previously published data unadjusted for age relating BMI to percent body fat determined by densitometry (Table 10–3). Thus, it is not yet clear whether electrical resistance measurements can provide a substantially better estimate of percent body fat in epidemiologic settings than simple combinations of weight and height (Houtkooper et al., 1996). Because electrical resistance measures of body composition are easier and more rapid than standard methods, such as densitometry and deuterium dilution, their validity deserves examination in greater detail from an epidemiologic perspective.

DISTRIBUTION OF BODY FAT

In recent years, considerable attention has been given to the possibility that the distribution of fat is related to certain diseases independent of overall obesity. For example, abdominal fat has been reported to be independently associated with risk of diabetes (Hartz et al., 1984). Similarly, Vague (1956) has reported that women having a high ratio of skinfold thickness of the posterior neck to thickness at the sacrum (which was termed *android obesity*) had a high probability of diabetes, gout, and atherosclerosis compared with women with a low ratio (termed *gynecoid obesity*). The approaches for measuring the distribution of body fat are many, as one can imagine a large number of ways in which the distribution of fat might vary, and these distributions may, in turn, be measured in different ways. For example, fat distribution can vary with respect to the proportions stored subcutaneously, intraabdominally, and within the muscle mass. Moreover, the subcutaneous distribution of fat itself can vary between persons; the relative thickness may differ between extremity and trunk and between upper extremity and lower extremity. Understandably, the many possibilities for measurement have led to a plethora of approaches that cannot be reviewed here; however, two of the most commonly employed measures, the waist-to-hip circumference ratio and the biceps-to-subscapular skinfold ratio, are discussed here.

Waist-to-Hip Circumference Ratio

Individuals with a predominance of abdominal (visceral) fat exhibit numerous metabolic differences, including insulin resistance and elevated free-fatty acid production, compared with those having fat primarily distributed subcutaneously over the lower extremities (Bjorntorp, 1987). These metabolic differences provide a conceptual rationale for examining risk of disease in relation to these different adipose distributions (Lapidus et al., 1984). The most commonly employed measure has been the waist-to-hip circumference ratio.

A standard protocol for measurement of waist-to-hip ratio has not been developed, in part because measurements have been made by personnel with different levels of training or by subjects themselves in studies conducted by mail. Trained personnel can use bony landmarks for measurements (e.g., half-way between the lower rib margin and the iliac crest), whereas less trained observers may simply be asked to measure the waist at its narrowest point. The specific location of these measurements does appear to provide different results; the correlations of waist-to-hip circumference ratios measured with different landmarks were 0.77 for women and 0.90 for men (Seidell et al., 1987). Factors, such as postprandial status, time of day, standing position, and depth of inspiration, also affect these measurements. Because the degree to which these factors may contribute error is uncertain, standardizing such factors within a study to the greatest degree possible is prudent. Moreover, abdominal circumference includes contributions of both intraabdominal and subcutaneous fat. Therefore, if only intraabdominal fat is metabolically distinct from overall fatness, as has been suggested, then even highly accurate circumference measurements will only indirectly reflect the variable of conceptual interest.

In a number of large epidemiologic studies, participants have been asked to measure their own body circumferences and report these on mailed questionnaires (Kushi et al., 1988; Rimm et al., 1990). In some studies a paper tape measure was provided, and in other cases participants were asked to use their own measure. Kushi and co-workers (1988) examined the reproducibility and validity of self-assessed circumference measurements among a sample from a large cohort of postmenopausal women. The intraclass correlations for repeated self-measurements (n=41) of the same circumference approximately 2 months apart were 0.96 for waist, 0.97 for hip, and 0.85 for waist-to-hip ratio. In a sample of 87 women also measured by a technician, correlations between technician and self-measurement were 0.97 for waist, 0.98 for hip, and 0.86 for waist-to-hip ratio. In a similar study, Rimm and coworkers (1990) compared self-assessed waist and hip circumference measurements of 123 male health professionals and 140 female nurses with measurements taken by a technician up to 9 months after the self-measurement and again 6 to 9 months later. Reproducibility correlation for waist, hip, and waist-to-hip ratio measurements by the technician at an average interval of 7.8 months were 0.89, 0.88, and 0.68 for men and 0.91, 0.88, and 0.78 for women. The correlations between self-measurement and an average of two technician measurements for the same variable were 0.95, 0.88, and 0.68 for men and 0.89, 0.84, and 0.68 for women.

The validity of the waist-to-hip circumference ratio as a measure of intraabdominal obesity was evaluated in several studies by comparing this ratio with abdominal fat measured by computed tomography (Ashwell et al., 1985; Seidell et al., 1987; Schreiner et al., 1996). Reasonably strong correlations were seen; in the Seidell study, the correlation coefficients were 0.55 for women and 0.75 for men. Age alone, however, predicted intraabdominal fat nearly as well as the waist-to-hip ratio so that after adjustment for age and BMI, the waist-to-hip ratio was not significantly correlated with intraabdominal fat. Because the focus of epidemiologic studies is usually the effect of abdominal fat independent of age and overall obesity, this analysis suggests that the errors associated with the use of waist-to-hip ratios as a measure of intraabdominal fat in epidemiologic studies may be substantial. In a similar study of 97 men and 60 women, Schreiner et al. (1996) found reasonably strong correlations between waist-to-hip ratio and intraabdominal fat (age-adjusted partial r approximately 0.60 for both men and women), and the correlations between waist circumference alone and intraabdominal fat were of similar magnitude. However, the correlations between waist circumference and subcutaneous fat were even stronger (0.84 in men and 0.77 in women) and were similar to the correlations between BMI and subcutaneous fat. The correlations between waist-to-hip ratio and subcutaneous fat were only slightly weaker (0.57 in men and 0.44 in women) than the correlations between waist-to-hip ratio and intraabdominal fat. Thus, although waist circumference and waist-to-hip ratio do provide information on intraabdominal fat, they do not appear to be very useful in distinguishing between intraabdominal and subcutaneous fat.

The interpretation of epidemiologic findings based on body circumferences (or other measures of fat distribution) must consider that neither total body fat (as assessed by BMI) nor fat distribution are measured perfectly and that the relative validities of these measurements can vary by age, gender, and race. Thus, it is possible that an apparent independent effect of abdominal circumference (or waist-to-hip ratio) in predicting disease risk after controlling for BMI could result from additional information about total body fat provided

by circumference rather than an effect of body fat distribution. As discussed earlier, the relative contribution of abdominal circumference to information on total fatness is likely to increase with age due to a reduced validity of BMI as a measure of fatness because of age-related variation in lean mass.

The interpretation of waist-to-hip ratio is further complicated because it is the ratio of two complex variables. Although waist circumference is a fairly unambiguous measure of abdominal fat, but less so of visceral fat, hip circumference reflects both muscle and fat, as well as bony structure. Indeed, the biologic justification for the ratio is somewhat obscure, but it seems in part an attempt to correct abdominal circumference for variation in body size (adjustment for height by regression analysis would have been one alternative). It is possible that both the numerator (waist) and denominator (hip) could contribute to disease prediction. For example, in predicting cardiovascular disease, adiposity is known to increase risk, but gluteal muscularity is likely to be associated with reduced risk because it reflects physical activity because greater muscularity reduces insulin resistance. Thus, rather than using only the ratio of these circumferences to predict disease, it may be informative to include waist and hip as separate terms in a multivariate model. In this situation, hip circumference will tend to reflect more its muscular component, as fatness will be represented by abdominal circumference.

Several investigators have compared various combinations of circumference with measures of coronary heart disease risk, such as blood pressure or blood lipids. Han et al. (1995) found that waist, waist-to-hip ratio, and BMI were similarly correlated with coronary heart disease factors. Hsieh and Yoshinaga (1995) found that the waist-to-height ratio was more strongly associated with coronary risk factors than was waist-to-hip ratio, but this ratio must be used cautiously because height itself has been inversely related to blood pressure and coronary heart disease incidence.

The value of having body circumference measurements in addition to weight and height was demonstrated in several recent analyses within the Health Professionals Follow-up Study. Among men younger than 65 years of age, a strong positive association was observed between BMI and risk of coronary heart disease (relative risk = 3.4, 95% confidence interval 1.7 to 7.1 for BMI of 33 kg/M² or more compared with less than 23), and waist-to-hip ratio did not add further to prediction of risk (Rimm et al., 1995). However, among men 65 years or older, BMI was minimally predictive of coronary disease, but waist and waist-to-hip ratio were strongly predictive of disease (for highest vs. lowest quintile of the ratio, the relative risk = 2.8, 95% confidence interval 1.2 to 6.2). Had only the weight and height measurements been available, it might have been concluded that excess body fat was an important risk factor for coronary disease only in young men. However, with the addition of circumference measurements, it is more likely that body fat is an important risk factor for coronary disease at all ages, but that the best methods for assessing fatness may vary by age. In this cohort, we also examined the relation of body fat with risk colon cancer (Giovannucci et al., 1995); this relation had been unclear or weak in previous studies based on weight and height indices. Although only a weak relationship was seen between BMI and risk of colon cancer in this cohort, the relation with waist circumference was clear and strong (relative risk = 2.56, 95% confidence interval 1.33 to 4.96). As the large majority of colon cancer cases occurred in men 65 years of age or older, we cannot be sure whether abdominal obesity per se is more important than overall obesity or whether waist circumference is just a better measure of fatness in this population. Regardless, this finding indicates an important role of body fatness in colon carcinogenesis.

It is notable that in a prospective study where the association of waist-to-hip circumference ratios with cardiovascular disease was both statistically significant and important (relative risks between 2 and 3), the difference in means between subjects who subsequently developed disease and those who remained healthy (0.938 vs. 0.925) was only about 1% (Larsson et al., 1984). (This can happen when the distribution of exposure is narrow, i.e., the standard deviation is small in relation to the mean.) Because even the smallest degree of systematic bias or an effect of disease on these measurements could obscure such a difference, it is uncertain whether valid case–control studies can be conducted using this ratio (see Chapter 2).

When either abdominal circumference or waist-to-hip ratio (both of which reflect total fatness as well as regional fatness) are included as independent variables in a multivariate model with BMI (which reflects weight due to both lean and fat mass), it is notable that the meaning of BMI may become counterintuitive. In this situation, BMI will tend to reflect lean mass to a greater degree because the component of weight due to fatness will be accounted for by abdominal circumference. Thus, BMI may be more an index of muscularity than fatness in this multivariate model. This will be particularly true in older persons because, as noted earlier, BMI reflects lean mass to a similar degree as fat mass in the elderly, even before adjustment for circumference measurements. To maintain the usual meaning of BMI as an indicator of overall fatness, the residual from the regression of abdominal circumference (or waist-to-hip ratio) on BMI (and height as well) could be computed to represent regional fatness independent of overall fatness, and then the residual could be included as an independent variable together with BMI in the prediction of disease. This procedure is analogous to the distinction between total energy and fat intake described in Chapter 11.

Triceps and Subscapular Skinfolds

The triceps and subscapular skinfold thicknesses have been used as relative measures of extremity and truncal obesity, respectively. In a number of studies it has been suggested that truncal obesity is more strongly related to disorders of carbohydrate and lipid metabolism and hypertension than is peripheral obesity (Blair et al., 1984). The use of triceps and subscapular skinfolds appears to be largely based on convention and convenience; it is possible that skinfolds measured at the other sites might be more representative of obesity in the extremities or trunk and, thus, stronger predictors of disease (Roche, 1984).

The distinction between intraabdominal and subcutaneous truncal adiposity with respect to disease occurrence is not well-defined at present. The interpretation of data relating to body fat distribution is difficult as the measurements at different areas tend to be strongly correlated. It is possible, for example, that subscapular skinfolds are simply acting as a surrogate for intraabdominal fat. To understand the physiologic effects of fat distribution, it is important to use a number of these measures simultaneously. The interpretation of such studies is likely to be further complicated as the strength of associations between various measures of fat distribution depend on the relative degree of measurement error associated with each of them, as well as the true strength of their biologic relationships.

SUMMARY

Most of our present information on the health effects of obesity is derived from data on weight and height. Because these variables are easy and inexpensive to collect and can be assessed quite accurately even by self-report, they continue to play a central role in epidemiologic studies. Height and other dimensions that potentially reflect early nutritional status could be exploited more fully than has been done thus far. When using combinations of weight and height to assess obesity, BMI (weight/height^2) is as strongly correlated with overall body fat as alternative indices and provides the considerable advantage of comparability across studies.

Despite the widespread use of obesity indices based on weight and height, their error in representing percent body fat is considerable, not because of failure to measure height and weight accurately but because the lean body mass can vary considerably among persons of the same height. The validity of BMI is likely to vary considerably by age because of substantial losses of lean mass by some, but not all, older persons. The validity of combinations of weight and height for epidemiologic applications has probably been overestimated in the past by artificially increasing the between-person variation in fatness by using study populations heterogeneous with respect to age and sex. On the other hand, the use of percent body fat as the criterion for assessing BMI is probably inappropriate because this index reflects absolute mass (as opposed to relative mass) and evidence exists that absolute fat mass adjusted for height is a better predictor of the adverse effects of excess body fat. BMI does appear to have excellent validity as a measure of absolute fat mass adjusted for height in young and middle-aged adults. The use of physiologic indicators of fatness, such as blood pressure, high-density lipoprotein cholesterol, and fasting blood glucose level can be useful to evaluate further the relative validities of various methods for measuring fatness as well as the biologic relevance of various ways of expressing fatness.

Errors associated with obesity indices as a measure of fatness imply that the health effects of obesity are underestimated in epidemiologic studies. This underestimation can be addressed by statistical corrections for measurement error, as discussed in Chapter 12, or by using improved methods to measure percent body fat in future studies. Among the alternative approaches, bioelectric impedance appears to be the only method sufficiently simple and inexpensive to be widely used epidemiologically. Sufficient data, however, do not exist to quantify the incremental validity it can provide among populations typically studied by epidemiologists.

The present interest in body fat distribution is likely to enhance our understanding of the pathophysiology of numerous diseases. Additional work, however, is needed to define what is actually being measured by the ratios that are commonly employed today, as they reflect both total fatness and fatness in specific locations.

REFERENCES

Abe, T., M. Kondo, Y. Kawakami, and T. Fukunga (1994). Prediction equation for body composition of Japanese adults by B-mode ultrasound. *Am J Hum Biol 6*, 161–170.

Allen, T. H., M. T. Peng, and K. Chen, et al. (1956). Prediction of total adiposity from skinfolds and the curvilinear relationship between external and internal adiposity. *Metabolism 5*, 346–352.

Anonymous (1996). Bioelectrical impedance analysis in body composition measurement. Proceedings of a National Institutes of Health Technology Assessment Conference, Bethesda, Maryland, December 12–14, 1994. *Am J Clin Nutr 64(suppl)*, 387S–532S.

Ashwell, M., T. J. Cole, and A. K. Dixon (1985). Obesity: New insight into the anthropometric classification of fat distribution shown by computed tomography. *BMJ Clin Res 290*, 1692–1694.

Baumgartner, R. N. (1996). Electrical impedance and total body electrical conductivity. In Roche, A. F., Heymsfield, S. B., and Lohman, T. G. (eds.): *Human Body Composition*. Champaign, IL: Human Kinetics Books, pp. 79–108.

Benn, R. T. (1971). Some mathematical properties of weight-for-height indices used as measures of adiposity. *Br J Prev Soc Med 25*, 42–50.

Bjorntorp, P. (1987). Classification of obese patients and complications related to the distribution of surplus fat. *Am J Clin Nutr 45(suppl)*, 1120–1125.

Blair, D., J. P. Habicht, E. A. Sims, D. Sylwester, and S. Abraham (1984). Evidence for an increased risk for hypertension with centrally located body fat and the effect of race and sex on this risk. *Am J Epidemiol 119*, 526–540.

Bray, G. A., F. L. Greenway, M. E. Molitch, W. T. Dahms, R. L. Atkinson, and K. Hamilton (1978). Use of anthropometric measures to assess weight loss. *Am J Clin Nutr 31*, 769–773.

Brinkley, D., R. G. Carpenter, and J. L. Haybittle (1971). An anthropometric study of women with cancer. *Br J Prev Soc Med 25*, 65–75.

Brozek, J., F. Grande, J. T. Anderson, and A. Keys (1963). Densitometric analysis of body composition: Revision of some quantitative assumptions. *Ann NY Acad Sci 110*, 113–140.

Clark, R. R., J. M. Kuta, and J. C. Sullivan (1993). Prediction of percent body fat in adult males using dual energy x-ray absorptiometry, skinfolds, and hydrostatic weighing. *Med Sci Sports Exerc 25*, 528–535.

Colliver, J. A., S. Frank, and A. Frank (1983). Similarity of obesity indices in clinical studies of obese adults: A factor analytic study. *Am J Clin Nutr 38*, 640–647.

Criqui, M. H., M. R. Klauber, E. Barrett-Connor, M. J. Holdbrook, L. Suarez, and D. L. Wingard (1982). Adjustment for obesity in studies of cardiovascular disease. *Am J Epidemiol 116*, 685–691.

de Waard, F. (1975). Breast cancer incidence and nutritional status with particular reference to body weight and height. *Cancer Res 35*, 3351–3356.

Evans, J. G., and I. A. Prior (1969). Indices of obesity derived from height and weight in two Polynesian populations. *Br J Prev Soc Med 23*, 56–59.

Fanelli, M. T., and R. J. Kuczmarski (1984). Ultrasound as an approach to assessing body composition. *Am J Clin Nutr 39*, 703–709.

Florey, C. du, V. (1970). The use and interpretation of ponderal index and other weight–height ratios in epidemiologic studies. *J Chronic Dis 23*, 93–103.

Frisancho, A. R. (1984). New standards of weight and body composition by frame size and height for assessment of nutritional status of adults and the elderly. *Am J Clin Nutr 40*, 808–819.

Frisch, R. E., and J. W. McArthur (1974). Menstrual cycles: Fatness as a determinant of minimum weight for height necessary for their maintenence or onset. *Science 185*, 949–951.

Gallagher, D., M. Visser, D. Sepulveda, R. N. Pierson, T. Harris, and S. B. Heymsfield

(1996). How useful is body mass index for comparison of body fatness across age, sex, and ethnic groups? *Am J Epidemiol 143,* 228–239.

Garn, S. M. (1979). Optimal nutritional assessment. In Jelliffe, D. B., and Jelliffe, E. F. P. (eds.): *Nutrition and Growth.* Vol. 2 of *Human Nutrition* (series). New York: Plenum Press, pp. 273–296.

Garn, S. M., W. R. Leonard, and V. M. Hawthorne (1986). Three limitations of the body mass index. *Am J Clin Nutr 44,* 996–997.

Garn, S. M., and S. D. Pesick (1982). Comparison of the Benn index and other body mass indices in nutritional assessment. *Am J Clin Nutr 36,* 573–575.

Giovannucci, E., A. Ascherio, E. B. Rimm, G. A. Colditz, M. J. Stampfer, and W. C. Willett (1995). Physical activity, obesity, and risk of colon cancer and adenoma in men. *Ann Intern Med 122,* 327–334.

Going, S. B. (1996). Densitometry. In Roche, A. F., Heymsfield, S. B. and Lohman, T. G. (eds.): *Human Body Composition.* Champaign, IL: Human Kinetics Books, pp. 3–24.

Goldbourt, U., and J. H. Medalie (1974). Weight-height indices. Choice of the most suitable index and its association with selected variables among 10,000 adult males of heterogenous origin. *Br J Prev Soc Med 28,* 116–126.

Grodin, J. M., P. K. Siiteri, and P. C. MacDonald (1973). Source of estrogen production in postmenopausal women. *J Clin Edocrinol Metab 36,* 207–214.

Habicht, J. P., C. Yarbrough, and R. Martorell (1979). Anthropometric field methods: Criteria for selection. In Jelliffe, D. B. and Jelliffe, E. F. P. (eds.): *Nutrition and Growth.* Vol. 2 of *Human Nutrition* (series). New York: Plenum Press, pp. 365–387.

Han, T. S., E. M. van Leer, J. C. Seidell, and M. E. J. Lean (1995). Waist circumference action levels in the identification of cardiovascular risk factors: Prevalence study in a random sample. *Br Med J 311,* 1401–1405.

Hansen, N. J., T. G. Lohman, S. B. Going, M. C. Hall, R. W. Pamenter, L. A. Bare, T. W. Boyden, and L. B. Houtkooper (1993). Prediction of body composition in premenopausal females from dual-energy X-ray absorptiometry. *J Appl Physiol 75,* 1637–1641.

Harsha, D. W., R. R. Frerichs, and G. S. Berenson (1978). Densitometry and anthropometry of black and white children. *Hum Biol 50,* 261–280.

Hartz, A. J., D. C. Rupley, and A. A. Rimm (1984). The association of girth measurements with disease in 32,856 women. *Am J Epidemiol 119,* 71–80.

Helenius, M. Y., D. Albanes, M. S. Micozzi, P. R. Taylor, and O. P. Heinonen (1987). Studies of bioelectric resistance in overweight, middle-aged subjects. *Hum Biol 59,* 271–279.

Hirayama, T. (1978). Epidemiology of breast cancer with special reference to the role of diet. *Prev Med 7,* 173–195.

Hodgdon, J. A., and P. I. Fitzgerald (1987). Validity of impedance predictions at various levels of fatness. *Hum Biol 59,* 281–298.

Houtkooper, L. B., T. G. Lohman, S. B. Going, and W. H. Howell (1996). Why bioelectrical impedance analysis should be used for estimating adiposity. *Am J Clin Nutr 64 (suppl),* 436S–448S.

Hsieh, S. D., and H. Yoshinaga (1995). Abdominal fat distribution and coronary heart disease risk factors in men-waist/height ratio as a simple and useful predictor. *Int J Obesity 19,* 585–589.

Insull, W. J., T. Oiso, and K. Tsuchiya (1968). Diet and nutritional status of Japanese. *Am J Clin Nutr 21,* 753–777.

Jebb, S. A., and M. Elia (1993). Techniques for the measurement of body composition: A practical guide. *Int J Obesity 17,* 611–621.

Katch, V. L., and P. S. Freedson (1982). Body size and shape: Derivation of the "HAT" frame size model. *Am J Clin Nutr 36,* 669–675.

Katch, V. L., P. S. Freedson, F. I. Katch, and L. Smith (1982). Body frame size: Validity of self appraisal. *Am J Clin Nutr 36,* 676–679.

Keys, A., F. Fidanza, M. Karvonen, N. Kimura, and H. L. Taylor (1972). Indices of relative weight and obesity. *J Chronic Dis 25,* 329–343.

Khosla, T., and C. R. Lowe (1967). Indices of obesity derived from body weight and height. *Br J Prev Soc Med 21,* 122–128.

Killeen, J., D. Vanderburg, and W. R. Harlan (1978). Application of weight–height ratios and body indices to juvenile populations— The National Health Examinations Survey data. *J Chronic Dis 31,* 529–537.

Kuczmarski, R. J., M. T. Fanelli, and G. G. Koch (1987). Ultrasonic assessment of body composition in obese adults: Overcoming the limitations of the skinfold caliper. *Am J Clin Nutr 45,* 717–724.

Kushi, L. H., S. A. Kaye, A. R. Folsom, J. T. Soler, and R. J. Prineas (1988). Accuracy and reliability of self-measurement of body girths. *Am J Epidemiol 128,* 740–748.

Kushner, R. F., and D. A. Schoeller (1986). Estimation of total body water by bioelectrical impedance analysis. *Am J Clin Nutr 44*, 417–424.

Lapidus, L., C. Bengtsson, B. Larsson, K. Pennert, E. Rybo, and L. Sjostrom (1984). Distribution of adipose tissue and risk of cardiovascular disease and death: A 12-year follow up of participants in the population study of women in Gothenberg, Sweden. *BMJ 289*, 1257–1261.

Larsson, B., K. Svardsudd, L. Welin, L. Wilhelmsen, P. Bjorntorp, and G. Tibblin (1984). Abdominal adipose tissue distribution, obesity, and risk of cardiovascular disease and death: 13 year follow up of participants in the study of men born in 1913. *BMJ 288*, 1401–1404.

Lee, J., L. N. Kolonel, and M. W. Hinds (1981). Relative merits of the weight-corrected-for-height indices. *Am J Clin Nutr 34*, 2521–2529.

Lew, E. A., and L. Garfinkel (1979). Variations in mortality by weight among 750,000 men and women. *J Chronic Dis 32*, 563–576.

Lohman, T. G. (1981). Skinfolds and body density and their relation to body fatness: A review. *Hum Biol 53*, 181–225.

Lohman, T. G. (1996). Dual energy x-ray absorptiometry. In Roche, A. F., Heymsfield, S. B. and Lohman, T. G. (eds.): *Human Body Composition*. Champaign, IL: Human Kinetics Books, pp. 63–78.

Lohman, T. G., A. F. Roche, and R. Martorell (1988). *Anthropometric Standardization Reference Manual*. Champaign, IL: Human Kinetics Books.

Lukaski, H. C. (1987). Methods for the assessment of human body composition: Traditional and new. *Am J Clin Nutr 46*, 537–556.

Lukaski, H. C., W. W. Bolonchuk, C. B. Hall, and W. A. Siders (1986). Validation of tetrapolar bioelectrical impedance method to assess human body composition. *J Appl Physiol 60*, 1327–1332.

Lukaski, H. C., and P. E. Johnson (1985). A simple, inexpensive method of determining total body water using a tracer dose of D2O and infrared absorption of biological fluids. *Am J Clin Nutr 41*, 363–370.

Lukaski, H. C., P. E. Johnson, W. W. Bolonchuk, and G. I. Lykken (1985). Assessment of fat-free mass using bioelectrical impedance measurements of the human body. *Am J Clin Nutr 41*, 810–817.

Manson, J. E., M. J. Stampfer, C. H. Hennekens, and W. C. Willett (1987). Body weight and longevity. A reassessment. *JAMA 257*, 353–358.

Mellits, E. D., and D. B. Cheek (1970). The assessment of body water and fatness from infancy to adulthood. In Brozek, J. (ed.): *Physical Growth and Body Composition: Papers from the Kyoto Symposium on Anthropological Aspects of Human Growth*. Chicago: University of Chicago Press, pp. 12–26.

Metropolitan Life Insurance Co. (1959). *New Weight Standards for Men and Women*. New York: Statistics Bulletin.

Michielutte, R., R. A. Diseker, W. T. Corbett, H. M. Schey, and J. R. Ureda (1984). The relationship between height–weight indices and the triceps skinfold measure among children age 5 to 12. *Am J Public Health 74*, 604–606.

Micozzi, M. S. (1985). Nutrition, body size, and breast cancer. *Yearbook Phys Anthropol 28*, 175–206.

Micozzi, M. S., D. Albanes, D. Y. Jones, and W. C. Chumlea (1986). Correlations of body mass indices with weight, stature, and body composition in men and women in NHANES I and II. *Am J Clin Nutr 44*, 725–731.

Micozzi, M. S., and T. M. Harris (1990). Age variations in the relation of body mass indices to estimates of body fat and muscle mass. *Am J Phys Anthropol 81*, 375–379.

Moore, F. D., K. H. Olesen, J. D. McMurrey, H. V. Parker, M. R. Ball and C. M. Boyden (1963). *The Body Cell Mass and Its Supporting Environment*. Philadelphia: W. B. Saunders.

Mueller, W. H., and L. Stallones (1981). Anatomical distribution of subcutaneous fat: Skinfold site choice and construction of indices. *Hum Biol 53*, 321–335.

Must, A., W. C. Willett, and W. H. Dietz (1993). Remote recall of childhood height, weight, and body build by elderly subjects. *Am J Epidemiol 138*, 56–64.

Palta, M., R. J. Prineas, R. Berman, and P. Hannan (1982). Comparison of self-reported and measured height and weight. *Am J Epidemiol 115*, 223–230.

Parizkova, J. (1961). Total body fat and skinfold thickness in children. *Metabolism 10*, 794–807.

Quetelet, L. A. (1869). *Physique Sociale*. Brussels: C Muquardt.

Revicki, D. A., and R. G. Israel (1986). Relationship between body mass indices and measures of body adiposity. *Am J Public Health 76*, 992–994.

Rhoads, G. G., and A. Kagan (1983). The relation of coronary disease, stroke, and mortality to weight in youth and middle age. *Lancet 1*, 492–495.

Rimm, E. B., M. J. Stampfer, G. A. Colditz, C. G. Chute, L. B. Litin, and W. C. Willett (1990). Validity of self-reported waist and hip circumferences in men and women. *Epidemiology 1*, 466–473.

Rimm, E. B., M. J. Stampfer, E. Giovannucci, A. Ascherio, D. Spiegelman, G. A. Colditz, and W. C. Willett (1995). Body size and fat distribution as predictors of coronary heart disease among middle-aged and older US men. *Am J Epidemiol 141*, 1117–1127.

Roche, A. F. (1984). Anthropometric methods: New and old, what they tell us. *Int J Obesity 8*, 509–523.

Roche, A. F. (1996). Anthropometry and ultrasound. In Roche, A. F., Heymsfield, S. B., and Lohman, T. G. (eds.): *Human Body Composition*. Champaign, IL: Human Kinetics Books, pp. 167–190.

Roche, A. F., R. N. Baumgarther, and S. Guo (1987). Population methods: Anthropometry or estimations. In Norgan, N. G. (ed.): *Human Body Composition and Fat Distribution. Report of an EC Workshop, London, December 10–12, 1985.* Den Haag, the Netherlands: CIP-gegevens Koninklijke Bibliotheek. pp. 31–47.

Roche, A. F., S. B. Heymsfield, and T. G. Lohman (eds.): (1996). *Human body composition.* Champaign, IL: Human Kinetics Books.

Roche, A. F., R. M. Sievogel, W. C. Chumlea, and P. Webb (1981). Grading body fatness from limited anthropometric data. *Am J Clin Nutr 34*, 2831–2838.

Rose, G. A., and H. Blackburn (1982). Cardiovascular survey methods. *WHO Monograph Series No. 58.* Geneva: World Health Organization.

Roubenoff, R., J. J. Kehayias, B. Dawson-Hughes, and S. B. Heymsfield (1993). Use of dual-energy x-ray absorptiometry in body-composition studies: Not yet a "gold standard." *Am J Clin Nutr 58*, 589–591.

Ruiz, L., J. R. Colley, and P. J. Hamilton (1971). Measurement of triceps skinfold thickness. An investigation of sources of variation. *Br J Prev Soc Med 25*, 165–167.

Schoeller, D. A. (1996). Hydrometry. In Roche, A. F., Heymsfield, S. B., and Lohman, T. G., (eds.): *Human Body Composition.* Champaign, IL: Human Kinetics Books, pp. 25–44.

Schreiner, P. J., J. G. Terry, G. W. Evans, W. H. Hinson, J. R. Crouse, III, and G. Heiss (1996). Sex-specific associations of magnetic resonance imaging-derived intra-abdominal and subcutaneous fat areas with conventional anthropometric indices. The Atherosclerosis Risk in Communities Study. *Am J Epidemiol 144*, 335–345.

Segal, K. R., B. Gutin, E. Presta, J. Wang, and T. B. van Itallie (1985). Estimation of human body composition by electrical impedance methods: A comparative study. *J Appl Physiol 58*, 1565–1571.

Seidell, J. C., A. Oosterlee, M. A. Thijssen, J. Burema, P. Deurenberg, J. G. Hautvast, and J. H. Ruijs (1987). Assessment of intra-abdominal and subcutaneous abdominal fat: Relation between anthropometry and computed tomography. *Am J Clin Nutr 45*, 7–13.

Seltzer, C. C., R. F. Goldman, and J. Mayer (1965). The triceps skinfold as a predictive measure of body density and body fat in obese adolescent girls. *Pediatrics 36*, 212–218.

Sheng, H. P., and R. A. Huggins (1979). A review of body composition studies with emphasis on total body water and fat. *Am J Clin Nutr 32*, 630–647.

Siri, W. E. (1961). Body composition from fluid spaces and density: Analysis of methods. In Brozek, J. and Henschel, A. (eds.): *Techniques for Measuring Body Composition.* Washington, DC: National Academy of Science, National Research Council, pp. 223–244.

Sorensen, T. I. A., A. J. Stunkard, T. W. Teasdale, and M. W. Higgins (1983). The accuracy of reports of weight: Children's recall of their parents' weights 15 years earlier. *Int J Obesity 7*, 115–122.

Spiegelman, D., R. G. Israel, C. Bouchard, and W. C. Willett (1992). Absolute fat mass, percent body fat, and body-fat distribution: Which is the real determinant of blood pressure and serum glucose? *Am J Clin Nutr 55*, 1033–1044.

Stevens, J., J. E. Keil, L. R. Waid, and P. C. Gazes (1990). Accuracy of current, 4-year, and 28-year self-reported body weight in an elderly population. *Am J Epidemiol 132*, 1156–1163.

Stewart, A. L. (1982). The reliability and validity of self-reported weight and height. *J Chronic Dis 35*, 295–309.

Stewart, A. W., R. T. Jackson, M. A. Ford, and R. Beaglehole (1987). Underestimation of relative weight by use of self-reported height and weight. *Am J Epidemiol 125*, 122–126.

Stunkard, A. J., and J. M. Albaum (1981). The accuracy of self-reported weights. *Am J Clin Nutr 34*, 1593–1599.

Troy, L. M., D. J. Hunter, J. E. Manson, G. A. Colditz, M. J. Stampfer, and W. C. Willett (1995). The validity of recalled height and past weight among younger women. *Int J Obesity 19*, 570–572.

Troy, L. M., K. B. Michels, D. J. Hunter, D. Spiegelman, J. E. Manson, G. A. Colditz, M. J. Stampfer, and W. C. Willett (1996). Self-reported birthweight and history of having been breastfed among younger women: An assessment of validity. *Int J Epidemiol 25*, 122–127.

Vague, J. (1956). The degree of masculine differentiation of obesity: A factor determining predisposition to diabetes, atherosclerosis, gout and uric-calculous disease. *Am J Clin Nutr 4*, 20–34.

Van Itallie, T. B., K. R. Segal, and R. C. Funk (1986). Total body electrical conductivity: A rapidly measured index of lean body mass. In Norgan, N. G. (ed.): *Human Body Composition and Fat Distribution. Euro-Nut Report No.8*. Washington, Holland: Euro-Nut, pp. 113–127.

Watson, P. E., I. D. Watson, and R. D. Batt (1980). Total body water volumes for adult males and females estimated from simple anthropometric measurements. *Am J Clin Nutr 33*, 27–39.

Womersley, J., and J. V. Durnin (1977). A comparison of the skinfold method with extent of "overweight" and various weight-height relationships in the assessment of obesity. *Br J Nutr 38*, 271–284.

World Health Organization (1983). *Measuring Change in Nutritional Status*. Geneva: World Health Organization.

World Health Organization (1995). *Physical Status: The Use and Interpretation of Anthropometry*. Technical Report Series No. 854. Geneva: World Health Organization, Expert Committee on Physical Status.

Zerfar, A. (1979). Anthropmetric field methods: General. In Jelliffe, D. B., and Jelliffe, E. F. P. (eds.): *Nutrition and Growth*. Vol. 2 of *Human Nutrition* (series) New York: Plenum Press, pp. 339–362.

11

Implications of Total Energy Intake for Epidemiologic Analyses

WALTER WILLETT AND MEIR STAMPFER

Total energy intake deserves special consideration in nutritional epidemiology for three reasons:

1. The level of energy intake may be a primary determinant of disease.
2. Individual differences in total energy intake produce variation in intake of specific nutrients unrelated to dietary composition because the consumption of most nutrients is positively correlated with total energy intake. This added variation may be extraneous, and thus a source of error, in many analyses.
3. When energy intake is associated with disease but is not a direct cause, the effects of specific nutrients may be distorted or confounded by total energy intake.

Before examining these three issues in detail, the physiologic aspects of energy utilization and the determinants of variation in energy intake in epidemiologic studies are discussed. In accordance with common practice, *total caloric intake* is used synonymously with *total energy intake* in this chapter, although use of joules as a unit of measurement is more correct.

PHYSIOLOGIC DETERMINANTS OF ENERGY UTILIZATION

Physiologists have partitioned energy expenditure into several components: resting metabolic rate, thermogenic effect of food, physical activity, and adaptive thermogenesis (Horton, 1983) (Fig. 11–1). Resting

Parts of this chapter are reproduced from Willett and Stampfer (1986) and Willett (1987) with permission of the original publishers. Several of the ideas on various analytic strategies evolved during a March 1988 workshop sponsored by the SEARCH program of the International Agency for Cancer Research, Lyon, France. Much is owed to discussions with James Marshall, Geoffrey Howe, Larry Kushi, and Larry Freedman, which are partly embodied in Willett et al., 1997.

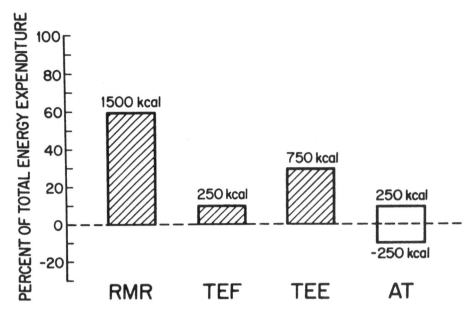

Figure 11–1. Components of energy expenditure. RMR, resting metabolic requirement; TEF, thermogenic effect of food; TEE, total energy expenditure; AT, adaptive thermogenesis. From Horton, 1983: reproduced with permission.)

metabolic requirements are quantitatively the most important, representing approximately 60% of total energy expenditure in most individuals. The thermogenic effect of food (which is the metabolic cost of absorbing and processing carbohydrate, protein, and fat) varies with the sources of energy (Donato and Hegsted, 1985), but is only about 10% of the total. Adaptive thermogenesis represents the capacity of an individual to conserve or expend energy in response to variable intake of food or, perhaps, temperature extremes. In humans, adaptive thermogenesis is defined differently by various investigators (Sjostrom, 1985) and is difficult to measure. It has been estimated to be less than ± 10% of calories. In a moderately active individual, physical activity accounts for approximately 30% of energy intake (Horton, 1983).

Determinants of Between-Person Variation in Total Energy Intake

Although it is helpful to consider the average values for physiologic components of energy expenditure, epidemiologists are primarily interested in the determinants of variation in energy intake between individuals. Although many specific factors influence energy intake, they can be considered as three general categories: body size, metabolic efficiency, and physical activity. Departures from energy balance, that is, change in body energy stores due to intake above or below expenditure, also account for part of the observed variation among persons (Fig. 11–2).

Body size affects the amount of energy needed for resting metabolic activity and to sustain physical exertion. On the basis of careful measurements, such as those by Jequier and Schutz (1983) using a specially designed respiratory chamber, it appears that body size is a primary determinant of energy expenditure (Fig. 11–3), particularly at low levels of physical activity. These authors found that 24-hour energy expenditure was a linear function of body weight, which accounted for 74% of the variance in expenditure. Using similar methods, it has further been demonstrated that energy

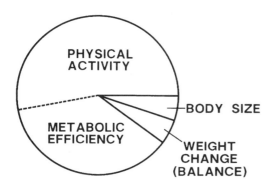

Figure 11–2. Components of between-person variation in energy intake. The relative sizes of these components vary depending on the population being studied.

expenditure is primarily related to lean body mass rather than to fat mass (Ravussin et al., 1986). It must be noted that these study groups were heterogeneous with respect to age and gender and were atypically enriched with obese subjects, all of which would tend to inflate variation attributable to weight or lean body mass. More important, as noted by these authors, the usual physical activity of subjects in these studies was constrained by their restriction to a small metabolic chamber.

Among free-living subjects of the same gender and similar size, neither height nor weight accounts for a major proportion of the between-person variation in total caloric intake (Thomson and Billewicz, 1961; Gordon et al., 1984). For example, neither measure of body size was significantly correlated with caloric intake among a group of 194 women aged 34 to 59 years who collected four 1-week weighed diet records over 1 year (Willett et al., 1985) (Spearman $r = 0.08$ for height and $r = -0.10$ for weight, unpublished data). Underreporting of intake by clearly obese subjects has been documented (Prentice et al., 1986) and could explain some of the lack of a positive association between weight and energy intake. Although body size does not appear to be the major determinant of variation in energy intake among free-living subjects within a specific age and sex group, if anal-

yses were conducted on groups markedly heterogeneous in size, which would be true if both men and women were included, then body size would become a more important determinant.

Although energy expenditure at rest accounts for the majority of absolute energy intake, resting energy expenditure does not vary greatly among individuals of similar age and sex. Thus, physical activity assumes a relatively large role in determining the *variation* in energy expenditure among individuals unconstrained by a metabolic chamber. The positive relationship between physical activity and energy intake has been appreciated for years (Johnson et al., 1956; Saltzman and Roberts, 1995) and has been clearly demonstrated by Morris and colleagues (1977) in an epidemiologic study among a population of bank clerks (Table 11–1). Among the 194 women previously mentioned, the correlation between a physical activity questionnaire and caloric intake based on 28 days of diet recording was 0.22 (unpublished data). The obese tend to be less physically active, and this relationship is sufficient to explain the weak inverse relation between relative weight and caloric intake that has been observed in most epidemiologic studies (Gordon et al., 1981; Romieu et al., 1988). The relationship also presumably underlies a long-term decline in per capita caloric intake in the United States despite an increasing prevalence of obesity (van Itallie, 1978; Abraham and Carroll, 1979; National Center for Health Statistics, 1979). The true proportion of variation in energy intake accounted for by physical activity varies substantially among populations and is likely to be seriously underestimated in most studies because of difficulty in accurately measuring physical activity. Ravussin and colleagues (1986) have demonstrated that even motor activity within the confines of a respiratory chamber ("fidgeting") varies dramatically between persons and can account for hundreds of kilocalories per day. Such differences in activity would not be detected by typical

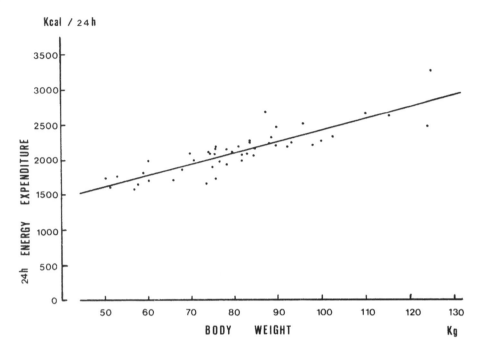

Figure 11–3. Relationship between body weight and 24-hour energy expenditure, based on respiration-chamber measurements. (From Je-quier and Schutz, 1983; reproduced with permission.)

questionnaires. Thus, it appears likely that physical activity, which includes both fine motor and major muscle movement, is the dominant explanation for between-person differences in energy intake. Indeed, in most instances total energy intake can be interpreted as a crude measure of physical activity, particularly after controlling for body size, age, and sex.

Metabolic efficiency may contribute to individual differences in caloric intake; metabolically inefficient persons require greater amounts of energy to maintain their level of activity and weight. The mechanisms and determinants of metabolic efficiency (including differences in absorption and the general category of thermogenesis) are poorly defined in humans and are beyond the scope of this chapter. Individual differences apparently exist, and under carefully controlled conditions some subjects gain weight more rapidly than others who have a similar caloric intake (Sims et al., 1973; Saltzman and Roberts, 1995). However, these differences in metabolic efficiency among individuals, particularly between obese and nonobese persons, are relatively small and inconsistently observed. In a number of studies increased energy intake has appeared to reduce metabolic efficiency, in other words to increase thermogenesis (Miller, 1973; Himms-Hagen, 1984; Woo et al., 1985; Leibel et al., 1995). However, recent work using doubly-labeled water indicates that extra calories added to the diets of most persons are mainly stored as fat, suggesting that these individuals are already operating at maximal thermogenesis (Roberts et al., 1993). However, some modest capacity to increase metabolic efficiency (reduce thermogenesis) exists during underfeeding, thus aggravating attempts to lose weight. This degree of adaptive thermogenesis is modest, probably less than 10% of total energy intake (Webb, 1985; Saltzman and Roberts, 1995).

Unfortunately, there is no practical method of measuring metabolic efficiency in an epidemiologic setting. The data of Jequier and Schutz (1983) (Fig. 11–3), however, suggest that there is relatively little between-person variation in energy expenditure after physical activity has been restricted and weight is accounted for. Thus, the contribution of metabolic efficiency to between-person variation in energy expenditure remains poorly defined but is not likely to be large.

The net balance of energy intake in relation to body size, metabolic efficiency, and physical activity determines whether a person gains or loses weight. In the absence of compensatory mechanisms, relatively small changes maintained over long periods would have a profound effect on body weight. For example, if an adult male who consumes 2,500 kcal per day increases his caloric consumption by only 2% and other factors remaining constant, over a 10-year period a theoretical 20-kg weight gain will result (theoretical weight change over 10 years = 2,500 kcal per day × 0.02 × 365 days per year × 10 years/9,000 kcal per kg of fat = 20.3 kg). In reality, the increase in weight will not be so dramatic, as the additional energy cost of maintaining and moving the added mass eventually equals the increment in energy intake and a new steady-state is obtained.

Hofstetter and colleagues (1986) have used the cross-sectional data in Figure 11–3, in which 1 kg in weight corresponds to about 20 kcal per day, to estimate the ultimate weight gain associated with a given change in energy availability. In this manner, the 2% change in energy intake (50 kcal/day) would result in an ultimate change of 2.5 kg, which is still readily measurable epidemiologically. (It must be noted that such calculations of projected weight changes from cross-sectional data are likely to be somewhat inaccurate for

Table 11–1. Association of leisure time physical activity and energy intake among London bus drivers

Thirds of distribution of men for energy intake	Physical activity in leisure time		
	Little	Moderate	Much
Low third	16	9	4
Middle third	9	12	3
High third	5	10	9

From Morris et al., 1977.

several reasons, including that weight in the cross-sectional data is largely lean body mass, whereas changes in weight caused by simple increases in caloric intake would be primarily due to adipose.) Careful, long-term studies of the effects of small increments in energy intake on body weight would be most useful because most studies have been done using large increments (Webb, 1985).

During short periods, such as months, the proportion of energy intake accounted for by balance (i.e., weight gain or loss) is larger if some persons are experiencing rapid weight change. Over the long-term, however, balance can account for only a very small part of between-person differences in energy intake. The true between-person variation in long-term caloric intake is poorly defined. Using 28 days of diet recording per subject (which minimizes variation within persons), we observed a standard deviation of 323 kcal/day (mean 1,620) among middle-aged women (Willett et al., 1985). This amount is somewhat less than the standard deviation of 473 kcal/day for women (mean 1,793) estimated by Beaton and coworkers (1979) from multiple 24-hour recalls using an analysis-of-variance model.

Because differences in total energy intake between individuals are largely determined by physical activity, body size, and metabolic efficiency, it is apparent that an epidemiologic study of only energy intake in relation to disease risk is difficult or impossible to interpret. Energy intake is measurable only crudely (errors being considerably larger than 2%) with standard questionnaires or interviews; physical activity is probably measured even more crudely than diet; and metabolic efficiency is essentially unmeasurable in an epidemiologic setting. Thus, it would be difficult if not impossible to partition an individual's total energy intake with sufficient precision so as to measure the balance available after accounting for physical activity and metabolic efficiency because this balance would be computed as the difference between two crudely measured variables minus an unmeasurable variable. It is therefore not surprising that the degree of obesity is not strongly correlated with energy intake in cross-sectional studies.

Although the interpretation of energy intake data in epidemiologic analyses may be difficult, simple and readily available measures of weight and height can be extremely useful as alternatives to direct measures of energy intake. The presence of high relative weight implies that, sometime in life, a positive balance between energy intake and energy expenditure has occurred. Even more useful, a change in weight implies a positive or negative energy balance during that time. The interpretation of data on weight and height, however, is potentially complicated because individuals apparently have some ability to compensate for increased or decreased caloric intake by changing their thermogenesis (i.e., reducing or increasing metabolic efficiency). Moreover, individuals may vary in their capacity to respond in this way (Miller, 1973). It is thus conceivable that excess caloric intake could increase disease risk in a manner that was mediated by a thermogenic response (i.e., related to increased metabolic rate) rather than by the accumulation of fat. The interpretation of epidemiologic data relating to weight and energy intake, therefore, depends in an important way on how body weight responds to increased energy intake. In model 1 (Fig.

11–4), increased energy intake is fully compensated by adaptive thermogenesis up to a certain point, and weight gain occurs only after a threshold increase in caloric intake is exceeded. In model 2, any long-term increase in energy intake causes weight gain; any compensatory increase in thermogenesis occurs only in conjunction with weight gain.

The implication of model 2 for epidemiologists is that the absence of a relationship between obesity and risk of disease implies that the disease is not caused by excess energy intake. Failure to observe an association between relative weight and risk of disease thus provides evidence that changes in energy intake alone do not influence disease occurrence. This may be appreciated by considering the hypothetical situation where even a small increase in energy intake, say 5%, with physical activity held constant raises the risk of disease. If model 2 applies, this difference in intake would produce an easily measurable weight gain; therefore, individuals who had increased their energy consumption would weigh more, and we would observe a positive association between relative weight and risk of disease. If model 1 were correct, an absence of association with obesity would not exclude the possibility that increased energy intake causes a higher risk of disease by inducing a fully compensating higher level of thermogenesis. Recognizing that individuals may vary in their response to energy intake, model 2 would need to apply only to an appreciable proportion of the population, not necessarily to all individuals, to be relevant epidemiologically.

The data of Donato and Hegsted (1985), based on rats, indicate that gain in body weight is a linear function of energy availability, that is, model 2 applies. Based on a review of metabolic studies among humans, Woo and colleagues (1985) suggested that any adaptive response in thermogenesis occurs only after some change in adiposity, and this has been supported by more recent evidence (Saltzman and Roberts, 1995). Thus, it seems appropriate to

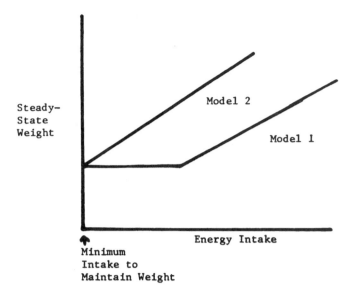

Figure 11–4. Alternate models of response to an increase in long-term energy intake. In model 1, increased thermogenesis prevents weight gain up to a certain increment in energy intake. In model 2, any compensatory increase in energy expenditure occurs only in conjunction with weight gain.

interpret a lack of association with relative weight in a specific study as evidence against a direct causal effect of total energy intake on risk of disease.

Relation of Energy Intake With Specific Nutrient Intake

Intakes of most nutrients in free-living populations tend to be positively correlated with total energy intake (Jain et al., 1980; Lyon et al., 1983; Gordon et al., 1984). Data based on four 1-week diet records were used to examine these correlations among 194 women (see Table 11–2, last row). Correlations were particularly strong for fat, protein, and carbohydrate (which contribute to energy intake); in this population alcohol intake was quite modest and was only weakly correlated with total energy consumption. Every other nutrient examined, however, was also correlated with total energy intake even though many did not contribute to energy. For example, the correlation with energy was 0.24 for fiber, 0.25 for vitamin A, and 0.19 for vitamin C. This tendency for all nutrients, even

minerals and vitamins, to be correlated with total energy intake results from the tendency of larger, more active, and less metabolically efficient persons to eat more food in general.

These interrelations are further complicated by the observation that the composition of diets may vary by level of total caloric intake, depending on the behavior of the population. For example, as shown in Table 11–3, women with lower energy intake tended to have a proportionally higher intake of fiber than women with higher energy intake. These correlations between caloric intake and specific nutrient intakes further highlight the need to consider total energy intake when interpreting associations between specific nutrients and disease in epidemiologic studies.

ADJUSTMENT FOR ENERGY INTAKE IN EPIDEMIOLOGIC ANALYSES

When relationships with disease are analyzed, nutritional factors may be examined in terms of absolute amount (crude intake)

Table 11–2. Correlations (Spearman r) between intakes of specific nutrients[a]

	Protein	Total fat	Saturated fat	Polyunsaturated fat	Total carbohydrate	Crude fiber	Vitamin A	Sucrose	Vitamin B$_6$	Vitamin C	Cholesterol	Alcohol
Protein	—	—	—	—	—	—	—	—	—	—	—	—
Total fat	0.44	—	—	—	—	—	—	—	—	—	—	—
	−0.13											
	−0.14											
Saturated fat	0.42	0.93	—	—	—	—	—	—	—	—	—	—
	−0.10	0.74										
	−0.10	0.74										
Polyunsaturated fat	0.28	0.73	0.52	—	—	—	—	—	—	—	—	—
	−0.08	0.56	0.02									
	−0.11	0.56	0.02									
Total carbohydrate	0.39	0.56	0.47	0.41	—	—	—	—	—	—	—	—
	−0.34	−0.48	−0.43	−0.15								
	−0.23	−0.52	−0.57	−0.14								
Crude fiber	0.36	0.01	−0.06	0.12	0.45	—	—	—	—	—	—	—
	0.32	−0.44	−0.51	−0.07	0.35							
	0.24	−0.45	−0.51	−0.08	0.45							

Vitamin A	0.45 / 0.40 / 0.37	0.08 / −0.33 / −0.32	0.03 / −0.38 / −0.36	0.10 / −0.08 / −0.08	0.66 / 0.13 / 0.19	0.66 / 0.64 / 0.61	—	—	—	—	—	—
Sucrose	0.21 / −0.54 / −0.45	0.53 / −0.18 / −0.21	0.46 / −0.19 / −0.25	0.37 / −0.13 / −0.11	0.18 / 0.60 / 0.56	0.18 / −0.17 / −0.05	0.14 / −0.20 / −0.12	—	—	—	—	—
Vitamin B$_6$	0.56 / 0.44 / 0.41	0.15 / −0.49 / −0.48	0.14 / −0.39 / −0.38	0.12 / −0.22 / −0.22	0.65 / 0.26 / 0.33	0.65 / 0.61 / 0.59	0.57 / 0.53 / 0.59	0.22 / −0.23 / −0.16	—	—	—	—
Vitamin C	0.34 / 0.32 / 0.26	0.002 / −0.47 / −0.45	−0.05 / −0.46 / −0.44	−0.00 / −0.14 / −0.15	0.61 / 0.17 / 0.34	0.61 / 0.62 / 0.59	0.13 / 0.60 / 0.58	0.13 / −0.12 / −0.04	0.55 / 0.53 / 0.51	—	—	—
Cholesterol	0.60 / 0.58 / 0.50	0.51 / 0.16 / 0.19	0.55 / 0.22 / 0.26	0.26 / −0.02 / −0.04	0.05 / −0.36 / −0.32	0.05 / −0.00 / −0.07	0.25 / −0.17 / 0.13	0.18 / −0.34 / −0.30	0.24 / 0.09 / 0.05	0.12 / 0.11 / 0.03	—	—
Alcohol	−0.03 / −0.16 / −0.13	0.04 / −0.12 / −0.12	0.12 / 0.06 / 0.05	−0.01 / −0.13 / −0.13	−0.15 / −0.50 / −0.54	−0.14 / −0.19 / −0.18	−0.03 / −0.10 / −0.07	−0.06 / −0.14 / −0.21	−0.06 / −0.16 / −0.14	−0.06 / −0.14 / −0.12	−0.04 / −0.15 / −0.12	—
Energy	0.59	0.86	0.81	0.59	0.82	0.24	0.25	0.71	0.40	0.19	0.47	0.15

[a] For each comparison, top r value is for crude nutrient intake, middle value is for nutrient density, and the bottom value is for calorie-adjusted (using regression analysis) nutrient intake. Data are based on the individual means of 28 days of diet recording by each of 194 women.

Table 11–3. Correlations (Pearson r) between total caloric intake, crude nutrient intake, nutrient densities, and calorie-adjusted nutrient intakes[a]

Nutrient	Calories vs. crude nutrient	Nutrient density[b] vs. crude nutrient	Calorie-adjusted vs. crude nutrient[c]	Calories vs. nutrient density[b]	Calories vs. calorie-adjusted[c]	Nutrient density[b] vs. calorie-adjusted[c]
Protein	0.60	0.31	0.80	−0.57	0.000	0.82
Total fat	0.88	0.52	0.48	0.05	0.000	0.99
Saturated fat	0.81	0.66	0.58	0.09	0.000	0.99
Polyunsaturated fat	0.64	0.77	0.77	−0.01	0.000	0.99
Sucrose	0.72	0.91	0.70	0.33	0.000	0.93
Cholesterol	0.47	0.70	0.88	−0.31	0.000	0.95
Carbohydrate	0.86	0.72	0.52	0.26	0.000	0.97
Fiber	0.34	0.82	0.94	−0.26	0.000	0.97
Vitamin A-ns	0.34	0.84	0.94	−0.23	0.000	0.97
Vitamin A-ws	0.25	0.90	0.97	−0.19	0.000	0.98
Vitamin B_6-ns	0.46	0.76	0.89	0.22	0.000	0.97
Vitamin B_6-ws	0.15	0.98	0.99	−0.06	0.000	0.99
Vitamin C-ns	0.28	0.88	0.96	−0.20	0.000	0.98
Vitamin C-ws	0.15	0.96	0.99	−0.13	0.000	0.99

[a] Data are based on the individual means of 28 days of dietary recording by each of 194 women and on four 1-week diet records. All values were transformed using natural logarithm to improve normality. ns, without supplements; ws, with supplements.

[b] Nutrient density is the nutrient divided by calories.

[c] Calorie-adjusted using regression analysis.

or in relation to total caloric intake. The analytic approach depends on both the nature of the biologic relationship and the public health considerations. If a nutrient is metabolized in approximate proportion to total caloric intake (such as the macronutrients and some vitamins), nutrient intake is most likely biologically important in relation to caloric intake. To the extent that energy intake reflects body size, adjustment for total energy intake is usually appropriate as an absolute amount of a specific nutrient tends to have less of an effect for a larger, higher energy-consuming person than for a smaller person. In some situations, we may be unsure whether it is the absolute amount of a nutrient or the amount in relation to total caloric intake that is most biologically relevant. (Of course, the biologically relevant relationship with caloric intake may actually be complex and nonlinear.) If a nutrient selectively affects an organ system that is uncorrelated with body size (e.g., the central

nervous system), or if physical activity does not affect its metabolism, absolute intake may be most relevant. For example, menstrual blood losses are not thought to increase with physical activity; thus iron requirements to prevent anemia among premenopausal women might be related to absolute intake.

It is interesting to note that if absolute nutrient intake rather than intake in relation to calories is biologically most relevant, caloric intake should be associated with disease, as intakes of virtually all nutrients are positively correlated with total caloric intake. For example, if higher absolute intake of a nutrient is a cause of disease, then those who consume more total food due to being large, active, or metabolically inefficient should be at higher risk of disease. In the example above, we would expect to see a greater risk of iron deficiency anemia among women with lower total energy intake due to lower physical activity. Conversely, a lack of association between total energy intake and disease can be taken as evidence against the importance of absolute nutrient intake, but not against the importance of nutrient composition of the diet.

Because a person's long-term total caloric intake is largely determined by body size, physical activity, and metabolic efficiency, even relatively small changes in caloric intake cannot be made unless changes in weight or physical activity also occur. In the absence of such changes, therefore, most alterations in absolute nutrient intake must be accomplished by changing the composition of the diet rather than the total amount of food. For this reason, Hegsted (1985) has suggested that dietary recommendations should be made in reference to total caloric intake; for example, it has been recommended that we reduce total fat intake to 30% of total caloric intake. Therefore, from a practical or public health standpoint, nutrient intake in relation to total caloric intake (i.e., the qualitative aspect or composition of diet) is most relevant. For this reason, in epidemiologic studies, nutrient intakes adjusted for total energy intake, rather than absolute nutrient intakes, are of primary interest in relation to disease risk. Adjusting nutrient intakes for total energy intake in epidemiologic studies can also be viewed as being analogous to animal experiments or metabolic studies in humans; to determine whether an effect is due to a nutrient per se, it is essential that the diets being compared are isocaloric.

As reports of diet and disease relationships have often been made without adjustment for total caloric intake, the implications of this approach are discussed first. Because body size, physical activity, and metabolic efficiency contribute to the variation of specific nutrient intakes, associations between nutrients and diseases that are actually independent of these factors are weakened. That is, differences in the levels of these factors cause variation in energy intake and, secondarily, variation in intake of specific nutrients that may be extraneous or irrelevant to occurrence of disease. For example, tall and physically active women tend to have high absolute fat intakes on the basis of their size and exercise level alone. If the relevant exposure for breast cancer risk is fat intake independent of body size and physical activity (i.e., the fat composition of the diet), failure to account for these factors results in misclassification of exposure that is likely to be largely random. The influence of removing extraneous variation can be appreciated in studies that have examined the correlation between nutrient intake, such as specific carotenoids, and levels of these nutrients in blood or adipose, which presumably are more directly reflective of biologic effects. In general, adjustment for total energy intake has increased associations between calculated nutrient intakes and levels in blood or adipose (Willett et al., 1983; London et al., 1991; Ascherio et al., 1992; Hunter et al., 1992), sometimes to only a small degree, but in other instances substantially. To partially address this issue, nutrient intakes are sometimes divided by a measure of body size, such as intake per kilogram of body weight (Sopko et al., 1984). Unfortunately, it is seldom possible to account for the effects of physical activity and metabolic efficiency in a similar manner because these are difficult to measure accurately.

When total caloric intake is associated with disease, the interpretation of individual nutrient intake is complex, and the consequences of failing to account for energy intake may be far more serious. As has been pointed out by Lyon and colleagues (1983), specific nutrients tend to be associated with disease simply on the basis of their correlation with caloric intake. For example, in nearly every study of diet and coronary heart disease, subjects who subsequently develop disease have lower total caloric intake on the average than do those who remain free of disease (Morris et al., 1977; Garcia-Palmieri et al., 1980; Gordon et al., 1981; Kromhout and de Lezenne Coulander, 1984; McGee et al., 1984b). As a result, intakes of specific nutrients also tend to be lower among cases than among noncases.

These relationships are illustrated in analyses of prospectively collected data on dietary intake and coronary heart disease incidence among men living in Honolulu, Puerto Rico, and Framingham (Gordon et al., 1981). Among the Honolulu men, for example, the crude intakes of 9 of 11 nutrients (including total calories) were lower among those with subsequent coronary heart disease, and for two nutrients there was no difference (Table 11–4). In this situation, it is helpful to consider possible reasons for an observed difference in caloric intake between men who developed coronary disease and those who remained free of disease. Difference in body size is an unlikely explanation as men who subsequently develop coronary heart disease tend, if anything, to weigh more than those who do not. Variation in level of metabolic efficiency is usually impossible to eliminate as an explanation. On the other hand, several investigators have clearly demonstrated that decreased physical activity is associated with an increased risk of coronary heart disease (Morris et al., 1977; Paffenbarger et al., 1978). Although differences in physical activity provide the most likely explanation for the low caloric intake associated with coronary heart disease, this explanation was not universally appreciated (Garcia-Palmieri et al., 1980; McGee et al., 1984a). Thus, an appropriate interpretation of the inverse association between total caloric intake and risk of coronary heart disease is not that one should increase food intake to avoid a myocardial infarction, but rather that an increase in physical activity may reduce the risk of disease. This example, incidentally, illustrates the need to be guided by an understanding of biologic relationships when interpreting statistical associations to avoid absurd conclusions.

Because variation in caloric intake be-

tween persons largely reflects physical activity, size, and metabolic efficiency, an association between a specific nutrient and disease is not likely to be of primary etiologic importance if that association is simply the result of a difference in caloric intake. For this reason, Morris and coworkers (1977) have pointed out that it "would not be instructive to present data relating crude nutrient intakes with disease in a situation in which caloric intake has an important relationship with the outcome."

It is, of course, possible that overeating or undereating (caloric excess or deficiency) is a primary cause of a disease. In this situation, higher intakes of nutrients that contribute to calories (proteins, fats, carbohydrates, and alcohol) might be considered as the primary exposures that lead to increased total caloric intake, which in turn causes disease. It could be argued that adjustment for caloric intake in this situation would represent "overcontrol" of a variable in the causal pathway. Before attributing an effect to a specific nutrient, however, the burden is on the epidemiologist to demonstrate that the association of this nutrient with disease is independent of caloric intake. For example, perhaps excessive caloric intake increases the risk of colon cancer, and dietary fat is associated with this disease because of its high caloric content. Before implicating fat per se as a specific cause, however, it would be essential to demonstrate that this effect is not shared by protein or carbohydrate when these are eaten in equicaloric amounts. Otherwise, a reduction in the fat content of the diet that was replaced by an increase in carbohydrate or protein on a calorie-by-calorie basis would have no effect on disease occurrence: This would only happen when the total caloric intake was also changed. The desirability of relating nutrient intake to total caloric intake has been discussed in a thoughtful correspondence with respect to studies of coronary heart disease (Kushi et al., 1985; Shekelle et al., 1985). Recognizing the need to adjust for the effect of total

Table 11–4. Age-adjusted means of crude nutrient intakes and nutrient intakes as a percentage of total calories according to subsequent coronary heart disease (CHD) death or myocardial infarction (MI)[a]

	Crude intakes		Intakes as % of calories	
	No CHD	MI or CHD death	No CHD	MI or CHD death
	(n=7,008)	(n=164)	(n=7,008)	(n=164)
Total calories (kcal)	2,319	2,149[b]		
Total protein (g)	95	93	16.6	17.4[c]
Total fat (g)	87	86	33.4	35.6[c]
Saturated fat (g)	32	31	12.3	12.9[c]
Monounsaturated fat (g)	33	32	12.8	13.6[b]
Polyunsaturated fat (g)	16	16	6.0	6.7
Total carbohydrate (g)	264	242[b]	46.2	45.4
Sugar (g)	46	46	7.9	8.2
Starch (g)	165	151[b]	29.2	28.5
Other carbohydrate (g)	52	45[c]	9.1	8.7
Cholesterol (mg)	555	530		
Alcohol (g)	14	5[b]	3.8	1.7[b]

[a] Data are based on a cohort of 7,172 Honolulu men aged 46–64 years initially free of CHD.
From Tables 4 and 8 of Gordon et al., 1981.
[b] $p < 0.01$.
[c] $p < 0.05$.

food consumption, a number of investigators have employed "nutrient densities" to control for the effect of total caloric intake.

Analyses of Diet–Disease Relationships by the Use of Nutrient Densities

Nutrient densities are measures of dietary composition computed by dividing nutrient values by total caloric intake; they provide a convenient way to describe foods or diets. An analogous approach for macronutrients is to express intake as a percentage of total caloric intake; for purposes of discussion, both approaches are referred to as *nutrient density*. Nutrient density has the appeal of simplicity and practicality; unfortunately, this is actually a complex variable that can lead to confusion when used to address diet–disease relationships. Such a variable has two components: the nutrient intake and the inverse of total caloric intake. The relative contributions of nutrient intake and total caloric intake to between-person differences in nutrient density are related to the ratio of their vari-

ability. Thus, as the between-person variation in the specific nutrient intake decreases, the nutrient density value approaches the inverse of caloric intake (multiplied by a constant).

When energy intake is unrelated to disease, dividing nutrient intakes by total calories may have the desired effect of reducing the variation in nutrient intake that is due to differences in size, activity, and metabolic efficiency. The division, however, also can create unwanted variation. Particularly when a specific nutrient has a weak correlation with total energy intake or has a low variability, dividing by total calories creates a variable that is, in fact, highly related to the factor whose effect we wish to remove, that is, caloric intake. In addition, methodologic error in measuring total energy intake could potentially contribute to variation in nutrient density as a result of this division. The basic principle involved is that dividing by a variable does not necessarily remove or "control for" the effect of that variable.

Like any ratio (or cross-product term), the nutrient density can also be viewed statistically as an interaction, which has troubled some persons. However, this ratio is in itself biologically meaningful; it would be expected that the effect on an absolute intake of a specific nutrient would be greater at low energy intakes (e.g., for a small person) than at high energy intakes (e.g., for a large person) (Willett, 1990).

As with absolute nutrient intakes, the use of nutrient densities has serious potential pitfalls when total energy intake is itself associated with disease. Because a nutrient density variable contains the inverse of energy intake as a component, nutrient densities tend to be associated with disease in the direction opposite to that of total caloric intake, even when the nutrient itself has no association with disease independent of energy intake. The data of Gordon and colleagues (1981), which present nutrient intakes as percentages of total calories, again illustrate this point. Because coronary heart disease is associated with low caloric intake, nutrient densities (or intakes as percentages of total calories) tend to be positively associated with disease (Table 11–4). In this instance, dividing by total calories has changed the direction of association with coronary heart disease for protein and total, saturated, monounsaturated, and polyunsaturated fat, and four of these differences become statistically significant. Differences between cases and controls have essentially disappeared for the three measures of carbohydrate intake that were statistically significant in the crude analysis. The potential for artifact created by the use of nutrient densities in this example can most vividly be appreciated by realizing that any random variable divided by total energy intake would be positively associated with risk of coronary heart disease.

In some studies, the reason for an association between energy intake and risk of disease may be obscure. In a carefully conducted Canadian case–control investigation of large bowel cancer by Jain and coworkers (1980), cancer patients reported higher caloric intake than did controls but did not weigh more than the controls (see crude intakes, Table 11–5). In addition, cancer cases consistently reported higher intakes of fat than did noncases, which was interpreted to "support the hypothesis that high dietary fat intake is causally associated with cancer of the colon and rectum." In interpreting these findings, it is again useful to consider possible explanations for the difference in caloric intake between cases and controls. It seems unlikely that higher physical activity by cancer cases would explain their higher energy intake; indeed, many studies to the contrary have been published (Garabrant et al., 1984; Vena et al., 1985; Giovannucci, 1995). We cannot dismiss the possibility that cases have a metabolic abnormality that renders them less efficient in their utilization of food energy. For example, it is conceivable that subjects who absorb food poorly present more substrate to their fecal flora, which metabolize this to carcinogenic substances and thus increases the risk of large bowel cancer. The case–control difference in caloric intake is unlikely to be the result of simple overeating in this study as cases did not weigh more than controls, even several years before diagnosis.

In addition to biologic factors, recall bias cannot be dismissed as an explanation for the findings of Jain and colleagues (1980) as this was a case–control study. Whatever biologic or methodologic factors contribute to the association of caloric intake with colon cancer, any differences in the intakes of specific nutrients between cases and controls that result from the strong association of caloric intake with cancer must be regarded as secondary. For illustrative purposes, we recalculated intakes as nutrient densities instead of crude values as originally presented; the findings were dramatically altered (Table 11–5). The association with total fat intake essentially disappears for men and is largely eliminated for women. On the other hand, strong inverse associations are seen for fiber and vitamin C intakes expressed as nutrient densities,

Table 11–5. Case minus control differences in crude and nutrient density intakes expressed as a percentage of case value[a]

	Case–control difference (%)							
	Crude intake (original analysis)				Nutrient density intake (recalculation)			
	Males		Females		Males		Females	
	Colon	Rectum	Colon	Rectum	Colon	Rectum	Colon	Rectum
Calories								
Neighborhood controls	9[b]	7	12[c]	17[c]				
Hospital controls	1	9[d]	6[d]	11[b]				
Total fat								
Neighborhood controls	8[b]	6	15[c]	22[c]	0	−1	4	7
Hospital controls	2	11[d]	10[d]	15[b]	2	2	4	5
Saturated fat								
Neighborhood controls	13[b]	8	16[c]	27[c]	4	1	5	12
Hospital controls	6	13[d]	9[d]	19[c]	5	4	2	8
Crude fiber								
Neighborhood controls	−5	−3	1	2	−15	−11	−12	−17
Hospital controls	−2	5	7	5	−3	−5	1	−7
Vitamin C								
Neighborhood controls	−3	4	−4	0	−13	−3	−18	−20
Hospital controls	−2	6	−2	−3	−3	−6	−9	−16

[a]Data are calculated from Table 5 of a case–control study of colon and rectal cancer conducted among Canadian men and women between 1976 and 1978 (Jain et al., 1980). No tests of statistical significance are available for nutrient density data.
[b]$p < 0.01$.
[c]$p < 0.002$.
[d]$p < 0.05$.

From Willett and Stampfer, 1986.

which had no association with cancer in the crude analysis. This nutrient density analysis, however, overstates the protective association of fiber and vitamin C and underestimates the effect of fat, because dividing by caloric intake produces inverse associations even when these nutrients are not independently associated with disease. Jain and colleagues (1980) recognized the potential for confounding by total caloric intake and stated that the effects of fat and total caloric intake were difficult to separate as it was not possible to enter both simultaneously in a logistic model because of their high correlation. Instead, they considered fat rather than calories to be the primary factor due to its stronger (albeit slight) association with cancer and the findings of previous animal studies. On the ba-

sis of the data presented in the original article, the findings for fat are difficult to interpret as the positive association of this and other nutrients is overstated in crude analyses and understated in nutrient density analyses. If it could be demonstrated that the positive association between caloric intake and colon cancer incidence is related to a real difference in metabolic efficiency between cases and noncases rather than to methodologic bias, this would be an important increment in knowledge, even though the association would not represent a primary etiologic effect of diet and, therefore, would have no direct implications for nutritional advice.

The study of Jain and coworkers (1980) is presented as an example; these authors have provided additional data from their study (Howe et al., 1986, 1997) demonstrating that saturated fat was positively associated with risk of colon cancer independent of energy intake, but fiber intake was not independently related to risk. In a meta-analysis of case–control studies (Howe et al., 1997), a strong and consistent positive association was again seen with total energy intake. After controlling for total energy, no association was seen with total or saturated fat, and a strong inverse association was seen with fiber intake. However, results from subsequent large prospective cohort studies do not support a positive relation between energy intake and risk of colon cancer. In all of these studies, the relationship of total energy intake with risk of colon cancer was inverse (Willett et al., 1990; Bostick et al., 1994; Giovannucci et al., 1994; Goldbohm et al., 1994); in two studies this was statistically significant (Bostick et al., 1994; Goldbohm et al., 1994). The prospective findings are thus consistent with the clear evidence of a protective effect of physical activity against colon cancer and strongly suggest that the case–control findings with total energy intake were due to methodologic bias. This discordance raises serious concerns regarding the validity of case–control studies of diet and cancer. Because both the meta-analysis of case–control studies and most cohort studies found little association between fat intake and colon cancer risk after adjusting for total energy intake, this adjustment may lead to correct conclusions by accounting for bias in reporting of overall food intake in some situations, but not necessarily in all circumstances.

ALTERNATE APPROACHES TO ADJUST FOR TOTAL ENERGY INTAKE

For reasons already discussed, it is usually desirable in epidemiologic analyses to employ a measure of nutrient intake that is independent of total energy intake, particularly when energy intake is associated with disease. In this section four analytic strategies and their relationships to each other are considered: the "energy-adjusted" method, the standard multivariate method, the "energy decomposition" method, and the multivariate nutrient density method.

Energy-Adjusted or Residual Method

"Energy-adjusted" nutrient intakes are computed as the residuals from the regression model with total caloric intake as the independent variable and absolute nutrient intake as the dependent variable (Fig. 11–5). The nutrient residuals by definition provide a measure of nutrient intake uncorrelated with total energy intake. Conceptually, this procedure isolates the variation in nutrient intake due only to the nutrient composition of the diet from the overall variation in nutrient intake, which is due to both composition and overall food consumption. For macronutrients, if expressed in units of calories (e.g., calories from fat), the residuals can also be conceptualized as the substitution of that nutrient for a similar number of calories from other sources (Kipnis et al., 1993). This model can also be viewed as analogous to animal or metabolic feeding studies in which total energy is held constant, but the amount of the nutrient being evaluated is varied between the groups being compared. For an energy-bearing nutrient, a decision needs to be made regarding the other dietary components for which the nutrient will be exchanged. Because residuals have a mean of zero and include negative values, they do not provide an intuitive sense of actual nutrient intake. It may, therefore, be desirable to add a constant; logical choices are the predicted nutrient intake for the mean energy intake of the study population or a round number for energy intake near the population mean (Fig. 11–5).

To illustrate adjustment for total energy intake by regression analysis, we have used daily intakes of total calories and total fat based on the means of four 1-week diet records kept by each of 194 women, as described previously (Willett et al., 1985).

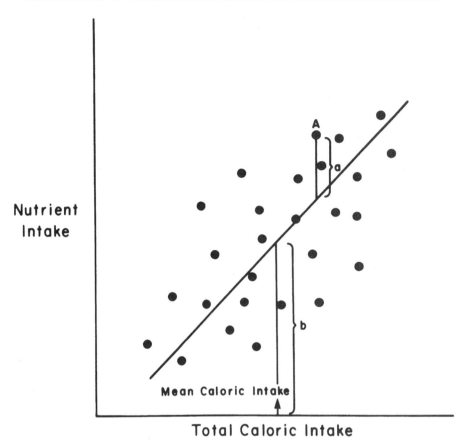

Figure 11–5. Calorie-adjusted intake = $a + b$, where a = residual for subject from regression model with nutrient intake as the dependent variable and total caloric intake as the independent variable and b = the expected nutrient intake for a person with mean caloric intake. (From Willett and Stampfer, 1986; reproduced with permission.)

With 28 days of recording per subject, the effect of day-to-day variation has been sufficiently dampened such that these values can be assumed to reasonably represent each subject's long-term intake. The unadjusted intake of total fat has a reasonably wide distribution (mean = 68.9, 1 standard deviation = 17.0 g per day; Fig. 11–6). Because total fat and total caloric intake are highly correlated (r = 0.86), adjustment for total caloric intake reduces the variation in fat intake substantially (mean = 68.9, 1 standard deviation = 8.7 g per day; shaded area in Fig. 11–6). Nevertheless, the degree of variation remaining is realistic in relation to current dietary recommendations; the 10th percentile (median

of the lowest quintile) represents 33% of calories from fat, and the 90th percentile represents 44% of calories from fat. Thus, sufficient variation exists in this population to test the effectiveness of a 25% reduction in the proportion of calories accounted for by fat, as recommended by the National Heart, Lung, and Blood Institute (Anonymous, 1985).

When total energy intake is an important predictor of disease, total caloric intake should be included in the model with the nutrient calorie-adjusted term (model 2, Table 11–6). This approach is preferable to entering only calorie-adjusted nutrient into a model, as the random error (and width of confidence limits for the effect of the nu-

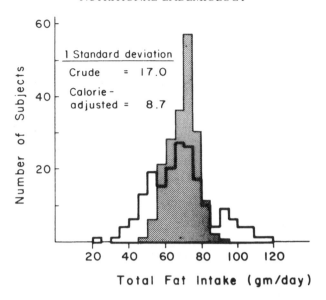

Figure 11–6. Distribution of total fat intake with *(shaded area)* and without *(dark line)* adjustment for total caloric intake. Data are based on four 1-week diet records completed by 194 Boston-area women aged 34 to 59 years. Calorie-adjusted values were calculated as described in the text, with residuals computed in the $\log_e$ scale to improve normality. (From Willett and Stampfer, 1986; reproduced with permission.)

trient) may be reduced if caloric intake has an important association with the outcome independent of nutrient intake. Gail and coworkers (1984) have also shown that uncorrelated variables can confound each other in nonlinear models, including logistic regression. Another advantage of using model 2 rather than model 1 is that the full effect of total caloric intake can be observed.

Shekelle et al. (1987) have calculated calorie-adjusted nutrient intakes using regression analysis and examined their correlations with nutrient densities; these correlations were consistently high (greater than 0.90). On this basis they suggested that, although the calorie-adjusted values were theoretically preferable, the use of nutrient densities may not necessarily lead to materially different conclusions in epidemiologic analyses. We observed similarly high correlations (Table 11–3), but were not confident that the difference between calorie-adjusted values and nutrient densities might not be important in some in-

stances, as the major concern is the potential for confounding by calories. As shown in Table 11–3, the correlations between calorie-adjusted values and calories is, by definition, zero. Several nutrient density values, however, particularly for those nutrients less strongly correlated with total energy intake, were moderately correlated with caloric intake. For example, the correlation of calories with protein/calories was −0.57 and with fiber/calories was −0.26, meaning that the potential for confounding by total calories is substantial if energy intake is related to disease. Because the magnitudes of these correlations are partly related to food choices rather than by laws of nature, these correlations will vary from one group to another. The degree of confounding depends on the strength of association between energy intake and disease as well as nutrient intake and disease; therefore, it seems that distinction between nutrient densities and regression-adjusted values is likely to have practical importance in some, although certainly not all, in-

Table 11–6. Alternative disease risk models for addressing the correlations of specific nutrient intakes with total energy intake in epidemiologic analyses

Model 1 (Residual Method) Disease=b_1 Nutrient residual[a]
Model 2 (Residual Method) Disease=b_1 Nutrient residual+b_2 Calories
Model 3 (Standard Multivariate Method) Disease=b_3 Calories+b_4 Nutrient
Model 4 (Energy Partition Method) Disease=b_5Cal$_{Nutrient}$[b]+b_6Cal$_{other}$[c]
Model 5 (Multivariate Nutrient Density Method) Disease=b_7 Nutrient/Calories+b_8Calories

[a] "Nutrient residual" is the residual from the regression of a specific nutrient on calories.

[b] Cal$_{nutrient}$ represents calories provided by the specific nutrient.

[c] Cal$_{other}$ represents calories from sources other than the specific nutrient.

stances. It appears that this distinction was of major importance for fiber intake in the case–control study by Jain and coworkers (1980) because the nutrient density data in Table 11–5 imply a protective association whereas the regression-adjusted analysis reportedly did not.

The Standard Multivariate Method

The residual approach of calorie adjustment (model 1, Table 11–6) is similar, although not identical, to including both caloric intake and absolute nutrient intake as terms in a multiple regression model with disease outcome as the dependent variable (model 3). The coefficient for the nutrient term in this multivariate model (b_4) is identical to that for the calorie-adjusted nutrient term in a univariate model (b_1). With total caloric intake also in the calorie-adjusted model (model 2), the standard error as well as the coefficient for the calorie-adjusted nutrient term (b_1) is identical to that for the nutrient term (b_4) in the standard multivariate model with nutrient and calories.

Although similar in some respects, the standard multivariate model (model 3) creates complexities in interpretation not shared by model 2. If calories and nutrient are simply entered as separate terms, the coefficient for calories (b_3) represents calories independent of the specific nutrient, which may have a meaning distinctly different from total energy intake. For example, if fat is the specific nutrient in model 3, then the term for calories has the meaning of carbohydrate plus protein (not considering the possible contribution of alcohol). Thus the inclusion of a specific nutrient together with calories in a model fundamentally changes the biologic meaning of calories. The coefficient for calories in this model (b_3) may, therefore, fail to attain significance when total energy intake, in fact, has a significant and important relation with disease. In contrast, the two terms in model 2 clearly address two distinct and clear questions: Is total energy intake associated with disease? Is the nutrient composition of the diet related to disease? The simple and clear meaning of the calorie-adjusted intakes also makes them attractive for bivariate analyses and data presentation. For example, if interest exists in the nutrient composition of the diet, represented by the nutrient residual, it is important to know more about this variable, such as the foods that contribute to its intake and the validity of its measurement as assessed in comparisons with other methods. These issues cannot be easily addressed unless the variable of interest is expressed as a single term.

The use of the standard multivariate model can also create confusion between the distributions of crude nutrient intake and the nutrient intake independent of energy intake. For example, if the nutrient is used as a continuous variable, a single coefficient is obtained; to convert this to a relative risk, a somewhat arbitrary increment in the nutrient intake is needed. Unless the residuals have been computed and examined, an increment based on the crude nutrient intake, for example the 90th versus the 10th percentile, might be chosen. However, this degree of variation in the nutrient intake independent of energy intake would probably not actually exist in the population, and the relative risk would thus be unrealistically large. A relative risk based on the 90th versus 10th percentile of the residual nutrient intake, which would be a smaller increment, would be more appropriate.

Some authors have voiced concern over the simultaneous inclusion of strongly correlated variables in the same model, which will frequently occur using the standard multivariate model in nutritional studies. McGee and colleagues (1984a) have noted that widely divergent results are obtained when highly correlated variables are entered in multiple logistic models using various inclusion criteria, and they suggest that variables with correlation coefficients of more than approximately 0.60 not be simultaneously included. The issue of collinearity is, however, better viewed in biologic rather than purely statistical terms. The first problem created by including two strongly correlated variables in a model is that their meaning may change in a manner that is not readily appreciated. The example of calories and fat is noted above, and the problem of height becoming a measure of body composition when weight is included in a model was noted in Chapter 10. The second problem resulting from collinearity is that one or both variables may have a markedly reduced degree of independent variation when they are entered simultaneously. Rather than using an arbitrary level of correlation as a criterion for unacceptable collinearity, however, a more informative approach is to examine the degree of residual variation in the variables of interest and judge whether the remaining differences among individuals are worthy of study. For example, even though the correlation between total energy and total fat intakes was 0.86 in the data displayed in Figure 11–5, the residual variation in fat after adjusting for total calories was found to be of potential interest. If the residual variation in the variable of interest, such as fat intake, is not large enough to be informative, the issue is not statistical but relates to the nature of the study population; the

only solution is to find another population with a wider residual variation. When faced with highly correlated nutritional variables, models 1 and 2 allow a clear specification of the meaning of the variables, as well as the opportunity to evaluate the residual variation in nutrient intake directly.

The "Energy Decomposition" or "Energy Partition" Method

Howe and colleagues (1986) have presented an alternative model in which they entered separate terms for energy from a specific macronutrient, such as fat, and for energy from other sources, meaning protein, carbohydrate, and alcohol (model 4, Table 11–6). To extend the comparison with animal or metabolic studies, this model implies that more of the nutrient would simply be added to one diet, keeping the other nutrients constant. Thus, this is not an "isocaloric" comparison, and any observed association with the nutrient can still be confounded by total energy intake. In this model, the coefficient for the specific macronutrient (b_5) represents the full effect of the nutrient unconfounded by other sources of energy (b_6), but this model does not directly address the question of whether energy from the specific nutrient has an association with disease not shared by other sources of energy. To address this issue would require determining whether the magnitude of the coefficient for the specific nutrient (b_5) was actually different from the coefficient for other sources of energy (b_6), in other words, the appropriate focus should be b_5–b_6. It is not adequate merely to note that the nutrient coefficient (b_5) is significant, whereas b_6 is not; even when all sources of energy have the same relation with disease on a calorie-for-calorie basis, the coefficient for other calories (b_6) might not be significant simply because of low between-person variation in this factor. In fact, it can be shown that the difference in these coefficients (b_5–b_6) and the standard error of this difference are identical to the coefficient and standard error for the nutrient residual (b_1) in model 2 (Howe, 1989; Pike et al., 1989).

Although the "energy decomposition" model may provide insight in some instances, its coefficients may be misleading unless interpreted with care, particularly when total energy intake has a noncausal relationship with disease. For example, use of this model in the example of coronary heart disease noted previously could easily indicate a protective association for fat intake as its effect would still be confounded by total energy consumption secondary to differences in physical activity. An additional limitation of this model is that it cannot be readily extended to nutrients that do not contribute to energy intake.

Multivariate Nutrient Density Model

Another approach, used in the study by Jain and colleagues (1980) to examine the effect of fiber, is to compute the nutrient density and then enter both this and the total energy in a multiple logistic regression model (model 5). The coefficient for the nutrient density term (b_7) represents the relation of the nutrient composition of the diet with disease, holding total energy intake constant; thus, this method is an "isocaloric" analysis and does control for confounding by energy intake. This model overcomes the primary statistical problem associated with the use of the nutrient density alone, while retaining its attractive features of general recognition and intuitive interpretation as a measure of dietary composition. The coefficient for calories in this model (b_8) will generally be interpretable as representing the effect of calories in the usual biologic sense because nutrient densities are not inherently part of or highly correlated with total energy intake.

The multivariate nutrient density model may be particularly advantageous when body size (and thus total energy intake) varies greatly among subjects because models 2 and 3 imply that the nutrient residual has a similar effect for subjects with high and low energy intake. That a given increment in nutrient intake would have the same effect in a very small subject (with low energy intake) as in a very large subject (with high energy intake) is not plausible. Among specific age–sex groups of human populations, variation in size and total energy is not great, so that this is usually not a major issue. However, among other species, such as dogs (Sonnenschein et al., 1991), body size can vary more than 10-fold, making the use of the multivariate nutrient density model particularly attractive.

The Energy Determinant Method

An alternative approach, in theory, would be to include the major determinants of energy intake (body size, physical activity, and metabolic efficiency) as separate variables in a multivariate model. Unfortunately, measurements of these variables are usually not available in epidemiologic studies. It could be informative, however, to include as many of these variables as possible along with total energy intake as independent variables. Because energy intake and disease outcome may differ in their relationships with body components such as lean mass and fat, it would be desirable to include both height and a measure of fatness uncorrelated with height as separate terms in a multivariate model. The residual of weight on height, computed as described previously for calorie-adjusted nutrients, provides a measure of weight uncorrelated with height. Modeled in this way, height represents lean body mass as it has a linear relationship with total body water in adults (Mellits and Cheek, 1970), and weight independent of height primarily represents fat in middle-aged subjects.

The interpretation of energy intake as an independent variable depends on which other terms are included. If one assumes a steady state of energy balance, energy intake adjusted for body size and physical activity has the meaning of metabolic efficiency. When adjusted for height and weight only, total energy intake has the meaning of physical activity and metabolic efficiency combined. In real applications, these interpretations must be tempered with the knowledge that physical activity is probably measured only crudely and, in case–control studies, that energy intake may also refelct an overall bias in the measurement of dietary intake.

Implications of Non-Normality and Heteroscedasticity

Actual dietary data generally do not have the simple, approximately normal distributions as in Figure 11–5. More typically, energy intake and the nutrient intake are skewed toward higher values, and the variation in nutrient intake (and thus the residuals) is greater at higher total energy intake (Fig. 11–7, for example, using saturated fat). The lack of constant variation in the residuals across level of the independent variable (heteroscedasticity) is in principle a violation of usual regression assumptions and, if ignored, has serious implications for the various methods of energy adjustment. It has been pointed out (M. Maclure, personal communication) that if the residuals from heteroscedastic data are divided into categories, subjects in both the highest and lowest categories will tend to have the highest energy intake. Even though the residuals are overall uncorrelated with energy intake, the residuals would still be confounded by energy intake; if energy intake was positively associated with disease risk, this would create a U-shaped relation between energy-adjusted intake (residuals) and disease risk. If energy were included in the model, this would control for its confounding effect, but the association with disease would be dominated by subjects with high energy intake because they would be overrepresented in the extreme quintiles. This is particularly worrisome because the more extreme energy intakes may represent the least reliable data. Transformations, such as taking logarithms of the variables, are typically used to create residuals with a more constant variance across the independent variable (see Fig. 11–8). As a result, subjects will contribute similarly to information on dietary composition and dis-

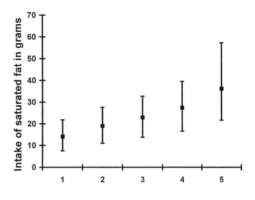

Quintiles of total energy intake
(Median and 95% upper and lower C.I.)

Figure 11–7. Intake of saturated fat by quintiles of total energy intake in the Health Professionals Follow-Up Study (n = 10,000).

ease risk regardless of their energy intake. However, the use of a logarithmic transformation means that nutrient intake is now expressed as a proportional difference (i.e., disease risk would be described for a percentage change in nutrient intake). As noted above, nutrients expressed as residuals have an unfamiliar scale (and even more so when logarithmically transformed); a back transformation can be made by adding a constant (e.g., the pre-

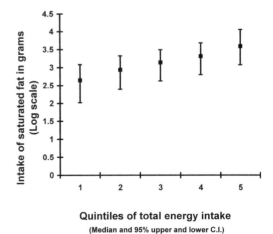

Quintiles of total energy intake
(Median and 95% upper and lower C.I.)

Figure 11–8. Log-transformed saturated fat intake energy data from Figure 11–7.

dicted value for log of 2,000 calories) and then taking the antilog. However, in the interpretation of data it must be remembered that the effect of the energy-adjusted nutrient intake will be expressed for the specified energy intake (e.g., 2,000 calories) and would vary with higher or lower intakes. That the effect of an absolute intake of a nutrient would vary by total energy intake (i.e., an interaction exists) is consistent with our general biologic understanding, as discussed in the context of nutrient density. Indeed, it is interesting that the logarithmically transformed nutrient residual has in common with the nutrient density the concept that its influence on disease risk is related to a relative change in intake.

Although the effects of heteroscedasticity are most transparent in the use of residuals as a measure of dietary composition, the same issues exist with the standard multivariate model, but may not be appreciated because the residuals from one independent variable regressed on another are not typically examined. In the "energy decomposition" model, the impact of non-normally distributed variables is less clear, but it is likely that variability in the nutrient of interest could differ by level of energy intake from other sources in some circumstances. These interrelationships deserve careful examination in any particular application.

More Complex Models
In the analytic approaches discussed previously, only one macronutrient at a time was considered in addition to total energy intake. In principle, these approaches could be extended to include other nutrients as well. For example, using the energy-adjustment approach (model 2), one can compute calorie-adjusted residuals for both protein and fat and include both along with total calories in the same model, or one can use the energy decomposition method to enter energy from fat, protein, and carbohydrate as three separate terms. The capacity to include multiple energy-adjusted nutrients in a model simultaneously will be limited by their intercorrelations and the size of the dataset; if the variables are substantially intercorrelated, the degree of independent variation will quickly become small. However, it will frequently be important to include at least two nutrients at a time. For example, in a study of fiber intake and coronary heart disease risk (Rimm et al., 1996), a critical part of the analysis was to demonstrate that the apparent protective effect of fiber was not explained by lower intake of saturated fat or higher intake of constituents of fruits and vegetables other than fiber. The inclusion of additional nutrient terms to these models should be done with caution as the interpretation of even the two-variable models can be complex.

In the simple multivariate nutrient density model that includes just one type of fat plus total energy intake, the coefficient estimates the effect of substituting that fat for the same amount of energy from the average mix of other macronutrients in that population. The mix would include other fats, proteins, and carbohydrates, which hardly provides a clear comparison. A more completely specified model can be used to make comparisons more explicit. For example, Hu et al. (1997) used a multivariate nutrient density model to study the effects of specific types of fat in relation to risk of coronary heart disease. The model included saturated fat, monounsaturated fat, polyunsaturated fat, *trans* fat, and protein (all expressed as percent of energy) as well as alcohol, total energy intake, and other established risk factors for coronary disease. Because carbohydrate was the only macronutrient not included in the model, the coefficient for a specific type of fat or protein estimated the effect of substituting a specified percentage of energy from that nutrient for the same percentage of energy from carbohydrate. Although the choice of the comparison macronutrient left unspecified is somewhat arbitrary, the comparison to carbohydrate is typical in metabolic studies because it is the largest source of energy in most diets. The same, more completely specified, model can also be used to estimate the effect of substituting one type of fat for another. As done by Hu et al. (1997) for example, the effect of substituting polyunsaturated fat for the same percentage of energy from saturated fat can be estimated as the difference between their coefficients. The confidence interval for this estimated effect can be calculated from the pooled variance derived from the variance-covariance matrix for the model.

Categorization of Nutritional Variables
In the preceding discussion of energy adjustment, nutrients have been considered as continuous variables. However, in many analyses nutrients are grouped by quartiles or other categories. Reasons for using categories include the capacity to compute relative risks for actual groups of subjects, the avoidance of imposing a dose–response relationship (such as linear) that does not actually exist, and the ability to avoid undue influences of outlier values. Alternative arguments exist for using continuous variables, including the maximization of statistical power; a thorough analysis will usually involve both approaches.

In conducting categorical nutrient analyses, it is important to recognize that the statistical interchangeability of the standard multivariate, energy partition, and residual models does not apply. This phenomena was demonstrated by Kushi and coworkers (1992) and was examined in detail by Brown and coworkers (1994). In the example provided by Kushi et al., it was noted that for quartiles of dietary fat the standard multivariate and energy partition models gave higher relative risks but wider confidence intervals than the residual method; the findings from the nutrient density method were similar to those from the residual method. This phenomenon arises for several reasons. The most basic difference is that the categories for the nutrient (say fat) in the standard multivariate model are based on the crude (marginal) distribution of fat intake, and the categories for residuals are made after removing variation

due to total energy intake. Thus, many individuals are no longer in the same category because someone can have a high crude fat intake but a low fat composition of their diet. Also, as shown earlier, the range in crude fat intake will be much wider than for energy-adjusted fat intake. Thus, the relative risk across quintiles from the standard multivariate categories will correspond to a greater difference in fat intake than for the residual quintiles; this will tend to create higher relative risks. However, because of the high collinearity between fat and total energy, the confidence intervals will be wider for the standard multivariate model. Brown and colleagues (1994) have shown that in the categorical analysis statistical power will be higher with the residual or nutrient density methods. For these reasons, categorical analyses based on the standard multivariate and energy partition models are probably best avoided.

Implications for Food-Frequency Questionnaire Data

The preceding discussion assumes that accurate, quantitative data are available for analysis. Because of the need for rapid, inexpensive methods to assess long-term intake in large numbers of subjects, many epidemiologists use simple or semiquantitative food-frequency questionnaires that are less than perfectly accurate. The meaning of energy intake computed from such questionnaires may be less clear than that from more quantitative methods. To the extent that subjects with higher caloric intakes simply consume larger portion sizes rather than more food items, nutrient intakes may be inherently adjusted for total caloric intake. This adjustment, however, is likely to be only partial at most because many food items (e.g., eggs, bread, and apples) come in predetermined units. With any method of assessing energy intake, subjects may either overestimate or underestimate their overall intake. As suggested by the greater standard deviation for total energy intake estimated from food-frequency questionnaires than from diet records (see Chapter 6), it is likely that these tendencies are greater with food-frequency questionnaires.

Although energy intake data from food-frequency questionnaires may be imperfect and thus not fully represent the effects of body size, activity, metabolism, and energy balance, it would still be appropriate to use this measure for the computation of energy-adjusted intakes as described previously. To the extent that this adjustment also reduces extraneous between-person variation due to general overreporting or underreporting of food intake, a further gain in accuracy may be obtained in some instances (see Chapter 6). However, improvement in validity by energy adjustment should be regarded as a secondary benefit rather than the primary justification for energy adjustment.

Energy intake measured by dietary records or 24-hour recall has repeatedly been found to be 10 to 30% lower in comparisons with total energy expenditure measured by doubly-labeled water, energy intake needed to maintain weight, or minimal estimates needed for survival (calculated from basal metabolic rates adjusted for age, gender, height, and weight) (Black et al., 1993; de Vries et al., 1994; Klesges et al., 1995). In general, underreporting has been greater among women and obese persons. Although some have used evidence of underreporting of energy intake to cast doubt on any measurements of dietary intake, total energy intake is rarely of direct interest in epidemiologic studies for reasons described above. Indeed, a major objective in analysis is typically to remove variation in nutrient intake due to energy intake. Moreover, systematic biases do not hinder the capacity to find important associations in epidemiologic studies. Whether underestimation of total energy intake is associated with dietary composition is of some importance to epidemiologists. In an Australian dietary survey, 29% of subjects had implausibly low energy intakes (Smith et al., 1994). However, mean nutrient intakes

expressed as nutrient densities did not change appreciably when underreporters were excluded, indicating that underreporting was not associated with dietary composition. Also, Nelson and Bingham (1997) found no relation between energy-adjusted intakes of fat, protein, and carbohydrate and underreporting of total energy intake assessed with doubly-labeled water. Similarly, Lissner and Lindroos (1994) and Martin and colleagues (1996) found substantial underreporting of total energy intake assessed by 24-hour recall among obese women, but there was no evidence of underreporting of macronutrients expressed as a percentage of energy. Thus, while underreporting of total energy intake is an important issue in some circumstances, it is not a major issue in epidemiologic analyses because dietary composition is the primary focus; moreover, the major correlates of underreporting such as age, gender, and body fat are accounted for in typical analyses.

Although adjustment for total energy intake based on a food-frequency questionnaire should reduce confounding by energy intake, because both the nutrient and the energy intake are imperfectly measured control of confounding may not be complete (Greenland, 1980). Data from a validation study can be extremely useful to evaluate the degree to which confounding has been controlled. For example, within the Nurses' Health Study a reasonably strong association was observed between risk of a certain disease and intake of both energy and total fat. The association with energy-adjusted fat was slightly less strong, but still potentially important. We were concerned, however, that the effect of energy-adjusted fat might be due to residual confounding by total energy intake, which was measured imperfectly by the questionnaire. Therefore, we examined the correlation between energy-adjusted fat intake measured by questionnaire and total energy intake measured by diet record in a validation study (presumably a very good measure of intake). The minimal correlation observed ($r = 0.01$) indicated that the association observed for energy-adjusted fat intake was not materially confounded by total energy intake. The control of confounding obtained, however, by energy adjustment was not complete for all nutrients, further indicating the usefulness of the validation study data as the degree and direction of confounding due to imperfectly measured total energy intake would have been difficult to predict.

SUMMARY

Associations between intakes of specific nutrients and disease cannot be considered primary effects of diet if they are simply the result of differences in total energy intake between cases and noncases resulting from differences in body size, physical activity, and metabolic efficiency. Epidemiologic studies of diet and disease should therefore be principally directed at the effects of the nutrient composition of the diet independent of total energy intake. This can be accomplished by the use of the nutrient density if total energy intake is also included as a covariate or by other methods that adjust nutrient intake for energy intake using regression analysis.

Although pitfalls in the manipulation and interpretation of energy intake data in epidemiologic studies have been emphasized, these considerations also highlight the importance of obtaining a measurement of total energy intake. For instance, if a questionnaire obtained information on only saturated fat intake in a study of coronary heart disease, it is possible that an inverse or no association would be found even if high saturated fat composition of the diet truly caused coronary disease, as the energy intake of cases is likely to be less than that of noncases. Such a finding could be appropriately interpreted if an estimate of total energy intake were available.

The relationships between dietary factors and disease are complex. Even with carefully collected measures of intake, consideration of the biologic implications of various analytic approaches is needed to avoid misleading conclusions.

REFERENCES

Abraham, S., and M. D. Carroll (1979). Food consumption patterns in the United States and their potential impact on the decline in coronary heart disease mortality. In Havlik, R. J., and Feinlieb, M. (eds.): *Proceedings of the Conference on the Decline in Coronary Heart Disease Mortality* (DHEW publication No. 79-1610). Washington, DC: National Institutes of Health, pp 253–281.

Anonymous (1985). Consensus Conference. Lowering blood cholesterol to prevent heart disease. *JAMA 253*, 2080–2086.

Ascherio, A., M. J. Stampfer, G. A. Colditz, E. B. Rimm, L. Litin, and W. C. Willett (1992). Correlations of vitamin A and E intakes with the plasma concentrations of carotenoids and tocopherols among American men and women. *J Nutr 122*, 1792–1801.

Beaton, G. H., J. Milner, P. Corey, V. McGuire, M. Cousins, E. Stewart, M. de Ramos, D. Hewitt, P. V. Grambsch, N. Kassim, and J. A. Little (1979). Sources of variance in 24-hour dietary recall data: Implications for nutrition study design and interpretation. *Am J Clin Nutr 32*, 2546–2549.

Black, A. E., A. M. Prentice, G. R. Goldberg, S. A. Jebb, S. A. Bingham, M. B. E. Livingstone, and W. A. Coward (1993). Measurements of total energy expenditure provide insights into the validity of dietary measurement of energy intake. *J Am Diet Assoc 93*, 572–579.

Bostick, R. M., J. D. Potter, L. H. Kushi, T. A. Sellers, K. A. Steinmetz, D. R. McKenzie, S. M. Gapstur, and A. R. Folsom (1994). Sugar, meat, and fat intake, and nondietary risk factors for colon cancer incidence in Iowa women (United States). *Cancer Causes Control 5*, 38–52.

Brown, C. C., V. Kiphis, L. S. Freedman, A. M. Harman, A. Schatzkin, and S. Wacholder (1994). Energy adjustment methods for nutritional epidemiology: The effect of categorization. *Am J Epidemiol 139*, 323–338.

de Vries, J. H., P. L. Zock, R. P. Mensink, and M. B. Katan (1994). Underestimation of energy intake by 3-d records compared with energy intake to maintain body weight in 269 nonobese adults. *Am J Clin Nutr 60*, 855–860.

Donato, K., and D. M. Hegsted (1985). Efficiency of utilization of various sources of energy for growth. *Proc Natl Acad Sci USA* 82, 4866–4870.

Gail, M. H., S. Wieand, and S. Pintadosi (1984). Biased estimates of treatment effect in randomized experiments with nonlinear regressions and omitted covariates. *Biometrika* 71, 431–444.

Garabrant, D. H., J. M. Peters, T. M. Mack, and L. Berstein (1984). Job activity and colon cancer risk. *Am J Epidemiol 119*, 1005–1014.

Garcia-Palmieri, M. R., P. Sorlie, J. Tillotson, R. Costas, Jr., E. Cordero, and M. Rodriguez (1980). Relationship of dietary intake to subsequent coronary heart disease incidence: The Puerto Rico Heart Health Program. *Am J Clin Nutr 33*, 1818–1827.

Giovannucci, E., E. B. Rimm, M. J. Stampfer, G. A. Colditz, A. Ascherio, and W. C. Willett (1994). Intake of fat, meat, and fiber in relation to risk of colon cancer in men. *Cancer Res 54*, 2390–2397.

Giovannucci, E., A. Ascherio, E. B. Rimm, G. A. Colditz, M. J. Stampfer, and W. C. Willett (1995). Physical activity, obesity, and risk for colon cancer and adenoma in men. *Ann Intern Med 122*, 327–334.

Goldbohm, R. A., P. A. van den Brandt, P. van't Veer, H. A. M. Brants, E. Dorant, F. Sturmans, and R. J. J. Hermus (1994). A prospective cohort study on the relation between meat consumption and the risk of colon cancer. *Cancer Res 54*, 718–723.

Gordon, T., M. Fisher, and B. M. Rifkind (1984). Some difficulties inherent in the interpretation of dietary data from free-living populations. *Am J Clin Nutr 39*, 152–156.

Gordon, T., A. Kagan, M. Garcia-Palmieri, W. B. Kannel, W. J. Zukel, J. Tillotson, P. Sorlie, and M. Hjortland (1981). Diet and its relation to coronary heart disease and death in three populations. *Circulation 63*, 500–515.

Greenland, S. (1980). The effect of misclassification in the presence of covariates. *Am J Epidemiol 112*, 564–569.

Hegsted, D. M. (1985). Dietary standards: Dietary planning and nutrition education. *Clin Nutr 4*, 159–163.

Himms-Hagen, J. (1984). Thermogenesis in brown adipose tissue as an energy buffer: Implications for obesity. *N Engl J Med 311*, 1549–1558.

Hofstetter, A., Y. Schutz, E. Jequier, and J. Wahren (1986). Increased 24-hour energy expenditure in cigarette smokers. *N Engl J Med 314*, 79–82.

Horton, E. S. (1983). Introduction: An overview of the assessment and regulation of energy balance in humans. *Am J Clin Nutr 38*, 972–7.

Howe, G. R. (1989). Re: "Total energy intake: Implications for epidemiologic analyses" (letter). *Am J Epidemiol 129*, 1314–1315.

Howe, G. R., A. B. Miller, and M. Jain (1986). Re: "Total energy intake: Implications for epidemiologic analyses" (letter). *Am J Epidemiol 124*, 157–159.

Howe, G. R., K. J. Aronson, E. Benito, R. Castelleto, J. Cornee, S. Duffy, R. P. Gallagher, J. M. Iscovich, J. Dengao, R. Kaaks, G. A. Kune, S. Kune, H. P. Lee, M. Lee, A. B. Miller, R. K. Peters, J. D. Potter, E. Riboli, M. L. Slattery, D. Trichopoulos, A. Tuyns, A. Tzonou, L. E. Watson, A. S. Whittemore, A. H. Wu Williams, et al. (1997). The relationship between dietary fat intake and risk of colorectal cancer-evidence from the combined analysis of 13 case-control studies. *Cancer Causes Control 8*, 215–228.

Hu, F. B., M. J. Stampfer, J. E. Manson, E. Rimm, G. A. Colditz, B. A. Rosner, C. H. Hennekens, and Walter C. Willett. (1997) Dietary fat intake and the risk of coronary heart disease in Women. *N Engl J Med, 337*, 1491–1499.

Hunter, D. J., E. B. Rimm, F. M. Sacks, M. J. Stampfer, G. A. Colditz, L. B. Litin, and W. C. Willett (1992). Comparison of measures of fatty acid intake by subcutaneous fat aspirate, food frequency questionnaire, and diet records in a free-living population of US men. *Am J Epidemiol 135*, 418–427.

Jain, M., G. M. Cook, F. G. Davis, M. G. Grace, G. R. Howe, and A. B. Miller (1980). A case–control study of diet and colorectal cancer. *Int J Cancer 26*, 757–768.

Jequier, E., and Y. Schutz (1983). Long-term measurements of energy expenditure in humans using a respiration chamber. *Am J Clin Nutr 38*, 989–998.

Johnson, M. L., B. S. Burke, and J. Mayer (1956). Relative importance of inactivity and overeating in the energy balance of obese high school girls. *Am J Clin Nutr 4*, 37–44.

Kipnis, V., L. S. Freedman, C. C. Brown, A. M. Hartman, A. Schatzkin, and S. Wacholder (1993). Interpretation of energy adjustment models for nutritional epidemiology. *Am J Epidemiol 137*, 1376–1380.

Klesges, R. C., L. H. Eck, and J. W. Ray (1995). Who underreports dietary intake in a dietary recall? Evidence from the Second National Health and Nutrition Examination Survey. *J Consulting Clin Psych 63*, 438–444.

Kromhout, D., and C. de Lezenne Coulander (1984). Diet, prevalence and 10-year mortality from coronary heart disease in 871 middle-aged men: The Zutphen Study. *Am J Epidemiol 119*, 733–741.

Kushi, L. H., R. A. Lew, F. J. Stare, C. R. Ellison, M. el Lozy, G. Bourke, L. Daly, I. Graham, N. Hickey, R. Mulcahy, and J. Kevancy (1985). Diet and 20-year mortality from coronary heart disease: The Ireland-Boston Diet-Heart study. *N Engl J Med 312*, 811–818.

Kushi, L. H., T. A. Sellers, J. D. Potter, C. L. Nelson, R. G. Munger, S. A. Kaye, and A. R. Folsom (1992). Dietary fat and postmenopausal breast cancer. *JNCI 84*, 1092–1099.

Leibel, R. L., M. Rosenbaum, and J. Hirsch (1995). Changes in energy expenditure resulting from altered body weight. *N Engl J Med 332*, 621–628.

Lissner, L., and A. K. Lindroos (1994). Is dietary underreporting macronutrient-specific? *Eur J Clin Nutr 48*, 453–454.

London, S. J., F. M. Sacks, J. Caesar, M. J. Stampfer, E. Siguel, and W. C. Willett (1991). Fatty acid composition of subcutaneous adipose tissue and diet in postmenopausal US women. *Am J Clin Nutr 54*, 340–345.

Lyon, J. L., J. W. Gardner, D. W. West, and A. M. Mahoney (1983). Methodological issues in epidemiological studies of diet and cancer. *Cancer Res 43(suppl)*, 2392–2396.

Martin, L. J., W. Su, P. J. Jones, G. A. Lockwood, D. L. Tritchler, and N. F. Boyd (1996). Comparison of energy intakes determined by food records and doubly labeled water in women participating in a dietary-intervention trial. *Am J Clin Nutr 63*, 483–490.

McGee, D., D. Reed, and K. Yano (1984a). The results of logistic analyses when the variables are highly correlated: An empirical example using diet and CHD incidence. *J Chronic Dis 37*, 713–719.

McGee, D. L., D. M. Reed, K. Yano, A. Kagan, and J. Tillotson (1984b). Ten-year incidence of coronary heart disease in the Honolulu Heart Program: Relationship to nutrient intake. *Am J Epidemiol 119*, 667–676.

Mellits, E. D., and D. B. Cheek (1970). The assessment of body water and fatness from infancy to adulthood. *Monogr Soc Res Child Dev 35*, 12–26.

Miller, D. S. (1973). Overfeeding in man. In Bray, G. A. (ed.): *Obesity in Perspective DHEW Publication No. 75–708*. Washington, DC: National Institutes of Health.

Morris, J. N., J. W. Marr, and D. G. Clayton (1977). Diet and heart: A postscript. *BMJ 2*, 1307–1314.

National Center for Health Statistics (1979). *Weight and Height of Adults 18–74 Years of Age: United States, 1971–74*. Hyattsville, MD: National Center for Health Statistics.

Nelson, M. and S. Bingham (1997). Food consumption and nutrient intake. In: Margetts, B. and Nelson, M. (eds.) *Design Concepts in Nutritional Epidemiology*, 2nd. ed., New York: Oxford University Press, pp. 123–170.

Paffenbarger, R. S., Jr., A. L. Wing, and R. T. Hyde (1978). Physical activity as an index of heart attack risk in college alumni. *Am J Epidemiol 108*, 161–175.

Pike, M. C., L. Bernstein, and R. K. Peters (1989). Re: "Total energy intake: implications for epidemiologic analyses" (letter). *Am J Epidemiol 129*, 1312–1315.

Prentice, A. M., A. E. Black, W. A. Coward, H. L. Davies, G. R. Goldberg, P. R. Murgatroyd, J. Ashford, M. Sawyer, and R. G. Whitehead (1986). High levels of energy expenditure in obese women. *Br Med J Clin Res 292*, 983–987.

Ravussin, E., S. Lillioja, T. E. Anderson, L. Christin, and C. Bogardus (1986). Determinants of 24-hour energy expenditure in man: Methods and results using a respiratory chamber. *J Clin Invest 78*, 1568–1578.

Rimm, E. B., A. Ascherio, E. Giovannucci, D. Spiegelman, M. J. Stampfer, and W. C. Willett (1996). Vegetable, fruit, and cereal fiber intake and risk of coronary heart disease among men. *JAMA 275*, 447–451.

Roberts, S. B., P. Fuss, W. J. Evans, M. B. Heyman, and V. R. Young (1993). Energy expenditure, aging, and body composition. *J Nutr 123*, 474–480.

Romieu, I., W. C. Willett, M. J. Stampfer, G. A. Colditz, L. Sampson, B. Rosner, C. H. Hennekens, and F. E. Speizer (1988). Energy intake and other determinants of relative weight. *Am J Clin Nutr 47*, 406–412.

Saltzman, E., and S. B. Roberts (1995). The role of energy expenditure in energy regulation: Findings from a decade of research. *Nutr Rev 53*, 209–220.

Shekelle, R. B., M. Z. Nichaman, and W. J. Raynor Jr. (1987). Re: Total energy intake: Implication for epidemiologic analyses (letter). *Am J Epidemiol 126*, 980–983.

Shekelle, R. B., O. Paul, and J. Stamler (1985). Diet and coronary heart disease (letter). *N Engl J Med 313*, 120.

Sims, E. A., E. Danforth, Jr., E. S. Horton, G. A. Bray, J. A. Glennon, and L. B. Salans

(1973). Endocrine and metabolic effects of experimental obesity in man. *Recent Prog Horm Res 29*, 457–496.

Sjostrom, L. (1985). *A Review of Weight Maintenance and Weight Changes in Relation to Energy Metabolism and Body Composition. Recent Advances in Obesity Research. Proceedings of the 4th International Congress on Obesity*. Wesport, CT: Food and Nutrition Press.

Smith, W. T., K. L. Webb, and P. F. Heywood (1994). The implications of underreporting in dietary studies. *Austral J Public Health 18*, 311–314.

Sonnenschein, E., L. Glickman, M. Goldschmidt, and L. McKee (1991). Body conformation, diet, and risk of breast cancer in pet dogs: A case–control study. *Am J Epidemiol 133*, 694–703.

Sopko, G., D. R. Jacobs, Jr., and H. L. Taylor (1984). Dietary measures of physical activity. *Am J Epidemiol 120*, 900–911.

Thomson, A. M., and W. Z. Billewicz (1961). Height, weight and food intake in man. *Br J Nutr 15*, 241–52.

Van Itallie, T. B. (1978). Dietary fiber and obesity. *Am J Clin Nutr 31(suppl)*, 43S–52S.

Vena, J. E., S. Graham, M. Zielezny, M. K. Swanson, R. E. Barnes, and J. Nolan (1985). Lifetime occupational exercise and colon cancer. *Am J Epidemiol 122*, 357–365.

Webb, P. (1985). The exchange of matter and energy in lean and overweight men and women: A calorimetric study of overeating, balanced intake and undereating. *Int J Obesity 9(suppl 2)*, 139–145.

Willett, W. C. (1987). Implications of total energy intake for epidemiologic studies of breast and large-bowel cancer. *Am J Clin Nutr 45(suppl)*, 354S–360S.

Willett, W. C. (1990). Total energy intake and nutrient composition: Dietary recommendations for epidemiologists. *Int J Cancer 46*, 770–771.

Willett W. C., Howe G. R., Kushi L. H. (1997) Adjustment for total energy intake in epidemiologic studies. *Am J Clin Nutr, 65(4 suppl s)*: 1220s–1228s.

Willett, W. C., L. Sampson, M. J. Stampfer, B. Rosner, C. Bain, J. Witschi, C. H. Hennekens, and F. E. Speizer (1985). Reproducibility and validity of a semiquantitative food frequency questionnaire. *Am J Epidemiol 122*, 51–65.

Willett, W. C., and M. J. Stampfer (1986). Total energy intake: Implications for epidemiologic analyses. *Am J Epidemiol 124*, 17–27.

Willett, W. C., M. J. Stampfer, G. A. Colditz, B. A. Rosner, and F. E. Speizer (1990). Relation of meat, fat, and fiber intake to the risk of colon cancer in a prospective study among women. *N Engl J Med 323*, 1664–1672.

Willett, W. C., M. J. Stampfer, B. A. Underwood, F. E. Speizer, B. Rosner, and C. H. Hennekens (1983). Validation of a dietary questionnaire with plasma carotenoid and alpha-tocopherol levels. *Am J Clin Nutr 38*, 631–639.

Woo, R., R. Daniels-Kugh, and E. S. Horton (1985). Regulation of energy balance. *Annu Rev Nutr 5*, 411–433.

12

Correction for the Effects of Measurement Error

All biologic and physical measurements in any branch of science have error; to a large extent, increments in knowledge depend on reducing this inexactness. It is therefore critical to improve continually the technical aspects of exposure measurement, whether based on questionnaires, biochemical assays, or anthropometry. At some level, however, it is difficult or impractical to reduce measurement error further. It is then important to measure the magnitude of the error and evaluate its effect on relationships under investigation. If the effect of measurement error is appreciable, then it may be appropriate to consider a statistical correction to better approximate the relationship that would have been observed if no measurement error had been present.

The correction of estimated associations for measurement error was rarely employed in the epidemiologic literature, but is now becoming a frequently used procedure. Because the methods for correction depend on the form of error, different types of errors and their impact on epidemiologic measures

of associations are discussed before considering alternatives for statistical correction. Additional reviews of the statistical effects of measurement error and methods to compensate for distortion have been published (Snedecor, 1968; Espeland and Hui, 1987; Byar and Gail, 1989; Chen, 1989).

TYPES OF ERRORS

The specific sources of error are innumerable; however, they can be thought of as two general types: random and systematic. For random error, the average value of many repeated measures approaches the true value, that is, the law of large numbers applies. For systematic errors, the mean of repeated measurements does not approach the true value. In epidemiologic studies, random or systematic errors, or both, can occur at two different levels: within a person and between persons. Thus at least four types of error can exist; these are depicted in Figure 12–1.

Random within-person error is typified

302

TYPE OF ERROR

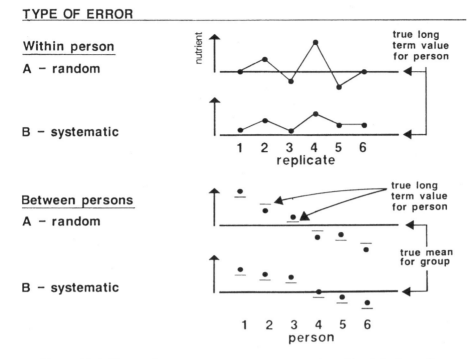

Figure 12–1. Types of exposure measurement errors in epidemiologic studies.

by the day-to-day fluctuation in dietary intake, discussed in Chapter 3. This apparently random variation is due both to the changes in food intake from day-to-day and to errors in the measurement of intake on any one day. Although it may be argued that true variation over time is not really error, it may be considered so if the long-term average intake for an individual is conceptually the true intake for that subject. The distinction between random measurement error and true random day-to-day change in diet is thus usually not important when considering their effects on epidemiologic associations.

In addition to random error, repeated measurements of diet within a subject may also be subject to systematic error. This can occur for many reasons; in open-ended methods, such as 24-hour recalls, persons may consciously or unconsciously tend either to deny or to exaggerate their food intake. Systematic within-person error is particularly likely to occur when standardized questionnaires are used: an important food

item for a subject (but not necessarily for all subjects) may have been omitted from a questionnaire or misinterpreted by a subject. If such a questionnaire is repeated, the same error is likely to recur; thus the mean of many replicate measurements for an individual will not necessarily approach that person's true mean.

Most literature addressing the issue of measurement error in nutritional epidemiology (and other fields) is based on the assumption that within-person error is strictly random. This is probably due to two principal reasons: (1) much of statistical theory is based on the assumption of random error and (2) systematic error is considerably more difficult to measure. Random within-person error can be measured simply with a single replicate measure for a sample of subjects, that is, a reproducibility study. The measurement of systematic error requires a second, superior measure of exposure, that is, a validation or calibration study. Unfortunately, no perfect measure of true long-term dietary intake exists, and the best measurements (e.g., diet recording or direct observation for many days) are laborious and expensive. Lack of a perfect gold standard is not unique to nutritional epidemiology. For example, it is generally assumed that within-person error in blood pressure measurement is purely random. It is likely, however, that systematic within-person error also occurs, as would happen if some individuals usually develop anxiety when their blood pressure is measured or have anatomic abnormalities in their arm that consistently causes an erroneous reading. A more direct measure of true long-term blood pressure would be continuous monitoring with an intraarterial catheter; however, this is obviously not practical in an epidemiologic setting.

When measuring dietary factors or other exposures among a group of persons, errors can also be either random or systematic. Random between-person error can be either the result of using only one or a few replicate measurements per subject in the presence of random within-person error or the consequence of systematic within-person errors that are randomly distributed among subjects. Random between-person error implies that an overestimation for some individuals is counterbalanced by an underestimation for others so that the mean for a large group of subjects is the true mean for the group. The standard deviation for the group is, however, exaggerated.

Systematic between-person error results from systematic within-person error that affects subjects nonrandomly. The mean value for a group of persons is thus incorrect. If the systematic error applies equally to all subjects and is simply additive, the observed standard deviation for the group is correct. If individuals, however, are affected to various degrees or the error is multiplicative (e.g., proportional to an individual's true level), the observed standard deviation will also not represent the true standard deviation. Systematic between-person errors are likely to be frequent and can have many causes: The omission of a commonly eaten food from a standardized questionnaire or the use of an incorrect nutrient composition value for a common food will affect all individuals in the same direction, but not to the same degree because the use of these foods will differ among subjects. As in these examples, it is probably uncommon that systematic within-person error affects all individuals equally. More commonly, random and systematic between-person errors are likely to exist in combination.

Because the ultimate focus of epidemiology is on associations with disease, the impact of exposure measurement error on measures of association, such as relative risk, is of greatest importance. As illustrated in Chapter 3, random within-person error tends to decrease correlation and regression coefficients toward 0 and bias relative risks toward 1. This effect applies to random between-person errors in general, even if it is the consequence of systematic within-person error that is unequally distributed among subjects. Systematic errors that affect all persons equally, however, do not affect measures of association.

In the later discussion we assume that all errors apply equally to cases and noncases in an epidemiologic study, that is, that errors are random in relation to disease. Systematic differences in measurement error between these two groups, that is, measurement errors that are biased with respect to disease, have serious consequences that are usually not amenable to correction. This topic is discussed in Chapter 1.

CORRECTION OF STANDARD DEVIATIONS

In dietary surveys, such as those used for monitoring national dietary intake, a major focus is typically the percentage of the population above or below a certain cut-point, such as the minimum intake to avoid deficiency. Because the standard deviation of a distribution is exaggerated in the presence of random within-person variation, the percentage of subjects below or above a specified cut-point will be seriously distorted (see Fig. 12–2 for an example).

Considerable attention has been given to methods for correcting the observed distributions of dietary intakes based on single 24-hour recalls for the effects of random within-person variation. A primary objective is to identify the true proportion of the population below a specified intake (i.e., proportion that may be deficient). All of these methods require that replicate measurements be made on all or a sample of the population. Analysis of variance can then be conducted as described in Chapter 3 to obtain the between-person variance ($S_b{}^2$). The square root of this variance (S_b) describes the true standard deviation for the population that would have been obtained with a large number of 24-hour measurements for each person. Because the mean is not affected by within-person variation, the corrected distribution can then be created (see Fig. 12–2), and the proportion of the population below the cut-point can be estimated using a table of standard deviates. Such calculations require a normally distributed variable or at least normality after appropriate transformation. Although based on the same principle, more complex methods have been developed that take into account departures from normality of distributions of dietary intakes (Nusser, 1996). Although the corrected distributions are useful on a population basis, they cannot be used to identify which *individuals* are below the cut-point.

Example: The example in Figure 12–2 can be considered in reverse. Based on 1 day of intake, the observed standard deviation was 35 units/day and the percentage of the population with intakes below 50 units/day was found to be 7.9%. In a sample of subjects, another day of dietary information was obtained and analysis of variance was used to separate the between-person and within-person variances (see Chapter 3). Both components of variance were 625 (thus, $s_w^2/s_b^2 = 1$). *Therefore, the true between-person standard deviation is*

$$\sqrt{625} = \text{units/day}$$

and, from a table of normal deviation, the true proportion of the population with intakes below 50/units/day (2.0 normal deviates = 50/25) is 2.3

CORRECTION OF EPIDEMIOLOGIC MEASURES OF ASSOCIATION FOR MEASUREMENT ERROR

Several methods are presented here for correcting correlation and regression coefficients and relative risks. Derivations of these formulas and those to compute confidence limits are beyond the scope of this book; the reader needs to refer to the original sources. In using these methods, careful attention must be given to assumptions regarding the type of error (whether it is random or systematic) and the distribution of exposure variables, as normality is often assumed.

Much of the literature related to error correction is based on the model

$$z = x + \varepsilon \qquad (12\text{–}1)$$

where x is the true measure of exposure, z is the surrogate measure that contains error, and ε is random measurement error (Kupper, 1984). This model thus assumes that error is simply added to (or subtracted from) the true measurement so that the standard deviation and variance of z are greater than that of x. In this model an assessment of the measurement error can be made by comparing these variances. The ratio of variances, the "reliability coefficient," can be calculated as

$$r^2{}_{zx} = s_x^2/s_z^2 \qquad (12\text{–}2)$$

The square root of the reliability coefficient (r_{zx}) is the correlation between the true and the surrogate measures.

Unfortunately, there is little reason to believe that the basic model for this approach to error correction is generally true. In the case of a dietary questionnaire, a very restricted list of foods that are commonly eaten by most people could produce a dis-

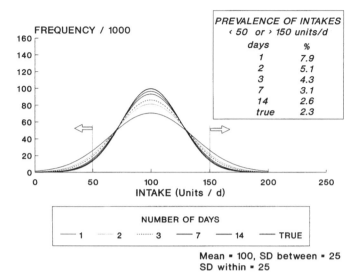

Mean = 100, SD between = 25
SD within = 25

Figure 12–2. Simulation of impact of random error on observed intake distributions. The assumptions are that both between- and within-person variations have a coefficient of variation of 25% (i.e., $s_w^2/s_b^2 = 1$) and that both are normally distributed. Also shown is the impact that days of data collected would have on the proportions of individuals with low (< 50 units) or high (> 150 units) intakes. (From Beaton, 1994; reproduced with permission.)

tribution of nutrient values with a standard deviation that was small, perhaps even smaller than the true distribution. Equation 12–2 would imply that this restricted questionnaire had little or no error, when in fact it could be providing no useful information. On the other hand, it is possible that a very complete and highly discriminating questionnaire could overestimate intake of those with truly high intake and underestimate intake of those with truly low intake. (This could happen, for example, with a food-frequency questionnaire that has multiple-choice responses if inappropriately high weights were assigned to the highest category and inappropriately low weights were assigned to the low category when computing nutrient intakes.) Equation 12–2 would suggest that this questionnaire had a high degree of error, even when discrimination among subjects was excellent. This model of measurement error is appropriate in some situations where the source of error is strictly random within persons and additive; however, it is unlikely to apply to many epidemiologic measures, in particular the assessment of diet by questionnaires. An alternative model relating true and surrogate measures using regression analysis that requires fewer assumptions is discussed later.

Correction of Correlation Coefficients

As discussed in Chapter 3, random within-person error in the measurement of one or both variables being compared tends to reduce correlation coefficients toward zero. This issue and approaches for correcting the correlation coefficients based on a partitioning of variance components have been discussed by Liu and colleagues (1978) and Beaton and colleagues (1979). When both variables, x and y, are subject to random within-person variation the relationship between the true correlation (r_t) and the observed correlation (r_o) can be written

$$r_t = r_o\sqrt{(1 + \lambda_x/n_x)(1 + \lambda_y/n_y)} \quad (12\text{–}3)$$

where:

$\lambda_x = s_w^2/s_b^2$ for x, that is, the ratio of the within- and between-person variances for x

$\lambda_y = s_w^2/s_b^2$ for y
n_x = the number of replicates per person for the x variable
n_y = the number of replicates per person for the y variable

If only one variable is considered to have within-person variance, this equation reduces to

$$r_t = r_o \sqrt{1 + \lambda_x/n_x} \qquad (12\text{--}4)$$

The within-person and between-person variances are obtained from an analysis of variance model as described in Chapter 3. Alternatively, λ_x and λ_y can be obtained from their respective intraclass correlations (r_I, the correlation describing the reproducibility of x or y, which can be thought of as the average correlation between pairs of replicate measurements):

$$\lambda = (1 - r_I)/r_I \qquad (12\text{--}5)$$

It should be noted that this method for error correction assumes that variation in x and y are independent (e.g., that they fluctuate randomly with respect to each other from day to day). This assumption does not appear to be seriously violated in most instances, but deserves consideration in any particular application. An additional term is required if variations in x and y are not independent (Beaton et al., 1979).

Example: In a study of dietary questionnaire validity (Willett et al., 1985), we examined the correlation between a self-administered food-frequency questionnaire and multiple diet records, assuming that the diet records represented true intake. Realizing that the within-person variation in diet is substantial, we collected 28 days per subject sampled over a 1-year period, with the assumption that the average of these days would reasonably represent an individual's true long-term intake. For cholesterol intake, the observed correlation between the questionnaire and the diet record intake was 0.51. We then sampled only 4 of the 28 days of diet records for each subject; the correlation between the questionnaire estimate of cholesterol intake and the

mean of these 4 days per subject was only 0.29. Based on these 4 days of dietary cholesterol intake per subject, an analysis of variance indicated that the within-person variance (s_w^2) was 3.43 and the between-person variance (s_b^2) was 0.50.

From Equation 12–4, the true correlation between a single questionnaire administration and true long-term cholesterol intake can be estimated as.

$$r_t = 0.29 \sqrt{1 + (3.43/0.50)/4} = 0.48$$

Thus, correcting the observed correlation for the attenuating effect of random within-person error provides a value similar to that obtained with a large number of replicates. The loss of information from using 4 rather than 28 days of dietary data is reflected in a wider confidence interval for the corrected coefficient. In this example, the 95% confidence interval for the original correlation of 0.51 was 0.39 to 0.61; for the corrected correlation of 0.48 this interval was 0.20 to 0.68. The calculation of confidence intervals for corrected correlation coefficients is more complex, as they reflect both error in the estimate of the observed correlation (which is a function of the number of subjects) and error in the estimation of the within-person and between-person variances (which is a reflection of the variability and number of replicates). A formula for this calculation is provided elsewhere (Rosner and Willett, 1988). From the example, it can be seen that the use of corrected correlation coefficients can provide a reasonable estimate of the true correlation with only a few replicate measures per subject (a minimum of two measurements for at least a subsample of subjects is necessary for an analysis of variance).

In making these corrections, it is important to consider carefully the true relationship that is of interest. In this example, the dietary questionnaire was administered twice so that we could have further corrected the observed correlation for within-person variation in the questionnaire using Equation 12–3. This, however, would have provided an estimate of the correlation between an infinite (or large) number of days of dietary record intake per subject with an infinite (or large) number of questionnaire administrations per subject. This is obviously not useful information as we generally have only one, or at most a few, questionnaire administrations per subject.

In designing a study to measure the correlation between two variables where one or both are subject to random within-person variation, the investigator must decide whether to enroll many subjects and collect few replicates per person or to enroll few subjects and collect many replicates for each person. An objective in designing such a study is to obtain the most precise estimate of the true correlation, that is, to minimize its standard error or confidence interval. The standard error of the corrected correlation (Rosner and Willett, 1988) thus provides a criterion for optimizing the trade-off between number of subjects and number of replicates per subject given a fixed number of measurements. The optimal solution is not simple as it depends on both the true correlation and on the intraclass correlation for the variable with random error. Table 12–1 provides variances of corrected correlations, assuming a total of 1,000 measurements, for various values of the true correlation (r_t) and the intraclass correlation (r_I). It can be seen, except for extreme situations, that the minimum variance occurs with only two replicates per subject. Even when the minimum variance is provided by a larger number of replicates, two replicates provide a variance that is close to optimal. The intuitive reason for this finding is that as replicate measures are correlated to at least some degree, each additional replicate adds progressively less new information. Although these particular calculations were based on the allocation of 1,000 total measurements (i.e., the number of subjects times the number of replicates per subject), the optimal number of replicates per subject was not sensitive to the total number of measurements. Further calculations using replicate samples for only a subset of the population indicated that it was generally most efficient (in minimizing the

standard error of the corrected correlation coefficient) to have at least two samples for all subjects; the exception occurred when the intraclass correlation was very high, in which case it can be most efficient to have more than one sample for only a subset of subjects. The number of replicates should be greater than two with a very low intraclass correlation. In addition to statistical efficiency, practical considerations also influence the optimal allocation of measurements. Applications of this approach have important implications for the design of validation studies; these are discussed in Chapter 6.

Systematic within-person error, as would typically characterize standardized dietary questionnaires, also tends to attenuate correlation coefficients toward zero as this error may not affect all persons equally. The methods used to correct for random within-person error, however, are not applicable, and it is not apparent that this issue has been formally addressed. Systematic between-person errors in which all subjects are measured too high or too low by the same amount do not affect the correlation coefficient; thus no correction is needed.

Correction of Regression Coefficients

The correction of regression coefficients for random within-person error has been discussed by Beaton and colleagues (1979), Liu and colleagues (1978), Madansky (1959), and others (Tukey, 1951; Riggs et al., 1978). When random error affects only the dependent variable (y), the regression coefficient is not attenuated and no correction is needed (of course, the precision of the estimated regression coefficient is reduced by measurement error). When such error affects the independent variable (x), a simple correction can be made as described by Beaton and coworkers (1979):

$$b_t = b_o(1 + \lambda_x/n_x) \qquad (12\text{--}6)$$

where b_t is the true regression coefficient, b_o is the observed regression coefficient,

Table 12–1. Variances of corrected correlation coefficients (r_t) multiplied by a fixed total number of measurements over the entire sample (n = subjects × measurements/subject = 1,000 in this example)[a]

r_t	r_I	Number of replicate measures per subject (n_y)								
		2	3	4	5	6	7	8	9	10
0.1	0.1	11.4	12.1	13.1	14.0	15.0	15.9	16.9	17.9	18.8
0.1	0.3	4.3	5.3	6.3	7.2	8.2	9.2	10.2	11.2	12.1
0.1	0.5	3.0	3.9	4.9	5.9	6.9	7.9	8.8	9.8	10.8
0.1	0.7	2.4	3.4	4.3	5.3	6.3	7.3	8.3	9.2	10.2
0.1	0.9	2.1	3.1	4.0	5.0	6.0	7.0	8.0	8.9	9.9
0.3	0.1	14.3	13.3	13.5	14.0	14.7	15.4	16.1	16.9	17.7
0.3	0.3	4.2	4.9	5.7	6.5	7.3	8.2	9.0	9.8	10.6
0.3	0.5	2.7	3.5	4.3	5.1	6.0	6.8	7.6	8.5	9.3
0.3	0.7	2.1	2.9	3.7	4.6	5.4	6.2	7.1	7.9	8.7
0.3	0.9	1.8	2.6	3.4	4.3	5.1	5.9	6.7	7.6	8.4
0.5	0.1	20.2	15.6	14.5	14.2	14.2	14.4	14.7	15.1	15.5
0.5	0.3	4.1	4.3	4.7	5.2	5.7	6.3	6.8	7.4	7.9
0.5	0.5	2.2	2.7	3.2	3.8	4.3	4.9	5.5	6.0	6.6
0.5	0.7	1.6	2.1	2.7	3.2	3.8	4.3	4.9	5.5	6.0
0.5	0.9	1.2	1.8	2.4	2.9	3.5	4.0	4.6	5.2	5.7
0.7	0.1	29.0	19.2	16.0	14.5	13.7	13.2	12.9	12.8	12.7
0.7	0.3	3.9	3.5	3.5	3.6	3.8	4.0	4.2	4.4	4.6
0.7	0.5	1.6	1.7	1.9	2.2	2.4	2.7	2.9	3.2	3.4
0.7	0.7	0.9	1.1	1.4	1.6	1.9	2.2	2.4	2.7	2.9
0.7	0.9	0.6	0.9	1.1	1.4	1.6	1.9	2.2	2.4	2.7
0.9	0.1	40.9	24.1	18.3	15.3	13.5	12.2	11.2	10.5	9.9
0.9	0.3	3.9	2.7	2.2	2.0	1.9	1.8	1.8	1.7	1.7
0.9	0.5	1.0	0.8	0.8	0.7	0.7	0.7	0.8	0.8	0.8
0.9	0.7	0.3	0.3	0.3	0.4	0.4	0.4	0.5	0.5	0.5
0.9	0.9	0.1	0.2	0.2	0.2	0.3	0.3	0.3	0.4	0.4

[a] Variances (×1,000) are shown for a given number of replicates per subject (n_y), a given intraclass correlation (r_I), and the corrected correlation coefficient (r_t).

From Rosner and Willett, 1988.

and the other notation is the same as for Equation 12–4. Again, this assumes that distributions are reasonably normal and that the within-person variation is random. Due to the measurement error, the true confidence interval is wider than the observed interval; the method of Rosner et al. (1990) can be used to estimate an expanded confidence interval that takes measurement error into account.

Example: Several authors have used the relationship of dietary cholesterol intake and serum cholesterol level to illustrate the attenuating effects of random within-person variation on regression coefficients (Liu et al., 1978; Beaton et al., 1979).

Based on metabolic ward feeding studies, Mattson and coworkers (1972) observed that serum cholesterol level increased by 12 mg/dl for each increase of 100 mg of cholesterol intake per 1,000 kcal daily. Thus b_t in this example is 0.12. From Table 3–3, it can be seen that the value for the ratio of within-person to between-person variances (λ) for cholesterol intake (divided by calories) is approximately 5 to 13. Assuming a value of 5 and that only 1 day of observation is obtained, the observed regression coefficient would be

$$b_o = b_t/(1 + \lambda_x/n_x = 0.12/ \\ (1 + 5/1) = 0.02$$

Because the attenuation is large and many factors other than dietary cholesterol intake affect serum cholesterol levels (e.g., laboratory error, genetic factors, physical activity, other dietary factors), it is not surprising that most studies based on a single or a few days of intake have failed to observe any association. Moreover, the data of Mattson and coworkers (1972) demonstrate that serum cholesterol is only weakly influenced by diet within the range that they studied; because a typical cholesterol intake would be 150 mg/1,000 calories and a typical serum level would be 250 mg/dl, a doubling of intake (to 300 mg/1,000 calories) would result in less than an 8% rise in serum cholesterol (18 mg/dl). For this reason, serum cholesterol cannot be considered a useful indicator of cholesterol intake or a reasonable standard for assessing the validity of any method for measuring cholesterol intake.

Analogous to the correction of correlation coefficients, methods for correcting regression coefficients based on the ratio of within-person to between-person variances are not applicable when systematic within-person error is present. In this case, a separate validation study employing an independent, more accurate measure of true exposure is necessary. A two-step process can be used. First, the "true" measure (x) is regressed on the surrogate measure (z) to obtain a regression coefficient (γ).

$$x = \alpha' + \gamma z + \varepsilon \qquad (12\text{--}7)$$

This coefficient (γ) thus describes the true change in exposure that corresponds to a given observed change in the surrogate exposure. As a second step, this information is used to correct the observed regression coefficient (b_o) describing the relationship between the surrogate exposure (z) and the dependent variable ($y = \alpha + b_o z + \varepsilon$). This relationship between the true and observed values of the regression coefficient is simply

$$b_t = b_o/\gamma \qquad (12\text{--}8)$$

Example: Using the relationship between dietary cholesterol and serum cholesterol described previously, let us assume, in a hypothetical cross-sectional study, that the observed relationship between cholesterol intake (in mg/1,000 kcal daily) measured by a dietary questionnaire and serum cholesterol (mg/dl) was 0.06. In a separate validation study comparing the questionnaire with a "true" measure of dietary intake (such as a large number of days of diet recording per subject), a 100 mg/1,000 kcal daily change in cholesterol intake measured by the questionnaire corresponded to a 50 mg/1,000 kcal daily change according to the true method, that is, $\gamma = 0.5$. The corrected regression coefficient would thus be $b_t = 0.06/0.5 = 0.12$.

Correction of Relative Risks

Random and systematic within-person errors that are unrelated to disease status tend to bias relative risks toward the null value of 1 in univariate models without confounding (see Chapter 3). Several methods are available to correct these attenuated relative risk estimates; methods are discussed first for categorical and then for continuous variables.

Categorical Variables
This discussion of measurement error has thus far only considered continuous variables as most dietary exposures are of this form. When computing relative risks, exposures may still be considered as continuous variables; the rates for two points on the distribution of exposure can be compared using a statistical model, such as a logistic or proportional hazards model. Often the continuous exposure is broken into categories, such as quintiles or 100-g units, and relative risks are computed comparing these groups. Also, some variables, such as the frequency of using a specific food or the use of a vitamin supplement, are inherently categorical. The

following example illustrates attenuation of the relative risk calculated as an odds ratio from a 2 × 2 table.

Example: Let the true relation between exposure and disease defined by a 2 × 2 table be as follows:

	Exposed (E)	Unexposed (U)	Total (E + U)
Diseased (D)	a = 400	b = 600	1,000
Well (W)	c = 200	d = 800	1,000

The odds ratio (OR) = $(a \div b)/(c \div d)$ = $(400 \div 600)/(200 \div 800)$ = 2.67.

If the true relationship is studied with an imperfect measurement method, the performance of the surrogate method can be described in terms of ϕ = sensitivity (the proportion of truly exposed subjects who are identified as exposed by the epidemiologic method) and ψ = specificity (the proportion of subjects who are truly unexposed who are identified as unexposed by the method). For this example, assume that an exposure measurement method having a sensitivity of 0.6 and a specificity of 0.9 is used to study the true exposure–disease relationship described previously. Therefore, of the 400 diseased and truly exposed subjects, only 400 × 0.6 = 240 would, on average, be measured as such and 400 − 240 = 160 would be measured as unexposed. Of the 600 diseased and truly unexposed subjects, only 600 × 0.9 = 540 would be measured as unexposed and 600 − 540 = 60 would be called exposed. Thus 240 + 60 = 300 diseased subjects would be measured as exposed and 540 + 160 = 700 as unexposed. With similar calculations for the well subjects, the observed 2 × 2 table would thus be

Observed OR = (300 ÷ 700)/(200 ÷ 800) = 1.71. In this example the observed OR (1.71) is appreciably lower than the true OR (2.67) due to measurement error.

Bross (1954) and Diamond and Lilienfeld (1962) provided a simple method for correcting relative risks for exposure misclassification in a 2 × 2 table and Barron (1977) extended this method for a 2 × 2 table when errors exist in the measurement of either (or both) exposure and disease. This method makes no assumptions regarding the nature of the measurement error, but does require an external validation study based on a "true" measure of exposure to define the probabilities of misclassification. The results of this external validation can be expressed in terms of sensitivity (ϕ) and specificity (ψ), as described previously. Barron (1977) has described his method in terms of matrix algebra. In the following example it is assumed that no error exists in the diagnosis of disease (this is often reasonably true in many epidemiologic studies), and the method of correction is presented in simple algebraic form. The use of this method is discussed in more detail by Kleinbaum and colleagues (1982).

The true relationship between exposure and disease can be described for a 2 × 2 table as using the notation:

	Exposed	Unexposed
Diseased	a*	b*
Well	c*	d*

Correspondingly, the observed relationship using an imperfect exposure measurement method can be expressed as

	Exposed	Unexposed	Total
Diseased	a	b	$a + b = n_D$
Well	c	c	$c + d = n_W$

	Exposed (E)	Unexposed (U)			Exposed (E)	Unexposed (U)
Diseased	240 + 60	540 + 160	→	Diseased	300	700
Well	120 + 80	720 + 80		Well	200	800

Given the sensitivity (ϕ) and the specificity (ψ) of the exposure measurement, the true values for a^*, b^*, c^*, and d^* corrected for measurement error can be written

$$a^* = (n_D\psi - b)/(\phi + \psi - 1)$$
$$b^* = (n_D\phi - a)/(\phi + \psi - 1)$$
$$c^* = (n_W\psi - d)/(\phi + \psi - 1)$$
$$d^* = (n_W\phi - c)/(\phi + \psi - 1)$$

Example: Referring back to the previous example that demonstrated how misclassification attenuated the correct relative risk, this method can be used to reconstruct the true relationship. If, from a separate validation study, we know that $\phi = 0.6$ and $\psi = 0.9$, then

$$a^* = (1,000 \times 0.9 - 700)/(0.6 + 0.9 - 1)$$
$$= 400$$
$$b^* = (1,000 \times 0.6 - 300)/(0.6 + 0.9 - 1)$$
$$= 600$$
$$c^* = (1,000 \times 0.9 - 800)/(0.6 + 0.9 - 1)$$
$$= 200$$
$$d^* = (1,000 \times 0.6 - 200)/(0.6 + 0.9 - 1)$$
$$= 800$$

Using these corrected cell numbers, OR = $400 \div 600/200 \div 800 = 2.67$, the same value as obtained for the original 2×2 table.

Although this method is straightforward and provides a simple estimate of the effects of misclassification, it has several important limitations. First, in practical epidemiologic applications we are seldomly interested in a single 2×2 table; typically age, gender, and other risk factors need to be controlled in any analysis. Furthermore, this does not provide corresponding confidence limits. However, more recently, this basic approach has been extended to multidimensional tables, and Greenland has developed a method for confidence intervals for corrected odds ratios (see Espeland and Hui, 1987; Greenland, 1988; Chen, 1989; Clayton, 1992).

Continuous Variables: Determination of True Standard Deviations

A simple approach can be based on an extension of Figure 3–6, which depicts how random within-person error reduces the true magnitude of association. For simplicity, it is assumed that variables are normally distributed and the variance is constant over the range of the data.

As described for the correction of standard deviation, replicate measurements from all or a sample of study subjects and analysis of variance can be employed to separate the within- and between-person components of variation (s_w^2 and s_b^2). The square root of the between-person variance (s_b) is the true standard deviation that would have been observed if no within-person variation had been present, that is, if we had used the mean of a large number of replicates per subject. Because the mean for cases and the mean for controls are not biased by this type of error, the true means and standard deviations for cases and controls can be described by the observed means $\pm$ s_b. If subjects above a cut-point (x) are considered exposed, then we can estimate the proportion of cases and controls above any specific cut-point using a table of normal deviates. These proportions can then be used to calculate the true relative risk or OR.

Example: The data employed to generate Figure 3–6B can be used in reverse to obtain a corrected relative risk. In this example, normal distributions for intake of a nutrient were observed for a case and a noncase group with the mean of the cases being 0.25 observed standard deviations above the mean of the noncases. A cut-point of 0.5 observed standard deviations above the mean of the noncase group was used to define exposed (above this point) and unexposed (below this point) subjects. Using a table of normal deviates to obtain the areas above and below the cut-point for cases and noncases, the proportions of exposed cases and noncases are

| | Nutrient Intake | |
	Exposed	Unexposed
Cases	0.40	0.59
Noncases	0.31	0.69

OR = 1.51

Now, let us assume that the error in the measure of exposure is strictly random within-person error and that a reproducibility study has been conducted in which it was determined that the within-person variance was three times the true between-person variance ($s_u^2/ s_b^2 = 3$). Thus, the total observed variance is $s^2_{obs} = s_b^2 + 3s_b^2 = 4s_b^2$. *Therefore, $s_{obs}/2 = s_b$.* That is, the true between-person standard deviation (s_b) is only one-half the observed standard deviation. Therefore, the same cut-point actually corresponds to 1.0 standard deviation unit above the noncase mean. Returning to the table of normal deviates to determine the areas above and below that cut-point, the following proportions are obtained:

| | Nutrient Intake | |
	Exposed	Unexposed
Cases	0.31	0.69
Noncases	0.16	0.84

OR = 2.36

The OR obtained after removing the effect of within-person variation is thus deattenuated and corresponds to the true value determined in Figure 3–6A.

This approach is intuitively simple and provides a conceptual cornerstone, but has several limitations, including the requirement for normally distributed variables (which may usually be approximated by transformation), the present lack of a method for obtaining confidence limits, and the inability to adjust simultaneously for confounding factors.

Approaches for correcting relative risks estimates obtained from multiple logistic regression models for random within-person exposure error have been provided by Carroll and colleagues (1984), Stefanski and Carroll (1985), Armstrong (1985),

Kaldor and Clayton (1985), and Rosner and colleagues (1992). A unified approach for linear, logistic, and Cox multivariate regression models has been provided by Spiegelman et al. (1997a). The basic principle underlying most of these techniques, regression calibration, provides a relatively simple method for providing approximate correction for measurement error, whether due to random or systematic within-person error.

The regression calibration approach provides an approximate correction for errors in continuous exposure variables. First, a validation or calibration study conducted among a subset of participants or similar subjects is used to correct the observed exposure value for each individual using regression analysis. Briefly, for individuals in the validation study, a simple linear regression model is fitted with x equal to the true value and z equal to the observed value (Eq. 12–7, see Fig. 6–7). The "corrected value" for each individual is their predicted value based on this model. These corrected values are then used in further analysis, whether they be stratified or multivariate analyses. It is apparent that relative risks based on ranked variable categories (e.g., percentile or quintiles) after the correction has been made are not altered by this method, because the relative rankings of individuals are unchanged. Relative risks based on absolute exposures, however, are corrected. For example, if we are interested in the relative risk of colon cancer for a 20-g difference in daily fat intake, this method would be appropriate. Carroll et al. (1995) have provided a method to obtain confidence intervals for this simple approach.

Rosner and colleagues (1989) have extended the regression calibration method for relative risk correction to multiple logistic regression. This approach accounts for both random and systematic within-person measurement error. Furthermore, the method provides tests and confidence limits that incorporate uncertainty due to both sample size in the main study and uncertainty in the estimation of validity. The latter component is important because, when validation studies are small, the degree of correction applied to the observed relative risk itself has error. Because this method is based on a multiple logistic regression model, measurement error can be accounted for while simultaneously adjusting for confounding by other variables. In common with the other methods to correct for systematic within-person error, this method requires data from a separate validation study. Because of the relative simplicity of this method and its ready applicability to epidemiologic data, it is discussed in detail.

The logistic model relating disease and observed exposure (z) can be written

$$ln[p/(1 - p)] = \alpha + \beta z \quad (12–9)$$

while the true relationship between disease and exposure can be written

$$ln[p/(1 - p)] = \alpha^* + \beta^* x \quad (12–10)$$

Using data from the separate validation study, the relationship between the observed exposure (z) and true exposure (x), as in Equation 12–7, can be written

$$x = \alpha' + \gamma z + \varepsilon \quad (12–11)$$

From substitution of Equation 12–11 into Equation 12–10,

$$\beta^* = \beta/\gamma \quad (12–12)$$

Because the antilog of the logistic regression coefficient is an estimate of the relative risk, the corrected relative risk (RR_t) is simply computed as

$$RR_t = \exp(\beta/\gamma) \quad (12–13)$$

It is of note that the corrected value for β^* in Equation 12–11 is an approximation rather than an exact equality, as the logistic model is not linear. For this reason the correction is not complete, and some bias toward the null remains. However, with small or modest relative risks (less than about 5) and a moderate degree of measurement error, the degree of residual bias is generally small and unimportant (Rosner et al., 1989; Carroll and Wand, 1991).

A formula for the variance of β^*, which incorporates error in β as well as error in the estimation in validity (γ), can be written

$$var(\beta^*) = (1/\gamma^2)(var\beta) + (\beta^2/\gamma^4)(var\gamma) \quad (12–14)$$

where $var\beta$ is obtained from Equation 12–9 and $var\gamma$ from Equation 12–11. It follows that the $100\% \times (1 - \alpha)$ confidence limits are given by

$$exp[\beta^* \pm Z_{1-\alpha/2}s.e.(\beta^*)] \quad (12–15)$$

In some instances, the estimate (x) of true exposure may be subject to random within-person error, such as when the average of a small number of replicate measures is used to estimate true exposure. Because the estimate of true exposure (x) is used in Equation 12–11 as the dependent variable, γ still provides an unbiased estimate of the regression coefficient of x on z when x is subject to random within-person variation. Because it appears that within-person errors based on diet records can be reasonably assumed to be random in some instances, the validation study could be conducted with as little as a single day of diet recording per subject (see Chapter 6). Random error inherent in x, however, results in increased variance of γ and, ultimately, in a wider confidence interval for the corrected relative risk.

Example: Relative risk of breast cancer in relation to calorie-adjusted saturated fat intake corrected for errors in measurement (continuous variable). In a previous study, we examined prospectively the relationship between dietary saturated fat intake and risk of breast cancer among a cohort of 89,538 women (Willett et al., 1987). To measure dietary fat in this study, we used a self-administered, semiquantitative food-frequency questionnaire that had been subjected to a detailed validation study (Willett et al., 1985) among 173 cohort members. To represent true dietary intake in the validation study, we used an average of four 1-week diet records based on weighed food intake collected by each subject at 3-month intervals over a 1-year period.

In the main study, we employed a multiple logistic model with breast cancer incidence as the dependent variable and calorie-adjusted saturated fat intake (a continuous variable) as the primary predictor variable. Age and alcohol intake were also included as covariates. In this model, the coefficient for calorie-adjusted saturated fat intake represents the effect on breast cancer incidence of a daily increase of 1 g of saturated fat with total calories held constant. Because the average saturated fat intake was approximately 25 g daily, 1 g is a very small increment. Thus, we computed the relative risk for a 10-g increase in daily calorie-adjusted saturated fat intake, which approximates the difference between the means of the top and bottom quintiles as assessed by the diet record data (Willett et al., 1985). To estimate γ, we used the data provided by the 173 women in the validation study: calorie-adjusted saturated fat intake measured by the average of four 1-week diet records (x) was regressed on the calorie-adjusted saturated fat intake measured by the questionnaire (z). The regression coefficient for the questionnaire measurement thus provides an estimate of γ, and var(γ) is obtained directly from this model; these two parameters were then used in Equations 12–13 and 12–14.

Based on the full 28 days of diet records, the estimated slope (γ) representing the change in diet record calorie-adjusted saturated fat intake (g/day) associated with a 1-g change in daily saturated fat intake measured by the questionnaire was 0.468, with a standard error of 0.048. Based on the actual data in the total cohort, the observed relative risk for a 10-g increase in

calorie-adjusted saturated fat intake was 0.92 (95% confidence interval [CI] = 0.80 to 1.05). Using Equation 12–13, the corrected relative risk was 0.83, with 95% confidence limits from 0.61 to 1.12 (Table 12–2), providing the best estimate of the effect due to a true 10-g difference in calorie-adjusted saturated fat intake given our main study data and allowing for measurement error. As expected, the point estimate of the corrected relative risk is further from unity than the observed relative risk, and the width of the 95% confidence limits has increased. For purposes of illustration, hypothetical examples are provided using different values for β but the same standard error of β and the same value for γ (Table 12–2).

In this example, we assumed that the 28 days of diet recording in the validation study were sufficient to dampen within-person variation and thus provide a close approximation to true intake for an individual. To provide an example of the situation where x (true exposure) is still subject to within-person variation, we sampled 2 days (one each from weeks 1 and 3) and 4 days (one from each week) from the total 28 days of diet record. In Table 12–2, we have provided corrected relative risk estimates using these 2 or 4 days of diet recording to estimate γ. As expected, the estimates of γ were similar, but their standard errors were larger; in this instance, however, the degree of variation in the standard error of γ had only a small influence on the confidence limits for the corrected relative risks. Because, by chance, the value for γ was somewhat lower using all 28 days, the confidence intervals were actually slightly narrower with fewer days. The application of this method of correction for exposure data based on ordinal categories (e.g., quintiles) is discussed in Rosner and colleagues (1989).

Ideally, the validation study would be conducted among a subsample of the main study participants to minimize concern regarding the generalizability of the validity estimate to the main study population. It

Table 12–2. Relative risks of breast cancer for a 10-g/day increase in calorie-adjusted saturated fat intake, adjusted for errors in measurement

Example	Validation study[a] Dietary questionnaire vs.	γ	SE	Main study[b]: RR for 10-g increase Observed RR	(95% CI)	Corrected RR	(95% CI)
1. Actual data	28 day record	0.468	(0.048)	0.92	(0.80, 1.05)	0.83	(0.61, 1.12)
$\beta = -0.0878$	4 day record	0.554	(0.073)	0.92	(0.80, 1.05)	0.85	(0.66, 1.10)
SE = 0.0712	2 day record	0.540	(0.090)	0.92	(0.80, 1.05)	0.85	(0.65, 1.11)
2. Hypothetical data	28 day record	0.468	(0.048)	1.00	(0.87, 1.15)	1.00	(0.74, 1.35)
$\beta = 0.000$	4 day record	0.554	(0.073)	1.00	(0.87, 1.15)	1.00	(0.78, 1.29)
SE = 0.0712	2 day record	0.540	(0.090)	1.00	(0.87, 1.15)	1.00	(0.77, 1.29)
3. Hypothetical data	28 day record	0.468	(0.048)	1.50	(1.30, 1.72)	2.38	(1.68, 3.36)
$\beta = 0.405$	4 day record	0.554	(0.073)	1.50	(1.30, 1.72)	2.08	(1.52, 2.85)
SE = 0.0712	2 day record	0.540	(0.090)	1.50	(1.30, 1.72)	2.12	(1.48, 3.02)

[a] Validation study data are based on 173 women participating in the Nurses' Health Study. Each woman completed four 1-week diet records over a 1-year period. The 4 days used in this analysis were sampled one from each week; the 2 days were sampled one from each of weeks 1 and 3.

[b] Main study data are based on 590 cases of breast cancer occurring among 89,538 women participating in the Nurses' Health Study, aged 34–59 years and folllowed for 4 years. Logistic model included calorie-adjusted saturated fat intake in g/day as a continous variable, age (34–39/40–49/50–54/55–59) and alcohol intake (0, 0.1–4.9, and 5+ g/day).

From Rosner et al. (1989).

may be possible, with caution, however, to use an estimate of validity from a completely external source if the populations are generally similar.

Equation 12–13 may be rearranged to compute the relative risk that would be observed given an estimated true relative risk and a particular level of validity (γ):

$$RR_o = (RR_t)^\gamma \qquad (12\text{–}16)$$

where RR_o is the observed relative risk and RR_t is the estimated true relative risk. In Table 12–3, examples of observed relative risks corresponding to estimated true relative risks of 1.5, 2.0, 3.0, and 5.0 and values of γ ranging from 0.2 to 1.0 are provided. There is no obvious threshold of γ below which a measure of exposure is useless; however, for true relative risks of 1.5 or 2.0, epidemiologic effects are difficult to detect if γ is substantially less than 0.5.

It will be apparent that the value of γ does not readily provide a generally interpretable measure of validity. For example, in Table 12–2, part of the correction is related to a change in scale because the

standard deviation of calorie-adjusted saturated fat intake measured by the questionnaire is larger than the standard deviation according to the diet record. Thus, even if the two measures were perfectly correlated, the larger standard deviation of the questionnaire would result in a value of γ less than 1. Although imperfect measures usually result in larger variances, this is not necessarily true, so that the value of γ can exceed 1 (this can also result simply from a change in units). If both the "true" (x) and surrogate (z) measures have the same standard deviation or are based on percentile rankings, such as quintiles, then the value for γ is equivalent to the correlation coefficient relating x and z and is comparable to the measure of misclassification discussed by Walker and Blettner (1985).

The effect of including covariates in a multiple logistic model on the correction of relative risks deserves comment. In principle, the measure of validity should be conditional on the same set of covariates that would be included in the logistic model; this would be particularly important for

Table 12–3. Observed relative risks for different levels of validity in the measurement of exposure[a]

γ^b	True relative risks			
	1.5	2.0	3.0	5.0
0.2	1.08	1.15	1.25	1.38
0.3	1.13	1.23	1.39	1.62
0.4	1.18	1.32	1.55	1.90
0.5	1.22	1.41	1.73	2.24
0.6	1.28	1.52	1.93	2.63
0.7	1.33	1.62	2.16	3.09
0.8	1.38	1.74	2.41	3.62
0.9	1.44	1.87	2.69	4.26
1.0	1.50	2.00	3.00	5.00

[a] $RR_o = (RR_t)^\gamma$ where RR_o is the observed relative risk and RR_t is the estimated true relative risk.

[b] The regression coefficient for the true measure on the surrogate measure or (when both measures have the same standard deviation) the correlation coefficient between them.

variables that are strongly associated with the primary exposure. Thus, both x and z should each be adjusted for relevant covariates before regressing x on z as in Equation 12–11 (this adjustment can also be accomplished by including these covariates as independent variables). For example, if the multiple logistic model in a nutritional analysis included gender, then the estimate of validity should be conditional on gender as men tend to eat more of most nutrients than women.

CORRECTION FOR MEASUREMENT ERROR IN CONFOUNDING VARIABLES

As demonstrated by Greenland (1980) and Kupper (1984), errors in the measurement of confounding variables can distort relative risk estimates in any direction. Kupper (1984) has provided a method to adjust partial correlation coefficients for such errors; the details are beyond the scope of this book.

Methods have been developed to correct relative risks from logistic regression models for measurement error in confounding variables (covariates) as well as the variable of primary interest, assuming either strictly

random within-person error (Rosner et al., 1992) or combinations of random and systematic within-person error (Rosner et al., 1990). The latter approach is a multivariate extension of the linear approximation method discussed above and requires a validation/calibration substudy with all of the predictor variables measured simultaneously. The method takes into account not only the error with which each variable is measured but also the correlation of errors. Thus, adjustments are made for the incomplete control of confounding by variables that are measured imperfectly. This approach can also be used for multiple linear and Cox regression models (Spiegelman et al., 1997a). The method has been applied to a prospective analysis of dietary fat and breast cancer in which dietary fat, energy, and alcohol were all considered to be measured imperfectly, and adjustments were made for all of these variables simultaneously (Willett et al., 1992).*

An example of adjustment for errors in the measurement of multiple covariates, assuming only random within-person variation, is provided in Table 12–4 using data from the Framingham Heart Study (Rosner et al., 1992). This analysis focused on the relation of body mass index to risk of coronary heart disease during a 10-year follow-up period. In this analysis, fasting blood glucose level, total serum cholesterol level, and blood pressure were considered as covariates that, along with body mass index, were measured with error; the errors were assessed using repeated measurements over time in the total study population. These covariates should not be considered as actual confounders because they are likely to be in the casual pathway between obesity and coronary heart disease. Rather, the analysis considers the degree to which these variables can *explain* the relation between obesity and coronary disease; mathematically, though, there is no distinction

*For software, contact Donna Spiegelman, D.Sc., at the Department of Epidemiology, Harvard School of Public Health, 677 Huntington Avenue, Boston, MA 02115 or at donna.spiegelman@channing.harvard.edu.

Table 12–4. Relation of selected coronary risk factors to 10-year incidence of coronary heart disease in multivariate analyses, uncorrected and corrected for measurement error[a]

	OR (95% CI)[b]	
Risk factor	Uncorrected	Corrected
Serum cholesterol (mg/dl)	2.21 (1.43–3.39)	2.93 (1.60–5.36)
Serum glucose (mg/dl)	1.27 (0.97–1.66)	1.51 (0.90–2.53)
Body mass index (kg/m²)	1.64 (1.04–2.58)	1.58 (0.97–2.56)
Systolic blood pressure (mmHg)	2.80 (1.85–4.24)	3.78 (2.16–6.62)

[a] The subjects were 1,731 men who were seen at examinations 4 to 9 of the Framingham Heart Study. All risk factors were assessed at baseline (examination 4), and all subjects were free of coronary disease at or before examination 4. Models also included age and cigarette smoking. Coronary heart disease included either nonfatal myocardial infarction or fatal coronary heart disease (No. of events = 163). OR, odds ratio; CI, confidence interval.

[b] Based on a comparison of men at the 10th and 90th percentiles of the observed distribution of specific risk factors at examination 4 (serum cholesterol, 185 vs. 285 mg/dl; serum glucose, 65 vs. 99 mg/dl; body mass index, 22.1 vs. 30.8 kg/m²; systolic blood pressure, 110 vs. 159 mmHg).

From Rosner and colleagues (1992)

between confounding and explanatory variables. As can be seen in the standard multivariate analysis that does not account for measurement error, body mass index has a significant independent association with coronary heart disease risk. In the model adjusted for measurement error, the coefficients for fasting blood glucose level, total serum cholesterol level, and blood pressure increase. In contrast, the coefficient for body mass index decreases and becomes nonsignificant because, once errors in measurement of covariates are accounted for, they explain a greater part of the effects of obesity.

Impact of Imperfect "True" Measurements in Regression Calibration

In using regression calibration methods to correct for measurement error, the validity of the assumed "true" or "gold standard" method should always be of concern. Because all measurements have errors, Spiegelman and colleagues (1997b) have ex-

amined the implications of imperfect "true" measurements. These authors confirmed the point made earlier that purely random errors in "true" measurements do not bias the regression coefficients from the validation/calibration study and thus do not bias the corrected relative risks. Hence, for example, only a single 24-hour recall can be used for measurement of "true" intake in a calibration study on the assumption that this is an unbiased estimate of true intake (see Chapter 6).

Biased corrections can occur when the errors in true and surrogate measurements are correlated. For example, if the same erroneous database is used to calculate nutrient intakes for the "true" and surrogate methods, the regression coefficient relating the two methods could be overstated. Spiegelman and colleagues (1997b) used a triangulation approach (see Chapter 6) employing a third measure with errors that can be assumed to be independent from the other measurements to estimate the correlation of errors for the "true" and surrogate measures. They then used the correlation of errors to develop an additional correction factor for adjusting relative risks for measurement error. Using the example from Chapter 6 in which food-frequency and diet record estimates of polyunsaturated fat intake were both compared with adipose measurements of polyunsaturated fat, the errors in dietary intake methods were found to be uncorrelated. However, when intakes of vitamin E from the two dietary methods were compared with blood levels, errors in the two dietary methods were found to be moderately correlated (0.37 for log vitamin E intake). However, correcting for this degree of correlated error had little impact on the relative risks corrected for measurement error. Although the potential for correlations in errors between methods used for regression calibration should always be considered, and should be assessed whenever possible, even moderate correlations in these errors do not appear to result in much bias if they are ignored when using standard error correction procedures.

ESTIMATION OF RELATIVE RISKS BASED ON DUAL RESPONSES

Marshall and Graham (1984) have described an approach to improve the estimation of relative risks based on two measures of exposure for all subjects, with the assumption that neither method is perfect. For dichotomous variables they suggest that subjects be categorized as exposed according to both measures, unexposed according to both measures, or exposed according to only one measure. The true relative risk would then be best approximated by comparing subjects classified as exposed by both methods with those classified as unexposed by both methods. This approach provides an opportunity to improve the estimation of effects in epidemiologic studies in the absence of known validity for either measurement. This lack of quantified measurement error, however, limits interpretation as relative risks still tend to be underestimated, although the magnitude of underestimation remains uncertain. Walter (1984) proposed a maximum likelihood method based on dual responses to provide an unbiased estimate of the true association between exposure and disease. This method is also more efficient because all the data are used, not just those with concordant exposures. Howe (1985) has conducted simulations of various approaches that use dual responses for all subjects and has confirmed that the additional information improves the estimate of the relative risk and the statistical power of tests under most circumstances. The use of repeated measurements of diet is discussed further in Chapter 13.

SUMMARY

A variety of methods exist to correct epidemiologic measures of association for error in the measurement of exposure. Newer methods can provide both relative risks and confidence intervals that are corrected for measurement error in the primary exposure variable as well as in covariates. Each method requires assumptions that are rarely perfectly satisfied. For example, many methods require that errors be strictly due to random within-person variation. Most methods based on a validation substudy assume that the true measure is indeed true (or at least an unbiased estimate of the truth). Despite these limitations, careful use of these adjustment procedures should provide better estimates of the quantitative relationships between nutritional factors and disease than analyses that ignore the effects of measurement error altogether.

REFERENCES

Armstrong, B. (1985). Measurement error in the generalized linear model. *Commun Statist Simul Comput 14*, 529–544.

Barron, B. A. (1977). The effects of misclassification on the estimation of relative risk. *Biometrics 33*, 414–418.

Beaton, G. H. (1994). Approaches to analysis of dietary data—Relationship between planned analyses and choice of methodology. *Am J Clin Nutr 59(suppl)*, S253–S261.

Beaton, G. H., J. Milner, P. Corey, V. McGuire, M. Cousins, E. Stewart, M. de Ramos, D. Hewitt, P. V. Grambsch, N. Kassim, and J. A. Little (1979). Sources of variance in 24-hour dietary recall data: Implications for nutrition study design and interpretation. *Am J Clin Nutr 32*, 2546–2549.

Bross, I. D. (1954). Misclassification in 2 × 2 tables. *Biometrics 10*, 478–486.

Byar, D. P., and M. H. Gail (1989). Errors-in-variables workshop. *Statist Med 8*, 1027–1029.

Carroll, R. J., D. Ruppert, and L. A. Stefanski (1995). *Measurement Error in Nonlinear Models*. London: Chapman & Hall.

Carroll, R. J., C. H. Spiegelman, and K. K. Gordon, et al. (1984). On errors in variables for binary regression models. *Biometrika 71*, 19–25.

Carroll, R. J., and M. P. Wand (1991). Semiparametric estimation in logistic measurement error models. *J R Statist Soc B 53*, 573–585.

Chen, T. T. (1989). A review of methods for misclassified categorical data in epidemiology. *Statist Med 8*, 1095–1106.

Clayton, D. G. (1992). Models for the analysis of cohort and case–control studies with inaccurately measured exposures. In Dwyer, J. H., Feinlieb, M., and Lipsert, P., et al. (eds.): *Statistical Models for Longitudinal*

Studies of Health. New York: Oxford Press, pp 301–331.

Diamond, E. L., and A. M. Lilienfeld (1962). Effects of errors in classification and diagnosis in various types of epidemiological studies. *Am J Public Health 52*, 1137–1144.

Espeland, M. A., and S. L. Hui (1987). A general approach to analyzing epidemiologic data that contain misclassification errors. *Biometrics 43*, 1001–1012.

Greenland, S. (1980). The effect of misclassification in the presence of covariates. *Am J Epidemiol 112*, 564–569.

Greenland, S. (1988). Variance estimation for epidemiologic effect estimates under misclassification. *Statist Med 7*, 745–757.

Howe, G. R. (1985). The use of polytomous dual response data to increase power in case–control studies: An application to the association between dietary fat and breast cancer. *J Chronic Dis 38*, 663–670.

Kaldor, J., and D. Clayton (1985). Latent class analysis in chronic disease epidemiology. *Statist Med 4*, 327–335.

Kleinbaum, D. G., L. L. Kupper, and H. Morganstern (1982). *Epidemiologic Research: Principles and Quantitative Methods.* Belmont, CA: Lifetime Learning Publications.

Kupper, L. L. (1984). Effects of the use of unreliable surrogate variables on the validity of epidemiologic research studies. *Am J Epidemiol 120*, 643–648.

Liu, K., J. Stamler, A. Dyer, J. McKeever, and P. McKeever (1978). Statistical methods to assess and minimize the role of intra-individual variability in obscuring the relationship between dietary lipids and serum cholesterol. *J Chronic Dis 31*, 399–418.

Madansky, A. (1959). The fitting of straight lines when both variables are subject to error. *J Am Statist Assoc 54*, 173–205.

Marshall, J. R., and S. Graham (1984). Use of dual responses to increase validity of case–control studies. *J Chronic Dis 37*, 125–136.

Mattson, F. H., B. A. Erickson, and A. M. Kligman (1972). Effect of dietary cholesterol on serum cholesterol in man. *Am J Clin Nutr 25*, 589–594.

Nusser, S. M., A. L Carriquiry, K. W. Dodd, and W. A. Fuller (1996). A semiparametric transformation approach to estimating usual daily intake distributions. *J Am Statist Assoc 91*, 1440–1449.

Riggs, D. S., J. A. Guarnieri, and S. Addelman (1978). Fitting straight lines when both variables are subject to error. *Life Sci 22*, 1305–1360.

Rosner, B., D. Spiegelman, and W. C. Willett (1990). Correction of logistic regression relative risk estimates and confidence intervals for measurements error: The case of multiple covariates measured with error. *Am J Epidemiol 132*, 734–745.

Rosner, B., D. Spiegelman, and W. C. Willett (1992). Correction of logistic regression relative risk estimates and confidence intervals for random within-person measurement error. *Am J Epidemiol 136*, 1400–1413.

Rosner, B., and W. C. Willett (1988). Interval estimates for correlation coefficients corrected for within-person variation: Implications for study design and hypothesis testing. *Am J Epidemiol 127*, 377–386.

Rosner, B., W. C. Willett, and D. Spiegelman (1989). Correction of logistic regression relative risk estimates and confidence intervals for systematic within-person measurement error. *Statist Med 8*, 1051–1069.

Snedecor, W. G. (1968). Error in measurement in statistics. *Technometrics 10*, 637–666.

Spiegelman, D., A. McDermott, and B. Rosner (1997a). Regression calibration method for correcting measurement-error bias in nutritional epidemiology. *Am J Clin Nutr 65 (suppl)*, 1179S–1186S.

Spiegelman, D., S. Schneeweiss, and A. McDermott (1997b). Measurement error correction for logistic regression models with an "alloyed gold standard." *Am J Epidemiol 145*, 184–196.

Stefanski, L. A., and R. J. Carroll (1985). Covariate measurement error in logistic regression. *Ann Statist 13*, 1335–1351.

Tukey, J. W. (1951). Components in regression. *Biometrics 7*, 33–69.

Walker, A. M., and M. Blettner (1985). Comparing imperfect measures of exposure. *Am J Epidemiol 121*, 783–790.

Walter, S. D. (1984). Commentary on "Use of dual responses to increase validity of case-control studies." *J Chronic Dis 37*, 137–142.

Willett, W. C., D. J. Hunter, M. J. Stampfer, G. A. Colditz, J. E. Manson, D. Spiegelman, B. Rosner, C. H. Hennekens, and F. E. Speizer (1992). Dietary fat and fiber in relation to risk of breast cancer: An 8-year follow-up. *JAMA 268*, 2037–2044.

Willett, W. C., L. Sampson, M. J. Stampfer B. Rosner, C. Bain, J. Witschi, C. H. Hennekens, and F. E. Speizer (1985). Reproducibility and validity of a semiquantitative food frequency questionnaire. *Am J Epidemiol 122*, 51–65.

Willett, W. C., M. J. Stampfer, G. A. Colditz, B. A. Rosner, C. H. Hennekens, and F. E. Speizer (1987). Dietary fat and the risk of breast cancer. *N Engl J Med 316*, 22–28.

13

Issues in Analysis and Presentation of Dietary Data

This chapter is a synthesis of selected issues relating to the analysis and presentation of dietary data, building on recent experiences of those working in this field. It is not a cookbook for data analysis as there is no single approach at any step; the area is in active evolution, and further creative efforts are needed. The underlying objectives of data analysis and presentation are to learn as much as possible from the available data and to present what has been learned to readers completely and with maximum clarity. Particularly for presentation, the approaches should vary depending on the intended readership. For example, simpler analytic approaches and greater use of figures may be appropriate for a general medical journal, whereas more complex methods and primarily tabular results may be best for an epidemiologic publication. Issues related to adjustment for total energy intake were addressed in Chapter 11; other issues that have arisen in the use of dietary data are discussed here.

DATA CLEANING: BLANKS AND OUTLIERS

Before analysis, careful consideration of criteria for acceptable data quality is important. A common issue with dietary data is the treatment of questionnaires in which some food items have been left blank. With a typical list of 100 to 150 foods, many subjects will leave one or more questions blank. The best solution is to prevent blank responses, for example, by reviewing forms immediately after completion and asking participants to complete the missing items. However, in large studies, particularly those conducted by mail, this is not possible. Two issues arise frequently: Should subjects with more than a specific number of blanks be excluded, and how should blanks be treated in calculating nutrient intakes?

In developing a strategy for dealing with blank food items, it is useful to understand why participants may not have completed a response for a specific food. This could be due to inattention or carelessness or because the participant did not eat the food (even though they should have answered "never"). When examining questionnaires with multiple blank items, several patterns can be seen. For many forms, blank items are interspersed with plausible and seemingly carefully completed responses to other foods and the "never" category is not used, suggesting that blanks meant that the food was not consumed. In occasional questionnaires, whole sections are left blank, suggesting that they were missed. Caan and colleagues (1991) have described their follow-up of subjects who left items blank; they found that items were generally left blank because the food was not consumed. Thus, in calculating nutrient intakes, it seems best to consider intermittent blanks as no consumption of the food.

In the Nurses' Health Study, we initially used an arbitrary criterion of 10 or more blanks to exclude questionnaires. However, after a detailed examination of this issue in the Health Professionals Follow-up Study, we modified this rule because most questionnaires with a higher number of blanks appeared plausible if the missing items were considered as zero. Thus, our usual criterion has allowed up to 70 blanks (out of about 130 items) as long as no whole sections or pages were blank. This criterion has been evaluated empirically within a validation study by examining the correlation between number of blanks on a questionnaire and measurement error, which was calculated for each person as the absolute value of the difference between the food-frequency questionnaire and diet record values (Rimm et al., 1992). For all nutrients examined there was no appreciable correlation. Although a small association between number of blanks and validity cannot be excluded, it did not appear to be substantial in this population. A firm rule for allowable number of blanks cannot be made for all situations, and it is desirable to conduct similar empirical evaluations of decision rules whenever possible.

Once nutrients are calculated, some responses will be implausibly high or low, necessitating additional decisions regarding allowable ranges (see Chapter 11 for a discussion of the general issue of underreporting of energy intake). The use of total energy intake as a primary criterion can be justified because it is the only nutrient for which intake is physiologically fixed within a fairly narrow and predictable range. For example, it is generally considered that total energy intakes below approximately 1.2 times the resting or basal metabolic rate estimated from age, gender, and weight are unlikely to be correct (FAO/WHO/UNU ad hoc Expert Consultation on Energy and Protein Requirements, 1985; James, 1985; Schofield, 1985a and b, Smith et al., 1994; Klesges et al., 1995; Pryer et al., 1995; Shetty et al., 1996), and intakes of more than 4,000 kcal/day are unlikely to be true for even relatively active men (see Appendix 13–1 for basal metabolic rate prediction equation). However, in most datasets, using energy intake less than 1.2 times the estimated resting metabolic rate as an exclusion criterion would result in a substantial loss of subjects due to some inevitable degree of measurement error. Thus we have usually used an arbitrary allowable range of 500 to 3,500 kcal/day for women and 800 to 4,000 kcal/day for men. Although the extremes within this range rarely are correct, adjustment of nutrient intakes for total energy intake will, to a large extent, compensate for overall under- or overreporting (see Chapter 11). Further work regarding the impact of various exclusion criteria on the validity of energy-adjusted nutrient intakes would be useful.

Dietary data are highly sensitive to coding and data entry errors because nutrients are calculated from large numbers of foods. Even low error rates can be devastating; for example, miscoding a teaspoon to a cup for one food on a questionnaire or in a 1 week food record can seriously misclassify an individual for many nutrients. Multiple-choice formats and machine-readable questionnaires are less prone to such errors, but if any hand-coded or open-ended questions are included, such errors may occur. Extreme values are primarily at the high end of the distribution due to the skewed distributions of most nutrients, and they can be heavily influential when nutrients are considered as continuous variables. For this reason, they should be examined carefully, even though it is difficult to create biologically justifiable exclusion rules. Sometimes such extreme values will be indicative of improper completion of questionnaires, such as marking the top category for all foods in a section; however, this pattern will also usually be detected as an outlier for total energy intake. In other cases, coding, data entry, or food composition database errors may be discovered. Some values, however, will just reflect unusual food intake patterns without obvious error. Various criteria for exclusion of outliers have been proposed for other applications (Rosner, 1983; Barnett and Lewis, 1994), but little work has been done specifically regarding dietary variables. Whatever decisions are made, it will be important to confirm that any conclusions are not sensitive to the inclusion of a small number of extreme nutrient values.

CATEGORIZED VERSUS CONTINUOUS PRESENTATION OF INDEPENDENT VARIABLES

Unlike many variables traditionally evaluated by epidemiologists, intakes of nutrients and food groups are primarily continuous. Data for individual foods, typically collected as frequencies of use, are inherently continuous but usually are collected as ordinal categorical or semicontinuous variables, which may still be treated as continuous variables. As the traditional presentation of epidemiologic data has been in the form of rate ratios and rate differences for levels of exposure, and statistical methods have been developed for such purposes, it is not surprising that most continuous dietary data have been categorized for analysis in nutritional epidemiologic studies. A variety of approaches have been used for

creation of categories including the use of arbitrarily defined quantiles (such as quartiles or quintiles), as by Willett et al. (1992), the use of standard round-numbered cutpoints, or the use of cut points that are determined a priori to have biologic relevance such as the Recommended Daily Allowance or the intake at which an enzyme is saturated (Stahelin et al., 1991). Each of these approaches has its advantages. The use of standard round-number cut-points potentially allows greater comparison among studies, although comparisons of absolute intake levels among various populations should be made only cautiously due to differences in dietary assessments or the responses of different populations to the same questionnaire. The most important point is that the primary analysis should be conducted using cut-points determined a priori rather than searching for cut-points to maximize the statistical significance. However, if carefully described, secondary analyses using alternative cut-points that best describe the biologic relationship can sometimes be justified, particularly if a significant overall relationship is seen in the primary analysis. Also, finer divisions of extreme categories may often be useful to extend an examination of the dose–response relationship.

The use of categorized variables has several advantages. First, the investigator can visualize directly how the actual numbers of cases and noncases vary by level of intake. Second, the use of multiple categories makes no assumptions about the dose–response relationship, and it is therefore possible to visualize whether this is most compatible with a linear trend or some nonlinear alternative. In nutritional epidemiology, simple linear dose–response relationships are probably unlikely if a sufficiently wide range of intake is examined because most dietary factors have limits in absorption, transport, metabolism, or storage, and their effects may be mediated by enzyme activities that can be saturated. Third, the use of categories constrains any undue influence of outlying datapoints, which are the observations most likely to be affected by errors in data collection or processing.

Arguments can also be made for using continuous variables. First, the greatest statistical power is provided by a continuous variable if the function reasonably fits the data, although this advantage may be slight with the use of five of more categories combined with an overall test for trend. Second, when used as a covariate, a crudely categorized variable may not fully account for the effect of that variable, resulting in possible residual confounding. This potential problem is particularly great when the primary variable is highly correlated with the confounder, as in the example of fat and total energy intake, which is discussed in Chapter 11. Third, the use of continuous variables may facilitate comparisons among studies because a single relative risk is reported for an arbitrarily specified increment of intake (e.g., relative risk for 100 mg of cholesterol per day) that does not depend on the distribution of the dietary factor in the particular population or on the choice of cut-points of individual studies. However, caution is warranted in making quantitative comparisons among studies for reasons noted above. The presentation of a single relative risk (with confidence interval), rather than relative risks for each category of intake, also provides a compact presentation of data, which is an issue when many dietary factors are examined. This can be particularly attractive when many foods (each with its own distribution) are analyzed; for example, the data can be summarized by providing relative risks for one serving per day (or week) for each food. Tests for nonlinearity, such as the addition of a quadratic term, can be used to evaluate the presence of nonlinearity. However, abundant data are needed to detect a statistically significant deviation from linearity; the use of only statistical tests to detect departure from linearity may lead to an inaccurate description of the data. For example, the analysis by quintiles could show that a substantial difference in risk exists between the first and second quintile, but none between quintiles two through five (a highly plausible biologic relationship). The test for a simple linear relationship using continuous data might be nonsignificant (leading to a report of no association), or it might be significant but an added exponential term might be nonsignificant (leading to the report of a linear relationship); neither correctly represents the findings. The use of locally smoothed regression curves represents an approach that combines some of the advantages of both categorical and continuous analysis (see below).

GRAPHIC PRESENTATION OF DATA

The central data of epidemiologic studies should be presented in numerical form to provide the actual numbers of exposed subjects and the numbers of endpoints, but judicious ancillary use of figures summarizing the primary findings can be helpful to many readers. (Also, a clear and attractive summary figure is likely to enhance the probability that others will include your data in their presentations.) A wide variety of methods can be used to present dietary data graphically, and a plethora of software has facilitated their implementation. A detailed discussion is beyond the scope of this chapter, but a few points are worth noting.

Single Variable Effects

For presenting the effects of one or a few dichotomous exposure variables, a graphic display provides little additional perspective and tables should be used. However, with multiple ordinal categories, a figure can assist in visualizing an overall relationship (Fig. 13–1). The use of histograms to present relative risks has generally been disfavored because this parameter is more correctly represented as a point, and confidence intervals are less readily presented. Some have argued that the relative risk on the vertical axis should be in the natural logarithm scale because this is statistically

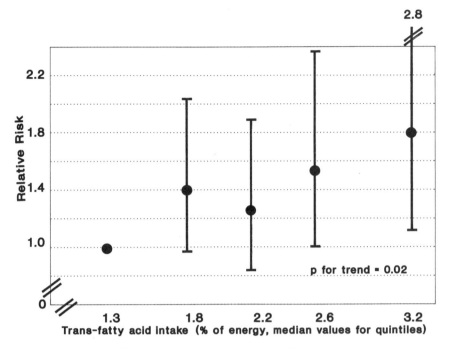

Figure 13–1. Relative risk of CHD by *trans*-fatty acid intake as percentage of total energy.

(From Willett et al., 1993; reproduced with permission.)

symmetric. However, a general medical audience would be more confused than enlightened by the meaning of ln relative risks. Also, the untransformed relative risk is proportional to absolute risk, which does relate to the public health importance of an effect (e.g., if a common reference category is used, a relative risk of 2 corresponds to a much greater absolute effect than a relative risk of 0.5). It might be argued that, if absolute risk is really of interest, then the dependent variable should be expressed as absolute risk. However, one reason that relative rather than absolute risks are generally utilized in epidemiologic studies is that age is usually the most powerful determinant; thus, absolute risks are usually arbitrary depending on the age to which the data have been standardized.

The actual width of categories of the exposure variable should be represented in the graphic display. For example, in Figure 13–1, *trans*-fatty acid intake was divided into quintiles; as typically seen, the dis-

tances between quintile medians were greater for the extreme quintiles than for the middle three quintiles. Thus, the distances between quintiles in the figure were made to be proportional to the differences between quantile medians. Similarly, tests for trends across categories should usually use the median values rather than a simple integer scale, such as 1 to 5.

Actual Versus Predicted Relationships

In graphic displays of the relationship between two variables, one issue that naturally arises is whether to provide the actual data or the prediction from a model derived from the data. For example, this could be the choice between providing the relative risks of disease (with confidence interval) for quintiles of dietary intake or the fitted logistic regression line (with confidence bands) relating intake to risk. Although not all may agree, many epidemiologists believe that the actual data should be provided so that the reader can

view the findings without being forced to
assume the appropriateness of any model
assumptions, such as whether a linear relationship adequately describes the relationship. However, the best solution may
be to do both; for example, provide the
data points for categories and superimpose
the fitted regression line (Fig. 13–2). One
clearly inappropriate approach is to analyze the data as continuous, but then present the findings as though they were categorical, for example, by displaying the
odds ratios (and confidence intervals) for
multiple discrete levels of intake that are all
based on a single regression coefficient (Table 13–1). This provides the potentially
misleading impression of a clearly monotonic relationship and confidence intervals
that are too narrow for a specific level because they are based on the overall data.

Display of Joint Effects

Widely available graphics software has created many ways to represent the joint
effects of two exposure variables. One
common approach is the three-dimensional
histogram (Fig. 13–3A). This has been criticized by some for the same reasons that
the use of histograms to present univariate
findings has been discouraged. An alternative display using points is shown in Figure
13–3B. A display of confidence intervals
is usually incompatible with the three-
dimensional histogram, but this may also
be problematic with the use of points as
their confidence intervals are frequently
overlapping. Thus, critical confidence intervals will usually need to be presented in
tabular form or in text. Although some
may wish to avoid the three-dimensional
histogram, I believe this often provides a
useful perspective of data that are inherently multidimensional.

Locally Smoothed Regression Curves and Regression Splines

Locally smoothed regression curves and regression splines have been used increasingly to display epidemiologic findings with
a continuous exposure variable (Hastie and

Tibshirani, 1987; Harrell et al., 1988;
Durrleman and Simon, 1989; Greenland,
1995). These can combine advantages of
both categorical and continuous analyses.
With smoothed regression curves, the values of the dependent variable, such as a relative risk, are estimated for a continuously
moving window of values of the independent variable. In using regression splines,
separate linear or nonlinear functions are
fit between specified points ("knots") on
the exposure distribution, and functions
are connected at the knots to produce a
smooth curve. Confidence bands for the
continuous function can also be calculated.
The principal advantages of these approaches are that *a priori* assumptions are
not imposed regarding the shape of the
dose–response relationship and that maximal use is made of the continuous nature
of the dependent variable. As an example,
data relating alcohol intake to risk of
breast cancer are described in Figure 13–4.
In this example, those data fit using regression splines provide a strong sense that the
relationship is approximately linear and
that a significant increase in risk is seen
even at about 10 g (approximately one
drink) per day. Whether this adds substantially to the perspective provided by the
traditional categorical data is not clear.

As another example, smoothing techniques were used to evaluate the relationship between vitamin A intake and risk of
neural crest congenital malformations
(Rothman et al., 1995) (Fig. 13–5). This
analysis suggested the existence of a threshold at approximately 10,000 IU, above
which risk increased substantially. One
possible concern is that inflection points
may be accepted too literally, especially
when the data are sparse; in this example,
for instance, the method does not provide
a confidence interval for the apparent
threshold, which would probably be quite
wide. This might be regarded as an over-
fitting of the data, analogous to an extreme
form of selecting optimal cut-points to
demonstrate a relationship. Also, the degree to which the conclusions are affected

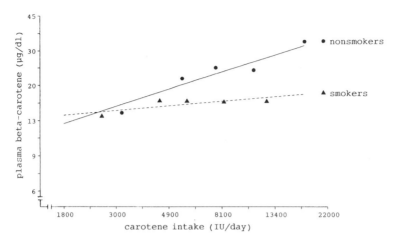

Figure 13–2. Plasma beta-carotene levels by quintile of intake, female smokers vs. nonsmokers, melanoma study controls, Boston, 1982–1985. Plasma beta-carotene levels are adjusted for plasma cholesterol, plasma triglycerides, age, Quetelet index, total energy intake, alcohol intake, and preformed total vitamin A intake by adding residual from a multiple regression model back to the overall mean (on the log scale) for plasma beta-carotene. (From Stryker et al., 1988; reproduced with permission.)

by somewhat arbitrary choices such as the width of the window used for smoothing and the number and spacing of knots deserves further consideration. Although smoothing methods and regression splines for analyses involving dietary intake may prove valuable, particularly in exploratory data analysis, their use deserves further evaluation.

EXAMINATION OF FOODS AND NUTRIENTS

As discussed in Chapter 2, a full evaluation of the relationship between diet and a disease should involve the analysis of data on both food and nutrient intakes. If an association with disease is found for a specific nutrient, it is important to examine and report whether the major foods contributing to this nutrient (as seen in the same dataset, defined in terms of either absolute contribution or contribution to between-person variance) are also related similarly to risk of disease. If so, this would lend support to the nutrient finding, but if major contributors are not similarly re-

lated, this would detract from the nutrient hypothesis. Again, as noted in Chapter 2, foods are of inherent importance in themselves, and findings based on foods can avoid the problem of being overly specific, which is a potential hazard when an effect is attributed to one of the many nutrients comprising foods.

One serious problem with analyses of specific foods is the large number of items on a typical questionnaire. The appropriate statistical procedure to use when multiple exposures are examined, a "multiple comparison" issue, has been a topic of debate in epidemiology. Some argue that the p value used for statistical significance should be adjusted according to the number of variables examined, but the general consensus in epidemiology is that this unduly reduces power and that individual associations should be evaluated on their own merits, and conclusions should be made in the light of consistency with other information internal and external to the study (Rothman, 1990; Savitz and Olshan, 1995). Nevertheless, when a large number of foods (or nutrients) are screened for as-

Table 13–1. Risk of primary cardiac arrest associated with red blood cell levels of long-chain n-3 polyunsaturated fatty acids.

Quartile	Mean % total fatty acid	OR	95% CI
1	3.3	1.0	
2	4.3	0.5	0.4–0.8
3	5.0	0.3	0.2–0.6
4	6.5	0.1	0.1–0.4

From a conditional logistic model that included the linear term for red blood cell membrane n-3 fatty acids. OR and CI were calculated using the mean value of each category (Siscovick et al, 1995)

sociations without a prior hypothesis, the likelihood that some statistically significant relationships will occur by chance must be considered when interpreting the findings. This issue is complicated by the large number of foods because an association with a food is generally more likely to be reported if statistically significant, particularly if consistent with prior expectations. Reporting the association for each food on a questionnaire, and possibly for groups of foods, is impossible in most journals. Thus, the literature on foods is likely to be highly biased, and any summary of the published literature cannot avoid this bias. As an example, an association between red meat consumption and the risk of breast cancer was seen in a prospective study that received wide media attention (Toniolo et al., 1994). This association was also examined in the much larger Nurses' Health Study, and no clear relation was seen; however, all we reported was that "we observed nonsignificant trends with consumption of meats and desserts" (Willett et al., 1992). It is likely that other authors who had reported on dietary fat and breast cancer in prospective studies also had examined this relationship and found it unremarkable, but had not reported the findings. Regardless of the ultimate truth, it is easy to appreciate that associations that arise by chance can lead to a biased view regarding the effects of specific foods. No simple solution exists for this source of bias, but the potential

problems require caution in presenting and interpreting such data. A partial solution may be to deposit data in the National Auxiliary Publications Service or on the Internet for all foods when an analysis on a particular disease is published*; at least such data will be available to others attempting to summarize the literature. If associations were found by routinely screening foods or nutrients without a prior hypothesis, this should be noted when reporting results. However, the best approach for avoiding publication bias on specific foods is probably to analyze collaboratively the primary data from all available studies on a topic (see section below on pooled analyses). Witte and colleagues (1994) have proposed a hierarchical regression method for analyzing foods and nutrients simultaneously that is likely to reduce wildly spurious results for individual foods that may occur by chance. Whether this approach will be useful for detecting associations that truly exist is presently unclear; concern exists because all foods are considered simultaneously in a model and the collinearity may be excessive.

The widespread use of multiple vitamins and other nutritional supplements adds complexity to dietary analyses, but can also provide important insight by greatly extending the range of observable nutrient intakes. Also, details on dose and duration of supplement use are usually obtainable with substantially greater precision than is possible for foods. When examining associations with foods or with nutrient intakes, not including supplements, it will be important to conduct analyses excluding supplement users, because any effects of nutrients from foods may be swamped by the relatively high levels of intakes from supplements. If similar associations are seen with a nutrient from foods among nonsupplement users and from supplements controlling for intake from foods, this can add

*Information and charges can be obtained from NAPS c/o Microfiche Publications, P.O. Box 3513, Grand Central Station, New York, NY 10163–3513.

A

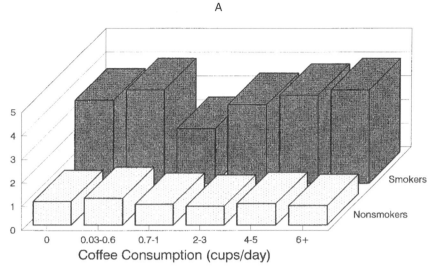

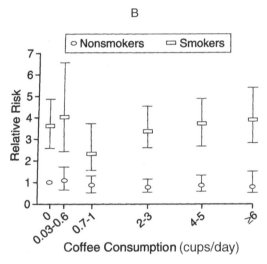

Figure 13–3. (A) Relative risk of coronary heart disease from 1980 to 1990 by level of coffee consumption and smoking status (never and past smokers combined). Reference category is nonsmokers who drank less than one cup of coffee per month. Data are adjusted for age, menopausal status, parental history of myocardial infarction before age 60, multiple vitamin use, vitamin E supplement use, alcohol consumption, and history of diabetes, hypertension and hypercholesterolemia. (Data from Willett et al., 1996.) (B) Relative risk (with 95% confidence interval) of coronary heart disease from 1980 to 1990 by level of coffee consumption and smoking status (never and past smokers combined). Reference category is nonsmokers who drank less than one cup of coffee per month. Data are adjusted as above.

substantially to support for causality because the potentially confounding dietary factors are usually quite different for nutrients from these two sources. Analyses of folic acid intake in relation to neural tube defects provide a good example (see Chapter 18). As discussed later in this chapter, stratification by nutrient intake from foods may also be important when examining the effect of the same nutrient from supplements because little effect of supplementa-

tion might be expected when intake from foods is high. The greatest contrast in risk would usually be expected when long-term supplement users with high intakes from diet are compared with nonsupplement users with low intakes from diet.

The Effect of Time

For most chronic diseases, the temporal relationship between diet and diagnosis is unknown. Sometimes we have leads from

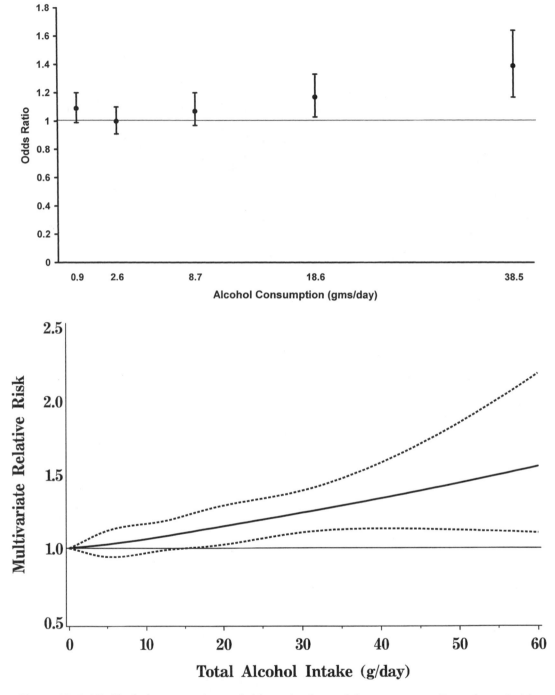

Figure 13–4. (A) Alcohol consumption and risk of breast cancer. (B) Nonparametric regression curve for the relationship between total alcohol intake and breast cancer. (Data from Smith-Warner et al., 1998.

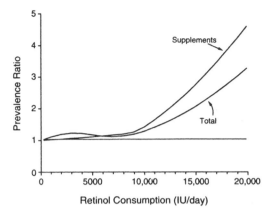

Figure 13–5. Estimated prevalence ratio for birth defects related to the cranial neural crest, according to retinol intake during the first trimester of pregnancy. The smoothed curves were fitted with unrestricted quadratic splines. The prevalence ratio is the ratio of the prevalence of defects among the babies born to women who consumed a given amount of vitamin A (from food and supplements [total] or from supplements alone) to the prevalence among the babies of women with a hypothetical intake of zero. (From Rothman et al., 1995; reproduced with permission. Copyright 1995 Massachusetts Medical Society. All rights reserved.)

other risk factors; for example, risk of breast cancer did not increase until more than 15 years after exposure to the atomic bomb blasts in Japan (Land, 1995), depending on age at exposure, and excess risk has persisted for several decades, which suggests a substantial induction period. However, the use of oral contraceptives or postmenopausal estrogen appears to increase risk of breast cancer within a shorter time, and excess risk dissipates almost entirely within several years after cessation, suggesting a rather short-term effect. These temporal differences are likely to be related to distinct effects at various stages in the sequence of events leading from normal cell growth to clinical cancer. Dietary factors may similarly operate at various stages of this sequence; for example, an antioxidant might reduce the effect of ionizing radiation (an early event), or alcohol may influence endogenous hormone metabolism (which is

likely to be most important later in carcinogenesis). The effect of diet may also be cumulative so that risk is related to a function of both dose and duration of exposure; such a relation would presumably characterize factors that elevate low-density lipoprotein cholesterol and thus the accumulation of atherosclerotic plaques. Dietary factors may also have effects at specific periods in life far removed from the time of diagnosis; for example, high growth rates before puberty appear to increase breast cancer risk by advancing the age at menarche, and effects of maternal diet during pregnancy on the offspring's risk of breast cancer have been hypothesized (Trichopoulos, 1990). Because our knowledge is often not sufficient to be confident that an effect of diet would be limited to only a particular period, it will usually be difficult to exclude an effect of a dietary factor until a fairly wide range of temporal relationships have been examined.

Ideally, a comprehensive dietary assessment would include a measurement of current diet and also diet at various times in the past, for example, at 5, 10, 15, 20, and 30 years ago. In either a case–control or cohort study this would provide an assessment of various latent periods as well as cumulative exposure. Unfortunately, a comprehensive assessment of even current diet is already a major burden on participants. Moreover, the validity of recall diminishes with time, and the reporting of past diet is heavily influenced by current diet (see Chapter 7), so that truly independent retrospective assessments of various periods appear impossible. In practice, in cohort studies an assessment of current diet (usually over the past year) is used, and in case–control studies a period in the past thought to be most plausibly relevant to the disease (typically 5 or 10 years ago for cancer) is the focus of recall. The possibility of finding true associations depends considerably on the consistency of diet within persons over time, but with increasing time this correlation will diminish. Some ancillary information can be useful. In the

Nurses' Health Study baseline questionnaire we asked, for each food, whether use
had greatly increased or had decreased over
the last 10 years (see Appendix 1 of Chapter 5). This has been used to exclude subjects who had unstable intake of foods that
were major sources of the dietary factor being studied; for example, exclusion of
women who changed their consumption of
margarine strengthened the association between intake of *trans*-fatty acids and risk
of coronary heart disease (Willett et al.,
1993). For intake of vitamin and mineral
supplements, information on duration of
use can be readily collected and can be critical; for example, and as expected biologically, for vitamin E supplements in relation
to coronary heart disease risk (Rimm et al.,
1993; Stampfer et al., 1993) and for vitamin C supplements in relation to risk of
cataracts (Hankinson et al., 1992) the associations were limited to longer term
users.

Prospective studies provide important
additional means of assessing temporal relationships with diet. As described by
Rothman (1986), baseline data on current
diet can be examined in relation to disease
incidence at various follow-up periods; under the reasonable assumption that diet
varies over time, the maximum relative risk
should provide information on the true induction period. The limitation of this approach is largely practical as few cohorts
will be sufficiently large to provide statistically stable estimates of risk during multiple time periods. For example, if only recent exposure is important, the study must
be sufficiently large to detect an association
within a few years of the dietary assessment. Prospective studies with replicate dietary assessment provide the opportunity
to examine various intervals between dietary intake and disease diagnosis with
much greater power; for example, the effect of recent exposure can be examined
during the several years after each dietary
assessment. Further use of multiple measurements is discussed below.

THE USE OF MULTIPLE
DIETARY ASSESSMENTS IN
PROSPECTIVE STUDIES

A powerful feature of cohort studies is the
opportunity to collect repeated dietary data
over time; in the Nurse's Health Study, for
example, five comprehensive dietary assessments were collected between 1980 and
1994. Such repeated measurements of dietary intake provide many possible analytic
opportunities to reduce the effects of measurement error and to evaluate various hypothesized temporal relationships between
the dietary factor and the disease outcome
(Table 13–2). For example, some distinction between short and long induction periods can be made by using either the earliest or the most recent questionnaire, thus
providing much greater power for short induction periods than would be available
with only a baseline questionnaire. A more
detailed evaluation of induction periods
can be made by relating each repeated
questionnaire to incidence of disease during specific categories of induction time
(i.e., 1 to 2 years, 3 to 4 years, 5–9 years,
and so forth), and then combining the results for each specific category from all
questionnaires. As discussed in Chapter 3,
measured changes in diets of individuals
over time are a mix of true variation and
measurement error. Thus, the comparison
of persons whose intakes are consistently
high with those whose intakes are consistently low can provide a strong test of cumulative exposure, as well as both long
and short latency, because it is highly likely
that these persons were truly high or truly
low over long durations. The major limitation of this strategy is the loss of power
due to the exclusion of the many persons
who changed categories and the need to exclude cases that occur before the repeated
measurement if the analyses are to be truly
prospective. To address partially this loss
of power, some intermediate strategies may
be useful; for example, if the hypothesis relates to short latency, those in the highest

Table 13–2. Choice of approaches for using repeated dietary assessments and related hypotheses

Strategy	Hypothesis
Use earliest measure only	Long latency
Use most recent measure	Short latency
Use consistently high vs. consistently low	Cumulative exposure
Use cumulative average measure	Cumulative exposure
Use change in exposure, controlling for baseline	Relatively short latency

category in the most recent assessment, as well as in the one or two highest categories on the previous assessment, can be compared with a similar grouping at low intake. The use of cumulative average measurements (i.e., the average of all measurements for an individual up to the start of each follow-up interval) takes advantage of all prior data and thus should provide a statistically more powerful test of an association of cumulative exposure. This approach deserves further methodologic development, though, to take into account the different degrees of measurement error and information provided at each interval. It is also likely that some of the latent class methods for the use of multiple measurements discussed in Chapter 12 can be applied to longitudinal data; these could also take full advantage of all available data, but this approach has not been fully developed.

Because our understanding of disease etiology is often inadequate to specify a temporal relationship with confidence, the use of several rather than just one analytic strategy to examine various temporal relationships will generally be appropriate. If an association is observed, we can be more confident that a true relationship exists if the relative risk increases with strategies that should provide maximum associations (such as when persons with consistently high intakes are compared with those

having consistently low intakes). Also, clear evidence that an association is strongest with a particular temporal relationship can provide important information on the pathogenetic process and possibilities for intervention. For example, if the strongest relative risk is seen when only the initial measurement is used, and if the association gets weaker when early follow-up is deleted, this would suggest that relatively short-term intervention trials might not be informative or that populations in older age groups might not be appropriate targets of prevention programs. If, on the other hand, no association is observed, the demonstration that this lack of relationship is seen when a full range of temporal relationships is examined provides the most compelling evidence that an important association has not been missed (for example, see Table 13–3 for analysis of the relationship between coffee consumption and risk of coronary heart disease in women).

MULTIVARIATE ANALYSES

Multivariate methods may be particularly important in nutritional epidemiology because dietary factors tend to be intercorrelated, sometimes strongly so. The use of multivariate methods has been discussed in relation to total energy intake (Chapter 11) and anthropometric measurements (Chapter 10). A thorough understanding of these relatively simple relationships can be enlightening because analogous approaches can be used in more complex analyses, and potential pitfalls can also be appreciated. For example, the addition of one variable to a model can dramatically change the biologic meaning of another variable; as noted in Chapter 10, the addition of weight changes the meaning of height to a measure of body composition rather than a measure of overall size. Some general approaches to analyses involving two or more dietary factors are discussed here.

A common reason for using multivariate analysis in a study of diet and disease is to

Table 13–3. Alternative analyses of coffee consumption in relation to risk of coronary heart disease (CHD) in multivariate analysis, relative risk, with 95% confidence interval in parenthesis[a]

Coffee consumption (cups/day)	Overall effect: 1980 coffee intake; total CHD, 1980–1990 (712 cases)	Fatal CHD: 1980 coffee intake; fatal CHD, 1980–1990 (181 cases)	Nonfatal CHD: 1980 coffee intake; nonfatal CHD, 1980–1990 (567 cases)	Long-term effect: 1980 coffee intake, excluding women who changed intake in previous decade; total CHD, 1980–1990 (531 cases)	Acute effect: most recent coffee intake; CHD within next 2 years (457 cases)	Lagged effect: 1980 coffee intake; total CHD, 1984–1990 (477 cases)
0	1.0	1.0	1.0	1.0	1.0	1.0
0.03–0.6	1.15(0.82–1.61)	1.14(0.60–2.16)	1.14(0.78–1.67)	1.22(0.83–1.81)	1.15(0.79–1.67)	1.03(0.67–1.58)
0.7–1	0.82(0.62–1.08)	0.92(0.56–1.50)	0.77(0.56–1.06)	0.75(0.54–1.03)	0.82(0.58–1.15)	0.92(0.66–1.27)
2–3	0.88(0.71–1.09)	0.72(0.48–1.09)	0.92(0.72–1.17)	0.78(0.61–1.00)	1.03(0.79–1.34)	0.85(0.66–1.11)
4–5	0.96(0.76–1.21)	0.68(0.42–1.10)	1.05(0.81–1.37)	0.91(0.69–1.19)	1.03(0.76–1.40)	1.04(0.78–1.37)
≥6	0.95(0.73–1.26)	0.81(0.48–1.39)	1.00(0.73–1.36)	0.91(0.66–1.24)	1.26(0.86–1.83)	0.84(0.59–1.18)
p, trend	0.77	0.11	0.65	0.26	0.48	0.47

[a]Model includes the following: age (5-year categories); time period; body mass index (five categories); cigarette smoking (never, past, and current smoking of 1 to 14, 15 to 24, and ≥25 cigarettes per day); menopausal status (premenopausal, postmenopausal without hormone replacement, postmenopausal with past hormone replacement, postmenopausal with current hormone replacement); parental history of myocardial infarction before 60 years of age; multiple vitamin use; vitamin E supplement use; alcohol consumption (four categories); and history of diabetes, hypertension, and hypercholesterolemia.

From Willett et al., 1996.

address the question of whether an observed association between a specific dietary factor and disease risk is only secondary to its correlation with another, truly causal dietary factor. A standard approach is simply to include both variables together in the same model; for example, vitamin C might be added to a model in which dietary fiber has been shown to be predictive of a disease. As the focus will typically be on dietary composition rather than on absolute amounts (see Chapter 11), the specific nutrients should usually be expressed as energy-adjusted residuals or nutrient densities, and total energy should be included as a term unless it is unrelated to disease risk. Often, many possible alternative dietary factors could be considered as potential confounding variables, and the temptation may be to simply include these all simultaneously in a model. For example, in addition to vitamin C, we might want to consider beta-carotene, folic acid, and vitamin E as potential confounders. A problem with including a large number of dietary factors simultaneously is that the remaining independent variation in the primary dietary factor (fiber in this case) may become quite small because, collectively, the other variables can account for almost all of its variation. This will be manifested by a large confidence interval, indicating that the analysis is essentially uninformative. The calculation of residuals can also be informative regarding the degree of independent variation (see Chapter 11. In this example, an ordinary multiple regression model could be fit with dietary fiber as the dependent variable and with demographic variables, standard risk factors, and vitamin C, beta-carotene, folic acid, and vitamin E as independent variables. The residuals for dietary fiber could then be examined to evaluate whether the degree of variation remaining was of interest; most likely it would not be.

An alternative strategy is to conduct a series of analyses including standard non-dietary risk factors (base model) and with two dietary factors at a time (i.e., dietary fiber and each of the other nutrients, one at a time. In this process, it may be possible to eliminate several or all alternative variables by showing that they have no independent association with disease and that the association with the primary variable remains. If several variables with independent association remain, models with three nutrients may be attempted. There is no clear limit as to the number of nutrients that may be included simultaneously as this will depend on their intercorrelation as well as size of the dataset. However, because many dietary variables are strongly correlated with many others, the maximum number is likely to be modest before confidence intervals became uninformatively wide.

Another common situation arises when one or more dietary factors are subcomponents of another, such as saturated, monounsaturated, and polyunsaturated fat, which are the components of total fat. Entering all four variables simultaneously is impossible as they are redundant; the various options depend on the question to be addressed. In some ways the analytic issues are analogous to those discussed in Chapter 11 relating to the adjustment of nutrients for total energy intake. However, the analogy is not complete because a central biologic argument for holding total energy intake constant (by including it as a term in the model) is that total energy intake for an individual is physiologically fixed within narrow limits unless activity and body size are changed. This does not apply here because intakes of fat (and other nutrients) have little physiological constraint.

Several options, using types of fat as an example, are listed in Table 13–4. In all of these models, total energy intake is accounted for, making them "isocaloric." Model 1a is a standard multivariate model and does address the independent effect of saturated fat. With total fat held constant, this may also be considered a substitution model (i.e., does substituting saturated fat for other types of fat influence disease

Table 13–4. "Isocaloric" models for assessing independent contributions of specific types of fat to disease risk

---

Is saturated fat intake related to disease risk independent of total fat intake? Or, does substituting saturated fat for other types of fat affect disease risk?

1a. Total fat + sat fat + energy
1b. Total fat$_{res\ E}$ + sat fat$_{res\ total\ fat}$ + energy
1c. Total fat/E + sat fat/E + energy
2a. Total fat + sat fat + poly fat + energy
2b. Total fat$_{res\ E}$ + sat fat$_{res\ total\ fat}$ + poly fat$_{res\ total\ fat}$ + energy
2c. Total fat/E + sat fat/E + poly fat/E + energy

Is saturated fat intake related to disease risk independent of monounsaturated or polyunsaturated fat intake?

3a. Sat fat + mono fat + energy
3b. Sat fat$_{res\ E}$ + mono fat$_{res\ E}$ + poly fat$_{res\ E}$ + energy
3c. Sat fat/E + mono fat/E + poly fat/E + energy

---

risk?). In this model, the term for total fat no longer has the biologic meaning of total fat because a major component, saturated fat, is included separately; its meaning then becomes mono-and polyunsaturated fat. In model 1b, the residual from the regression of energy-adjusted saturated fat on energy-adjusted total fat is included. This will provide the same coefficient for saturated fat as in model 1a, but the full biologic meaning of total fat is retained. Thus, this model describes disease risk in relation both to the total fat composition of the diet and to the type of fat. In model 1c, the term for saturated fat, expressed as a nutrient density, can be interpreted as substituting a certain percentage of energy from saturated fat for the same amount of other types of fat. Here, the term for total fat as a nutrient density reflects primarily the energy density of mono- and polyunsaturated fats.

Models 2a, 2b, and 2c are analogous to the above, but more specifically address the substitution of saturated fat for monounsaturated fat because polyunsaturated fat is included as a separate term. By exchanging monounsaturated fat for poly-

unsaturated fat in the models, the effect of substituting saturated for polyunsaturated fat can be addressed. These models can also be used for testing the general question: Does the type of fat add independently to the prediction of disease above and beyond total fat? The formal test statistic is calculated from the difference in log likelihoods for the models with and without the terms for the specific types of fat.

Models 3a, 3b, and 3c are not fat substitution models because the total fat composition of the diet is not constrained. These models address a somewhat different issue: Are each of the types of fat, substituted for other sources of energy, independently associated with disease risk? If two or more types of fat are predictive of disease, this would strengthen the hypothesis that fat per se is predictive of disease. This is a much stronger, positive statement than could be derived from a nonsignificant coefficient for saturated fat in models 1a–c because the lack of significance could be due to inadequate power. The difference in coefficients for saturated and monounsaturated fats in these models would be equal to the coefficient for saturated fat in the analogous models 2a–c. Also, a formal test for the difference in coefficients for saturated and monounsaturated fat in these models (which would require a calculation of the pooled variance of the difference using the variance–covariance matrix from the model) would be equivalent to the test of significance for saturated fat in models 2a–c.

Another common example of a dietary factor with nested subcomponents is alcohol intake, where the question frequently arises whether an observed association is due to a certain type of alcoholic beverage. This application, including complexities arising from nonlinear relationships between alcohol consumption and disease risk, has been discussed by Kimball et al. (1992) and Kimball and Friedman (1992).

The interpretation of multivariate analyses including two or more dietary factors should always be tempered by knowledge that none of the dietary variables are measured perfectly. Moreover, the degree of measurement error may vary among different dietary factors. Because of imperfect measurement, there will be less certainty about the independent effects of specific dietary factors than there appears to be in traditional multivariate analyses (Clayton, 1992). Moreover, one dietary factor may appear to be the true predictor and the other a confounder only because the former is better measured. If data are available from validation studies, these problems can be addressed using the multivariate measurement error methods discussed in Chapter 12.

EMPIRICAL DIETARY SCORES

Two traditional methods of combining data on intakes of various foods have been (1) to compute nutrient intakes using food composition tables and (2) to create food groups based on similarities in nutrient content. Use of global scores to describe dietary patterns or quality has also been suggested (Kant et al., 1995; Kennedy et al., 1995; Kant, 1996). A variety of strategies based on empirical observations are possible.

Factor Analysis

Factor analysis can be used to identify two or more uncorrelated dietary patterns based on foods that tend to be used (or avoided) by the same persons (Jacobson and Stanton, 1986). A score is created for each person for each factor by assigning weights to their frequency of use of each food. Once the scores are computed for each person, their relation to risk of disease can be examined. Using this approach, Randall et al. (1990) identified nine factors based on responses to a 110-item food-frequency questionnaire. An examination of the foods contributing to each factor reveals that both nutritional similarities and behavioral patterns determine their content. For example, the factor labeled "fruit" contains beer as an item (with a negative coefficient), and the factor labeled

"staple vegetables" contains hot dogs. When applied to a case–control study of diet and colon cancer, several factors were more strongly associated with risk in men than were nutrient intakes (Randall et al., 1992). However, the findings were not consistent across gender.

The role of factor analysis or other multivariate methods, such as principal components or cluster analysis, to create scores for dietary patterns in nutritional epidemiology remains unclear. In contrast to calculations of nutrient intakes, there is no biologic basis for these scores, their use is unlikely to enhance biologic understanding of diet and disease relationships, and the scores may not even be sufficiently clear to provide dietary guidance. This approach may be useful for describing the intercorrelation of foods and thus the identification of potential confounders. It is most likely to be helpful, if at all, in preliminary data exploration, particularly when few a priori hypotheses exist.

Empirically Selected Variable Score

A tempting strategy for developing a prediction score is to examine the relation of each food (or nutrient) with risk of disease, pick the significant associations, and create a summary score comprised of these variables. Such a strategy has been used by Farchi et al. (1994) and Manousos et al. (1983). The problem with this approach can be appreciated by considering that, if 100 foods are examined as disease predictors, by chance alone about five will be statistically significant. A score based on these five variables will be extremely significantly predictive of disease, all on the basis of chance. A similar problem arises using stepwise regression to create a predictive score from a large number of potential variables. Of course, the scores derived from these procedures may have some true predictive value, but this requires confirmation in a separate dataset. One common strategy for cross-validation is to divide the dataset into halves, create an empirical prediction score in one half (training set) and evaluate the score in the other half (test or validation set). More statistically efficient alternatives for cross-validation exist, such as the jack knife, which involve successively leaving out one observation and fitting the model with the remaining data to predict the omitted observation. As with factor analysis, these approaches may not lead to enhanced biologic understanding or even clear dietary guidance.

Nutrient Prediction Models Using an Independent Gold Standard

In calculating nutrient intakes from a food-frequency questionnaire, foods are weighted by their frequency of use and their nutrient content using a food composition database. Ideally, the weight would also take into account the validity with which intake of each food was assessed and the bioavailability of the nutrient from each food. This additional weighting can, in principle, be accomplished by using an independent quantitative assessment of nutrient intake or a biochemical indicator of nutrient intake in a sample of the population.

Diet records, which are often used to assess the validity of a food-frequency instrument, could be used as an independent estimate of true nutrient intake to develop a prediction score from foods on a food-frequency questionnaire. To do so, the nutrient intake from the diet record would be used as the independent variable in a multiple regression analysis with all foods from the food-frequency questionnaire being allowed to enter in a stepwise multiple regression analysis. Foods that explain the most between-person variance in the nutrient intake enter first. However, if the validity of a food item on the questionnaire is low, for example, if it was worded poorly, it should not contribute appreciably to the prediction of the nutrient. The nutrient score based on the coefficients from the stepwise regression could then be computed for each person and used in analyses predicting disease. Although this is an attractive approach, a main limitation is that

a large number of subjects are needed to provide stable estimates of regression coefficients, probably considerably larger than most validation studies. Also, the regression coefficients will reflect in part the respondent characteristics—which is a desirable feature because they may influence validity—but this means that they may not be generalizable to other populations. In one evaluation of this approach (Feskanich et al., 1994), the nutrients calculated with empirical regression coefficients did not perform as well in a different population as those derived from food composition tables when compared with another independent estimate of nutrient intake. However, the approach needs further evaluation. A related strategy would be to conduct the analysis on the basis of foods (i.e., to regress intake of each food [one at a time] from the diet record on intake of that food from the food-frequency questionnaire to derive an additional weighting factor). Foods with perfect validity would have a weight of 1, and those with poor validity would be weighted lower. Intakes of nutrients would then be calculated incorporating the weighting factor, as well as frequency and nutrient content. This approach does not appear to have been used or evaluated.

Instead of using diet records or recalls as a standard to develop a prediction score from foods on a food-frequency questionnaire, a biochemical indicator could serve as the standard. Such an approach would take into account factors such as the bioavailability of the nutrient in each food and the validity of each food item. This method was used by Romieu and colleagues (1990) to develop prediction scores for vitamin E (alpha-tocopherol) and beta-carotene using plasma levels of these nutrients as the standard. Using a cross-validation approach, the empirical prediction for beta-carotene did not outperform the calculated intake using the standard food composition database approach, thus providing support for the validity of the database. However, for vitamin E, the empirical coefficients were superior, raising doubts about the adequacy of the database. Giovannucci and colleagues (1995) used such an approach to develop a prediction score for lycopene intake using plasma lycopene levels as a standard. Based on other data, there was reason to believe that lycopene from raw tomato products is poorly absorbed, but its bioavailability is enhanced by cooking, particularly in the presence of fat. Indeed, Giovannucci et al. (1995) found that cooked tomato products predicted plasma lycopene levels better than did raw tomato products; so this was incorporated into the empirical prediction equation. When this empirical score was used to examine the relation between lycopene intake and risk of prostate cancer in the total cohort, a stronger association was observed than using the standard calculation of intake. These approaches deserve further evaluation as they may greatly enhance the value of biochemical validation studies by using them to improve, as well as to assess, the validity of dietary questionnaires. As noted above, the size of the substudy is a critical issue because it determines the precision of coefficients, but the desirable size is not clear.

SUBGROUP ANALYSES AND INTERACTIONS

Although the overall main effects of dietary factors will generally be the primary focus of analyses in nutritional epidemiology, we know from extensive metabolic and experimental evidence that the effects of most dietary factors are likely to vary among subgroups, depending on the intake of other dietary factors and characteristics of the subjects. This issue, generally known as *effect modification* or *interaction*, has been discussed extensively in the epidemiologic literature (Rothman, 1986; Thompson, 1991). A fundamental issue is whether the interaction should be assessed on an absolute scale (whether the rate difference is constant across categories of the third variable) or relative scale (whether the rate ra-

tio or relative risk is constant across these categories); this is not discussed here (for further detail, see Rothman, 1986).

One general concern has been that an extensive search for interactions and associations within subgroups of other variables creates a high likelihood of statistically significant associations arising by chance. Indeed, the epidemiologic literature is replete with subgroup findings that have, in the end, not been reproducible. An example of how this can arise was observed in the pooled analysis of prospective studies of dietary fat and breast cancer described in Chapter 16 (Hunter et al., 1997). In one cohort study, a strong positive association between dietary fat and breast cancer was noted among women with an early age at first birth and an inverse association was seen in those with a later age at first birth; a formal test for interaction was highly statistically significant. The investigators could have easily been tempted to publish a report based on this interaction, which would have required multiple additional publications to confirm or refute the finding. Fortunately, the same interaction was being evaluated in all seven cohorts simultaneously, and it was immediately apparent that the finding was not reproducible. Indeed, in one other study a nearly significant interaction was seen for the same covariate, but in the opposite direction. As noted in the earlier discussion of multiple comparisons, various strategies have been suggested, such as requiring smaller p values for statistical significance. Although there is no simple solution for evaluating subgroups with confidence, this should not deter investigators from examining them. Some subgroup analyses are so important a priori that they must be examined, and failure to find evidence of effect modification may even cast doubt on an association. For example, if vitamin A reduces the risk of breast cancer, a protective effect of vitamin A supplements should be greatest among those with low vitamin A intakes from their diets (this was the case in the study of Hunter and colleagues, 1993).

Also, if obesity increases the risk of breast cancer among postmenopausal women by raising endogenous estrogen levels, the effect should be strongest among women who never used estrogen replacement therapy (Huang et al., 1997).

When two dietary factors act by a similar mechanism, it may be difficult to observe an association by examining only one of these variables at a time; an examination of joint exposures may be most powerful. As an example, risk of noninsulin-dependent diabetes was found to be particularly high among men who consumed both a high glycemic load and a low cereal fiber intake (Salmeron et al., 1997a); this finding was reproduced in women (Salmeron et al., 1997b). Purely exploratory analysis of associations among subgroups of known risk factors is also a good practice even when little a priori reason exists because new knowledge may be gained. However, such explorations without strong prior expectations should be clearly described as such, and the reader should be skeptical of any findings. Some would suggest not reporting p values in such circumstances. Ultimately, the only fail-safe protection against spurious conclusions based on subgroups is demonstration of reproducibility, perhaps over time within the same study and, most importantly, in other independent datasets.

ERROR CORRECTION

Methods to correct observed associations for errors in measurement of exposure variables, discussed in Chapter 12, are becoming more widely employed in nutritional epidemiology. These methods require data on either reproducibility or validity; this information is now being collected as part of many large studies, so future reports will even more routinely include analysis accounting for measurement error.

The most common use of error correction procedures is the de-attenuation of correlation coefficients, probably because this only requires replicates of one or both

measurements being compared. This procedure has become quite routine in validation studies, where a small number of days of diet records or 24-hour recall data are collected as an independent representation of true long-term intake. Studies of diet in relation to blood pressure have also used such methods; in this case, both variables are often subject to substantial within-person variation (Dyer et al., 1997).

In studies of disease incidence, the calculation of relative risks and confidence intervals adjusted for measurement error has usually been done as a secondary analysis (Willett et al., 1992; Hunter et al., 1996; Rimm et al., 1996). These analyses address three interrelated objectives: first, to obtain the best estimate of the relative risk after accounting for attenuation due to imperfect measurement of the primary exposure; second, to obtain the best estimate of the true confidence interval, which is particularly important when little association is seen, because the central question becomes whether the adjusted confidence intervals are sufficiently narrow to be informative; and third, to account for residual confounding by imperfectly measured covariates. These issues are so central to nutritional epidemiology, and to epidemiology in general, that it is possible that the adjustment procedures may eventually be incorporated in the primary analyses. It is important, however, that these are not done in a purely mechanical manner as the measurements of true intake used in validation studies are never perfect measurements themselves, and the degree to which they are imperfect should always be considered.

ROLE OF META-ANALYSIS AND POOLED ANALYSIS IN NUTRITIONAL EPIDEMIOLOGY

The role of meta-analysis for systematically combining the results of published randomized trials has become routine (Sacks et al., 1992; Mosteller and Colditz, 1996), but its place in epidemiology has been controversial (Greenland, 1994; Petitti, 1994; Shapiro, 1994a,b) despite widespread use in social sciences. Some have argued that the combining of data from randomized trials is appropriate because statistical power is increased without concern for validity since the comparison groups have been randomized, but that in observational epidemiology the issue of validity is determined largely by confounding and bias rather than limitations of statistical power. Thus, the great statistical precision obtained by the combining of data may be misleading because the findings may still be invalid. On the other hand, the combining of all available epidemiologic data can be of great value, particularly when a body of evidence becomes substantial and difficult to assimilate at once and if the potential for bias is not ignored. Greenland (1993) has emphasized the potential value for meta-analyses that do not simply compute a summary measure of association, but rather that also examine possible explanations for heterogeneity among studies according to characteristics of study populations or design features. For example, Longnecker et al. (1988) found that the association between alcohol consumption and breast cancer tended to be stronger in prospective than in case–control studies. Colditz and colleagues (1995) have expanded on the use of meta-analysis to examine possible reasons for heterogeneity and also noted that these summaries can address questions not posed in the original studies, such as details of dose–response relationships.

An alternative to the combining of published epidemiologic data is to pool and analyze the primary data from all available studies on a topic that meet specified criteria (Howe et al., 1989; Whittemore et al., 1992; Hunter et al., 1996). Ideally, this should involve the active collaboration of the original investigators, who are fully familiar with the data and its limitations. Because of the complexity of dietary data, this approach has great advantages in nu-

tritional epidemiology and can address many limitations of individual studies. Any attempt to combine published data on diet and disease is immediately confronted with the problem that various investigators have usually used different approaches for presenting their findings that make them difficult to combine. Sometimes relative risks are given for arbitrary quantiles and other times for specified increments using continuous variables. Adjustments for total energy intake are often done using a variety of methods or not at all, and the inclusion of other covariates typically differs among studies. When individual foods are examined, those with significant and expected associations are much more likely to be reported, in part because the large number of foods precludes reporting on all. A major advantage of pooling primary data is that all data can be analyzed simultaneously using common approaches and definitions of exposure. This can produce insight that could not be achieved from published reports. For example, in a pooled analysis of case–control studies of diet and colon cancer, it was found that total and saturated fat intakes were not associated with disease risk when adjusted for total energy intake (Howe et al., 1997); this was not apparent from the published reports. Using a variety of approaches for all datasets simultaneously can also potentially facilitate consensus among investigators regarding complex issues.

In a pooled analysis, the range of dietary factors that can be addressed can be considerably greater than in the separate analyses because any one study will have few subjects in the extremes of intake and, sometimes, because the studies will vary in distribution of dietary factors. For example, in the pooled analysis of prospective studies of diet and breast cancer, it was possible to evaluate associations from less than 15% to more than 45% of energy from fat, which was a far greater range than possible in the individual studies. Although few pooled analyses have been conducted at the level of specific foods, this can provide a less biased assessment of relationships based on the total body of evidence. As already discussed, evaluation of the consistency of findings in subgroup analyses across studies will reduce the likelihood of overinterpreting findings that may have occurred by chance.

The data quality may differ among studies due to differences in the questionnaires used, study designs, or populations. As discussed in Chapter 12, this can be addressed if each study includes a validation/calibration substudy so that corrections can be made for the study-specific measurement error, and the studies with more valid assessments of diet can be given more weight (Hunter et al., 1996). The advantages of pooled analyses in nutritional epidemiology are so substantial that this should become common practice for important issues.

SUMMARY

Datasets on diet and disease are rapidly growing in number, size, and complexity, which creates many challenges and opportunities for analysis and the presentation of findings. Use of dietary data as both categorical and continuous variables will be helpful, and carefully conducted multivariate analyses can provide additional insight into the effects of diet. Nutrients and foods should be evaluated and presented simultaneously. The temporal relation between dietary intake and diagnosis of disease is likely to be critical; specific examination of alternative temporal relationships will reduce the likelihood that important associations are missed and can provide insight into the pathogenesis of disease. Error correction should become a standard part of analysis; this will require the collection of necessary data on validity and reproducibility. Finally, pooled analyses of important diet and disease relationships using all data meeting specified criteria can greatly enhance understanding of the effects of diet on disease.

REFERENCES

Barnett, V., and T. Lewis (1994). *Outliers in Statistical Data*. New York: Wiley & Sons.

Caan, B., R. A. Hiatt, and A. M. Owen (1991). Mailed dietary surveys: Response rates, error rates, and the effect of omitted food items on nutrient values. *Epidemiology 2*, 430–436.

Clayton, D. G. (1992). Models for the analysis of cohort and case-control studies with inaccurately measured exposures. In Dwyer, J. H., Feinlieb, M., and Lipsert, P., et al. (eds.): *Statistical Models for Longitudinal Studies of Health*. New York: Oxford Press, pp. 301–331.

Colditz, G. A., E. Burdick, and F. Mosteller (1995). Heterogeneity in meta-analysis of data from epidemiologic studies: A commentary. *Am J Epidemiol 142*, 371–382.

Durrleman, S., and R. Simon (1989). Flexible regression models with cubic splines. *Statist Med 8*, 551–561.

Dyer, A., P. Elliott, D. Chee, and J. Stamler (1997). Urinary biochemical markers of dietary intake in the INTERSALT Study. *Am J Clin Nutr 65(suppl)*, S1246–S1253.

FAO/WHO/UNU ad hoc Expert Consultation on Energy and Protein Requirements (1985). *Energy and Protein Requirements. Report of a Joint FAO/WHO/UNU Expert Consultation*. WHO Technical Report No. 724. Geneva: World Health Organization.

Farchi, G., F. Fidanza, S. Mariotti, and A. Menotti (1994). Is diet an independent risk factor for mortality? 20 year mortality in the Italian rural cohorts of the Seven Countries Study. *Eur J Clin Nutr 48*, 19–29.

Feskanich, D., J. Marshall, E. B. Rimm, L. B. Litin, and W. C. Willett (1994). Simulated validation of a brief food frequency questionnaire. *Ann Epidemiol 4*, 181–187.

Giovannucci, E., A. Ascherio, E. B. Rimm, M. J. Stampfer, G. A. Colditz, and W. C. Willett (1995). Intake of carotenoids and retinol in relation to risk of prostate cancer. *JNCI 87*, 1767–1776.

Greenland, S. (1993). A meta-analysis of coffee, myocardial infarction, and coronary death. *Epidemiology 4*, 366–374.

Greenland, S. (1994). Can meta-analysis be salvaged? *Am J Epidemiol 140*, 783–787.

Greenland, S. (1995). Dose–response and trend analysis in epidemiology: Alternatives to categorical analysis. *Epidemiology 6*, 356–365.

Hankinson, S. E., M. J. Stampfer, J. M. Seddon,

G. A. Colditz, B. A. Rosner, F. E. Speizer, and W. C. Willett (1992). Nutrient intake and cataract extraction in women: A prospective study. *BMJ 305*, 335–339.

Harrell, F. E. Jr., K. L. Lee, and B. G. Pollock (1988). Regression models in clinical studies: Determining relationships between predictors and response. *JNCI 80*, 1198–1202.

Hastie, T., and R. Tibshirani (1987). Generalized additive models: Some applications. *J Am Statist Assoc 82*, 371–386.

Howe, G. R., K. J. Aronson, E. Benito, R. Castelleto, J. Cornee, S. Duffy, R. P. Gallagher, J. M. Iscovich, J. Dengao, R. Kaaks, G. A. Kune, S. Kune, H. P. Lee, M. Lee, A. B. Miller, R. K. Peters, J. D. Potter, E. Riboli, M. L. Slattery, D. Trichopoulos, A. Tuyns, A. Tzonou, L. E. Watson, A. S. Whittemore, and A. H. Wu Williams, et al. (1997). The relationship between dietary fat intake and risk of colorectal cancer—Evidence from the combined analysis of 13 case–control studies. *Cancer Causes Control 8*, 215–228.

Howe, G. R., J. D. Burch, A. M. Chiarelli, H. A. Risch, and B. C. K. Choi (1989). An exploratory case–control study of brain tumors in children. *Cancer Res 49*, 4349–4352.

Huang Z. P., S. E. Hankinson, G. A. Colditz, M. J. Stampfer, D. J. Hunter, J. E. Manson, C. H. Hennekens, B. Rosner, F. E. Speizer, W. C. Willett, (1997). Dual effects of weight and weight gain on breast cancer risk, *JAMA, 278*, 1407–1411.

Hunter, D. J., J. E. Manson, G. A. Colditz, M. J. Stampfer, B. Rosner, C. H. Hennekens, F. E. Speizer, and W. C. Willett (1993). A prospective study of the intake of vitamins C, E and A and the risk of breast cancer. *N Engl J Med 329*, 234–440.

Hunter, D. J., D. Spiegelman, H. O. Adami, L. Beeson, P. A. van den Brandt, A. R. Folsom, G. E. Fraser, R. A. Goldbohm, S. Graham, G. R. Howe, L. H. Kushi, J. R. Marshall, A. McDermott, A. B. Miller, F. E. Speizer, A. Wolk, S.-S. Yaun, and W. C. Willett (1996). Cohort studies of fat intake and the risk of breast cancer: A pooled analysis. *N Engl J Med 334*, 356–361.

Hunter, D. J., D. Spiegelman, H. O. Adami, P. A. van den Brandt, A. R. Folsom, R. A. Goldbohm, S. Graham, G. R. Howe, L. H. Kushi, J. R. Marshall, A. B. Miller, F. E. Speizer, W. C. Willett, A. Wolk, and S. S. Yaun (1997). Non-dietary factors as risk factors for breast cancer, and as effect modifiers of the association of fat intake and

risk of breast cancer. *Cancer Causes Control 8*, 49–56.

Jacobson, H. N., and J. L. Stanton (1986). Pattern analysis in nutrition research. *Clin Nutr 5*, 249–253.

James, W. P. (1985). Basal metabolic rate: Comments on the new equations. *Hum Nutr Clin Nutr 39(suppl 1)*, 92–96.

Kant, A. K. (1996). Indexes of overall diet quality: A review. *J Am Diet Assoc 96*, 785–791.

Kant, A. K., A. Schatzkin, and R. G. Ziegler (1995). Dietary diversity and subsequent cause-specific mortality in the NHANES I Epidemiologic Follow-Up Study. *J Am Coll Nutr 14*, 233–238.

Kennedy, E. T., J. Ohls, S. Carlson, and K. Fleming (1995). The Healthy Eating Index: Design and applications. *J Am Diet Assoc 95*, 1103–1108.

Kimball, A. W., and L. A. Friedman (1992). Alcohol consumption regression models for distinguishing between beverage type effects and beverage preference effects. *Am J Epidemiol 135*, 1279–1286.

Kimball, A. W., L. A. Friedman, and R. D. Moore (1992). Nonlinear modeling of alcohol consumption for analysis of beverage type effects and beverage preference effects. *Am J Epidemiol 135*, 1287–1292.

Klesges, R. C., L. H. Eck, and J. W. Ray (1995). Who underreports dietary intake in a dietary recall? Evidence from the Second National Health and Nutrition Examination Survey. *J Consult Clin Psych 63*, 438–444.

Land, C. E. (1995). Studies of cancer and radiation dose among atomic bomb survivors. The example of breast cancer. *JAMA 274*, 402–407.

Longnecker, M. P., J. A. Berlin, M. J. Orza, and T. C. Chalmers (1988). A meta-analysis of alcohol consumption in relation to risk of breast cancer. *JAMA 260*, 652–656.

Manousos, O., N. E. Day, D. Trichopoulos, F. Gerovassilis, A. Tzanou, and A. Polychronopoulou (1983). Diet and colorectal cancer: A case–control study in Greece. *Int J Cancer 32*, 1–5.

Mosteller, F., and G. A. Colditz (1996). Understanding research synthesis (meta-analysis). *Annu Rev Public Health 17*, 1–23.

Petitti, D. B. (1994). Of babies and bathwater. *Am J Epidemiol 140*, 779–782.

Pryer, J., E. Brunner, P. Elliott, R. Nichols, H. Dimond, and M. Marmot (1995). Who complied with COMA 1984 dietary fat recommendations among a nationally representative sample of British adults in 1986–7 and what did they eat? *Eur J Clin Nutr 49*, 718–728.

Randall, E., J. R. Marshall, J. Brasure, and S. Graham (1992). Dietary patterns and colon cancer in western New York. *Nutr Cancer 18*, 265–276.

Randall, E., J. R. Marshall, S. Graham, and J. Brasure (1990). Patterns in food use and their associations with nutrient intakes. *Am J Clin Nutr 52*, 739–745.

Rimm, E. B., A. Ascherio, E. Giovannucci, D. Spiegelman, M. J. Stampfer, and W. C. Willett (1996). Vegetable, fruit, and cereal fiber intake and risk of coronary heart disease among men. *JAMA 275*, 447–451.

Rimm, E. B., E. L. Giovannucci, M. J. Stampfer, G. A. Colditz, L. B. Litin, and W. C. Willett (1992). Reproducibility and validity of a expanded self-administered semiquantitative food frequency questionnaire among male health professionals. *Am J Epidemiol 135*, 1114–1126.

Rimm, E. B., M. J. Stampfer, A. Ascherio, E. Giovannucci, G. A. Colditz, and W. C. Willett (1993). Vitamin E consumption and the risk of coronary heart disease in men. *N Engl J Med 328*, 1450–1456.

Romieu, I., M. J. Stampfer, W. S. Stryker, M. Hernandez, L. Kaplan, A. Sober, B. Rosner, and W. C. Willett (1990). Food predictors of plasma beta-carotene and alpha-tocopherol: Validation of a food frequency questionnaire. *Am J Epidemiol 131*, 864–876.

Rosner, B. (1983). Percentage points for a generalized ESD many-outlier procedure. *Technometrics 25*, 165–172.

Rothman, K. J. (1986). *Modern Epidemiology.* Boston, MA: Little, Brown and Company.

Rothman, K. J. (1990). No adjustments are needed for multiple comparisons. *Epidemiology 1*, 43–46.

Rothman, K. J., L. L. Moore, and M. R. Singer, et al. (1995). Teratogenicity of high vitamin A intake. *N Engl J Med 333*, 1369–1373.

Sacks, H. S., J. Berrier, D. Reitman, D. Pagano, and T. C. Chalmers (1992). Meta-analysis of randomized control trials: An update of the quality and methodology. In Bailar, J. C., and Mosteller, F. (eds.): *Medical Uses of Statistics.* Boston MA: NEJM Books, pp. 427–442.

Salmeron, J., A. Ascherio, E. B. Rimm, G. A. Colditz, D. Spiegelman, D. J. Jenkins, M. J. Stampfer, A. L. Wing, and W. C. Willett (1997a). Dietary fiber, glycemic load, and risk of NIDDM in Men. *Diabetes Care 20*, 545–550.

Salmeron, J., J. E. Manson, M. J. Stampfer, G. A. Colditz, A. L. Wing, and W. C. Willett (1997b). Dietary fiber, glycemic load,

and risk of non-insulin–dependent diabetes mellitus in women. *JAMA 277*, 472–477.

Savitz, D. A., and A. F. Olshan (1995). Multiple comparisons and related issues in the interpretation of epidemiologic data. *Am J Epidemiol 142*, 904–908.

Schofield, C. (1985a). An annotated bibliography of source material for basal metabolic rate data. *Hum Nutr Clin Nutr 39(suppl 1)*, 42–91.

Schofield, W. N. (1985b). Predicting basal metabolic rate, new standards and review of previous work. *Hum Nutr Clin Nutr 39(suppl 1)*, 5–41.

Shapiro, S. (1994a). Is there is or is there ain't no baby?: Dr. Shapiro replies to Drs. Petitti and Greenland. *Am J Epidemiol 140*, 788–791.

Shapiro, S. (1994b). Meta-analysis/Shmeta-analysis. *Am J Epidemiol 140*, 771–778.

Shetty, P. S., C. J. K. Henry, A. E. Black, and A. M. Prentice (1996). Energy requirements of adults: An update on basal metabolic rates (BMRs) and physical activity levels (PALs). *Eur J Clin Nutr 50(suppl)*, S11–S23.

Siscovick, D. S., T. E. Raghunathan, I. King, S. Weinman, K. G. Wicklund, J. Albright, V. Bovbjerg, P. Arbogast, H. Smith, L. H. Kushi, L. A. Cobb, M. K. Copass, B. M. Psaty, R. Lemaitre, R. Retzlaff, M. Childs, and R. H. Knopp (1995). Dietary intake and cell membrane levels of long-chain N-3 polyunsaturated fatty acids and the risk of primary cardiac arrest. *JAMA 274*, 1363–1367.

Smith, W. T., K. L. Webb, and P. F. Heywood (1994). The implications of underreporting in dietary studies. *Austral J Public Health 18*, 311–314.

Smith-Warner, S. A., D. Spiegelman, S.-S. Yaun, H. O. Adami, P. A. van den Brandt, A. R. Folsom, R. A. Goldbohm, S. Graham, G. R. Howe, J. R. Marshall, A. B. Miller, J. D. Potter, F. E. Speizer, W. C. Willett, A. Wolk, and D. J. Hunter (1998). Alcohol and breast cancer in women: A pooled analysis of cohort studies. *JAMA 279*, 535–540.

Stahelin, H. B., K. F. Gey, M. Eichholzer, E. Ludin, F. Bernasconi, J. Thurneysen, and G. Brubacher (1991). Plasma antioxidant vitamins and subsequent cancer mortality in the 12-year follow-up of the prospective Basel Study. *Am J Epidemiol 133*, 766–775.

Stampfer, M. J., C. H. Hennekens, J. E. Manson, G. A. Colditz, B. Rosner, and W. C. Willett (1993). Vitamin E consumption and the risk of coronary disease in women. *N Engl J Med 328*, 1444–1449.

Stryker, W. S., L. A. Kaplan, E. A. Stein, M. J. Stampfer, A. Sober, and W. C. Willett (1988). The relation of diet, cigarette smoking, and alcohol consumption to plasma beta-carotene and alpha-tocopherol levels. *Am J Epidemiol 127*, 283–296.

Thompson, W. D. (1991). Effect modification and the limits of biological inference from epidemiologic data. *J Clin Epidemiol 44*, 221–232.

Toniolo, P., E. Riboli, R. E. Shore, and B. S. Pasternack (1994). Consumption of meat, animal products, protein, and fat and risk of breast cancer: a prospective cohort study in New York. *Epidemiology 5*, 391–397.

Trichopoulos, D. (1990). Is breast cancer initiated in utero? *Epidemiology 1*, 95–96.

Whittemore, A. S., R. Harris, and J. Itnyre (1992). Characteristics relating to ovarian cancer risk: Collaborative analysis of 12 U.S. case–control studies. II. Invasive epithelial ovarian cancers in white women. *Am J Epidemiol 136*, 1184–1203.

Willett, W. C., D. J. Hunter, M. J. Stampfer, G. A. Colditz, J. E. Manson, D. Spiegelman, B. Rosner, C. H. Hennekens, and F. E. Speizer (1992). Dietary fat and fiber in relation to risk of breast cancer: An 8-year follow-up. *JAMA 268*, 2037–2044.

Willett, W. C., M. J. Stampfer, J. E. Manson, G. A. Colditz, B. A. Rosner, F. E. Speizer, and C. H. Hennekens (1996). Coffee consumption and coronary heart disease in women: A ten-year follow-up. *JAMA 275*, 458–462.

Willett, W. C., M. J. Stampfer, J. E. Manson, G. A. Colditz, F. E. Speizer, B. A. Rosner, L. A. Sampson, and C. H. Hennekens (1993). Intake of *trans* fatty acids and risk of coronary heart disease among women. *Lancet 341*, 581–585.

Witte, J. S., S. Greenland, R. W. Haile, and C. L. Bird (1994). Hierarchical regression analysis applied to a study of multiple dietary exposures dietary exposures and breast cancer. *Epidemiology 5*, 612–621.

APPENDIX 13–1.

Equations for predicting basal metabolic rate from body weight (W) in kg[a]

Age range (yr)	kcal/day	SD[b]
Males		
0–3	$60.9 \, W - 54$	53
3–10	$22.7 \, W + 495$	62
10–18	$17.5 \, W + 651$	100
18–30	$15.3 \, W + 679$	151
30–60	$11.6 \, W + 879$	164
>60	$13.5 \, W + 487$	148
Females		
0–3	$61.0 \, W - 51$	61
3–10	$22.5 \, W + 499$	63
10–18	$12.2 \, W + 746$	117
18–30	$14.7 \, W + 496$	121
30–60	$8.7 \, W + 829$	108
>60	$10.5 \, W + 596$	108

[a]Note: Addition of height to equation did not appreciably improve the prediction of basal metabolic rate.

[b]Standard deviation of differences between actual basal metabolic rates predicted estimates.

From FAO/WHO/UNU ad hoc Expert Consultation on Energy and Protein Requirements, 1985.

14

Nutrition Monitoring and Surveillance

TIM BYERS

Monitoring and surveillance efforts are intended to discern population subgroup differences and/or trends in a population over time in diet or nutritional status by making systematic measures that can be repeated. Some reasons to discern trends or to contrast population subgroups require precise measures of population nutritional parameters, while others require only crude nutrition indicators (Thompson and Byers, 1994). The measures that are useful for monitoring and surveillance at the population level are often quite different from those that are useful for assessing the diet or nutritional status of individuals. For example, even though within-person variance might cause a single 24-hour diet recall or a single measure of blood concentration of a nutrient to be an unreliable indicator of the diet or nutritional status of an individual, such measures can produce precise estimates of diet or blood nutrient concentrations that can be useful for contrasting the dietary or nutritional status of population subgroups or for examining trends over time.

Nutrition monitoring and surveillance are more properly seen as goals than as specific methods. The fundamental question of why data are being collected in the first place should drive the design and conduct of any monitoring or surveillance effort. What difference would be made by the data collected? What would be done differently even with perfect knowledge of the nutritional status of everyone? Are there any policy options or nutrition interventions that would be instituted or modified as a result of such knowledge? Honest reflection on the answers to these questions can lead to the development of useful systems for dietary monitoring and surveillance. The methods used for nutrition monitoring and surveillance in various countries, with emphasis on systems now in use in the United States, are reviewed in this chapter.

The distinction between monitoring and

surveillance is subtle. *Monitoring* implies the collection and analysis of quantitatively precise measures from representative samples of a population for the purpose of precisely tracking trends. *Surveillance* implies a system of collection of less precise measures intended to trigger timely interventions in response to the detection of meaningful trends (Thacker and Berkelman, 1988). Nutrition monitoring systems therefore usually assess large, representative samples of the population with accurate measures, such as direct measures of body weight and precise diet recalls, whereas nutrition surveillance systems usually assess samples that are not necessarily representative of the entire population, using more cursory measures, such as self-reported weight and brief food-frequency questioning. Nutrition monitoring data tend to be analyzed as direct estimates of nutritional parameters of larger, national populations in the time frame of years, whereas nutrition surveillance data tend to be analyzed as indirect indicators of nutritional parameters of smaller, local populations in the time frame of months. The distinction, then, between nutrition monitoring and nutrition surveillance is defined by differences in the quantitative accuracy of the measures, by differences in the size of the population studied, and by differences in the timeline of the analysis. These distinctions are subtle, however. In the context of a variety of nutritional data systems, the two terms are understandably often used interchangeably.

NUTRITION MONITORING

Information about dietary determinants and behaviors of people in specific populations is needed by those who wish to make nutrition policy and by those who wish to carry out effective nutrition intervention programs (Kohlmeier et al., 1990; Interagency Board for Nutrition Monitoring and Related Research, 1992; Briefel, 1994; Kuczmarski et al., 1994). On the national level, data from the nutrition

monitoring system provide information to guide policy development for food production and distribution as well as for the setting and tracking of national health goals. At the crudest level, dietary trends can be followed using aggregate data from food production, imports, and exports. This is the so-called food disappearance method, which is based on the "food balance sheets" compiled by the United Nations Food and Agricultural Organization (the United Nations Food and Agricultural Organization publishes the *Agricultural Economics Statistics*, a monthly bulletin). The most important limitations of this method are its dependence on assumptions regarding food wastage and its inability to link food consumption to any characteristics of individuals within the population.

Many nutrition monitoring systems are based on the availability of foods at the household level. In Japan, representative samples of the population have been asked annually since 1950 to complete 3-day records of all foods purchased at the level of the household. Both foods and nutrients are reported every 5 years (Ministry of Health and Welfare [Japan], 1992). In Great Britain, the National Food Survey has employed a food accounting method since 1952 to annually measure food use at the household level (Margetts and Nelson, 1991). In this survey, all foods brought into the sampled households are recorded by survey respondents for a 7-day period. The advantages of the Japanese and British monitoring systems are that similar methods have been used for the past 45 years, but the disadvantages are that intake information for individuals within the household is not known, and food wastage and foods consumed outside the household are not fully accounted. The Total Diet Study is an annual survey by the U.S. Food and Drug Administration to monitor the chemical composition of foods (Interagency Board for Nutrition Monitoring and Related Research, 1992). Diets based on 234 foods purchased from stores selected to be representative of the diets of Americans are blenderized and then assayed for minerals and selected organic and elemental contaminants. Though the Total Diet Study is not a system intended to monitor food choices, it does contribute to information on the composition of foods as purchased and hence reflects trends in the availability of selected minerals and food contaminants.

In the United States, nutritional surveys are based increasingly on individual rather than on household measures (Table 14–1). Nutrition monitoring systems based on measures of individuals generally employ repeated cross-sectional surveys that collect quantitatively precise point-in-time measures, such as anthropometric measures, blood nutrient levels, and dietary intake as reflected by food records or 24-hour diet recalls. The past U.S. Department of Agriculture Nationwide Food Consumption Surveys measured both individual consumption, using recalls and records, and household food use, using a 7-day food record. However, the current on-going U.S.D.A dietary survey (Continuing Survey of Food Intake of Individuals) measures only individual consumption. The use of food records has been dropped from surveys in the United States in recent years, with greater reliance on 24-hour recalls, as these are thought to be more cost efficient and less likely to affect the dietary choices being measured. Although a single 24-hour recall cannot reliably estimate the usual intake of an individual, it can generate a valid estimate of the average intake of a population. The use of at least two 24-hour recalls from survey respondents provides sufficient information to estimate both the central tendencies and the variances of the intakes of foods and nutrients (see Chapter 12).

There are some formidable problems in the interpretation of even the best nutritional monitoring data. The utility of the food-frequency questions in national surveys has been a source of considerable controversy (Block and Subar, 1992; Briefel et al., 1992). Even with the 24-hour re-

call method, changes over time in even subtle details of the methods of data collection or in the nutrient databases that are used can create artifactual changes that are difficult to distinguish from true trends. Caloric intake increased, for instance, by about 200 kcal between National Health and Nutrition Examination Surveys (NHANES) II (1976–1980) and phase I of NHANES III (1989–1991), but because of changes in the probing and coding schemes used in the diet recalls it is not clear whether this represents a true increase in caloric intake in the U.S. population (McDowell et al., 1994).

In the United States, there are many interconnected efforts to systematically collect information about the nutritional status of the population. Since 1990 these activities have been coordinated by the National Nutrition Monitoring System, which is a joint program of the Department of Health and Human Services and the Department of Agriculture (Interagency Board for Nutrition Monitoring and Related Research, 1992; Briefel, 1994; Kuczmarski et al., 1994).

NUTRITION SURVEILLANCE

From the perspective of those at local levels, national nutritional monitoring data lack both representativeness and timeliness. National surveys produce dietary intake estimates that are representative of the national population, but they are not designed to provide measures that are representative of any particular locality. Moreover, analyses of national survey data are often not conducted until several years after data collection. Local dietary surveillance is necessary to provide locally representative and timely measures of any behaviors or nutritional determinants that are needed for planning, targeting, and evaluating nutrition intervention programs.

There is no better example of the immediate utility of high-quality, timely local information than for the purpose of assessing the problems of nutritional deficiencies

Table 14–1. A summary of the major dietary intake surveys conducted in the United States[a]

Survey	Years	Approximate number interviewed	Dietary assessment method
National Health and Nutrition Examination Surveys			
NHANES I	1971–74	28,000	24-hr recall, 19-item food frequency
NHANES II	1976–80	25,000	24-hr recall, 26-item food frequency
NHANES III	1988–94	35,000	24-hr recall, 62-item food frequency
Hispanic Health and Nutrition Examination Survey	1982–84	14,000	24-hr recall, 22-item food frequency
National Health Interview Survey			
HIS, 1987	1987	22,000	60-item food frequency
HIS, 1992	1992	12,000	68-item food frequency
Nationwide Food Consumption Survey			
NFCS, 77–78	1977–78	30,000	7-day household record, 24-hr recall, 2-day record
NFCS, 87–88	1987–88	10,000	24-hr recall, 2-day record
Continuing Survey of Food Intakes of Individuals			
CSFII, 85–86	1985–86	9,000	Six 24-hr recalls
CSFII, 89–91	1989–91	15,000	24-hr recall, 2-day record
CSFII, 94–96	1994–96	15,000	Two 24-hr recalls

[a] Additional information about these surveys can be obtained from the following sources:

Health and Nutrition Examination Surveys: Division of Health Examination Statistics, National Center for Health Statistics, 6525 Belcrest Road, Room 900, Hyattsville, MD 20782

Health Interview Surveys: Division of Health Interview Statistics, National Center for Health Statistics, 6525 Belcrest Road, Room 860, Hyattsville, MD 20782

USDA surveys (NFCS and CSFII): Food Composition Research Branch, Human Nutrition Information Service, USDA, 6505 Belcrest Road, Hyattsville, MD 20782

Data from these surveys can also be obtained directly from the National Technical Information Service, 5285 Port Royal Road, Springfield, VA 22161 (703-487-4650)

Data are from Kuczmarski et al., 1994, and Thompson and Byers, 1994.

of macronutrients or micronutrients in populations of developing countries. The methodology of rapid assessment for protein-calorie malnutrition among refugee populations and during famines has been used successfully in many settings to mobilize resources for humanitarian aid (Habicht et al., 1982; Uvin, 1994; Jerome and Ricci, 1997). Systems of surveillance designed to detect nutritional crises before protein-calorie malnutrition becomes epidemic have also been instituted in many countries at nutritional risk. These systems use repeated measures of the height, weight, and other anthropometric indicators of undernutrition. In addition, surveillance of the availability and distribution of

food and projecting effects of weather and crop yields have been used as early-warning systems for impending famines. Deficiencies of vitamin A, iodine, and iron have been increasingly targeted by intervention programs in developing countries. Surveillance systems for these deficiencies have employed markers of biologic deficiency (e.g., blood levels of vitamin A, thyroid stimulating hormone, and hemoglobin) to contrast population subgroups and to examine trends over time in micronutrient sufficiency.

In the United States, nutritional surveillance has been largely targeted to populations served by maternal and child health programs, with the purpose to watch over trends in undernutrition and iron deficiency (Table 14-2). Increasingly, however, surveillance efforts have been used to watch over trends in nutritional factors related to chronic disease risk, including obesity, dietary fat intake, and inadequate intake of fruits and vegetables. Local data are very much needed for these purposes, as national data lack both representativeness and timeliness. For instance, phase I of NHANES III (1989–1991) sampled subjects from only 21 states, and the first standard tables for intakes of nutrients were not published until about 5 years after the survey midpoint (McDowell et al., 1994). Local nutritional data are useful for catalyzing local interest in nutrition intervention programs, contributing to program design, and assessing intervention effectiveness (Byers et al., 1997).

Height, weight, and blood hemoglobin levels have been monitored from public health clinics offering services to children and pregnant women as part of two nutrition surveillance systems operated jointly by state departments of health and the Centers for Disease Control and Prevention (CDC) (Trowbridge et al., 1990). The Pediatric Nutrition Surveillance System (PedNSS) has been examining data from children since 1973, and the Pregnancy Nutrition Surveillance System (PNSS) has been examining data from pregnant women since 1979. Data are analyzed locally on a monthly basis and/or at the CDC on a quarterly basis to identify and track individual cases exhibiting indicators of nutritional inadequacy (e.g., anemia or low weight-for-height), as well as to watch over the populations of specific clinics and localities for changes in the prevalences of such indicators. Dietary recalls are often conducted by nutritionists for the purposes of program eligibility determination or for clinical nutritional counseling, but this information is not now collected or recorded in a systematic way, so dietary intake is not now a part of these surveillance systems. Food-frequency methods are being developed and tested, however, for possible future use in public health clinical settings (U.S. Department of Agriculture, 1992).

State health agencies, in collaboration with the CDC, operate the Behavioral Risk Factor Surveillance System (BRFSS), a telephone-based surveillance system designed to measure the major behavioral causes of chronic diseases and injuries in each state (Remington et al., 1988). These measures of health-related behaviors are used by state health departments to design, target, and evaluate prevention programs. Telephone interviews of approximately 2,000 individuals per state per year are conducted on an ongoing basis using random-digit telephone sampling. Questions on body weight and weight control practices have been included in the BRFSS since its beginning in the early 1980s. The participation rate in the BRFSS in recent years has been approximately 80% of sampled adults from residential households who answered their phones. Dietary measures were first included in 1990 when two sets of optional questions were offered to participating BRFSS states: 6 questions designed to assess fruit and vegetable intake and 13 questions designed to assess dietary fat intake. Validation studies have shown that the brief BRFSS methods perform similarly to longer food-frequency methods (Serdula et al., 1993; Coates et al., 1995). Between 1990 and 1993, 28 states chose to include the fruit and vegetable questions, and 28 states chose to include the dietary fat questions during one or more years. The fruit and vegetable questions will have been asked in all states every other year from 1994 forward. In the future, the BRFSS instruments should be helpful in tracking states' progress toward health goals related to fruits and vegetables, dietary fat, and weight control. Because 24-hour recall data can be collected on the telephone (see Chapter 4), some state health agencies have explored the use of BRFSS-type random-digit dialing to collect dietary recall data in samples representative of state or local populations.

The Youth Risk Behavior Surveillance

Table 14–2. A summary of dietary surveillance systems in use in the United States[a]

System	Responsible agencies	Year system began	Nutrition assessment method
Pediatric Nutrition Surveillance System (PedNSS)	CDC, state health agencies	1973	Anthropometry, blood hemoglobin
Pregnancy Nutrition Surveillance System (PNSS)	CDC, state health agencies	1979	Anthropometry, blood hemoglobin, smoking, alcohol
Behavioral Risk Factor Surveillance System (BRFSS) weight control module	CDC, state health agencies	1982	Height, weight, intention to control weight
Behavioral Risk Factor Surveillance System (BRFSS) dietary fat module	CDC, state health agencies	1990	13 food-frequency questions on high fat foods
Behavioral Risk Factor Surveillance System (BRFSS) fruit and vegetable module	CDC, state health agencies	1990	6 food-frequency questions on fruits and vegetables
Youth Risk Behavior System (YRBS)	CDC, state education departments	1991	Weight control, yesterday's intake of fruits, vegetables, and high fat foods

[a]Additional information about these surveys can be obtained from the following sources:

PedNss and PNSS: Division of Nutrition, National Center for Chronic Disease Prevention and Health Promotion, Mail Stop K-26, 4770 Buford Highway, Atlanta, GA 30341

BRFSS: Division of Surveillance, National Center for Chronic Disease Prevention and Health Promotion, Mail Stop K-30, 4770 Buford Highway, Atlanta, GA 30341

YRBS: Division of Adolescent and School Health, National Center for Chronic Disease Prevention and Health Promotion, Mail Stop K-32, 4770 Buford Highway, Atlanta, GA 30341

Data are from Thompson and Byers, 1994.

(YRBS) system examines health-related behaviors of American adolescents, based on self-reported data from questionnaires completed by children in classrooms that are drawn as a representative sample of ninth to twelfth grades (Kolbe et al., 1993). The national YRBS survey was first conducted in 1991 and is conducted every 2 years, but the same survey instrument is used at the discretion of state and local education departments to generate annual state- and city-specific estimates. In 1993, for example, 24 states and 9 cities conducted their own YRBS surveys in addition to the 1993 national survey. The YRBS measures tobacco, alcohol, and drug use, behaviors related to accidents and violence, high-risk sexual behaviors, and weight control practices. Selected dietary behaviors are measured by questions referencing each student's recall of the intake of nine specific foods on the previous day. These questions do not provide quantitatively precise estimates of individual diets, but they are designed to provide crude measures of subgroup differences and trends in dietary intakes of adolescents based on foods that are indicators of fruit and vegetable and fat intake.

MONITORING AND SURVEILLANCE OF KNOWLEDGE, ATTITUDES, AND BELIEFS ABOUT NUTRITION

Because many interventions are usually designed to target the prebehavioral determinants of dietary choices, measuring knowledge, attitudes, and beliefs should be included in both the design and evaluation of nutrition intervention programs. Such measures can help to develop targeting strategies for dietary messages and can provide additional endpoints to assess the efficacy of nutrition intervention messages (Campbell et al., 1994). Nonetheless, national nutrition surveys have typically assessed only dietary behavior, providing little information about dietary knowledge, attitudes, and beliefs.

Both the Health Interview Surveys and the periodic Health and Diet Surveys (by the Food and Drug Adminstration) have included questions about dietary knowledge, attitudes, and beliefs of American adults, but these surveys have not also included quantitatively precise measures of dietary intake (Kuczmarski et al., 1994). Conversely, national surveys that were designed to collect high-quality dietary intake data have in the past inquired little about knowledge, attitudes, and beliefs. The ongoing Continuing Survey of Food Intakes of Individuals, however, now includes both diet recalls and a module of questions on knowledge and beliefs of diet that is asked of all respondents. Behavioral research in smoking cessation has suggested that there are several "stages of change" through which people move as they progress toward cessation (Prochaska et al., 1992). This paradigm of "stages of change" may also apply to dietary change (Glanz et al., 1994). More routine assessment of the status of populations according to this paradigm of readiness for making dietary changes could help us to better design and target programs and to better assess program effects.

EMERGING METHODS FOR NUTRITIONAL SURVEILLANCE

A major barrier to the collection of dietary data for states and localities has been the high burden on resources demanded by the collection of quantitatively precise dietary data. This is why small surveys and brief methods have typically been used for state and local dietary surveillance. Although these systems are useful for some surveillance purposes, they cannot provide the quantitatively precise estimates of dietary intake that are required for some monitoring purposes, such as for estimating the population distribution of percentage of calories from fat, or for providing dietary estimates that are sensitive enough to measure small effects that are expected from population-level interventions intended to improve diet. For that reason, state and local health agencies have been interested in learning how to include more quantitatively precise methods of dietary assessment, such as 24-hour recalls, in dietary surveillance for their populations. In many cases, public health nutritionists are already collecting 24-hour recall data for program eligibility or clinical counseling. This information, however, is often incomplete, and it has limited utility for the intended purpose—to characterize the diet of an individual. Such data could be better used if higher quality recalls were to be collected, computerized, and analyzed as indicators of the dietary status and trends of the clinical population being served by the program.

There are many barriers to the collection of quantitatively precise dietary intake data in localities. Public health nutritionists are not well trained to collect and computerize recall data, and appropriate computer hardware and software are often not available in public health agencies. With improved technology for personal computer (PC)–based dietary assessment, more states and localities are capable of choosing and applying methods appropriate for their needs for assessing dietary intake of their populations both in clinical settings and, using telephone surveys, in whole communities. PC-based programs can also be written to provide automated analyses of outputs from PC-based dietary assessments. Methods are also needed that are reasonably standardized and comparable to other survey data, especially national surveys. Using software that links food reports to a common nutrient database, such as the U.S.D.A. nutrient database, also helps to enable comparability.

Localities need to identify methods of measuring nutritional indicators that are valid, yet feasible with limited resources. In recent years, states have begun to identify additional resources for dietary assessments from various sources, such as preventive block grants, funds supporting categorical programs (e.g., heart disease, diabetes, or cancer prevention), and funds

directly supporting public health surveillance and nutrition intervention projects. Resources for state and local surveillance could also be identified through public and private partnerships with food companies and marketers. Some commercial food marketing surveys (e.g., A. C. Nielsen, MRCA) provide very detailed information on food product purchases and consumption. These surveys often impanel survey cohorts to record detailed information over time, with brand specificity. The information from these commercial sources is therefore very detailed and timely, but also tends to be very expensive to purchase.

Other indicators of dietary practices in communities have also been explored for use in nutritional surveillance. For instance, simple measures of the proportion of shelf space dedicated to more healthful foods in grocery stores have been shown to be indicative of dietary changes in the community (Cheadle et al., 1995). Community-level indicators of diet could be generated as well by examining food sales data. Most large food retailers keep computerized records of food label codes ("bar codes") read by laser scanners at retail points of purchase. Such sales data could be used for surveillance of specific indicator foods in particular regions or neighborhoods. For example, the ratio of low fat milk to whole milk sold in stores could be assessed in different neighborhoods in response to a nutrition education campaign to reduce dairy fat intake. The use of food sales data such as these for surveillance is currently limited, however, by the data management burden of working with large datasets. The Universal Product Codes (UPC) used as a basis for the bar codes on foods are also difficult to analyze both because they are not categorized according to logical food groups of interest to nutritionists and because the UPC codes change over time. Just within the dairy case, for instance, there are over 40,000 different UPC codes now in use. In the future, if UPC food codes could be automatically linked to a food in the U.S.D.A. nutrient databank (or to a nutrient database containing manufacturer-specified information), food sales data could be used for community-wide surveillance and intervention evaluation for specific foods and nutrients.

Many different methods are now in use or in development for nutritional monitoring and surveillance. It is important to remember that the intended uses of the information should determine the design and implementation of any monitoring or surveillance system. Although it may seem axiomatic that monitoring and surveillance efforts need to be tied directly to considerations about how the information will be used, monitoring and surveillance systems often acquire an institutional life of their own, and they become less useful than they should be. The timely feedback of information to affect nutrition policy is the key feature of successful nutritional monitoring, and the timely feedback of information to target and evaluate nutrition intervention programs needs to be the key feature of successful nutritional surveillance.

REFERENCES

Block, G., and A. F. Subar (1992). Estimates of nutrient intake from a food frequency questionnaire: The 1987 National Health Interview Survey. *J Am Diet Assoc 92,* 969–977.

Briefel, R. R. (1994). Assessment of the U.S. diet in National nutrition surveys: National collaborative efforts and NHANES. *Am J Clin Nutr 59(suppl),* 164S–167S.

Briefel, R. R., K. M. Flegal, D. M. Winn, C. M. Loria, C. L. Johnson, and C. T. Sempos (1992). Assessing the nation's diet: Limitations of the food frequency questionnaire. *J Am Diet Assoc 92,* 959–962.

Byers, T., M. Serdula, S. Kuester, J. Mendlein, C. Ballew, and S. McPherson (1997). Dietary surveillance for states and localities. *Am J Clin Nutr 65(suppl),* 1210s–1214s.

Campbell, M. K., B. M. DeVellis, V. J. Strecher, A. S. Ammerman, R. F. DeVellis and R. S. Sandler (1994). Improving dietary behavior: The effectiveness of tailored messages in primary care settings. *Am J Public Health 84,* 783–787.

Cheadle, A., B. M. Psaty, P. Diehr, T. Koepsell, E. Wagner, S. Curry, and A. Kristal (1995). Evaluating community-based nutrition programs: Comparing grocery store and individual-level survey measures of program impact. *Prev Med 24,* 71–79.

Coates, R., M. Serdula, and T. Byers (1995). The performance of a brief, telephone-administered food frequency questionnaire for surveillance of dietary fat intakes of Americans. *J Nutr 125,* 1473–1483.

Glanz, K., R. E. Patterson, A. R. Kristal, C. C. DiClemente, J. Heimendinger, L. Linnan, and D. F. McLerran (1994). Stages of changes in adopting healthy diets: Fat, fiber, and correlates of nutrient intake. *Health Educ Q 21,* 499–519.

Habicht, J. P., L. D. Meyers, and C. Brownie (1982). Indicators for identifying and counting the improperly nourished. *Am J Clin Nutr 35,* 1241–1254.

Interagency Board for Nutrition Monitoring and Related Research (1992). *Nutrition Monitoring in the United States: The Directory of Federal and State Nutrition Monitoring Activities.* Hyattsville, MD: Department of Health and Human Services, Public Health Service.

Jerome, N., and J. Ricci (1997). Food and nutrition surveillance: An international overview. *Am J Clin Nutr 65 (suppl),* 1198s–1202s.

Kohlmeier, L., E. Helsing, A. Kelly, O. Moreiras-Varela, A. Trichopoulou, C. E. Wotecki, D. H. Buss, E. Callmer, R. J. Hermus, and J. Sznajd (1990). Nutritional surveillance as the backbone of national nutrition policy: Recommendations of the IUNS committee on nutritional surveillance and programme evaluation in developed countries. *Eur J Clin Nutr 44,* 771–781.

Kolbe, L. J., L. Kann, and J. L. Collins (1993). Overview of the Youth Risk Behavior Surveillance System. *Public Health Rep 1,* 2–10.

Kuczmarski, M. F., A. Moshfegh, and R. Briefel (1994). Update on nutrition monitoring activities in the United States. *J Am Diet Assoc 94,* 753–760.

Margetts, B. M., and M. Nelson (1991). *Design Concepts in Nutritional Epidemiology.* New York: Oxford University Press.

McDowell, M. A., R. R. Briefel, K. Alaimo, A. M. Bischof, C. R. Caughman, and M. D. Carroll, et al. (1994). *Energy and Macronutrient Intakes of Persons Ages 2 Months and Over in the United States: Third National Health and Nutrition Examination Survey, Phase I 1988–1991.* DHHS Publication No. (PHS) 95–1250). National Center for Health Statistics, Centers for Disease Control, Public Health Service. Hyattsville, MD. Department of Health and Human Services.

Ministry of Health and Welfare (Japan) (1992). *National Nutrition Survey, 1966, 1970, 1975, 1980, 1985, 1990.* Tokyo: Daiichi Shuppan Publishers.

Prochaska, J. O., C. C. DiClemente, and J. C. Norcross (1992). In search of how people change. Applications to addictive behaviors. *Am Psychol 47,* 1102–1114.

Remington, P. L., M. Y. Smith, D. F. Williamson, R. F. Anda, E. M. Gentry, and G. C. Hogelin (1988). Design, characteristics, and usefulness of state-based behavioral risk factor surveillance: 1981–87. *Public Health Rep 103,* 366–375.

Serdula, M., R. Coates, T. Byers, A. Mokdad, S. Jewell, N. Chavez, J. Mares-Perlman, P. Newcomb, C. Ritenbaugh, F. Treiber, and G. Block (1993). Evaluation of a brief telephone questionnaire to estimate fruit and vegetable consumption in diverse study populations. *Epidemiology 4,* 455–463.

Thacker, S. B., and R. L. Berkelman (1988). Public health surveillance in the United States. *Epidemiol Rev 10,* 164–190.

Thompson, F. E., and T. Byers (1994). Dietary assessment resource manual. *J Nutr 124 (suppl),* 2245S–2317S.

Trowbridge, F. L., F. L. Wong, T. E. Byers, and M. K. Serdula (1990). Methodological issues in nutrition surveillance: The CDC experience. *J Nutr 11,* 1512–1518.

U.S. Department of Agriculture, F. A. N. S. (1992). *Dietary Assessment Methodology for Use in the Special Supplemental Food Program for Women, Infants, and Children (WIC).* U.S. Government Printing Office (311-367-602213). Washington, DC: U.S. Department of Agriculture.

Uvin, P. (1994). The state of world hunger. *Nutr Rev 52,* 151–161.

Prologue to Chapters 15–18: In the next four chapters, concepts described in the earlier sections are discussed in relation to specific topics of current epidemiologic interest: vitamin A intake and lung cancer, dietary fat and breast cancer, the diet-heart hypothesis, and folate intake and neural tube defects. Since space precluded a detailed review of all potentially important relationships between dietary factors and specific diseases, these topics were selected largely because a sufficient literature exists for each to illustrate some of the important principles in nutritional epidemiology. The substance of these chapters may become outdated rather quickly as these are areas of active investigation. Nevertheless, the lessons learned trying to unravel these complex relationships should be useful to investigators and consumers of the scientific literature who address these and other problems in the future.

15

Vitamin A and Lung Cancer

WALTER WILLETT AND GRAHAM COLDITZ

Vitamin A has long been recognized to play a central physiologic role in the regulation of cell differentiation (Wolbach and Howe, 1925; De Luca et al., 1972). Because loss of differentiation is a basic feature of malignancy, vitamin A may be related to cancer incidence. In numerous animal studies, naturally occurring preformed vitamin A and synthetic analogues have inhibited the occurrence of induced tumors and even reversed metaplastic changes (Hill and Grubbs, 1982; Sporn and Roberts, 1983). This inhibitory effect is present even when retinol is administered after the cancer has been induced (McCormick et al., 1981), a feature of major potential epidemiologic and public health importance. Under some laboratory conditions, however, the same compounds have not inhibited carcinogenesis and can actually increase the incidence of tumors (Schroder and Black, 1980; Moon et al., 1992).

Interest in vitamin A as a potential inhibitor of human cancer increased substantially with a report by Bjelke (1975) based on the follow-up of 8,278 Norwegian men who had earlier completed a mailed dietary questionnaire. After adjusting for the effects of cigarette smoking, Bjelke (1975) observed that the rate of lung cancer among men whose calculated intake of vitamin A was above average was only one-third that of men with intakes below average (Table 15–1).

The interpretation of Bjelke's important finding was complicated by the diversity of vitamin A sources. Natural preformed vitamin A, frequently referred to as retinol even though it is usually consumed in the form of retinyl esters, is found only in foods from animal sources. Plants, principally green leafy vegetables and yellow fruits and vegetables, contain not preformed vitamin A but a series of carotenoid compounds, some of which can be metabolized to form retinol, the physiologically active form of vitamin A. Beta-carotene, the most plentiful carotenoid with potential vitamin A activity, is a dimer that can be cleaved after absorption to form two

Table 15–1. Age-adjusted rates of lung cancer among men with high versus low vitamin A index[a]

| Cigarette smoking status | Rate of lung cancer[b] | | Relative risk: vitamin A index ≥5 vs.<5 |
	Vitamin A index ≤ 5	Vitamin A index ≥ 5	
Ever smoked	10.6	4.2	0.40[c]
Current smoker, >20 cigarettes/day	21.0	7.4	0.35
Current smoker, 1–19 cigarettes/day	12.8	5.7	0.44
Ex-smoker	6.1	1.5	0.25
Never smoked	1.1	1.2	1.01
Total, smoking adjusted	7.3	2.8	0.38[d]

[a] Data are based on 53 cases occurring during a 5-year follow-up study of 8,278 Norwegian men.
[b] Age-adjusted 5-year cumulative incidence/1,000 men.
[c] $p < 0.05$.
[d] $p < 0.01$.
From Bjelke, 1975.

molecules of retinol (Fig. 15–1). The majority of carotenoids in our food supply, such as lycopene, which is found in tomatoes and egg yolks, contribute yellow and red colors, but not vitamin A activity, to our diet. Some animal products contain modest amounts of beta-carotene and other carotenoids; without them, butter, egg yolks, and chicken fat would appear white. Vitamin A supplements and fortified foods, such as breakfast cereals, were until recently based on preformed vitamin A; now beta-carotene is frequently used in combination with preformed vitamin A. The availability of beta-carotene as specific supplements is also a recent phenomenon. Foods that provide large amounts of vitamin A activity from preformed vitamin A and carotenoids in the U.S. diet are described in Table 15–2.

Although some carotenoids share common physiologic functions with preformed vitamin A by virtue of their potential conversion to retinol, carotenoids may have other actions that are unique. The carotenoids efficiently quench singlet oxygen and free radicals that could otherwise initiate reactions such as lipid peroxidation (Peto et al., 1981; Krinsky and Deneke, 1982). Beta-carotene is a potent free radical scavenger under physiologic conditions of ox-

ygen tension, a characteristic not shared by retinol or other carotenoids (Burton and Ingold, 1984). Also, some carotenoids are specifically localized to certain tissues or organs. For example, lutein and zeaxanthin are concentrated in the macular region of the retina, where they appear to play a critical role in protection from excessive light (Schalch, 1992). It is thus important to distinguish between the effects of preformed vitamin A, derived from animal products and supplements, and carotenoids, obtained largely from plant products (Peto, 1983), as well as among the many specific carotenoids.

ADDITIONAL PROSPECTIVE STUDIES

The original findings of Bjelke (1975) were confirmed by a second report with extended follow-up of the same cohort (Kvale et al., 1983) that also provided more information on specific foods. The protective effect against lung cancer was primarily attributable to carrots and other vegetables with some additional contribution from milk. This study thus provided stronger evidence for a beneficial effect of carotenoids than for preformed vitamin A.

The first epidemiologic study in which the independent effects of carotenoids and

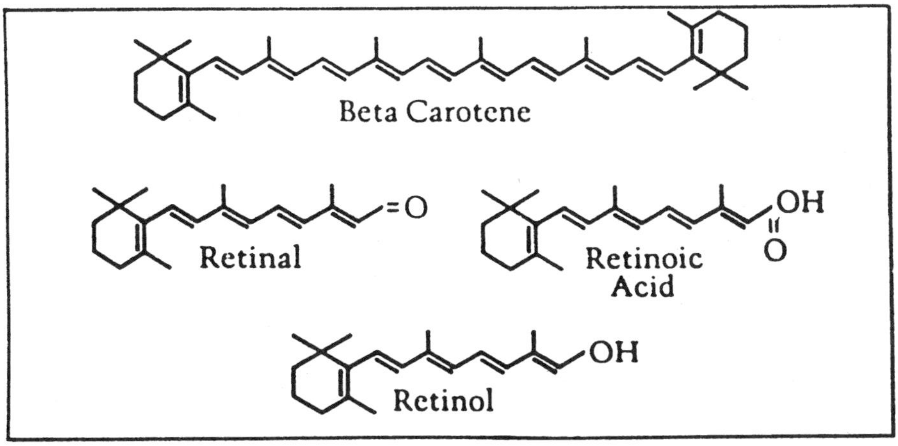

Figure 15–1. Beta-carotene and retinol. Some of the beta-carotene may be cleaved after absorption to form two molecules of retinol, and some circulates unchanged. (Reproduced with permission from Hoffmann-LaRoche.)

Table 15–2. Preformed vitamin A and vitamin A activity from carotenoids in several commonly consumed foods[a]

	Typical serving	Preformed vitamin A	Carotenoids
Major sources of preformed vitamin A			
Liver	3½ oz	52,033	298
Breakfast cereal, typical	½ cup	1,250	0
Margarine	1 pat (5 g)	97	58
Hard cheese	1 oz	183	117
Eggs	1	260	0
Low fat milk	8 oz glass	499	0
Butter	1 pat (5 g)	95	58
Skim milk	8 oz glass	499	0
Whole milk	8 oz glass	190	117
Major sources of carotenoids			
Carrots	1 carrot	0	19,152
Spinach	½ cup, cooked	0	7,371
Tomatoes	1 fruit	0	1,394
Yellow squash	½ cup	0	3,628
Broccoli	½ cup	0	1,099
Orange juice	6 oz glass	0	310
Mixed peas and carrots	½ cup	0	3,892
Canteloupe	4 oz slice	0	4,304
Tomato paste, sauce	4 oz	0	1,528

[a]Data from total vitamin A activity based on U.S.D.A. Handbook No. 8 (U.S. Department of Agriculture, 1989) and provisional tables. For foods containing both preformed vitamin A and carotenoid, the total vitamin A activity has been partitioned based on data from Paul and Southgate (1978).

preformed vitamin A were formally examined was the 19-year follow-up of 2,107 men enrolled in the Western Electric Study (Shekelle et al., 1981). Preformed vitamin A intake was not related to the incidence of lung cancer, which was diagnosed among 33 men. In striking contrast, intake of vitamin A from carotenoids was strongly associated with lower risk of this disease (Fig. 15–2). No significant relationship was observed between intake of either form of vitamin A and cancers other than lung cancer in this cohort, but the number of cases with these cancers was small.

The relationships of vitamin A intake with risk of lung cancer have been examined in other prospective studies, some of which had very limited dietary information or few cases (Table 15–3). Hirayama (1979) examined the association between intake of green and yellow vegetables, assessed with a single question, and the occurrence of 807 lung cancer deaths during 10 years of follow up among a cohort of 265,118 Japanese men and women. A reduced risk of lung cancer was observed for both smokers and nonsmokers who ate these vegetables daily compared with those who did not. The relative risks ranged from 0.4 to 0.8, depending on gender and smoking habits.

In 1 million men and women enrolled in the American Cancer Society cohort; 2,952 deaths due to lung cancer occurred during 10 years of follow up (Wang and Hammond, 1985). The details of analysis were quite incomplete; however, a strong protective effect was observed for those who consumed green salad and fruit or fruit juice five to seven times per week compared with those who consumed these foods fewer than three times per week. Although this and the Japanese studies provide support for the hypothesis that carotenoids reduce the risk of lung cancer, the very limited nature of the data did not provide an opportunity to explore alternate hypotheses, for example, that vitamin C may be the responsible factor. Furthermore, they do

not address the potential effect of preformed vitamin A.

Inverse associations with calculated intake of vitamin A from carotenoids have generally been observed in other prospective studies (Kromhout, 1987; Knekt et al., 1991; Chow et al., 1992; Shibata et al., 1992; Steinmetz et al., 1993), but these have sometimes been weak and not statistically significant. The dietary assessment used by Steinmetz and colleagues (1993) was quite complete and allowed a detailed examination of a variety of nutrients and foods. Although a weak inverse relationship was seen for both beta-carotene and vitamin C intake, stronger inverse relationships were observed for fruits plus vegetables or vegetables alone, suggesting that factors in these foods other than, or in addition to, beta-carotene might be protective against lung cancer.

CASE-CONTROL STUDIES

The relationship between vitamin A intake and risk of lung cancer has been examined in more than 20 case–control studies, which are summarized in Table 15–4. An explicit distinction between preformed vitamin A and carotenoid intake was made in most of the recent studies. Because data on the content of specific carotenoids has only recently become available, in almost all of these studies "carotene" or "carotenoid" intake was estimated indirectly by using the vitamin A activity (which has been routinely available for many years in most food composition databases) in fruits and vegetables, plus a small contribution from dairy products.

As a whole, the case–control investigations are remarkably consistent in suggesting that intake of preformed vitamin A has little or no relationship with the incidence of lung cancer within the range of intakes that were studied. In contrast, these studies have been remarkably consistent in providing support for a protective relationship between carotenoid sources of vitamin A and

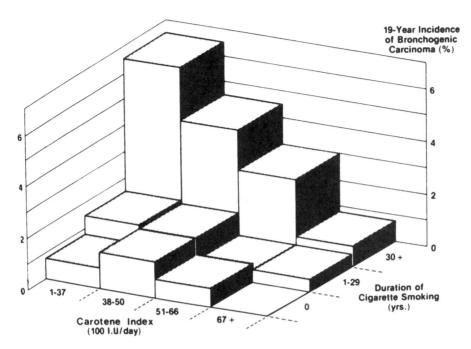

19-Year Incidence of Bronchogenic Carcinoma (%)

Duration of Cigarette Smoking (yrs.)
30 +
1-29
0

Carotene Index (100 I.U/day)
1-37
38-50
51-66
67 +

Figure 15–2. Association of carotene index and cigarette smoking with 19-year incidence of bronchogenic carcinoma. (From Shekelle et al., 1981; reproduced with permission.)

Table 15–3. Propective studies of vitamin A intake and lung cancer

	Populations	No. of cases	Relative risks for high vs. low intake categories		
			Total vitamin A	Preformed vitamin A	Carotenoid vitamin A
Bjelke (1975)	Norwegian men	53	0.4	—	—
Shekelle et al. (1981)	U.S. men	33	—	2.0	0.1
Kvale et al. (1983)	Norwegian men	168	0.5	—	—
Paganini-Hill et al. (1987)	California men and women	37 men	1.0	0.9	0.7
		18 women	0.9	0.7	0.7
Kromhout (1987)	Dutch men	63	—	—	0.7
Knekt et al. (1991)	Finnish men	18 nonsmokers	—	0.7	0.4
		99 current smokers	—	1.4	0.9
Shibata et al. (1992)[a]	California men and women	94 men	1.0	1.1	—
		70 women	0.7	0.6	—
Chow et al. (1992)	U.S. men	219	0.8	0.9	0.8
Steinmetz et al. (1993)	Iowa women	179	—	—	0.8

Update of Paganini-Hill et al. (1987).

Table 15-4. Case–control studies of vitamin A intake and lung cancer

			Relative risks for high vs. low intake categories		
Study	Populations	No. of Cases	Total vitamin A	Preformed vitamin A	Carotenoid vitamin A
MacLennan et al. (1977)	Chinese men and women in Singapore	233	—	—	0.6–0.7
Mettlin et al. (1979)	New York men	292	0.4	—	—
Gregor et al. (1980)	U.K. men and women	100	0.5 (men) 1.9 (women)	—	—
Hinds et al. (1984)	Men and women in Hawaii	364	0.7	—	—
Ziegler et al. (1984)	New Jersey white men	763	1.1	1.3	0.8
Samet et al. (1985)	New Mexico men and women	332 Anglos 125 Hispanics	0.6 1.1	1.1 1.7	0.7 1.1
Wu et al. (1985)	U.S. women	220	— —	0.8[a] 1.0[b]	0.4[a] 0.7[b]
Byers et al. (1987)	U.S. women	296 men 154 women	0.7 0.8	— —	0.6 0.8
Pastorino et al. (1987)	Italian women	47	—	0.4	0.3
Fontham et al. (1988)	U.S. men and women	1,253	—	0.9	0.9
Koo (1988)	Chinese women in Hong Kong	88	—	0.5	0.7
Ho et al. (1988)	Chinese men in Singapore	50	0.6	—	0.3
Le Marchand et al. (1989)	Men and women in Hawaii	230 men 102 women	0.6 0.4	1.1 1.0	0.5 0.4
Dartigues et al. (1990)	French men and women	106	—	0.2	0.2
Jain et al. (1990)	Toronto men and women	839	1.2	1.2	0.9
Kalandidi et al. (1990)	Non smoking Greek women	160	—	1.3	1.0
Harris et al. (1991)	U.K. men	96	—	—	0.5
Chengyu et al. (1992)	Chinese men and women	135	—	—	0.4 (per 2 SD)
Candelora et al. (1992)	Nonsmoking U.S. women	124	—	1.2	0.4
Mayne et al. (1994)	U.S. men and women	413			
	men	—	0.9	0.6
	women	—	1.0	0.8

[a] Adenocarcinoma

[b] Squamous cell carcinoma

the occurrence of lung cancer. However, most of these studies did not attempt to distinguish among the various carotenoids, including those without potential vitamin A activity, which tend to be correlated in the diet. In one of the few case–control studies to examine intake of specific carotenoids, Le Marchand and colleagues (1993) examined intakes of alpha-carotene, beta-carotene, and lutein/zeaxanthin and found that each was significantly associated with reduced risk of lung cancer. Ziegler and colleagues (1996) have also reanalyzed their case–control data with newer food composition data; inverse associations were seen with the same three carotenoids, but not with beta-cryptoxanthin and lycopene. The strongest apparent protective effect was for alpha-carotene; when alpha- and beta-carotene were controlled for each other, only alpha-carotene was inversely associated with lung cancer risk.

Associations of carotenoid sources with other cancers have been observed in some case–control studies, but consistent findings have not emerged; a review of this literature is outside the scope of this chapter.

STUDIES OF BLOOD VITAMIN A LEVELS AND RISK OF LUNG CANCER

Using a different approach, a number of investigators have examined the relationship between blood levels of vitamin A and lung cancer. The specific measurements that have been employed are discussed in further detail in Chapter 9; these have included serum or plasma levels of retinol, retinol-binding protein, total carotenoid, and beta-carotene.

Because the relationships between biochemical measurements and disease are usually much easier to investigate using a case–control study than a prospective design, it was natural that the early investigators of vitamin A and lung cancer used this approach. For example, Atukorala and

colleagues (1979) reported levels of serum total vitamin A and beta-carotene (probably this was actually total carotenoids, as they used an older spectrophotometric assay) among 26 patients with newly diagnosed lung cancer and 21 control subjects. They found that vitamin A levels were approximately 25% lower in the cases ($p < 0.001$); however, the difference in carotenoid levels was less and did not reach statistical significance. As the authors pointed out, this type of study could not distinguish the possibility that the low vitamin A levels might be a consequence of the tumor rather than a cause of the malignancy.

To avoid the possibility that the cancer might affect the level of vitamin A or other biochemical indicators, the specimens should be collected before the occurrence of disease. Although it would be ideal to analyze all the specimens at the time of collection and then follow the cohort to ascertain the occurrence of cancer, this is usually prohibitive in terms of cost and time. Thus, a number of investigators have conducted nested case–control studies using collections of sera that had been obtained and stored for other purposes, usually as part of studies of cardiovascular disease. Wald and colleagues (1980) followed a cohort of about 16,000 men and identified 86 cancers that occurred within 3 years of having provided a blood specimen that was frozen and stored. Sera for each case of cancer and two control subjects from this population matched by age, smoking habit, and date of blood collection were retrieved and analyzed for retinol. Overall, serum retinol levels in these specimens, collected before diagnosis, were 7% lower among the case subjects compared with levels among the controls (Table 15–5). This difference was statistically significant and translated into a dose–response relationship across quintiles with a relative risk of 0.6 for men in the highest category of serum retinol compared with those in the lowest category. At approximately the

Table 15–5. Studies of retinol levels in prospectively collected sera in relation to risk of lung cancer

Study	Population	No. of cases	Mean retinol level (μg/dl) Cases	Controls		Relative risk, high vs. low category
Wald et al. (1980)	English men	14 lung cancers	56.1	68.7	$p < 0.005$	—
		86 total cancers	64.2	68.7	$p < 0.025$	0.5
Kark et al. (1981)	Evans Co. men and women	12 lung cancers		(cases 9.1 μg/dl lower)		—
		85 total cancers	41.3	46.9	$p = 0.003$	0.2
Willett et al. (1984)	U.S. men and women, hypertensive	17 lung cancers		(cases 7.4 μg/dl higher)		—
		111 total cancers	67.3	68.7		1.1
Stahelin et al. (1984)	Swiss	35 lung cancers (other sites displayed separately)	286 IU/dl	280 IU/dl		—
Peleg et al. (1984)	Evans Co. men and women	17 lung cancers		(cases 6.4 μg/dl lower)		—
		135 total cancers	48.9	48.9		1.2
Salonen et al. (1985)	Finnish men and women	15 lung cancers	48.0	56.8	$p < 0.05$	—
		51 total cancers	48.3	52.4		1.1
Nomura et al. (1985)	Japanese-Hawaiian men	74 lung cancers	63.8[a]	59.6[a]		—
Friedman et al. (1986)	California men and women	151 lung cancers	82.2	82.4		0.8
Menkes et al. (1986)	Washington Co. men and women	99 lung cancers	60.6	61.3		0.9
Wald et al. (1986)	English men	41 lung cancers	65.6	66.3		—
		227 total cancers	67.0	68.8		0.8
Stahelin et al. (1991)[b]	Swiss	68 lung cancers	82.2	82.5		—
		204 total cancers	82.5	82.5		—

[a]Median value.

[b]Includes Stahelin et al. (1984).

same time, Kark and colleagues (1981) reported data from a similar study conducted in Evans County, Georgia. They found that the prediagnostic retinol levels in the cases averaged 12% lower than those of the control subjects, which corresponded to a dose–response relationship with a relative risk of 0.2 for those in the highest compared with the lowest quintile. In both the Wald and Kark studies, the difference between cases and controls was particularly large for lung cancer, which seemed apparently consistent with the case–control data on total vitamin A intake. These findings generated great interest in the area of cancer research as it appeared that retinol might be to cancer what serum cholesterol is to the field of cardiovascular epidemiology.

Despite the initial optimism that serum retinol levels might be a strong and potentially modifiable risk factor for cancer overall and lung cancer in particular, further studies did not confirm the original findings. In a preliminary report from Switzerland based on sera that were actually analyzed at the time of specimen collection, Stahelin and colleagues (1982) did not find lower levels of retinol among men who subsequently developed lung or all cancers combined (120 total cases). Willett and colleagues (1984) used a nested case–control design and sera that had been collected as part of a national multicenter trial of hypertension treatment to evaluate the hypothesis that low serum retinol levels are associated with an increased risk of cancer. No association was seen with the overall incidence of cancer, and for lung cancer the levels were actually somewhat higher for cases than controls. A similar lack of any protective relationship was seen for retinol-binding protein. In a small study conducted in Finland, Salonen and colleagues (1985) found no relationship between retinol levels and overall risk of cancer; however, the levels among the lung cancer cases were somewhat lower than among the control subjects. Four studies have been conducted with a sufficient number of total cancers to

examine lung cancer alone with substantial power (Nomura et al., 1985; Friedman et al., 1986; Menkes et al., 1986; Stahelin et al., 1991). In all four of these studies, the retinol levels of subjects who later developed lung cancer were nearly identical to those who remained free of cancer. In addition, Peleg and colleagues (1984) have published additional follow-up data from the Evans County study, and Wald and colleagues (1986) have reported on further experience within the English cohort. In both of these extensions of the two original studies in which a protective relationship was found, there no longer existed any material association between serum retinol and incidence of lung cancer. Indeed, during the extended follow-up in the English study, the relationship between retinol level and risk of lung cancer and total cancers was actually positive, although not significantly so. The body of evidence relating serum retinol levels to risk of lung cancer as well as overall cancer incidence is thus now overwhelmingly null, although the possibility cannot be excluded that an association exists with some less common specific malignancy.

In retrospect, it may be informative to consider whether preventable methodologic weaknesses were responsible for the initial inverse relationships. Wald and colleagues (1986) have considered this issue in detail (Table 15–6). In their second paper based on additional follow-up study, they confirmed with new data that an inverse relationship existed during the first 3 years following collection of the blood samples. As noted above, however, the inverse relationship did not persist beyond 3 years and actually reversed its direction. Wald and coworkers concluded that the initial finding was not likely to be due to chance; rather, it is more likely that preclinical malignancy, which would have been present at the time of blood collection for tumors diagnosed during the early follow-up period, was reducing the level of retinol by some unknown metabolic mechanism. This is analogous to the apparent inverse rela-

Table 15–6. Relative risks of cancer (all sites) according to quintile of serum retinol in preliminary report and during different follow-up intervals in the extended study[a]

Quintile of retinol	Relative risks (vs. lowest quintile)			
	Preliminary study (86 cases)	Second Study < 1 yr (66 cases)	Second study 1–2 yr (45 cases)	Second study 3+ yr (116 cases)
1 low	1.00	1.00	1.00	1.00
2	0.77	0.38	1.26	0.86
3	0.73	0.49	0.49	1.35
4	0.48	0.14	0.33	0.82
5 high	0.45	0.32	0.25	1.87
Test for trend in relative risks	$p < 0.025$	$p < 0.01$	$p < 0.025$	NS

[a] NS, not significant.

From Wald et al., 1980, and 1986.

tionship between serum cholesterol and cancer risk, which is largely manifested during the early follow-up period after blood collection (Rose and Shipley, 1980). Although it is not surprising that case–control studies of serum markers of nutritional status and cancer should provide misleading results, a sobering point raised by these studies of serum retinol and cancer is that even prospective studies may not be prospective enough. No single approach can provide absolute assurance that this problem will not be repeated. Extending the follow-up period, careful screening of subjects at the time of blood collection to eliminate prevalent disease, using early, superficial, or premalignant endpoints, and employing biochemical indicators that are less sensitive to recent metabolic or dietary changes, such as nails or subcutaneous fat, however, will reduce the likelihood of bias due to existing malignancies.

Although preclinical disease may have distorted the relationship between serum retinol and cancer in the initial study of Wald and colleagues, this phenomenon is not likely to explain the findings of Kark and colleagues, because subjects were followed up to 14 years. In this study, however, the sera for cases were handled in a systematically different manner from those

of controls as the specimens for cases but not controls had been thawed and refrozen as part of another investigation. The authors were aware of this potential problem and conducted a substudy to learn whether thawing and refreezing specimens would reduce the retinol levels; they detected no such effect. It is impossible, however, to reproduce exactly the procedures that the case sera had experienced, leaving concern that this differential treatment explained the observed inverse association.

The underlying issue in these two early studies is that relationships between nutritional factors and disease are likely to be exquisitely sensitive to methodologic distortion as small differences in mean values, which can be due to seemingly minor systematic biases, can translate into important relative risks. It is reassuring, however, that the nested case–control studies of serum retinol and cancer that have not been limited to only a short follow-up period and in which case and control specimens were handled identically have been remarkably consistent.

In retrospect, it also appears that the apparent convergence between the studies of vitamin A intake and serum retinol in relation to lung cancer was based on a misunderstanding of the relationship of vitamin A intake and serum retinol (see Chapter 9). Although serum retinol levels are clearly depressed with intakes sufficiently low to produce signs of clinical deficiency, over the range of diets in generally well-nourished populations, serum retinol levels are only very minimally related to vitamin A intake. For example, in one study in which 25,000 IU of preformed vitamin A (more than five times the usual dietary intake) was taken as a daily supplement for 8 weeks, no detectable increase in blood level was observed (Willett et al., 1983). Similarly, large supplements of beta-carotene have no material effect on blood levels of retinol (Willett et al., 1983; Costantino et al., 1988). In another randomized trial among women with initially low values of plasma retinol, a daily supplement of 10,000 IU increased blood levels by only 9%, which was marginally statistically significant (Willett et al., 1984). Therefore, the failure to observe an association between serum retinol level and lung cancer incidence reveals little about the relationship between dietary vitamin A and this disease.

NESTED CASE–CONTROL STUDIES OF BLOOD CAROTENE LEVELS AND LUNG CANCER

Based on the data from studies of dietary intake, it would be expected that blood levels of beta-carotene would be related to risk of lung cancer. This relationship has been more difficult to study than the association with serum retinol for two reasons. First, assays to measure specific carotenoids in large numbers of blood specimens became available only in the late 1980s; the older spectrophotometric methods could not distinguish, for example, beta-carotene from the other more plentiful carotenoids. Second, beta-carotene is far less stable in frozen sera than retinol so that ultra-low temperatures (e.g., $-80°C$) are needed to avoid degradation if specimens are to be held for more than a few months (see Chapter 9). Because a number of serum banks did not use ultra-low conditions, many studies were not able to measure carotenoid levels.

At the time that the nested case–control study reported by Willett and colleagues (1984) was conducted, an assay was not available for beta-carotene, which is only about 10% to 15% of total serum carotenoids, so that total carotenoids were measured instead; no significant association was observed either for lung or total cancers. Subsequently, Stahelin and colleagues (1984) reported significantly lower prediagnostic levels of serum beta-carotene in 35 lung cancer patients than in controls. These findings were confirmed with extended follow-up (Stahelin et al., 1991) (Table 15–5). After adjusting for age and the number of cigarettes smoked daily, Nomura and colleagues (1985) observed a significant inverse relationship between serum beta-carotene levels and incidence of lung cancer; the relative risk was 0.5 for men in the highest compared with the lowest quintile. In a similar analysis, Menkes and colleagues (1986) found that higher serum beta-carotene levels were associated with a lower risk of lung cancer among the Washington County cohort; the relative risk for subjects in the extreme quintiles was also 0.5. Similar inverse associations were observed by Connett and colleagues (1989), Wald and colleagues (1988), and in the ATBC Trial (The Alpha-Tocopherol Beta-Carotene Cancer Prevention Study Group, 1994).

In studies that have been able to measure beta-carotene in blood samples collected before the diagnosis of lung cancer, an inverse relationship has thus been consistently observed. Although this adds support to the hypothesis that higher intakes of beta-carotene reduce the risk of lung cancer, these findings also need to be interpreted cautiously. Studies based on biochemical measurements of beta-carotene have little advantage over those based on dietary intake with respect to control of potentially confounding factors. For example, in the dietary intake studies, it is possible that some factor in the green and yellow fruits and vegetables other than beta-carotene is responsible for the reduced risk of lung cancer. Similarly, it is possible that some other aspect of lifestyle among persons who consume higher amounts of these fruits and vegetables is responsible for the lower cancer incidence. The same limitations apply to the biochemical studies because the higher blood levels of beta-carotene could be only incidental to the increased intake of other protective factors in these plant products or to protective behavioral characteristics associated with diet. (Even the assay for beta-carotene used in the above studies was not specific for beta-carotene as the values also included alpha-carotene [Stahelin et al., 1991].) Although it is useful to obtain similar answers using different approaches, the value of these studies lies more in their prospective nature rather than their means of measuring exposure. Indeed, even the simple questionnaire employed in the study of Bjelke (1975) provided more opportunity than the biochemical studies to evaluate alternative explanations for the inverse association with "vitamin A" because these authors could calculate an index of vitamin C intake and demonstrate that it did not account for the association with vitamin A. (Vitamin C cannot be measured in routinely stored blood samples—see Chapter 9.) If the biochemical assay for beta-carotene also provides independent values for other carotenoids, these could be similarly examined as potential determinants of disease. Studies using biochemical markers can sometimes be informative when dietary intake studies are not; if beta-carotene were difficult or impossible to measure by questionnaire, then the biochemical marker could provide unique information. Because carotene intake derived from a questionnaire is correlated with blood levels of beta-carotene or total carotenoids (Willett et al., 1983; Russell-Briefel et al., 1985; Stryker et al., 1988), the biochemical marker does not provide special information.

The interpretation of data on blood levels of beta-carotene and lung cancer is also complicated by evidence that cigarette smoking may have a metabolic effect that reduces blood levels of beta-carotene. Although blood levels of total carotenoids and beta-carotene have been found in a number of studies to be lower among cigarette smokers than among nonsmokers, it is possible that this is simply the result of reduced intake of fruits and vegetables among smokers. Russell-Briefel and colleagues (1985), however, found that these differences in carotenoid levels could not be accounted for by dietary intake as measured by a simple food-frequency questionnaire. This finding was confirmed by Stryker and colleagues (1988), who also found that the slope of the regression line relating carotene intake to plasma beta-carotene was significantly reduced among smokers compared with nonsmokers. This implies that smoking has a direct metabolic effect on blood beta-carotene level and renders those studies of blood beta-carotene level and lung cancer risk, viewed on their own, almost uninterpretable. In theory, these studies have controlled for the confounding effects of smoking by adjusting for the reported number of cigarettes smoked daily. In reality, this is a rather crude measure of the actual physiologic impact of cigarette smoking as persons smoking exactly the same number of cigarettes per day can differ in unmeasurable details of the cigarette smoked, depth of inhalation, and the anatomic structure of their lungs. To the extent that these factors determine the concentration of tobacco combustion products in lung tissue and thus influence both the risk of lung cancer and blood levels of beta-carotene, confounding due to the actual physiologic intensity of smoking is not fully controllable in epidemiologic analyses. This problem could be particularly intractable because of the overwhelmingly strong relationship between cigarette smoking and lung cancer.

Fortunately, evidence for a relationship between beta-carotene and lung cancer is not solely based on the biochemical data. The consistent observation between intake of carotenoids and this disease strongly suggests that the higher risk of lung cancer among persons with low serum beta-carotene levels is not merely due to a metabolic effect of smoking on the blood levels, although it is possible that the magnitude of the relationship with serum levels may still be exaggerated. This issue illustrates one of the potential limitations of biochemical markers of diet. It has been frequently said that an advantage of such markers is that they provide a measure of exposure that is more proximal to the disease process than measurements based on dietary intake. If the question being addressed is the relation of dietary intake to risk of disease, however, then the biochemical indicators are less direct measures of exposure than diet itself. As such, they may be influenced by nondietary factors that can add extraneous variation. More seriously, the biochemical indicators are subject to the same sources of confounding as the dietary intake measures, plus additional sources of confounding that affect the biochemical levels independent of dietary intake. Thus these two general approaches of measuring exposure should be viewed as complementary, rather than one being a substitute for the other.

FURTHER CONSIDERATIONS

The remarkable consistency of the association between carotenoid intake and lung cancer seen in the case–control and cohort studies as well as those investigations based on prediagnostic blood specimens strongly suggests that this relationship is not due to chance or to methodologic artifact. What has remained less certain is whether this finding represents a true causal effect of beta-carotene or a confounding effect of another dietary or nondietary factor associated with carotene intake. It is particularly difficult to exclude the possibility that

another component of certain fruits and vegetables, such as a carotenoid other than beta-carotene or an indole compound (Wattenberg and Loub, 1978), is the truly protective factor. Indeed, the analysis of Ziegler et al. (1996) suggests that beta-carotene is not the responsible factor. The available data are, therefore, probably best interpreted as providing strong support for a protective effect of fruits and vegetables against lung cancer.

Ideally, the issue of confounding is best resolved in a randomized trial, as discussed later. Additional insight, however, can be gained by examining the relationships between individual food items and risk of lung cancer. The observations that carrots and yellow-range vegetables (Mettlin et al., 1979; Kvale et al., 1983; Ziegler et al., 1996), as well as green leafy vegetables (MacLennan et al., 1977; Ziegler et al., 1984; Steinmetz et al., 1993; Mayne et al., 1994), are associated with reduced risk provide some additional suggestion that a carotenoid may be the active agent as these distinctly different types of vegetables both have high concentrations of this nutrient. Unfortunately, the data from many studies have not been fully exploited by carefully examining the associations of specific foods or food groups with risk of lung cancer. In conducting such analyses it is important to control the effects of one food for use of other foods related to risk of disease as their consumption is typically correlated (Le Marchand et al., 1989).

RANDOMIZED TRIALS

A clear demonstration of an anticancer effect of beta-carotene in animal experiments would add substantially to the likelihood that this agent accounts for the observed inverse associations between consumption of fruits and vegetables and lung cancer risk in epidemiologic studies. Although many experiments have been conducted addressing the effect of preformed vitamin A and its synthetic analogues on the occurrence of tumors in animals, beta-carotene has been studied far less extensively in this manner (Krinsky, 1993). Beta-carotene, as well as other carotenoids without potential vitamin A activity, protect mice against skin tumors induced by ultraviolet light and chemical carcinogens (Mathews-Roth, 1982). It is not clear, however, whether this represents a specific protective effective against ultraviolet light, which beta-carotene is known to possess (Mathews-Roth et al., 1977). In one animal model neither beta-carotene nor preformed vitamin A inhibited lung tumors when given alone, but they were effective when administered together (Moon et al., 1992). In a short-term mouse lung tumor model, beta-carotene did not have any effect, whereas other plant extracts did (Yun et al., 1995). Beta-carotene caused a nonsignificant increase in respiratory tract tumors in another tumor model (Wolterbeek et al., 1995). When compared directly, alpha-carotene has appeared more potent than beta-carotene in preventing skin and lung cancers in other animal models (Murakoshi et al., 1992; Nishino, 1995). Thus, evidence from animal studies does not add clear support for a preventive role of beta-carotene against lung cancer, but alpha-carotene seems more promising.

The most rigorous test of the hypothesis that beta-carotene or another specific carotenoid reduces lung cancer risk in humans would be a randomized trial. Compared with trials of other dietary factors this is relatively easy to implement as the active agent can be formulated as a capsule that can be compared with a placebo in a double-blind manner. This is somewhat less straightforward than a typical drug trial, however, as all participants are consuming some of the active agent and have ready access to more through their diet or as a supplement from their local health food store. Because the effect of a supplement may well be greatest among persons with low initial dietary intakes of carotene, it would be important to at least measure dietary intake at baseline and, ideally, to screen potential participants and enroll only those with lower intake. Further considerations for design of such trials are discussed elsewhere (Stampfer et al., 1988).

Three large trials of beta-carotene supplementation have been completed, with findings that were largely unanticipated. In the first study, conducted among smoking men in Finland (The Alpha-Tocopherol Beta-Carotene Cancer Prevention Study Group, 1994), the follow up was stopped prematurely at approximately 6 years because incidence of lung cancer was about 18% *higher* in men receiving beta-carotene supplements than among those who did not. Rates of coronary heart disease and total mortality were also increased. In the CARET study (Omenn et al., 1996), conducted among mainly men who were at high risk due to smoking or asbestos exposure, a combination of beta-carotene and preformed vitamin A (25,000 IU daily) was compared with placebo. Follow up was also stopped prematurely because of a significant 28% increase in incidence of lung cancer among men receiving the supplements. Total mortality was also significantly elevated. In the third large randomized trial (Hennekens et al., 1996), U.S. physicians who received beta-carotene supplements for approximately 12 years experienced neither an increase nor a decrease in lung cancer (relative risk = 0.93). Since only 11% of these physicians smoked at baseline, the rate of lung cancer was low, and the 95% confidence interval (0.69 to 1.26) did not exclude a modest decrease in lung cancer risk or an increase of the magnitude seen in the other studies. Beta-carotene was included together with antioxidant nutrients in a randomized trial of cancer prevention in China (Blot et al., 1994); the incidence of stomach cancer was reduced, and a nonsignificantly lower risk of lung cancer was also seen.

These randomized trials collectively provide strong evidence against the hypothesis that high doses of beta-carotene supplementation can substantially reduce the risk of lung cancer. However, the increased incidence of lung cancer in two of the studies was highly unsuspected and raises further questions. When only the Finnish data were available, the possibility existed that chance explained the increase in risk (even though statistically significant) and that the trial had not been of sufficient duration to observe a realistic protective effect. However, the similar results in the CARET study strongly increase the likelihood that beta-carotene supplements do cause an increase in lung cancer in men at high risk due to cigarette smoking. Although the lack of any protective effect in the Physicians' Health Study, which lasted for 12 years, decreases the probability that an important protective effect was missed due to insufficient follow up, this still remains possible. Lung cancer risk does not appreciably increase until after several decades of smoking, so that a protective effect against the early stages of carcinogenesis would not have been detected in any of these trials.

The increase in risk of lung cancer among smoking men supplemented with high doses of beta-carotene strongly suggests that carotenoids are in some way related to carcinogenesis, although these relations are likely much more complex than anticipated. That beta-carotene per se is directly carcinogenic remains unlikely given the abundant literature indicating inverse associations with both intake and blood levels. Even in the Finnish trial, baseline serum levels of beta-carotene were inversely related to risk (Albanes et al., 1995). One speculative explanation could be that some other carotenoid, or combination of carotenoids, is actually protective and that the pharmacologic dose of beta-carotene given as a supplement interfered with the absorption or metabolism of the critical related factor. Such a hypothesis would be consistent with the observations that intake of other carotenoids has been more strongly associated with reduced lung cancer risk than beta-carotene (Ziegler et al., 1992,

1996). Also, beta-carotene has been shown to interfere with absorption of other carotenoids when given simultaneously (Micozzi et al., 1992; Kostic et al., 1995). The lack of an adverse (or beneficial) effect of beta-carotene in the Physicians' Health Study could possibly be related to the higher levels of blood carotenoids at baseline due to greater dietary intake in this health-conscious population, together with a low prevalence of smoking. Although only beta-carotene levels were measured, the median levels at baseline were 170 ng/ml in the Finnish trial (The Alpha-Tocopherol Beta-Carotene Cancer Prevention Study Group, 1994), 221 ng/ml in the Physicians' Health Study (preliminary data, personal communication from C. Hennekens), and 152 ng/ml in the CARET study (M. Thornquist, personal communication). In the recent investigation of an outbreak of optic neuritis in Cuba, the combination of low lycopene and cigarette smoking was particularly strongly related to increased risk, compatible with both an increased oxidative stress and lack of antioxidant protection (Anonymous, 1995). Collectively, these trials suggest that carotenoids have biologic activity but that their relation with lung cancer risk is far more complex than initially hypothesized.

SUMMARY

The inverse relationship between intake of vegetables and fruits and risk of lung cancer, which has been found in many case–control and cohort studies using both questionnaire and biochemical measurements of intake, represents one of the best established associations in the field of nutritional epidemiology. Both epidemiologic studies and randomized trials now indicate that this is unlikely to be due to a protective effect of beta-carotene. These randomized trials would have provided definitive information regarding the effect of beta-carotene if a reduction in cancer had been seen. Had they been totally null, it would have been difficult to exclude the possibility that the treatment was not continued for an adequate time or that study populations did not include a sufficient number of persons who were susceptible by virtue of low dietary carotenoid intake to observe an effect of supplementation. The unanticipated increase in risk among supplement users in populations of smokers greatly reduces the likelihood that beta-carotene is the protective factor in fruits and vegetables and thus makes it more likely that other carotenoids or unrelated constituents are the active agents.

We are left with the knowledge that intake of fruits and vegetables is associated with lower risk of lung cancer. The National Research Council and other bodies have recommended an increased intake of fruits and vegetables (Committee on Diet Nutrition and Cancer Assembly of Life Sciences, National Research Council, 1982; U.S. Department of Agriculture, U.S. Department of Health and Human Services, 1995). However, which fruits and vegetables are beneficial and what should be the optimal intake of these products remains unclear. The customary advice to eat a variety of fruits and vegetables is reasonable given our state of knowledge but leaves much to chance. For example, if a specific carotene is actually an active anticancer agent, it is quite possible to eat a variety of these products, such as cucumbers, iceberg lettuce, eggplant, and onions, and still have a low intake of carotenoids.

Thus, more specific and detailed analyses of observational data could be of great value. Maximal information should be extracted by conducting data analyses for individual foods and for known nutrients and other phytochemicals hypothesized to reduce cancer risk. In investigations using biochemical measurements, it will be helpful to measure a wide variety of nutritional factors, including other specific carotenoids. The most powerful information would be derived from prospective studies that employ both questionnaire and biochemical assessments.

REFERENCES

Albanes, D., O. P. Heinonen, J. K. Huttunen, P. R. Taylor, J. Virtamo, B. K. Edwards, J. Haapakoski, M. Rautalahti, A. M. Hartman, J. Palmgren, and P. Greenwald (1995). Effects of alpha-tocopherol and beta-carotene supplements on cancer incidence in the Alpha-Tocopherol Beta-Carotene Cancer Prevention Study. *Am J Clin Nutr 62 (suppl 6)*, S1427–S1430.

Anonymous (1995). Epidemic optic neuropathy in Cuba—Clinical characterization and risk factors. The Cuba Neuropathy Field Investigation Team. *N Engl J Med 333*, 1176–1182.

Atukorala, S., T. K. Basu, J. W. Dickerson, D. Donaldson, and A. Sakula (1979). Vitamin A, zinc, and lung cancer. *Br J Cancer 40*, 927–931.

Bjelke, E. (1975). Dietary vitamin A and human lung cancer. *Int J Cancer 15*, 561–565.

Blot, W. J., J. Y. Li, P. R. Taylor, and B. Li (1994). Lung cancer. and vitamin supplementation (letter). *N Engl J Med 331*, 614.

Burton, G. W., and K. U. Ingold (1984). Beta-carotene: An unusual type of lipid antioxidant. *Science 224*, 569–573.

Byers, T. E., S. Graham, B. P. Haughey, J. R. Marshall, and M. K. Swanson (1987). Diet and lung cancer risk: Findings from the Western New York Diet Study. *Am J Epidemiol 125*, 351–363.

Candelora, E. C., H. G. Stockwell, A. W. Armstrong, and P. A. Pinkham (1992). Dietary intake and risk of lung cancer in women who never smoked. *Nutr Cancer 17*, 263–270.

Chengyu, H., Z. Xiuquan, Q. Zhongkai, G. Li, P. Shusheng, L. Jiangrong, X. Ruming, and Z. Li (1992). A case–control study of dietary factors in patients with lung cancer. *Biomed Environ Sci 5*, 257–265.

Chow, W.-H., L. M. Schuman, J. K. Mc-Laughlin, E. Bjelke, G. Gridley, S. Wacholder, H. T. Co Chien, and W. J. Blot (1992). A cohort stdy of tobacco use, diet, occupation, and lung cancer mortality. *Cancer Causes Control 3*, 247–254.

Committee on Diet, Nutrition, and Cancer, Assembly of Life Sciences, National Research Council (1982). *Diet, Nutrition, and Cancer*. Washington, D.C: National Academy Press.

Connett, J. E., L. H. Kuller, M. O. Kjelsberg, B. F. Polk, G. Collins, A. Rider, and S. B. Hulley (1989). Relationship between carotenoids and cancer. The Multiple Risk Factor Intervention Trial (MRFIT) Study. *Cancer 64*, 126–134.

Costantino, J. P., L. H. Kuller, L. Begg, C. K. Redmond, and M. W. Bates (1988). Serum level changes after administration of a pharmacologic dose of β-carotene. *Am J Clin Nutr 48*, 1277–1283.

Dartigues, J. F., F. Dabis, N. Gros, A. Moise, G. Bois, R. Salamon, J. M. Dilhuydy, and G. Courty (1990). Dietary vitamin A, beta-carotene, and risk of epidemoid lung cancer in south-western France. *Eur J Epidemiol 6*, 261–265.

De Luca, L., N. Maestri, F. Bonanni, and D. Nelson (1972). Maintenance of epithelial cell differentiation: The mode of action of vitamin A. *Cancer 30*, 1326–1331.

Fontham, E. T., L. W. Pickle, W. Haenszel, P. Correa, Y. Lin, and R. T. Falk (1988). Dietary vitamin A and C and lung cancer risk in Louisiana. *Cancer 62*, 2267–2273.

Friedman, G. D., W. S. Blaner, D. S. Goodman, J. H. Vogelman, J. L. Brind, R. Hoover, B. H. Fireman, and N. Orentreich (1986). Serum retinol and retinol-binding protein levels do not predict subsequent lung cancer. *Am J Epidemiol 123*, 781–789.

Gregor, A., P. N. Lee, and F. J. C. Roe, et al. (1980). Comparison of dietary histories in lung cancer cases and controls with special reference to vitamin A. *Nutr Cancer 2*, 93–97.

Harris, R. W., T. J. Key, P. B. Silcocks, D. Bull, and N. J. Wald (1991). A case–control study of dietary carotene in men with lung cancer and in men with other epithelial cancers. *Nutr Cancer 15*, 63–68.

Hennekens, C. H., J. E. Buring, J. E. Manson, M. J. Stampfer, B. Rosner, N. R. Cook, C. Belanger, F. LaMotte, J. M. Gaziano, P. M. Ridker, W. C. Willett, and R. Peto (1996). Lack of effect of long-term supplementation with beta carotene on the incidence of malignant neoplasms and cardiovascular disease. *N Engl J Med 334*, 1145–1149.

Hill, D. L., and C. J. Grubbs (1982). Retinoids as chemopreventive and anticancer agents in intact animals. *Anticancer Res 2*, 111–124.

Hinds, M. W., L. N. Kolonel, J. H. Hankin, and J. Lee (1984). Dietary vitamin A, carotene, vitamin C, and risk of lung cancer in Hawaii. *Am J Epidemiol 119*, 227–237.

Hirayama, T. (1979). Diet and cancer. *Nutr Cancer 1*, 67–81.

Ho, S. C., S. P. Donnan, W. C. Martin, and S. Y. Tsao (1988). Dietary vitamin A, beta-carotene and risk of epidermoid lung cancer among Chinese males. *Singapore Med J 29*, 213–218.

Jain, M., J. D. Burch, G. R. Howe, H. A. Risch, and A. B. Miller (1990). Dietary factors and risk of lung cancer: Results from a case–control study, Toronto, 1981–1985. *Int J Cancer 45*, 287–293.

Kalandidi, A., K. Katsouyanni, N. Voropoulou, G. Bastas, R. Saracci, and D. Trichopoulos (1990). Passive smoking and diet in the etiology of lung cancer among non-smokers. *Cancer Causes Control 1*, 15–21.

Kark, J. D., A. H. Smith, B. R. Switzer, and C. G. Hames (1981). Serum vitamin A (retinol) and cancer incidence in Evans County, Georgia. *JNCI 66*, 7–16.

Knekt, P., R. Jarvinen, R. Seppanen, A. Rissanen, A. Aromaa, O. P. Heinonen, D. Albanes, M. Heinonen, E. Pukkala, and L. Teppo (1991). Dietary antioxidants and the risk of lung cancer. *Am J Epidemiol 134*, 471–479.

Koo, L. C. (1988). Dietary habits and lung cancer risk among Chinese females in Hong Kong who never smoked. *Nutr Cancer 11*, 155–172.

Kostic, D., W. S. White, and J. A. Olson (1995). Intestinal absorption, serum clearance, and interactions between lutein and beta-carotene when administered to human adults in separate or combined oral doses. *Am J Clin Nutr 62*, 604–610.

Krinsky, N. I. (1993). Actions of carotenoids in biological systems. *Annu Rev Nutr 13*, 561–587.

Krinsky, N. I., and S. M. Deneke (1982). Interaction of oxygen and oxy-radicals with carotenoids. *JNCI 69*, 205–210.

Kromhout, D. (1987). Essential micronutrients in relation to carcinogenesis. *Am J Clin Nutr 45(suppl)*, 1361–1367.

Kvale, G., E. Bjelke, and J. J. Gart (1983). Dietary habits and lung cancer risk. *Int J Cancer 31*, 397–405.

Le Marchand, L., J. H. Hankin, L. N. Kolonel, G. R. Beecher, L. R. Wilkens, and L. P. Zhao (1993). Intake of specific carotenoids and lung cancer risk. *Cancer Epidemiol Biomarkers Prev 2*, 183–187.

Le Marchand, L., C. N. Yoshizawa, L. N. Kolonel, J. H. Hankin, and M. T. Goodman (1989). Vegetable consumption and lung cancer risk: A population-based case–control study in Hawaii. *JNCI 81*, 1158–1164.

MacLennan, R., J. Da Costa, N. E. Day, C. H. Law, Y. K. Ng, and K. Shanmugaratnam (1977). Risk factors for lung cancer in Singapore Chinese, a population with high female incidence rates. *Int J Cancer 20*, 854–860.

Mathews-Roth, M. M. (1982). Antitumor activity of beta-carotene, canthaxanthin and phytoene. *Oncology 39*, 33–37.

Mathews-Roth, M. M., M. A. Pathak, T. B. Fitzpatrick, L. H. Harber, and E. H. Kass (1977). Beta-carotene therapy for erythro-poietic protoporphyria and other photo-sensitivity diseases. *Arch Dermatol 113*, 1229–1232.

Mayne, S. T., D. T. Janerich, P. Greenwald, S. Chorost, C. Tucci, M. B. Zaman, M. R. Melamed, M. Kiely, and M. F. McKneally (1994). Dietary beta carotene and lung can-cer risk in U.S. nonsmokers. *JNCI 86*, 33–38.

McCormick, D. L., F. J. Burns, and R. E. Albert (1981). Inhibition of benzo[a]pyrene-induced mammary carcinogenesis by reti-nyl acetate. *JNCI 66*, 559–564.

Menkes, M. S., G. W. Comstock, J. P. Vuilleu-mier, K. J. Helsing, A. A. Rider, and R. Brookmeyer (1986). Serum beta-carotene, vitamins A and E, selenium, and the risk of lung cancer. *N Engl J Med 315*, 1250–1254.

Mettlin, C., S. Graham, and M. Swanson (1979). Vitamin A and lung cancer. *JNCI 62*, 1435–1438.

Micozzi, M. S., E. D. Brown, B. K. Edwards, J. G. Bieri, P. R. Taylor, F. Khachik, G. R. Beecher, and J. C. Smith, Jr. (1992). Plasma carotenoid response to chronic intake of se-lected foods and beta-carotene supplements in men. *Am J Clin Nutr 55*, 1120–1125.

Moon, R. C., K. V. Rao, C. J. Detrisac, and G. J. Kelloff (1992). Animal models for chemoprevention of respiratory cancer. *JNCI Monogr 13*, 45–49.

Murakoshi, M., H. Nishino, Y. Satomi, J. Tak-ayasu, T. Hasegawa, H. Tokuda, A. Iwash-ima, J. Okuzumi, H. Okabe, H. Kitano, et al. (1992). Potent preventive action of al-pha-carotene against carcinogenesis: Spon-taneous liver carcinogenesis and promoting stage of lung and skin carcinogenesis in mice are suppressed more effectively by al-pha-carotene than by beta-carotene. *Can-cer Res 52*, 6583–6587.

Nishino, H. (1995). Cancer chemoprevention by natural carotenoids and their related compounds. *J Cell Biochem 33 (suppl)*, 231–235.

Nomura, A. M., G. N. Stemmermann, L. K. Heilbrun, R. M. Salkeld, and J. P. Vuilleu-mier (1985). Serum vitamin levels and the risk of cancer of specific sites in men of Jap-anese ancestry in Hawaii. *Cancer Res 45*, 2369–2372.

Omenn, G. S., G. E. Goodman, M. D. Thorn-quist, J. Balmes, M. R. Cullen, A. Glass, J. P. Keogh, F. L. Meyskens, B. Valanis, J. H.

Williams, S. Barnhart, and S. Hammar (1996). Effects of a combination of beta carotene and vitamin A on lung cancer and cardiovascular disease. *N Engl J Med 334*, 1150–1155.

Paganini-Hill, A., A. Chao, R. K. Ross, and B. E. Henderson (1987). Vitamin A, beta-carotene, and the risk of cancer: A pro-spective study. *JNCI 79*, 443–448.

Pastorino, U., P. Pisani, F. Berrino, C. Andreoli, A. Barbieri, A. Costa, C. Mazzoleni, G. Gramegna, and E. Marubini (1987). Vita-min A and female lung cancer: A case–con-trol study on plasma and diet. *Nutr Cancer 10*, 171–179.

Paul, A. A., and D. A. T. Southgate (1978). *McCance and Widdowson's the composi-tion of foods*, 4th ed. London: Her Maj-esty's Stationery Office.

Peleg, I., S. Heyden, M. Knowles, and C. G. Hames (1984). Serum retinol and risk of subsequent cancer: Extension of the Evans County, Georgia, study. *JNCI 73*, 1455–1458.

Peto, R. (1983). The marked differences be-tween carotenoids and retinoids: Method-ological implications for biochemical epi-demiology. *Cancer Surv 2*, 327–340.

Peto, R., R. Doll, J. D. Buckley, and M. B. Sporn (1981). Can dietary beta-carotene materially reduce human cancer rates? *Na-ture 290*, 201–208.

Rose, G., and M. J. Shipley (1980). Plasma lip-ids and mortality: A source of error. *Lancet 1*, 523–526.

Russell-Briefel, R., M. W. Bates, and L. H. Kuller (1985). The relationship of plasma carotenoids to health and biochemical fac-tors in middle-aged men. *Am J Epidemiol 122*, 741–749.

Salonen, J. T., R. Salonen, R. Lappetelainen, P. H. Meanpaa, G. Alfthan, and P. Puska (1985). Risk of cancer in relation to serum concentrations of selenium and vitamins A and E: Matched case–control analysis of prospective data. *BMJ Clin Res Ed 290*, 417–420.

Samet, J. M., B. J. Skipper, C. G. Humble, and D. R. Pathak (1985). Lung cancer risk and vitamin A consumption in New Mexico. *Am Rev Respir Dis 131*, 198–202.

Schalch, W. (1992). Carotenoids in the retina: A review of their possible role in preventing or limiting damage caused by light and ox-ygen. In Emerit, I., and Chance, B. (ed.): *Free Radicals and Aging*. Basel, Switzer-land: Birkhauser Verlag, pp 280–298.

Schroder, E. W. and P. H. Black (1980). Reti-noids: Tumor preventers or tumor enhanc-ers. *JNCI 65*, 671–674.

Shekelle, R. B., M. Lepper, S. Liu, C. Maliza, W. J. J. Raynor, A. H. Rossof, O. Paul, A. M. Shryock, and J. Stamler (1981). Dietary vitamin A and risk of cancer in the Western Electric Study. *Lancet 2*, 1186–1190.

Shibata, A., A. Paganini-Hill, R. K. Ross, and B. E. Henderson (1992). Intake of vegetables, fruits, beta-carotene, vitamin C and vitamin supplements and cancer incidence among the elderly: A prospective study. *Br J Cancer 66*, 673–679.

Sporn, M. B., and A. B. Roberts (1983). Role of retinoids in differentiation and carcinogenesis. *Cancer Res 43*, 3034–3040.

Stahelin, H. B., E. Buess, and F. Rosel, et al. (1982). Vitamin A, cardiovasular risk factors, and mortality (letter). *Lancet 1*, 394–395.

Stahelin, H. B., K. F. Gey, M. Eichholzer, E. Ludin, F. Bernasconi, J. Thurneysen, and G. Brubacher (1991). Plasma antioxidant vitamins and subsequent cancer mortality in the 12-year follow-up of the prospective Basel Study. *Am J Epidemiol 133*, 766–775.

Stahelin, H. B., F. Rosel, E. Buess, and G. Brubacher (1984). Cancer, vitamins, and plasma lipids: Prospective Basel Study. *JNCI 73*, 1463–1468.

Stampfer, M. J., W. C. Willett, and C. H. Hennekens (1989). Choice of population for cancer prevention trials. In Moon, T., and Micozzi, M. (eds.): *Nutrition and Cancer Prevention.* New York: Marcel Dekker, pp 473–482.

Steinmetz, K. A., J. D. Potter, and A. R. Folsom (1993). Vegetables, fruit, and lung cancer in the Iowa Women's Health Study. *Cancer Res 53*, 536–543.

Stryker, W. S., L. A. Kaplan, E. A. Stein, M. J. Stampfer, A. Sober, and W. C. Willett (1988). The relation of diet, cigarette smoking, and alcohol consumption to plasma beta-carotene and alpha-tocopherol levels. *Am J Epidemiol 127*, 283–296.

The Alpha-Tocopherol Beta-Carotene Cancer Prevention Study Group (1994). The effect of vitamin E and beta carotene on the incidence of lung cancer and other cancers in male smokers. *N Engl J Med 330*, 1029–1035.

U.S. Department of Agriculture (1989). *Composition of foods—Raw, Processed, and Prepared, 1963–1988. Agricultural Handbook No. 8 Series.* Washington, DC: Department of Agriculture, Government Printing Office.

U.S. Department of Agriculture, U.S. Department of Health and Human Services (1995). *Nutrition and Your health: Dietary Guidelines for Americans. Homes and Garden Bulletin No. 232.* Washington, DC: U.S. Printing Office.

Wald, N., J. Boreham, and A. Bailey (1986). Serum retinol and subsequent risk of cancer. *Br J Cancer 54*, 957–961.

Wald, N., M. Edle, and J. Boreham (1980). Low serum-vitamin A and subsequent risk of cancer. Preliminary results of a prospective study. *Lancet 2*, 813–815.

Wald, N. J., S. G. Thompson, J. W. Densem, J. Boreham, and A. Bailey (1988). Serum beta-carotene and subsequent risk of cancer: Results from the BUPA Study. *Br J Cancer 57*, 428–433.

Wang, L. D., and E. C. Hammond (1985). Lung cancer, fruit, green salad and vitamin pills. *Chin Med J 3*, 206–210.

Wattenberg, L. W., and W. D. Loub (1978). Inhibition of polycyclic aromatic hydrocarbon-induced neoplasia by naturally occurring indoles. *Cancer Res 38*, 1410–1413.

Willett, W. C., M. J. Stampfer, B. A. Underwood, L. A. Sampson, C. H. Hennekens, J. C. Wallingford, L. Cooper, C. C. Hsieh, and F. E. Speizer (1984). Vitamin A supplementation and plasma retinol levels: A randomized trial among women. *JNCI 73*, 1445–1448.

Willett, W. C., M. J. Stampfer, B. A. Underwood, F. E. Speizer, B. Rosner, and C. H. Hennekens (1983). Validation of a dietary questionnaire with plasma carotenoid and alpha-tocopherol levels. *Am J Clin Nutr 38*, 631–639.

Wolbach, S. B., and P. R. Howe (1925). Tissue changes following deprivation of fat-soluble A vitamin. *J Exp Med 42*, 753–777.

Wolterbeek, A. P., E. J. Schoevers, J. P. Bruyntjes, A. A. Rutten, and V. J. Feron (1995). Benzo[a]pyrene-induced respiratory tract cancer in hamsters fed a diet rich in beta-carotene. *J Environ Pathol Toxicol Oncol 14*, 35–43.

Wu, A. H., B. E. Henderson, M. C. Pike, and M. C. Yu (1985). Smoking and other risk factors for lung cancer in women. *JNCI 74*, 747–751.

Yun, T.-K., S.-H. Kim, and Y.-S. Lee (1995). Trial of a new medium-term model using Benzo[a]pyrene induced lung tumor in newborn mice. *Anticancer Res 15*, 839–846.

Ziegler, R. G., E. A. Colavito, P. Hartge, J. McAdams, J. B. Schoenberg, T. J. Mason, and J. F. Fraumeni Jr (1996). Importance of α-carotene, β-carotene, and other phytochemicals in the etiology of lung cancer. *JNCI 88*, 612–615.

Ziegler, R. G., T. J. Mason, A. Stemhagen, R. Hoover, J. B. Schoenberg, G. Gridley, P. W. Virgo, R. Altman, and J. F. Fraumeni Jr (1984). Dietary carotene and vitamin A and risk of lung cancer among white men in New Jersey. *JNCI* 73, 1429–1435.

Ziegler, R. G., A. F. Subar, N. E. Craft, G. Ursin, B. H. Patterson, and B. I. Graubard (1992). Does beta-carotene explain why reduced cancer risk is associated with vegetable and fruit intake? *Cancer Res* 52 *(suppl)*, 2060S–2066S.

16

Dietary Fat and Breast Cancer

The relationship of dietary fat intake with incidence of breast cancer illustrates issues involved in the synthesis of information from animal studies, correlational data based on population groups, studies of individual subjects, and the interpretation of null findings from epidemiologic data. The subject is also of major public health importance because a putative association has been an important rationale for recent recommendations to reduce fat consumption.

Nearly 50 years ago, it was shown that the amount of dietary fat could markedly influence the occurrence of mammary tumors in rodents (Tannenbaum and Silverstone, 1953). For decades this knowledge was largely limited to laboratory scientists, and sometimes regarded as a nuisance variable to those investigating more interesting carcinogens. The publication by Armstrong and Doll (1975) of striking correlations among countries between national per capita fat consumption and both incidence and mortality rates of breast cancer attracted widespread attention in the larger scientific community (Fig. 16–1 for a display of similar data by Carroll, 1975). The international differences in breast cancer rates are particularly great for postmenopausal women, suggesting the hypothesis that diet should be most strongly associated with breast cancer among these women (de Waard et al., 1964). The strong enthusiasm for this hypothesis was reflected in the abstract of a case–control study in which a positive, but not statistically significant, relationship was observed between fat intake and risk of breast cancer (Miller et al., 1978): "The Study has produced evidence of an association between an increased intake of nutrients, especially total fat, in both pre-menopausal and post-menopausal women with breast cancer. Reasons why a weak association might have been anticipated are discussed, and it is concluded that in reality the association is stronger. Furthermore, its consistency with other evidence, both experimental and international, suggests that it is causal."

After reviewing the published data, a

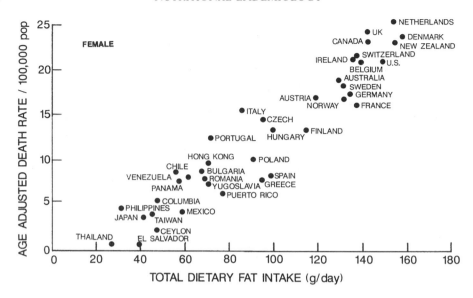

Figure 16–1. Relationship of national per capita fat intake with risk of breast cancer mortality.

(From Carroll, 1975; reproduced with permission.)

committee of the National Research Council issued a provisional recommendation that the fat content of the U.S. diet be reduced from an average of 40% to an average of 30% of calories, largely based on an anticipated reduction in breast cancer rates (Committee on Diet Nutrition and Cancer, Assembly of Life Sciences, National Research Council, 1982). This subsequently became the focus of a major health promotion campaign by the National Cancer Institute (1984). In this instance, epidemiologic findings were translated into public policy with remarkable speed. For purposes of illustration, the epidemiologic data addressing this relationship are examined in some detail.

ECOLOGIC STUDIES

The extremely strong international correlation between national per capita total fat "disappearance" and breast cancer rates has been noted; this correlation is primarily due to animal fat ($r = 0.83$), as the correlation for vegetable fat is considerably lower ($r = 0.18$) (Hems, 1978). The limitations of such data have been discussed

earlier. In particular, the association is potentially confounded by lean body mass, obesity, sedentary lifestyle, reproductive factors, and other correlates of economic development, because the high incidence countries tend to be westernized populations, whereas the low incidence countries tend to be nonindustrialized. Indeed, the correlation between gross national product and breast cancer mortality rate is 0.72 (Armstrong and Doll, 1975). Although Japan may appear to be an exception, because it is an industrialized country with low rates of disease, until recently its population largely consisted of peasant farmers; even in 1950 more than half of its population was rural (Nukada, 1975). Prentice and colleagues (1988, 1990) have examined the relationship between fat disappearance and breast cancer rates for 21 countries and were not able to explain the positive correlation on the basis of standard risk factors, but they did not have data on variables such as body composition and physical activity.

An examination of fat consumption in the analysis of Carroll (1975) reveals some of the problems of data quality using this approach (Fig. 16–1). The fat consumption estimate for the United States is 150 g/day; if this represents 40% of calories (approximate U.S. average in the 1960s and 1970s; National Research Council, Committee on Diet and Health, 1989), then total energy intake would be about 3,400 kcal per individual, including men, women, and children. A more reasonable estimate of a true intake would be 2,600 kcal for men and 1,800 kcal for women (Beaton et al., 1979). To the extent that wastage of fat is greater in the wealthy, industrialized countries, these international correlations are likely to at least in part represent a relationship between food wastage and breast cancer risk.

Other geographic correlations between fat intake and breast cancer risk are less striking. Chen and colleagues (1990) conducted a correlational study among 65 counties in China using a standardized method of dietary assessment in samples of men and women from each county, thus avoiding many of the problems associated with the use of food "disappearance" data. In addition, the potential for confounding by factors associated with affluent lifestyles was considerably reduced because all units of observation were within China. Although the mean fat intake for various counties varied considerably, ranging from 6% to 25% of energy, intake was only weakly associated with breast cancer mortality rates among women over 55 years of age (Marshall et al., 1992). The observation that fat intake was approximately 25% of energy in several counties and thus similar to intakes among women with low fat intake in the United States (Willett et al., 1992), despite a breast cancer mortality rate of approximately one-fifth of that in the United States, provides strong evidence that factors other than fat intake are the major determinants of the international differences in breast cancer. Because total energy intake among Chinese women was high (2,600 kcal/day) compared with older U.S. women, presumably reflecting high levels of physical activity, the overlap in

absolute fat intake was even greater; intake in the highest quintile of Chinese women (72 g/day) was similar to the fourth quintile of U.S. women (Willett et al., 1992) (Fig. 16–2). For geographic areas within England, a positive correlation between per capita consumption of dairy fat and breast cancer rates has been noted, but fat intake from other sources was inversely related to breast cancer rates (Stocks, 1970).

MIGRANT STUDIES

Migrant studies have demonstrated that the large differences in breast cancer rates among countries are not attributable to genetic factors. Buell (1973) observed that the offspring of immigrants from Japan to the United States, but not the immigrants themselves, have breast cancer rates that are similar to those of the general American population. Polish women, however, who migrate to the United Kingdom or the United States (Staszewski and Haenszel, 1965; Adelstein et al., 1979), and Italian women who migrate to Australia (McMichael and Giles, 1988), themselves attain rates of breast cancer that are similar to the higher rates among women born in these countries, suggesting that the delayed effect among Japanese-Americans may be due to a slower acculturation process. This distinction is potentially important for dietary studies, because an exposure that acts only in childhood but is manifested decades later will be difficult to investigate. More recently, Ziegler and colleagues (1993) used a case–control study design to examine risk of breast cancer among Asian-Americans in relation to age at migration. A sixfold gradient in risk was seen comparing women who had migrated from rural areas in Asia after age 36 years to women who had always lived in the United States. Although increases in risk were seen among the migrants themselves, the full impact of living in the United States was not manifested until three generations of U.S. residence. Thus, the potential periods of susceptibility to a western lifestyle appear

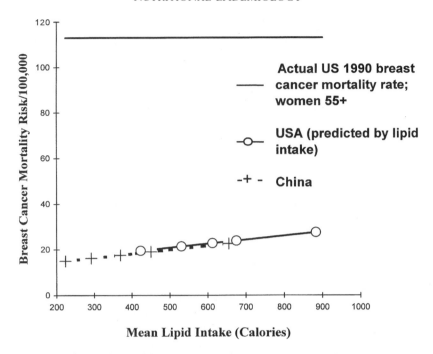

Figure 16–2. Dietary fat intake and breast cancer mortality rates in 65 Chinese counties. Also shown are predicted mortality rates for quintiles of fat intake in the Nurses' Health Study, showing the relationship between fat intake and breast cancer mortality in China. Note the considerable overlap of absolute fat intake and large differences between predicted and actual U.S. breast cancer mortality rate. (Adapted from Marshall et al., 1992.)

to include midlife and later, and effects of lifestyle may also be transmitted across generations.

SPECIAL POPULATIONS

The rates of breast cancer among special populations who have been consuming unique diets for long periods are of interest because an influence of diet should not be missed due to error in the measurement of individual diets or to a limited follow-up period in a cohort study. When compared with that for a U.S. white population of similar socioeconomic level, breast cancer mortality rates among a large group of Seventh-day Adventists were only slightly and nonsignificantly lower than expected (standardized mortality rate = 0.85) (Phillips et al., 1980). In striking contrast, the colon cancer mortality rate among the Seventh-day Adventists was only about half that of

the comparison population. Although total fat intake of Seventh-day Adventists (36% of energy) has been only slightly lower than the general U.S. population, vegetable fat is largely substituted for animal fat (Mills et al., 1988); thus these data do not support the hypotheses that animal fat or meat intakes are specifically related to breast cancer.

Kinlen (1982) compared rates of breast cancer among orders of nuns who either were vegetarians or ate only small amounts of meat with rates among single British women (thus presumably controlling for parity); no significant differences were found. Because these women had typically entered their convent before age 20, a contrast in diet had existed for many decades. Although the conclusions of this study were limited by the modest number of cases of breast cancer among the nuns (n = 62) and the limited quantitative data on their diets, this study illustrates the potential value of special exposure groups to evaluate dietary hypotheses. We cannot be certain that an unknown risk factor among the vegetarian nuns compensated for a protective effect of their diet, but this would require a complex hypothesis. If the rates of breast cancer had been different, the interpretation would be more difficult because many factors other than fat intake, both dietary and nondietary, differed between the groups of women.

The very strong correlation between dietary fat intake and breast cancer rates among five ethnic groups living in Hawaii (Kolonel et al., 1981) (Fig. 16–3) has been interpreted by some as evidence of an etiologic relationship. An examination of the scale of this figure, however, indicates that a 34% increase in fat is associated with a 200% increase in breast cancer incidence. Although it is possible that dietary fat intake explains some of the differences in rates, the implausibly strong relationship, which is much stronger than suggested by the international correlations, increases the likelihood that the association observed in this study is confounded by some other factors.

SECULAR TRENDS

Major changes in breast cancer rates within one country provide further strong evidence that nongenetic factors have an important influence on the occurrence of this disease. For example, dramatic changes in breast cancer incidence have occurred in Iceland during this century (Bjarnason et al., 1974). This increase was primarily in women 45 years of age and older (Fig. 16–4), which provides evidence to support the hypothesis of de Waard and coworkers (1964) that environmental factors differentially affect premenopausal and postmenopausal disease. Because the diet of the Icelandic population changed substantially over that period of time, becoming high in fat composition like other Western countries, these data are consistent with the

hypothesis that fat intake causes breast cancer, but do not exclude other possible explanations, including changes in reproductive factors, physical activity, and an increase in total energy availability in relation to requirements.

Since 1960, breast cancer incidence rates have increased in virtually all countries where data are available, including developing countries (Ursin et al., 1994). Prentice and Sheppard (1990) have reported that changes in absolute fat disappearance and changes in breast cancer incidence rates within countries are positively correlated. However, such analyses illustrate the potential pitfalls in using disappearance data. For example, in the United States, the apparent increase in fat intake resulted from a physiologically implausible increase in total energy disappearance (probably due to greater wastage of food); in actuality, fat intake as a percentage of energy has been declining since about the 1960s (Stephen and Wald, 1990; Willett and Stampfer, 1990; Centers for Disease Control and Prevention, National Center for Health Statistics, 1994). Because breast cancer incidence has steadily risen over this period, the secular trend does not support a causal role of fat intake.

Enig and colleagues (1978) have related consumption of different types of fats to the apparent increase in incidence of breast and other cancers in the United States. They have reported that the strongest association is that with the consumption of *trans*-fatty acids, which are fatty acids created in processes that convert liquid vegetable oils to margarine and solid vegetable shortening. Although this analysis should encourage further examination of the relationship between intake of *trans*-fatty acids and breast cancer risk, such data are far from conclusive because other aspects of lifestyle have also changed over time.

Famines or other sudden changes in national diets due to war and social upheavals may potentially be useful to examine the latent period between change in diet

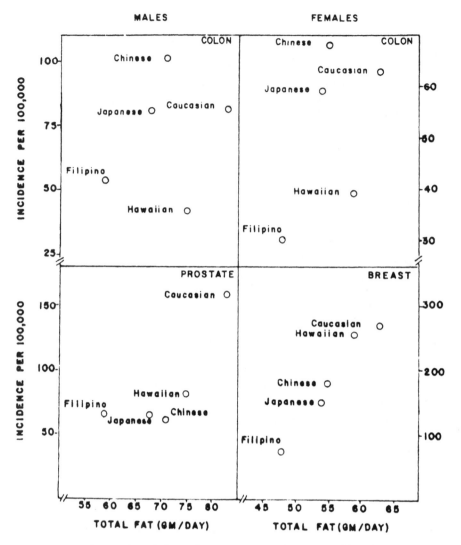

Figure 16–3. Dietary fat intake of five ethnic groups in Hawaii in relation to age-adjusted cancer incidence among men and women 45 years of age or older. (From Kolonel et al., 1981; reproduced with permission.)

and change in breast cancer rates. Ingram (1981) used this approach to examine the breast cancer mortality rates in England and Wales in relation to the marked changes in diet that occurred during World War II. He found positive correlations between breast cancer mortality and intake of meat, fat, and sugar, with maximal associations for a lag interval of 12 years. The marked differences in breast cancer mortality observed by Ingram, however, appear

to be an artifact due to a change in procedures for coding deaths (Key et al., 1987). Thus it appears that the changes in diet during and after World War II in England had no important effect on breast cancer mortality. More recently, Tretli and Gaard (1996) conducted a birth cohort analysis of breast cancer mortality rates in Norway (Fig. 16–5); women born in 1930 to 1932, who were thus exposed to famine during World War II, experienced an over-

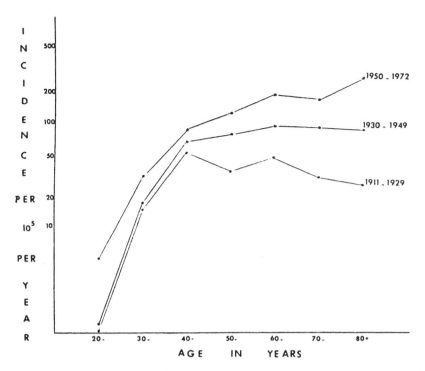

Figure 16–4. Age-specific incidence of breast cancer in Iceland for the three time periods 1911–1929, 1930–1949, and 1950–1972.

(From Bjarnason et al., 1974; reproduced with permission.)

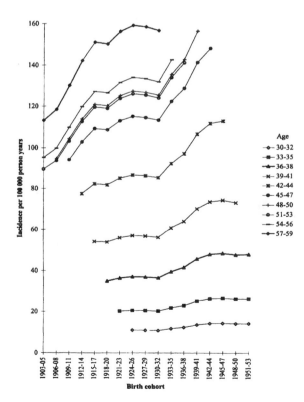

Figure 16–5. The estimated incidence of breast cancer in Norwegian women by age at diagnoses and birth cohort. (From Tretli and Gaard, 1996; reproduced with permission.)

all 13% lower risk of subsequent breast cancer, which has been manifested at all ages as these women have passed through the menopausal years. This finding provides strong support for an important role of diet during the period of sexual maturation but cannot distinguish between effects of total energy, fat, or meat, as these, as well as other aspects of diet, were greatly altered during the famine.

CASE–CONTROL STUDIES

The relationship between fat intake and risk of breast cancer has been examined in many case–control studies. This design can potentially allow for control of the many variables that could confound international comparisons. In the first detailed case–control study, Miller and colleagues (1978) compared the diets of 400 Canadian women with breast cancer with those of 400 neighborhood controls. Because of the exceptional quality of the data and the prominence this study has received as support for the dietary fat and breast cancer hypothesis (see the beginning of this chapter), the findings are examined in detail.

In the study conducted by Miller and colleagues (1978) three methods were used to measure dietary intake. A 24-hour recall was administered to familiarize subjects with the process of reporting food intake; a 4-day dietary record was completed to serve as a standard for validating their diet history questionnaire; and the dietary history questionnaire was completed during an interview that referred to a 2-month period 6 months earlier, with the intent of avoiding any influence of the cancer diagnosis or treatment on the report of diet. In their companion paper (Morgan et al., 1978), the authors state that they "believe that both the 24-hour recall and the 4-day diary are inherently less reliable for individual estimates of usual intake, and that when such estimates are required, the diet history should be used." They further appropriately note that in a case–control study there is reason to be concerned that

the diagnosis or treatment of cancer could alter diet or its recall; this is an additional reason to believe that data based on a 24-hour recall or on a diet record collected after the diagnosis of cancer will not be relevant to disease etiology.

Although Miller and colleagues (1978) presented their data in several ways, for purposes of illustration the means for cases and controls are shown here. Epidemiologists typically divide continuous exposures into categories, use one of these categories as a reference, and compare rates or relative risks of disease for the other categories to those for the reference. Analyzed in this way, it frequently becomes apparent that substantial and important effects of the exposure are present even when the differences in mean values for cases and controls seem trivial (see Chapter 3). Although a thorough analysis will include a display of relative risks according to exposure level, it is useful to recognize that these data are derived from the continuous distributions for cases and controls and that comparisons of mean values for the two groups, given that they are approximately normal and have similar variances, can provide a concise and informative summary of the data. Moreover, the potential for any systematic error or bias between cases and controls to distort the association can often be best appreciated by comparing means because the impact of even small and highly plausible degrees of bias becomes clear.

The primary findings from the study of Miller and colleagues (1978) are displayed in Table 16–1; although the authors provided information for other dietary lipid fractions, the data for calories, total fat, and saturated fat form the basis of their conclusions. It is apparent that the only statistically significant results are for data based on the 24-hour recall, which the authors appropriately believe is likely to be both unreliable (subject to major random error) as well as potentially biased in the context of this case–control study because it reflects diet (for the cases) after the di-

Table 16–1. Mean nutrient intake based on 24-hour recall, 4-day diet record, and diet history questionnaire for breast cancer cases and controls, premenopausal and postmenopausal women combined

Nutrients and series	Dietary method		
	24-hour recall	4-day record	History
Total calories			
Cases	1,697	1,805	2,280
Controls	1,587	1,785	2,230
Difference[a]	109	20	50[d]
(n)[b]	(396)	(309)	(388)
	($p = 0.01$)[c]		
Total fat (g)			
Cases	73.2	81.9	99.1
Controls	69.4	80.0	96.6
Difference	3.7	1.9	2.5
(n)	(386)	(309)	(395)
Saturated fat (g)			
Cases	28.0	32.0	38.3
Controls	26.2	30.3	37.1
Difference	1.8	1.7	1.2
(n)	(383)	(306)	(397)

[a] Mean difference for matched pairs.

[b] Number of pairs.

[c] One-sided p values; other comparisons not statistically significant.

[d] Difference erroneously given as 150 in original table.

Data from Miller et al., 1978.

agnosis of breast cancer. For their preferred method of assessment, the dietary history questionnaire, the differences between cases and controls are small and not statistically significant, even by their one-sided test. Moreover, the magnitude of the difference in total or saturated fat intake between cases and controls is almost exactly proportional to that of total caloric intake. From these data it can be calculated that the cases reported 39.1% of their calories from fat and the controls 39.0% of calories from fat. For saturated fat, the values are 15.1% for cases and 15.0% for controls. (As discussed in Chapter 11, this is not the optimal method to adjust for total caloric intake in an epidemiologic context, but will be close because of the minimal association between total energy intake and breast cancer risk. The optimal analysis would require the original raw data.) Thus, this study actually provides no support for the

hypothesis that the fat composition of the diet affects risk of breast cancer; furthermore, it illustrates the potential for bias when collecting information about diet after the 24-hour recall rather than before the diagnosis of disease.

Although the overall data of the study by Miller and coworkers (1978) do not support the hypothesis that dietary fat increases the risk of breast cancer, it is possible that a positive association exists within a subgroup that is obscured by only examining the total group. Many believe that diet would have the strongest relationships with breast cancer among postmenopausal rather than premenopausal women because the international differences and secular changes within some countries are substantially greater for older than younger women. Miller and colleagues (1978), therefore, examined women separately according to menopausal status (Table 16–2).

Table 16–2. Mean nutrient intake based on the diet history questionnaire for breast cancer cases and controls according to menopausal status

Nutrient and series	Premenopausal women	Postmenopausal women	Women aged 70 or more years
Total calories			
Cases	2,373	2,170	1,614
Controls	2,339	2,115	1,996
Difference	34	55	−383
(n)	(85)	(210)	(13)
Total fat			
Cases	109.4	91.8	58.9
Controls	104.2	90.7	71.7
Difference	5.2	1.1	−12.8
(n)	(88)	(213)	(13)
Saturated fat			
Cases	42.0	34.3	21.9
Controls	40.6	34.5	25.2
Difference	1.4	0.8	−3.4
(n)	(88)	(214)	(13)

Data from Miller et al., 1978.

Although none of the differences are statistically significant, the small overall differences in absolute total and saturated fat intake are almost entirely attributable to premenopausal women, in contrast with expectation. For postmenopausal women over the age of 70, the cases actually reported substantially lower fat intake than controls (see Table 4 of Miller et al., 1978). For total fat as a percentage of calories, cases reported 38.1% and controls 38.6%, whereas for saturated fat, cases reported 14.6% and controls 14.7%. The authors of this report also provided relative risks for different levels of fat intake. Although some of the relative risks were greater than 1.0 (1.6 for total fat and 1.4 for saturated fat, comparing highest and lowest thirds), none approached statistical significance, and no suggestions of any dose–response relationships were observed. Moreover, none was adjusted for total caloric intake, which would have reduced the observed associations.

In summary, this carefully conducted study does not support the hypothesis that the fat composition of the diet is associated with breast cancer incidence. It is reasonable to suggest that observed associations are likely to have been underestimated due to an imperfect measure of exposure. It seems inappropriate to conclude, however, that the use of an imperfect measure of diet means that a true association exists when no association, or one that is readily compatible with chance, is observed (see excerpt from abstract of Miller et al. [1978] at the beginning of this chapter).

Howe (1985) has published an important methodologic paper on the use of dual response measures to improve the estimates of relative risks when both measures are imperfect. However, the data used to illustrate his methods were the 24-hour recall and diet history information from the study by Miller and colleagues (1978) described earlier. The very strong imputed relative risks for saturated fat obtained by Howe (5.9 for high vs. low intake) has been cited as support for the fat and breast cancer hypothesis. It will be readily appreciated that these strong relative risks are largely due to the association based on the 24-hour recall, which the original authors appropriately recognized as artifactual. Sophisticated statistical manipulation cannot correct for primary data that are inherently biased.

The largest case–control study to date of dietary fat intake and breast cancer incidence was reported by Graham and colleagues (1982). Fat intake, estimated with a simple food-frequency questionnaire, among 2,024 women with breast cancer was essentially identical to that reported by 1,463 control women attending a hospital for a variety of benign conditions.

Howe and colleagues (1990) used the original data from 12 case–control studies (not including the large study by Graham et al. [1982] to conduct a pooled analysis of dietary fat and risk of breast cancer. Although no significant association between fat intake and breast cancer risk was seen in most of the individual studies, overall a statistically significant positive association was seen. Using the energy partition model (Chapter 11), the relative risk was 1.35 for an increment of 1,000 calories per day from fat. However, this is an extremely large and unrealistic increment as it corresponds to approximately 110 g of fat per day, whereas the average intake for women is typically 70 to 80 g per day. Using the same data converted to nutrient density, this would correspond to a relative risk of only 1.07 for 40% compared with 30% of energy from fat. The analysis was criticized by Marshall and Graham (1993) for having deleted studies that contributed to statistical heterogeneity in the findings (i.e., that a claim of consistency was made only after the inconsistent findings were deleted).

A number of additional case–control studies have been published subsequent to the pooled analysis of Howe and colleagues (1990). In general, they have provided little support for an association between fat intake and breast cancer risk (Zaridze et al., 1991; Kato et al., 1992; Malik et al., 1993; Holmberg et al., 1994; Katsouyanni et al., 1994; Landa et al., 1994; Martin-Moreno et al., 1994; La Vecchia et al., 1995; Yuan et al., 1995; Franceschi et al., 1996).

Studies conducted among the general populations of western countries share the constraint that few women consume a diet with less than 30% of calories from fat. For this reason the Japanese case–control study of Hirohata and colleagues (1985) conducted among 212 women with breast cancer and an equal number of each of hospitalized and neighborhood controls is of special interest. In this study, the mean daily total fat intake reported by cases was 51 g, by hospital controls was 52 g, and by neighborhood controls was 52 g. A similar lack of any substantial difference was seen for both animal fat and vegetable fat.

Several other case–control studies of breast cancer have contained assorted questions about the use of specific high fat foods, but these were not extensive enough to provide an estimate of total fat intake. One of these studies (Lubin et al., 1981) was interpreted as support for the fat and breast cancer hypothesis. Five hundred seventy-seven women hospitalized with breast cancer were asked about their frequency of use of eight foods. Apparently as an afterthought, it was decided to obtain similar information from a series of control women. This required hiring a new interviewing staff, which then administered the questionnaire at home to the 72% of a general population sample who were willing to participate. The associations found for the use of beef, pork, and sweet desserts were striking (Table 16–3). If these relationships were truly this strong, one would expect that Seventh-day Adventists or vegetarian nuns would have markedly lower rates of breast cancer and that associations for these foods would be obviously apparent in the case–control studies of Graham and co-workers (1982) and Miller and coworkers (1978) and in the prospective data described later including those of Phillips and Snowdon (1983) and Willett and colleagues (1992). In retrospect, it seems unlikely that these associations can be correct and that they are much more likely to be artifacts of the noncomparable manner in which the data were collected. The findings

Table 16–3. Age-adjusted relative risk of breast cancer for various food items categorized by tertiles

	Level[a]	Cases	Controls	RR	95% CI
Beef	6	87	127	1.53[b]	(1.1, 2.1)
	5	274	301	2.25	(1.8, 2.9)
	1–4	197	397	1.00	
Pork	4–6	320	398	2.16[b]	(1.6, 2.9)
	3	120	181	1.76	(1.3, 2.5)
	1–2	112	246	1.00	
Fowl	4–6	368	621	0.87	(0.6, 1.4)
	3	151	151	1.54	(0.9, 2.5)
	1–2	39	53	1.00	
Fish	4–6	288	438	1.02	(0.8, 1.3)
	3	141	185	1.26	(0.9, 1.7)
	1–2	129	201	1.00	
Eggs	6–5	160	254	0.84	(0.6, 1.2)
	4	293	449	0.88	(0.6, 1.2)
	1–3	105	121	1.00	
Cheese	6	199	310	1.11	(0.9, 1.4)
	5	126	159	1.37	(1.0, 1.9)
	1–4	232	354	1.00	
Creams (full, sour, ice, whipped)	5–6	79	120	0.92	(0.7, 1.2)
	4	184	307	0.90	(0.7, 1.2)
	1–3	290	301	1.00	
Sweet desserts	5–6	183	224	1.45[c]	(1.1, 1.9)
	4	189	286	1.26	(1.0, 1.6)
	1–3	176	316	1.00	

[a] Food frequency levels are defined as 6, daily; 5, 4–6 days/week; 4, 1–3 days/week; 3, >1 day/month and <1 day/week; 2, ≤1 day/month; 1, never.

[b] Test for linear trend, p <0.001.

[c] Test for linear trend, p =0.01.

From Lubin et al., 1981.

of this study suggest that adherence to the basic epidemiologic principles of comparability in data collection procedures for cases and controls is not merely a hypothetical issue.

In other case–control studies that included a limited list of foods, Phillips (1975) found a significant association between fried potatoes and the risk of breast cancer in a Seventh-day Adventist population, but apparently found no association with meat. In an Italian case–control study, Talamini and coworkers (1984) reported a positive association with intake of milk and dairy products, but not meat. In a French case–control study, Le and coworkers

(1986) found positive associations with the use of cheese and full cream milk, but not with the use of butter or yogurt. In Pakistan, no significant associations were found with meat and dairy products (Malik et al., 1993), and no association was seen with high fat foods in Japan (Kato et al., 1992).

PROSPECTIVE STUDIES

The potential for biased associations due to selective participation or differential recall of past diet inherent in case–control studies is eliminated in prospective studies of the fat and breast cancer relationship. Only recently have data from several prospective studies been published, which is largely because of the cost and time involved in conducting such studies. In a prospective study from Japan based on a very limited number of dietary questions, Hirayama (1978) reported a higher incidence of breast cancer among women consuming meat daily; however, the total number of cases among women who ate meat daily was only 14, which precluded any detailed analysis.

Phillips and Snowdon (1983) examined the relationship between meat consumption and mortality due to breast cancer during a 21-year follow-up period of California Seventh-day Adventists. During this period 186 women died of this disease; the breast cancer mortality rates (per 100,000 person-years) were 47.8 for no use of meat, 58.3 for meat use one to three times per week, and 56.9 for use of meat four or more times per week (p for trend = 0.28). These data are of particular value because of the large portion of the population that consumed no meat at all. This Seventh-day Adventist population also provided a rare opportunity to evaluate the effects on breast cancer risk of dietary changes at various ages because the age at adopting a vegetarian lifestyle can usually be determined. Mills and colleagues (1988) found that meat, cheese, milk, and eggs all were unrelated to risk of death due to breast cancer. Moreover, among women who did not eat meat, those who adopted a vegetarian lifestyle earlier in life tended to have a higher, rather than lower, risk of breast cancer.

The largest prospective study to date with a calculation of total fat intake was based on a dietary questionnaire (see Appendix 1 of Chapter 5) completed by 89,538 registered nurses aged 34 to 59 years in 1980 (Willett et al., 1987a, 1992). During the first 4 years of follow up, 601 cases of breast cancer were diagnosed among the participants. After adjustment for known determinants of breast cancer, the relative risk of breast cancer among women in the highest quintile of calorie-adjusted total fat intake, as compared with women in the lowest quintile, was 0.82 (95% confidence interval, 0.64 to 1.05), and for saturated fat intake the corresponding relative risk was 0.84 (0.66 to 1.08). Similar nonsignificant inverse trends were seen for calorie-adjusted linoleic acid and cholesterol and for the same dietary lipids not adjusted for caloric intake (Table 16–4) (unpublished data).

This study included a validation component that provided an assessment of the distribution of fat intake independent of the study questionnaire. Based on 28 days of diet records completed by 173 participants, the mean values for lowest and highest quintiles of absolute fat intake in this population were 47 and 98 g/day. Expressed as percentage of total caloric intake, the means for extreme quintiles were 32% and 44%. Ideally, one would like to examine the effect of fat intake below 30% of calories; however, at that time, there was insufficient follow up to provide enough cases to evaluate risk among the small percentage of women with lower fat intake. Nevertheless, this degree of variation in fat intake with the study population is of interest as it corresponds closely to the advice to decrease fat intake by one-fourth from about 40% of calories to 30% of calories. For saturated fat intake, most highly suspected because of the international correlations, the variation in intake was greater; the means of lowest and highest quintiles for absolute intake were 16 and 35 g/day (a 117% increase from lowest to highest) and in relation to caloric intake were 11% 17% (a 55% increase).

Even if adequate variation in dietary fat exists within the cohort, useful findings will be obtained only if the dietary questionnaire employed can discriminate among individuals. In this case, information on the performance of the questionnaire was provided by the validation study (Willett et al., 1985b) (see also Chapter 6). Briefly, the correlation between the dietary questionnaire completed at the end of the year of

Table 16–4. Age-adjusted relative risk (RR) of breast cancer according to quintile of calorie-adjusted intake of total and saturated fat, linoleic acid, and cholesterol

Measurement	(Low) 1	2	3	4	(High) 5	χ, trend (p value)
Total Fat						
No. of cases	145	112	122	110	112	
No. of women	17,841	17,909	17,924	17,929	17,935	−1.57
Multivariate RR[a]	1.0	0.80	0.88	0.80	0.82	(0.11)
(95% confidence limits)	—	(0.62, 1.02)	(0.69, 1.12)	(0.63, 1.03)	(0.64, 1.05)	
Saturated Fat						
No. of cases	146	112	126	105	112	
No. of women	17,848	17,910	17,938	17,915	17,927	−1.86
Multivariate RR[a]	1.0	0.80	0.91	0.77	0.84	(0.06)
(95% confidence limits)	—	(0.63, 1.03)	(0.72, 1.16)	(0.60, 1.00)	(0.66, 1.08)	
Linoleic acid						
No. of cases	151	119	103	115	113	
No. of Women	17,848	17,875	17,909	17,961	17,945	−1.42
Multivariate RR[a]	1.0	0.84	0.75	0.86	0.88	(0.16)
(95% confidence limits)	—	(0.65, 1.07)	(0.58, 0.97)	(0.67, 1.10)	(0.69, 1.12)	
Cholesterol						
No. of cases	118	129	119	129	106	
No. of women	17,916	17,935	17,878	17,920	17,889	−0.76
Multivariate RR[a]	1.0	1.06	1.02	1.07	0.91	(0.43)
(95% confidence limits)	—	(0.82, 1.38)	(0.79, 1.32)	(0.83, 1.38)	(0.70, 1.18)	

[a]The model includes indicator variables for quintiles 2 to 5 of fat intake, age (five catagories), a maternal history of breast cancer, a sister with a history of breast cancer, nulliparity, age at first birth <23 years, current smoking, highest quintile for relative weight, history of benign breast disease, postmenopausal status, and alcohol consumption (three categories).

diet record keeping and the average intake from the 28 days of diet records completed by each participant was 0.53 for calorie-adjusted total fat and 0.59 for calorie-adjusted saturated fat.

This degree of validity in measuring dietary fat is certainly not perfect, but appears to be comparable to many measurements used in epidemiology, such as blood pressure and physical activity (Chasan-Taber et al., 1996). How does this degree of error affect the findings? In general, error in the measurement of exposure that is random with respect to disease status has two implications. One is that the observed relative risk is closer to 1.0 than the true relative risk, and the other is that the usual calculated confidence intervals are narrower than the true confidence intervals (see Chapter 12). In this instance, where no significant association was ob-

served, the focus of interest is on the upper bound of the confidence interval. In other words, what is the upper limit of the plausible relative risks that are compatible with the observed data from the study? It is also of interest that the observed relative risks in this instance were less than 1.0, in the opposite direction of the hypothesis. As pointed out by Potter (1987), a correction for measurement error will, therefore, move the relative risk further from unity; for total fat intake he estimated the corrected relative risk would be approximately 0.6 to 0.7. Statistical methods developed after the original report (Rosner et al., 1989) were used to correct the observed confidence intervals for measurement error (which includes uncertainty due to the measurement error itself as well as uncertainty in the estimation of the measurement error) based on correction of logistic regression coefficients and their standard errors (see Chapter 12). Using this method and the data from the validation study, the observed relative risk (adjusted for age, alcohol intake, and calories) for the highest versus the lowest quintiles of saturated fat intake was 0.85 (95% confidence intervals, 0.67 to 1.07), which was corrected to 0.76 (95% confidence intervals, 0.50 to 1.13). Note that the point estimate moved away from one and the width of the confidence intervals increased. The upper bound was still only slightly above unity, indicating that, after accounting for error in the measure of fat intake, the data are compatible with only a weak positive association. Even if the relative risk was centered on the observed relative risk, only weak positive associations would lie within the expanded confidence interval. Further evidence that dietary fat varied within the cohort and that the questionnaire was capable of measuring this variation was provided by the observation that, in the same population, total and animal fat intake were positively associated with risk of colon cancer (Willett et al., 1990) (Fig. 16–6), and saturated fat intake was associated with risk of coronary heart disease in age-adjusted analyses (unpublished data). Short of finding a significant inverse association, it is difficult for any study to exclude the possibility of a very small positive association. However, that the failure of this study to find the substantial positive association between fat intake and breast cancer incidence predicted by the international correlations cannot simply be explained by imperfect measurement of exposure.

It is quite possible that the latent period between exposure and disease was not represented in the 4-year follow up of the Nurses' Health Study and that fat intake, therefore, might still influence breast cancer risk. This possibility cannot be eliminated as the latency period for breast cancer is unknown. In laboratory animals, however, dietary fats acts as a promoter, having an effect during the later stages of carcinogenesis (Hopkins and Carroll, 1979). More-

over, even though the follow-up period was limited, dietary intake tends to be correlated over time so that the baseline assessment also reflected previous intake over an extended period of years. As described in Chapter 6, we found that the validity of a food-frequency questionnaire was similar when compared with diet record data over a previous 1-year or 6-year period. This study, however, did not address the possible influence of fat intake much earlier in life, such as during childhood. Indeed, it is unclear whether the influence of diet composition in youth on risk of breast cancer can be effectively studied in adults because the validity of recall of remote diet has not been demonstrated.

Another limitation of that study was that the age distribution was truncated; the oldest participant was 59 years of age in 1980 when the dietary data were collected. Although there appeared to be no suggestion of any positive association between dietary lipid intake and risk of breast cancer in either premenopausal or postmenopausal women, an association among older postmenopausal women could not be excluded.

The Nurses' Health Study illustrates a major advantage of a prospective study as it is possible, with additional follow up, to examine the relationship of the same dietary exposure data with risk of breast cancer at different latent periods. Thus, the same relationship was examined after 8 years of follow up, during which 1,439 cases of breast cancer had been diagnosed (Willett et al., 1992); a similar lack of evidence for any positive association with total or any type of fat was observed. With the longer follow-up period most of the cases were postmenopausal, and there was no evidence of association among either pre- or postmenopausal women. The large number of cases afforded the opportunity to examine risks among extreme deciles of fat intake; for the lowest decile of fat intake in 1980 (median intake was 27% of energy) no suggestion of any reduction in risk was seen. A prospective study also provides the opportunity to repeat measurements of

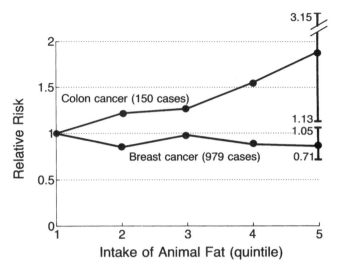

Figure 16–6. Relative risks of colon and breast cancer according to intake of animal fat, adjusted for total energy intake, during 6 years of follow-up. The bars represent 95% confidence intervals for the women in the highest quintile. (From Willett et al., 1990; reproduced with permission. Copyright 1990 Massachusetts Medical Society. All rights reserved.)

dietary intake; thus follow-up dietary questionnaires, which were longer and more detailed, were collected in 1984, 1986, 1990, and 1994. By 1984, dietary fat intake had decreased in the study population so that the median of the lowest decile was 23% of energy; for these women the risk of breast cancer from 1984 to 1988 was, if anything, slightly increased (relative risk, 0.83; 95% confidence interval, 0.56 to 1.21 for the highest vs. lowest decile of total fat intake). Using various combinations of the 1980 and 1984 questionnaires (e.g., comparing women who were consistently in the highest with those consistently in the lowest categories or using the mean of the two questionnaires) also produced no suggestion of any positive association (for women consistently in the highest vs lowest quintile, the relative risk was 0.84, 95% confidence interval, 0.57 to 1.24). Using the more detailed 1984 dietary data, a higher intake of monounsaturated fat was significantly associated with reduced risk of breast cancer. Analysis of the 12-year follow up also indicated no evidence for a positive association between fat intake and

breast cancer incidence (unpublished data). Ultimately, the repeated questionnaires can be used to examine the relationship between change in diet and change in risk of breast cancer, which has obvious public health implications.

The relationship between dietary fat and breast cancer risk has now also been examined in five other large prospective studies (Table 16–5). In all of these studies little or no association with risk of breast cancer was seen for total or saturated fat or among pre- or postmenopausal women. In none of these studies was the risk for the highest compared with the lowest quintiles statistically significant. Several smaller prospective studies (with fewer than 200 incident cases) have also been reported with variable results, but in none was there a significant positive association (Jones et al., 1987; Knekt et al., 1990; Toniolo et al., 1994). In another prospective study with 248 cases of breast cancer, no significant association was seen for total fat intake, but information on standard reproductive risk factors was not available (Gaard et al., 1995).

Table 16–5. Large prospective studies of total and saturated fat intake and risk of breast cancer

Study	Total no. in cohort	Years of follow-up	No. of cases	RR (95% CI)[a] (High vs. low category)	
				Total fat	Saturated fat
Nurses' Health Study (Willett et al., 1992)	89,494	8	1,439	0.86 (0.67–1.08)	0.86 (0.73–1.02)
Canadian Study (Howe et al., 1991)	56,837	5	519	1.30 (0.90–1.88)	1.08 (0.73–1.59)
New York State Cohort (Graham et al., 1991)	17,401	7	344	1.00 (0.59–1.70)	1.12 (0.78–1.61)[b]
Iowa Women's Study (Kushi et al., 1992)	32,080	4	408	1.13 (0.84–1.51)	1.10 (0.83–1.46)
Dutch Health Study (Van den Brandt et al., 1993)	62,573	3	471	1.08 (0.73–1.59)	1.39 (0.94–2.06)
Adventists' Health Study (Mills et al., 1989)	20,341	6	193	—	1.21 (0.81–1.81)

[a]RR, relative risk; CI, confidence interval.
[b]Animal fat.

A collaborative pooled analysis has been conducted of all the prospective studies included in Table 16–5 plus an additional recently published study from Sweden (Wolk et al., 1998); this included a total of 4,980 cases of breast cancer occurring among 337,819 women (Hunter et al., 1996). In addition to providing great statistical power and precision, the pooled analysis allowed standard analytic approaches to be applied to all studies (which had been analyzed in a variety of ways), an examination of a wider range of fat intake, and a detailed evaluation of interactions with other breast cancer risk factors. Overall, no association was observed between intake of total, saturated, monounsaturated, or polyunsaturated fat and risk of breast cancer (Table 16–6). Validation/calibration studies were available for each cohort, and these were used to adjust the relative risks and confidence for measurement error. For a 25g/day increment in total fat (approximately the difference between top and bottom quintiles assessed by multiple dietary records after accounting for total energy intake) the relative risk of energy-adjusted total fat intake was 1.02 (95% confidence interval, 0.94 to 1.11). After accounting for measurement error, the relative risk was 1.07 (95% confidence interval, 0.86 to 1.34). (The pooled and measurement error-corrected relative risk also weighted studies according to the validity of their respective dietary questionnaire because this error is accounted for in the variance of the corrected relative risk from each study—see Chapter 12.) No evidence of a positive association was seen when the data were limited to postmenopausal women (premenopausal breast cancer was more difficult to define because menopausal status was not updated in most cohorts).

The mean level of fat intake varied somewhat among cohorts; coupled with the large number of cases, this provided the chance to examine a wide range of fat intakes. In the pooled analysis, each cohort was first analyzed separately to make maximal use of available confounding covariates and allow for possible differences in their influence among the various cohorts. Then, a weighted average of the study-specific coefficients for fat intake was calculated using standard meta-analysis approaches. With this approach, information comparing the highest versus the lowest categories of fat intake would be lost if, as customary, the lowest category of fat intake were to be used for the reference

Table 16–6. Pooled relative risks of breast cancer and 95% confidence intervals for quintiles of energy-adjusted nutrient intake in the pooled analysis of cohort studies[a]

Nutrient	Quintile 1[b]	Quintile 2	Quintile 3	Quintile 4	Quintile 5	p Value for trend
Total fat	1.00	1.01 (0.89–1.14)	1.12 (1.01–1.25)	1.07 (0.96–1.19)	1.05 (0.94–1.16)	0.21
Saturated fat	1.00	1.03 (0.93–1.14)	1.04 (0.94–1.14)	1.00 (0.90–1.11)	1.07 (0.95–1.20)	0.41
Monounsaturated fat	1.00	1.07 (0.97–1.18)	1.11 (1.01–1.23)	1.10 (0.99–1.22)	1.01 (0.88–1.16)	0.73
Polyunsaturated fat	1.00	1.07 (0.97–1.18)	1.03 (0.94–1.14)	1.06 (0.96–1.16)	1.07 (0.97–1.17)	0.32
Cholesterol	1.00	1.04 (0.94–1.15)	1.02 (0.89–1.16)	1.05 (0.93–1.18)	1.08 (0.97–1.21)	0.19
Energy	1.00	1.01 (0.91–1.12)	1.13 (1.02–1.25)	1.04 (0.92–1.17)	1.11 (0.99–1.25)	0.15

[a]Relative risks are adjusted for the following variables: age at menarche ($\leq$11, 12, 13, 14, or $\geq$15 years), menopausal status (premenopausal, postmenopausal), parity (0, 1 to 2, $\geq$3), age at birth of first child ($\leq$20, 21–25, 26–30, $\geq$31 years), body mass index (the weight in kilograms divided by the square of the height in meters) ($\leq$21, >21 to $\leq$23, > 23 to $\leq$25, >25 to $\leq$29, >29), height (<1.60, 1.60 to <1.64, 1.64 to <1.68, $\geq$1.68 m), education (<high school graduation, high school graduation, >high school graduation), history of benign breast disease (no, yes), maternal history of breast cancer (no, yes), history of breast cancer in a sister (no, yes), oral contraceptive use ever (no, yes), fiber intake (quintiles), alcohol intake (0, >0 to <1.5, 1.5 to <5, 5 to <15, 15 to <30, $\geq$ 30 g per day), and energy intake (on a continuous scale).

[b]Quintile 1 values are the reference values.

From Hunter et al., 1996.

group because the study population with the lowest fat intake would include few if any women in the highest category of fat intake, and vice versa. Therefore, 30% to 35% percent of energy from fat was chosen as the reference category as this contained the largest number of women and would thus provide the most stable comparison group. As shown in Figure 16–7, no evidence of any trend of decreasing risk of breast cancer with lower fat intake was observed, even with fat intakes less than 20% of energy. Unexpectedly, when the relatively few women with fat intakes less than 15% of energy were examined, risk of breast cancer was actually increased (relative risk, 2.12; 95% confidence interval, 1.34 to 3.36). This increase in risk was seen among all four cohorts with women reporting less than 15% of energy from fat and could not be accounted for by other dietary or nondietary factors.

In calculations based on a series of theoretical assumptions, Prentice (1996) has argued that the pooled analysis of fat and breast cancer failed to detect a positive association due to measurement error that was not accounted for because the measurement error model did not include body mass index (BMI) as a covariate. However, one of his central assumptions, that the percentage of energy from fat is substantially underreported by women who underreport energy intake, is not supported by actual data (see Chapter 12). Moreover, including BMI in the measurement error model had little effect on the findings, and the other prediction based on his assumptions (strong associations between BMI and breast cancer incidence and between dietary fat and BMI) were not supported by the data (Hunter et al. 1998). Thus, these theoretical concerns appear groundless.

Interactions between fat intake and standard risk factors for breast cancer were systematically examined in each of the large prospective studies (Hunter et al., 1996). In some instances, highly significant interactions were seen in one study, but this was never confirmed in the other cohorts. When

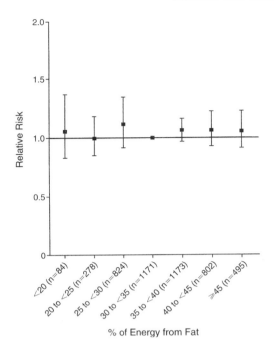

% of Energy from Fat

Figure 16–7. Relative risk of breast cancer by percentage of energy from fat in pooled analysis off prospective studies. (From Hunter et al., 1996); reproduced with permission. Copyright 1996 Massachusetts Medical Society. All rights reserved.)

summarized across all of the cohorts, no significant interactions were seen. These observations emphasize the substantial contribution that chance can play when examining multiple interactions. The investigators of the studies with a clearly significant interaction could easily have been tempted to report these as important observations, which then would have required multiple additional publications to refute these findings.

On the basis of limited animal studies, high intake of omega-3 fatty acids from fish has been hypothesized to reduce breast cancer incidence (Karmali, 1987). However, an inverse relation between extra long chain omega-3 fatty acids or fish consumption, the major source of these fats, was seen in only 1 of 13 case–control studies (Willett, 1997b). Also, little support for a protective

effect was seen in the Nurses' Health Study cohort (Stampfer et al., 1987) or in Norwegian or New York cohorts (Vatten et al., 1990; Toniolo et al., 1994). Also, no relationship was seen between omega-3 fatty acid levels in prospective blood specimens and breast cancer risk among a Scandinavian population (Vatten et al., 1993) or when measured in adipose in a U.S. case–control study (London et al., 1993).

Relatively little has been reported from the large prospective studies on associations between specific foods high in fat intake. Toniolo and colleagues (1994) reported a strong and significant association between consumption of red meat and breast cancer. Individual foods were all examined in each of the reports on fat intake and breast cancer from the Nurses' Health Study, but only one sentence was included in the text noting the general absence of associations with individual foods (including the findings for meat, which are included in Table 16–7). It is likely that other investigators also examined their data and did not find a remarkable finding for meat intake and thus did not make this the object of a report. Thus, the positive finding by Toniolo and colleagues (1994) most likely represents a chance observation. The tendency to report only statistically significant findings is understandable, as it is difficult to report data for the more than 100 foods on a questionnaire; however, this practice may contribute to a confusing literature. There is no simple solution to this reporting bias problem, because it is important to examine specific foods as well as nutrients; however, findings from any single study should be interpreted with extreme caution. Ultimately, the best solution is to conduct pooled food–based analyses of all available studies, as is done for dietary fat in the prospective studies noted above, to examine the overall results and to evaluate consistency among the individual studies. As with interactions, many false starts and unneeded confirmatory or refutation analyses could probably be avoided.

Table 16–7. Relation of meat-eating with incidence of breast cancer among 89,538 women during 4 years of follow-up[a]

	Frequency of eating				
	<1/wk	1/wk	2–4/wk	5–6/wk	Daily or more
Beef, pork, or lamb as a main dish					
Cases	67	186	258	45	33
Total women	11,416	27,301	36,453	8,820	5,305
Age-adjusted RR	1.00	1.21	1.26	0.90	1.05
χ, trend = −0.24					
Beef, pork, or lamb as a sandwich or mixed dish					
Cases	52	141	227	134	31
Total women	8,885	22,903	30,234	22,609	4,920
Age-adjusted RR	1.00	0.98	1.25	0.98	1.00
χ, trend = 0.27					

[a] Numbers add to slightly less than 89,538 due to missing data. RR, relative risk.
Data based on study of Willett et al., 1987.

INTEGRATION OF FINDINGS FROM CASE–CONTROL AND PROSPECTIVE STUDIES

The separate pooled results of the case–control and cohort studies of dietary fat and breast cancer appear to have provided somewhat different results, the case–control studies being positive and the cohort studies being null. One possibility is that the dietary assessment methods used in the case–control studies were more precise than those used in the cohort studies. However, the dietary assessment methods were generally similar in the case–control and cohort studies except that they were usually interview administered in the case–control studies. Although few of the dietary assessments used in the case–control studies were evaluated for validity, in the case–control study of Miller and colleagues (1978) there was no evidence of a higher degree of validity than generally found in cohort studies (Morgan et al., 1978). Furthermore, because it is likely that diet immediately before the diagnosis of breast cancer is not etiologically relevant, the reporting of current diet in the cohort studies may be more valid than the recall of past diets in case–control studies. The most likely explanation for the discordance is that in some, but not necessarily all, of the case–control studies, selection bias due to nonresponse resulted in an inappropriate control group or that recall bias due to the diagnosis of breast cancer or its treatment differentially affected the recall of past diet. The possibility of reporting bias was examined in two of the cohort studies by asking incident breast cancer cases and a sample of noncases to report their previous diet, as would be done in a case–control study. In the Canadian case–control study (Friedenreich et al., 1991), a similar lack of association with fat intake was seen when diet was assessed retrospectively and prospectively. Different results were seen in a study of similar design conducted within the Nurses' Health Study (Giovannucci et al., 1993). In this analysis, fat intake was positively associated with risk of breast cancer in the retrospectively collected data (the magnitude of association was similar to that in the pooled analysis of case–control studies), but was weakly inversely associated with risk in the data provided prospectively by the same women. Both selection and recall bias contributed to the positive association in the retrospective data (Friedenreich et al., 1994; Giovannucci and Willett, 1994). These analyses indicate that the positive association in the pooled analysis of case–control studies is compatible with methodologic bias in at least some of the studies, although this cannot be proven directly. However, it is also important to recognize that the case–control and cohort studies are not widely divergent; as noted above, the relative risk in the pooled case–control analysis was small (1.07) when expressed for a realistic contrast in fat intake, 40% compared with 30% of energy from fat.

In summary, the large prospective studies of dietary fat and breast cancer have been remarkably consistent in indicating little or no association between fat intake during adult life. The pooling of prospective studies has provided the opportunity to examine a wide range of fat consumption, and no evidence of an increased risk was seen at levels well below 30% of energy. The unexpected increase in risk among women with a very low fat intake is based on small numbers of women, but bears further examination in other data (which will continue to accrue rapidly as the existing cohorts age and more recently established cohorts begin to be published). The metabolic effects of very low fat intake also deserve further consideration. The possibility that dietary fat earlier in life, and even the exposure to maternal diets while in utero (Trichopoulos, 1990), can influence later breast cancer risk cannot be excluded by the present data and thus deserves further consideration. Also, the observations of inverse associations between olive oil consumption and breast cancer incidence with breast cancer incidence internationally and in multiple case–control studies (Cohen and Wynder, 1990; Katsouyanni et al., 1994; Landa et al., 1994; Martin-Moreno et al., 1994), together with suggestive animal studies (see below), indicate the need for further consideration of this relationship.

Sporadic associations have been observed between meat and dairy products in some case–control and cohort studies with a limited dietary assessment. These associations, however, have not been consistently observed in these limited studies or in the more comprehensive studies and are inconsistent with the rates of breast cancer in Seventh-day Adventists (Phillips et al., 1980) and vegetarian nuns (Kinlen, 1982). Moreover, if true, these positive associations with meat intake should have been readily observable in the prospective studies of Phillips and Snowdon (1983) and Willett and colleagues (1987a). It is, thus, most likely that these sporadic findings represent the play of chance combined with a tendency for positive findings within a study to be emphasized.

Randomized trials of fat reduction have been proposed as the ultimate means of resolving the uncertainty about the association between dietary fat and breast cancer. The Women's Health Trial, sponsored by the U.S. National Institutes of Health, has commenced with the goal of enrolling and randomizing several tens of thousands of women, half of whom will be trained to reduce their total fat intake to 20% calories derived from fat. Such a trial does not address the most promising modification of the dietary fat hypothesis (that dietary fat reduction at an early age may reduce breast cancer risk decades later). Furthermore, a number of problems may severely compromise the ability of any trial to address the effect of reducing the percentage of fat derived from calories to 20% (Michels and Willett, 1992). These include the difficulty of maintaining compliance with a diet incompatible with prevailing food consumption habits, as well as the fact that the gradual secular decline in total fat consumption already under way may reduce the size of the contrast of fat intakes between intervention groups and controls. This may be a particular problem among the health-conscious women willing to enroll in this long-term study. In addition, women in the dietary intervention group will be counseled to adopt a dietary pattern that is high in fruits, vegetables, and grain products and low in total fat and saturated fat (Freedman et al., 1993). Thus, the intervention is not a simple reduction in total fat intake, but a replacement of fat with other specific foods. In other words, the trial will be unable to distinguish between the effect of fat reduction and that of increasing intake of fruit, vegetables, and grain products (Hunter and Willett, 1993).

BIOLOGIC PLAUSIBILITY

Some support for the hypothesis that high levels of dietary fat increase the rate of breast cancer is derived from studies that have related diet to estrogen levels, which are, in turn, thought to be related to breast cancer risk (Pike et al., 1983). Among postmenopausal women, omnivores on a high fat, low fiber diet had higher urinary excretion of estriol and total estrogens (Armstrong et al., 1981) and higher plasma levels of estrone and estradiol (Goldin et al., 1981) than vegetarian women. The relatively low plasma levels of estrogen among postmenopausal vegetarians in the last-cited study were shown to be at least partly the result of greatly enhanced fecal excretion of estrogens. Feeding a high fat, western diet to postmenopausal black South African women who typically consumed a low-fat vegetarian diet caused an apparent decrease in levels of luteinizing hormone, follicle-stimulating hormone, and prolactin (Hill et al., 1980). In this study only a small increase in estradiol level was observed, and other estrogen fractions were apparently not measured. Hagerty and colleagues (1988) conducted a crossover trial of a high fat diet (46% of calories) versus a low fat diet (25% of calories) among six women. No effect was seen on plasma or urinary levels of estrone, estradiol, or plasma progesterone or prolactin. Also, in postmenopausal women, Prentice et al.

(1990) observed a 17% decrease in serum estradiol levels over a period of 2 to 6 months, but no change in estrone sulfate, among women assigned to a low fat diet. However, the study did not include a concurrent control group, and many of the women were only several years postmenopausal, a time when endogenous estrogens are steadily decreasing.

Rose and colleagues (1993) reported what appears to be the only randomized trial of a low fat diet and hormone levels in postmenopausal women; for this reason, the findings are of considerable interest. The authors reported that patients with higher baseline estradiol concentration (at least 10 pg/ml, below which measurements were thought to be less reliable) "showed a significant reduction in serum estradiol after 6 months on the low-fat diet (average 20%; $p < 0.005$); this was sustained over the 18-month study period." However, this interpretation appears to be the result of inappropriate analysis combined with the well-known statistical phenomenon of "regression to the mean" (Figure 16–8). The appropriate statistical approach in a randomized trial such as this is to compare change in one group with change in the other group, not to conduct separate tests for change in each study group. It is easily possible that a change in one group may be statistically significant and the change in the other group only slightly less great and not statistically significant, so that the changes in the two groups would not be significantly different from each other. This problem is compounded in the present example because the groups were divided according to high and low baseline values, which created regression toward the mean in all groups. Because of variation in serum levels of estradiol over time, due to both true variation and laboratory error, the values that were initially high will tend to be lower on follow up and those that were initially low will tend to be higher. As seen in Figure 16–8, this is what happened. Among women with baseline estradiol lev-

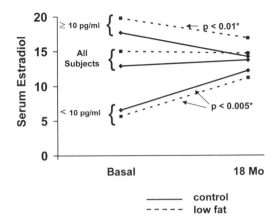

Figure 16–8. Low fat dietary intervention and serum estradiol in postmenopausal breast cancer patients. Data for 6 and 12 months are not shown as patterns were similar to 18 months (Adapted from Rose et al., 1993).

els of 10 pg/ml or higher, estradiol levels declined by an average of 15% in the low fat group and by 20% in the control group. Presumably because of some differences in variances, the change in the low fat group was statistically significant, but that in the control group was not. In an appropriate analysis, there would certainly have been no significant difference between groups. As expected from regression to the mean, among women with initially low estradiol levels, 18-month levels were substantially higher than at baseline; this increase was significant in both the low fat and control groups, but the changes were clearly not different between groups. In this study, dietary fat had little apparent effect on estrone sulfate level, although the levels at 18 months tended to be somewhat higher with the low fat diet. Contrary to the authors' conclusions, this study failed to support their hypothesis that a reduction in dietary fat decreases estrogen levels in postmenopausal women.

Among premenopausal women, inconsistent associations of diet and sex hormones have been observed. Studies among vegetarian and nonvegetarian Seventh-day Adventist teenagers (Gray et al., 1982b) and among teenage girls in four countries with large differences in breast cancer rates (Gray et al., 1982a) found no meaningful associations between plasma or urinary estrogen levels and dietary factors. Although premenopausal American women who were omnivores were found to have higher levels of plasma estrone and estradiol than vegetarians (Goldin et al., 1981), an apparent decrease in estradiol level was caused by feeding a high fat, western diet to premenopausal South African women (Hill et al., 1980). A decrease in fat intake from 35% to 21% of calories among women with cystic breast disease was associated with a reduction in estrone, estradiol, and estriol levels (Rose et al., 1987a), as well as prolactin level (Rose et al., 1987b); however, total caloric intake among participants was also reduced by an average of 23%. Bennett and Ingram (1990) randomized 39 premenopausal women to either omnivore, fish, or a vegetarian diet low in fat and higher in fiber. Although this was one of the few randomized trials of diet and endogenous hormone levels, it was also not appropriately analyzed, because only within-group, not between-group, changes were evaluated statistically. Nonprotein-bound estradiol level declined with the vegetarian diet when expressed as absolute level, but not when expressed as a percentage of total estradiol. Cross-sectional correlations indicated a positive association between complex carbohydrate intake and the proportion of estradiol that was not protein bound.

At this time, the relationship between dietary fat and endogenous estrogen levels remains unclear. This is troublesome because, in principle, there should be little difficulty in defining such relationships; studies require only a few dozen women and several months duration, which would allow good control of dietary intake. Unfortunately, very few studies have included a concurrent control group whose fat intake did not change, a weakness of study design that would not be tolerated in investigations of diet and blood lipids. As we know little about determinants of variations in endogenous hormones, this is particularly problematic. Furthermore, even in major research laboratories, endogenous hormone levels can be measured with great imprecision (Hankinson et al., 1994). Despite awareness by the laboratories that they were being evaluated, the coefficients of variation for repeated blinded samples from the same tube of blood were consistently higher, and sometimes much higher, than published values from the same laboratory (Hankinson et al., 1994). This imprecision greatly complicates the interpretation of published data as it is difficult to know which studies are truly informative. Also, there are many fractions of endogenous estrogens and ways that they can be measured, such as free and unbound, and in premenopausal women levels vary greatly over the menstrual cycle. Also, there is no clear evidence regarding which measurements, if any, are important determinants of breast cancer risk. Large prospective studies of endogenous estrogens are few and inconsistent; in the largest study (Toniolo et al., 1995), strong positive associations were seen with several estrogen fractions, but little relationship was seen in another reasonably large study (Helzlsouer et al., 1994). A number of large epidemiologic studies with archived blood specimens are presently underway that will examine the relationship of specific endogenous estrogen fractions to breast cancer risk; these should provide greater focus for metabolic studies. If dietary fat were shown to clearly increase endogenous estrogen levels and these levels were clearly predictive of breast cancer, this would provide plausibility for a causal relationship between dietary fat and breast cancer, but would not prove the relationship. Fat reduction, and the corresponding increase in carbohydrate intake, has other metabolic effects, including the elevation of

blood insulin levels and possibly growth hormone levels (Jenkins et al., 1990), which in turn increases insulin-like growth factor levels; it has been suggested that such changes might increase risk of several cancers (Giovannucci, 1995).

In addition to the possibility of acting on estrogen metabolism, several other mechanisms have been proposed by which dietary fat may increase the risk of breast cancer. Wynder and colleagues (1976) have suggested that fat may affect breast cancer risk by altering prolactin secretion. Such a mechanism is supported by some animal studies (Chan and Cohen, 1974), although it has not been established that prolactin secretion is related to breast cancer in humans. Another potential mechanism relates to the intake of polyunsaturated fats, which are subject to in vivo peroxidation. Highly reactive radicals generated in this process may damage DNA and other macromolecules, ultimately leading to neoplasia (Ames et al., 1995). In one study higher fat intake appeared to increase a biomarker of oxidative DNA damage in human white blood cells (Djuric et al., 1991), but information on the effects of specific types of fat is not available. Moreover, the international correlations that underlie the fat and breast cancer hypothesis are based on an association with animal fats, not vegetable fats, which are the primary source of polyunsaturated fatty acids in most countries. For example, Japanese diets differ from those in the United States in their saturated fat content, but not in the amount of polyunsaturated fatty acids (Insull et al., 1968).

It has also been suggested that dietary fat may be linked to breast cancer through increased caloric intake and the development of obesity. Adipose tissue can convert androstenedione to estrone (Grodin et al., 1973) and thus makes an important contribution to circulating levels in postmenopausal women (Hankinson et al., 1995). However, obesity is primarily a function of total energy intake and expenditure; the percentage of energy from fat in the diet appears to have little if any long-term effect on obesity (Willett, 1994, 1997a). Moreover, the association between obesity and incidence of breast cancer is complex (discussed later in this chapter).

Construction of a plausible mechanism whereby fat may affect the risk of breast cancer is seriously hindered by our basic ignorance of the pathophysiology of this disease. We do not really understand the steps that lead to breast cancer and lack an established measurable intermediary factor analogous to serum cholesterol or glucose level in the case of coronary heart disease. Without an established biochemical or molecular precursor lesion, the search for a plausible mechanism may be problematic and premature, particularly as the evidence suggests that high fat diets do not increase the risk of human breast cancer.

A RE-EXAMINATION
OF THE ANIMAL DATA

Although the hypothesis that high fat diets cause breast cancer in humans has been heavily based on animal studies, the interpretation of these laboratory findings is controversial. This issue cannot be reviewed in detail here, but is discussed at length by Birt (1986) and in the proceedings of a symposium (Pariza and Boutwell, 1987). A central question is whether fat intake has an effect on mammary cancer apart from its contribution to total energy intake; this issue is analogous to that facing epidemiologists discussed in Chapter 11.

There is little question that restriction of energy intake dramatically lowers the incidence of mammary tumors (Tannenbaum and Silverstone, 1953). Because fat is uniquely dense in its energy content, a low fat diet can be confounded by a reduction in energy intake unless strict care is undertaken to ensure that the available energy intake is held constant. This issue has been studied by Boissonneault and coworkers (1986), who found, like many others, that rats on a low fat ad libitum diet had lower tumor incidence than those on a high-fat ad libitum diet (Table 16–8). When the high fat diet was restricted so that total energy intake was about 20% lower than the ad libitum intake, however, the tumor incidence was reduced by 90%. This issue is further complicated by the finding that the net energy available to living organisms from macronutrients is not strictly proportional to the classic values obtained by bomb calorimetery (4 kcal/g of carbohydrate or protein and 9 kcal g of fat). Because more energy is required for the absorption and metabolic processing of carbohydrate and protein, in at least some situations these may provide approximately 20% less available energy than has been used in typical calculations (Donato, 1987).

Albanes (1987) has performed a meta-analysis of diet and mammary cancer experiments in mice over the last 50 years. An extremely strong overall positive association was seen for total energy intake; however, after adjustment for total energy intake, the fat composition was actually weakly inversely related to incidence of mammary tumors. In other reviews of animal experiments, Birt (1986) and Freedman et al. (1990) concluded that evidence did exist for an effect of dietary fat independent of total energy intake. In more recent animal studies specifically designed to determine the independent effects of fat and energy intakes, the effect of fat was either weak in relation to energy intake (Ip, 1990) or nonexistent (Beth et al., 1987).

A fundamental question related to the laboratory findings is whether any particular rodent model has relevance to human breast cancer. Ironically, this is a difficult issue to prove or disprove without firm human data. In toxicity studies, the analogy with humans is more direct as it involves fewer assumptions to presume that the different species will respond similarly; even in this situation many exceptions can be found. In many studies of diet and cancer in animal models, however, one is exam-

Table 16–8. Mammary tumor incidence in rats fed a diet with different fat contents

	Dietary regimen		
	High fat, ad lib	Low fat, ad lib	High fat, restricted
kcal consumption per day	41	42	34
Fat consumption per day (g)	2.7	0.6	2.2
Body weight (g)	217	190	182
Body composition			
% body fat	24	16	25
% body protein	20	23	20
Retained energy (kcal)	752	532	634
Tumor incidence (%)	73	43	7

From Boissonneau et al., 1986

ining the effect of diet on a cancer that is caused by high doses of an inducing agent that may be irrelevant to humans. Conditions that may more closely resemble human experience were used by Appleton and Landers (1986) to examine dietary fat in relation to spontaneously occurring breast tumors in rats and mice. As part of a large toxicologic screening program, two series of control animals, totaling over 10,000 animals, were used: those receiving and not receiving large daily doses of corn oil. Despite a large difference in fat and energy intakes (the corn oil animals gained more weight), there was little difference in mammary tumor incidence.

Using a quite different approach, Sonnenschein and colleagues (1991) conducted a case–control study of breast cancer in dogs by interviewing owners about the usual foods consumed by their animals. Compared with human populations, an extremely wide intake in the fat composition of the diet was observed among these animals (from 10% to 70% of energy) that varied little from day to day. Compared with controls having other cancers, and also a series of cancer-free controls, no association was observed with the fat composition of the diet. Although the total fat composition of the diet does influence the

risk of mammary tumors in some animal models, it does not appear to do so in other circumstances; thus, the existence of such a relationship in animals cannot be used as an argument that a similar effect should exist in humans.

SPECIFIC TYPES OF FAT AND BREAST CANCER

Apart from possible effects of total fat intake on the occurrence of breast cancer, the results of animal studies have suggested that the fatty acid composition of the diet has an independent relationship with this malignancy. In particular, it has been suggested that polyunsaturated fat may be most deleterious (Carroll and Hopkins, 1979; Hopkins and Carroll, 1979). This appears to be inconsistent with human data based on the international correlations that exist for animal but not vegetable fat in case–control studies (Howe et al., 1990) and in prospective analyses (Hunter et al., 1996). Also, Ip (1987) has suggested that little relationship exists in rodents once the essential requirements for linoleic acid have been met.

Some animal studies have suggested that monounsaturated fat, in the form of olive oil, may be protective relative to other sources of energy (Cohen et al., 1991; Carroll, 1987). In a Spanish study specifically undertaken because of the high consumption of olive oil and low breast cancer rates in this population, no association was observed with total fat intake (Martin-Moreno et al., 1994). However, higher intake of olive oil was associated with reduced risk of breast cancer. Similar inverse associations with olive oil or monounsaturated fat were seen in case–control studies in Greece (Katsouyanni et al., 1994), Italy (La Vecchia et al., 1995), and elsewhere in Spain (Landa et al., 1994); in the Italian study, polyunusaturated oils were also related to lower risk.

High intake of omega-3 fatty acids from marine oils has inhibited the occurrence of mammary tumors in animals (Karmali, 1987). However, case–control and cohort studies have in general found little relation between intake of omega-3 fatty acids or fish (the major source of extra long chain omega-3 fatty acids) and risk of breast cancer (Willett, 1997b).

ALTERNATIVE HYPOTHESES

The failure of most case–control and cohort studies to confirm the hypothesis that a diet high in total or saturated fat composition increases the incidence of human breast cancer leaves the large differences in breast cancer rates among countries unexplained. Many alternative hypotheses exist, including differences in reproductive risk factors (Spicer et al., 1995), intake of selenium and other minerals (Schrauzer et al., 1977), marine oils (Karmali, 1987), alcohol (Schatzkin et al., 1987; Willett et al., 1987b; Longnecker, 1994), specific vegetables (Knox, 1977; Kamiyama and Michioka, 1982; Steinmetz and Potter, 1991), phytoestrogens (Horn-Ross, 1995; Yuan et al., 1995), the use of hormone replacement therapy (Colditz et al., 1995), and physical activity (Bernstein et al., 1994). Although a combination of these factors may contribute to differences in rates between

countries, another alternative explanation for the large differences is that the powerful protective effect of energy restriction found consistently in animal studies also applies to humans. More specifically, one aspect of this hypothesis suggests that energy intake sufficiently restricted during childhood so as to reduce adult height will decrease the incidence of breast cancer in humans. This hypothesis has been suggested by de Waard (1975) to explain the low rates of breast cancer in Japan, and Gray and colleagues (1979) have shown that differences in body size can explain a large portion of the variation in national rates of breast cancer. Micozzi (1985) has used adult height as an index of energy balance during development and examined the correlation between mean national heights and breast cancer incidence rates (Fig. 16–9); a correlation very similar to that for per capita fat intake was observed.

Within some populations, use of height as an index of childhood energy balance appears to be legitimate. For example, the substantial gain in stature by offspring of Japanese emigrants to the United States provides clear evidence that caloric restriction has occurred in Japan (Insull et al., 1968). As not all members of a society are likely to have been equally restricted, the energy restriction hypothesis would lead us to expect a positive association between height and risk of breast cancer within countries, such as Japan, that have experienced a major secular change in adult height over this century. The positive association between height and breast cancer observed in Greece (Valaoras et al., 1969) and in Holland (de Waard, 1975) may be related to limited energy availability for some girls during periods of social disruption.

The interpretation of height in case–control or cohort studies within countries with a prolonged period of relative affluence is less clear. In the United States, caloric restriction sufficiently severe to limit attained height is likely to be less common

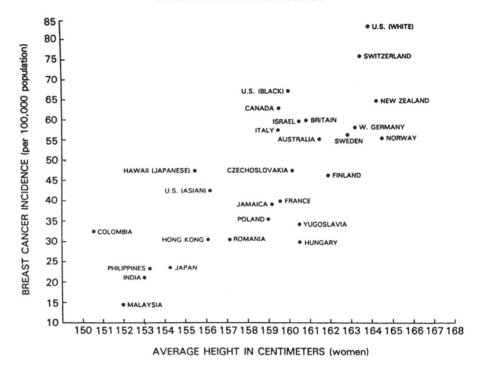

Figure 16–9. Correlation of average adult height in women with breast cancer incidence for 30 countries ($r = 0.8$). (From Micozzi, 1985; reproduced with permission.)

so that variability in height probably largely reflects genetic factors rather than nutritional status during development. Nevertheless, height generally appears to be a risk factor for breast cancer in affluent countries (Swanson et al., 1988; Hunter and Willett, 1989), although the findings have not been entirely consistent. Thus, height per se may be a risk factor (perhaps reflecting levels of endogenous growth factors) rather than simply serving as an indirect marker of earlier nutritional experiences. However, in Norway, the association between height and breast cancer risk was strongest among the cohort of women who were preadolescents during the World War II period of nutritional deprivation (Vatten and Kvinnsland, 1990), suggesting that the nutritionally determined component of height is particularly important.

Total energy intake almost certainly has an etiologic role in breast cancer risk that is mediated by age at menarche, which is a well-established risk factor. Both greater height and greater adiposity predict an earlier age at menarche (Meyer et al., 1990; Maclure et al., 1991); average age at menarche is approximately at 17 years in rural China (Chen et al., 1990) and in the United States has declined from a similar age 200 years ago to about 12 years at present (Wyshak and Frisch, 1982). Energy balance in childhood may also act by additional mechanisms because height appears to be a risk factor for cancers of the colon and other sites (Swanson et al., 1988). It is possible that restriction of other critical nutrients, such as protein or essential fatty acids, sufficient to inhibit growth rates may similarly delay menarche and reduce risk of breast cancer.

The relation between relative weight, which reflects energy balance throughout life, and breast cancer incidence is particularly complex (Willett, 1987; Hunter and Willett, 1993). Among premenopausal women in affluent countries, risk of breast cancer has been inversely related to indices of obesity, whether measured at age 18 or several years before diagnosis (Choi et al., 1978; Paffenbarger et al., 1980; Willett et al., 1985a; Le Marchand et al., 1988). This finding is seemingly at odds with the energy-restriction hypothesis, but the observation that irregular menstrual periods are more frequent among women with a higher relative weight (Willett et al., 1985a) is compatible with the hypothesis of Pike and colleagues (1983) that repeated ovulatory menstrual cycles and the accompanying cell division of breast tissue increases the likelihood of breast cancer. The relationship of higher relative weight to anovulation has been confirmed by the finding that the risk of anovulatory infertility is lowest among women with a BMI of 18 to 23 kg/m² (relatively lean by U.S. standards) and rises progressively among the few women with lower BMI and the far larger group with higher relative weights (Rich-Edwards et al., 1994).

Among postmenopausal women, a positive association has generally been observed between relative weight and risk of breast cancer (Valaoras et al., 1969; Brinton et al., 1979), although this relationship has been nonexistent or extremely weak in affluent populations with the high rates of breast cancer (Hunter and Willett, 1989; Tretli, 1989; Howe et al., 1990; Pathak and Whittemore, 1992). The lack of a stronger relation in high-risk populations has been perplexing because among postmenopausal women the levels of endogenous estrogens rise substantially with greater adiposity (Hankinson et al., 1995). Recent data from the Nurses' Health Study suggest that the weak overall relationship between BMI in postmenopausal women results in part because the protective effect of higher BMI in early adulthood against premenopausal breast cancer also extends

to protection after menopause. However, weight gain as an adult (which would result in higher estrogens levels after menopause) substantially increases risk of postmenopausal breast cancer, thus counterbalancing the benefit of earlier adiposity (Huang et al., 1997). Furthermore, the adverse effect of weight gain (and also the association with BMI after menopause) is considerably stronger among women who never used estrogen replacement therapy after menopause; among those who use estrogen replacements, the influences of adipose on endogenous estrogen levels appear to be masked by pharmacologic doses of estrogens. Together, weight gain after age 18 and use of estrogen therapy after menopause appeared to account for one-third of the postmenopausal breast cancer incidence in the Nurses' Health Study. The opposing effects of early adiposity and weight gain probably account for the stronger association between BMI and postmenopausal breast cancer in low-incidence countries than in high-risk regions. In low-incidence areas (e.g., developing Asian countries and Southern European countries), few women are likely to have sufficient adiposity to cause anovulation during the premenopausal years, and thus weight gain in midlife would be unopposed, resulting in a strong positive association between BMI and breast cancer after menopause. Of course, postmenopausal breast cancer rates reflect early adult exposures decades ago, and relationships with BMI in countries with historically low rates are likely to evolve toward those of high-incidence areas with increasing adiposity.

The energy-restriction and dietary fat-composition hypotheses are not mutually exclusive, and, in the extreme, they may converge. In traditional societies of physically active peasants who experienced chronic parasitic diseases and recurrent bouts of diarrhea and other infections during childhood, it would be difficult to avoid energy restriction on a rice or other staple diet that contained only 10% of calories as fat. A sedentary lifestyle, relative control of infectious diseases, and ready availability of refined carbohydrates, however, make it easy to obtain excess energy on what would be considered to be low fat diets, that is, 20% or 25% of calories as fat. Even if it is true that energy restriction sufficiently severe to limit adult height reduces breast cancer incidence, this is unlikely to provide a practical approach to the prevention of human breast cancer. Although a risk factor for breast cancer, tallness has also been consistently associated with lower risk of cardiovascular disease (Rich-Edwards et al., 1995). Being physically active and lean throughout life appears to be desirable for many reasons, including the possible delay of menstruation and reduction in risk of postmenopausal breast cancer (Frisch et al., 1985; Bernstein et al., 1994), as well as total mortality (Manson et al., 1995). Although a small increase in risk of breast cancer during the premenopausal years appears to be associated with leanness, breast cancer mortality is not increased among lean women, presumably because tumors are more easily detected and effectively treated (Tretli, 1989; Huang et al., 1996).

SUMMARY

There are good reasons to reduce intake of animal and partially hydrogenated fat. Existing data, however, provide little support for the hypothesis that reduction in dietary fat composition even to 20% of energy during adulthood will lead to a substantial reduction in breast cancer in western cultures. Some evidence suggests that substituting monounsaturated fat for other sources of energy may even reduce risk of breast cancer; this deserves further examination. Also, the avoidance of weight gain during adulthood has many benefits, which are likely to include an important reduction in risk of postmenopausal breast cancer.

REFERENCES

Adelstein, A. M., J. Staszewski, and C. S. Muir (1979). Cancer mortality in 1970–1972 among Polish-born migrants to England and Wales. Br J Cancer 40, 464–475.

Albanes, D. (1987). Total calories, body weight, and tumor incidence in mice. Cancer Res 47, 1987–1992.

Ames, B. N., L. S. Gold, and W. C. Willett (1995). The causes and prevention of cancer. Proc Natl Acad Sci USA 92, 5258–5265.

Appleton, B. S., and R. E. Landers (1986). Oil gavage effects on tumor incidence in the national toxicology program's 2-year carcinogenesis bioassay. Adv Exp Med Biol 206, 99–104.

Armstrong, B., and R. Doll (1975). Environmental factors and cancer incidence and mortality in different countries, with special reference to dietary practices. Int J Cancer 15, 617–631.

Armstrong, B. K., J. B. Brown, H. T. Clarke, D. K. Crooke, R. Hahnel, J. R. Masarei, and T. Ratajczak (1981). Diet and reproductive hormones: A study of vegetarian and nonvegetarian postmenopausal women. JNCI 67, 761–767.

Beaton, G. H., J. Milner, P. Corey, V. McGuire, M. Cousins, E. Stewart, M. de Ramos, D. Hewitt, P. V. Grambsch, N. Kassim, and J. A. Little (1979). Sources of variance in 24-hour dietary recall data: Implications for nutrition study design and interpretation. Am J Clin Nutr 32, 2546–2549.

Bennett, F. C., and D. M. Ingram (1990). Diet and female sex hormone concentrations: An intervention study for the type of fat consumed. Am J Clin Nutr 52, 808–812.

Bernstein, L., B. E. Henderson, R. Hanisch, J. Sullivan-Halley, and R. K. Ross (1994). Physical exercise and reduced risk of breast cancer in young women. JNCI 86, 1403–1408.

Beth, M., M. R. Berger, M. Aksoy, and D. Schmahl (1987). Comparison between the effects of dietary fat level and of calorie intake on methylnitrosourea-induced mammary carcinogenesis in female SD-rats. Int J Cancer 39, 737–744.

Birt, D. F. (1986). Dietary fat and experimental carcinogenesis: A summary of recent in vivo studies. Adv Exp Med Biol 206, 69–83.

Bjarnason, O., N. Day, G. Snaedal, and H. Tulinius (1974). The effect of year of birth on the breast cancer age-incidence curve in Iceland. *Int J Cancer 13*, 689–696.

Boissonneault, G. A., C. E. Elson, and M. W. Pariza (1986). Net energy effects of dietary fat on chemically induced mammary carcinogenesis in F344 rats. *JNCI 76*, 335–338.

Brinton, L. A., R. R. Williams, R. N. Hoover, N. L. Stegens, M. Feinleib, and J. F. Fraumeni, Jr. (1979). Breast cancer risk factors among screening program participants. *JNCI 62*, 37–44.

Buell, P. (1973). Changing incidence of breast cancer in Japanese-American women. *JNCI 51*, 1479–1483.

Carroll, K. K. (1975). Experimental evidence of dietary factors and hormone-dependent cancers. *Cancer Res 35*, 3374–3383.

Carroll, K. K. (1987). Summation: Which fat/how much fat—Animals. *Prev Med 16*, 510–515.

Carroll, K. K., and G. J. Hopkins (1979). Dietary polyunsaturated fat versus saturated fat in relation to mammary carcinogenesis. *Lipids 14*, 155–158.

Centers for Disease Control and Prevention, National Center for Health Statistics (1994). Daily dietary fat and total food-energy intakes—Third National Health and Nutrition Examination Survey, Phase 1, 1988–91. *Morbid Mortal Weekly Rep 43*, 116–117.

Chan, P. C., and L. A. Cohen (1974). Effect of dietary fat, antiestrogen, and antiprolactin on the development of mammary tumors in rats. *JNCI 52*, 25–30.

Chasan-Taber, S., E. B. Rimm, M. J. Stampfer, D. Spiegelman, G. A. Colditz, E. Giovannucci, A. Ascherio, and W. C. Willett (1996). Reproducibility and validity of a self-administered physical activity questionnaire for male health professionals. *Epidemiology 7*, 81–86.

Chen, J., T. C. Campbell, L. Junyao, and R. Peto (1990). *Diet, Life-Style and Mortality in China: A Study of the Characteristics of 65 Chinese Counties*. Oxford: Oxford University Press.

Choi, N. W., G. R. Howe, A. B. Miller, V. Matthews, R. W. Morgan, L. Munan, J. D. Bunch, J. Feather, M. Jain, and A. Kelly (1978). An epidemiologic study of breast cancer. *Am J Epidemiol 107*, 510–521.

Cohen, L. A., M. E. Kendall, E. Zang, C. Meschter, and D. P. Rose (1991). Modulation of N-nitrosomethylurea-induced mammary tumor promotion by dietary fiber and fat. *JNCI 83*, 496–501.

Cohen, L. A., and E. I. Wynder (1990). Do dietary monounsaturated fatty acids play a protective role in carcinogenesis and cardiovascular disease? *Med Hypoth 31*, 83–89.

Colditz, G. A., S. E. Hankinson, D. J. Hunter, W. C. Willett, J. E. Manson, M. J. Stampfer, C. Hennekens, B. Rosner, and F. E. Speizer (1995). The use of estrogens and progestins and the risk of breast cancer in postmenopausal women. *N Engl J Med 332*, 1589–1593.

Committee on Diet Nutrition and Cancer, Assembly of Life Sciences, National Research Council (1982). *Diet, Nutrition, and Cancer*. Washington, DC: National Academy Press.

de Waard, F. (1975). Breast cancer incidence and nutritional status with particular reference to body weight and height. *Cancer Res 35*, 3351–3356.

de Waard, F., E. A. Baanders-van Halewijn, and J. Huizinga (1964). The bimodal age distribution of patients with mammary carcinoma: Evidence for the existence of 2 types of human breast cancer. *Cancer 17*, 141–151.

Djuric, Z., L. K. Hielbrun, B. A. Reading, A. Boomer, F. A. Valeriote, and S. Martino (1991). Effects of a low-fat diet on levels of oxidative damage to DNA in human peripheral nucleated blood cells. *JNCI 83*, 766–769.

Donato, K. A. (1987). Efficiency and utilization of various energy sources for growth. *Am J Clin Nutr 45(suppl)*, 164–167.

Enig, M. G., R. J. Munn, and M. Keeney (1978). Dietary fat and cancer trends—a critique. *Fed Proc 37*, 2215–2220.

Franceschi, S., A. Favero, A. Decarli, E. Negri, C. La Vecchia, M. Ferraroni, A. Russo, S. Salvini, D. Amadori, E. Conti, M. Montella, and A. Giacosa (1996). Intake of macronutrients and risk of breast cancer. *Lancet 347*, 1351–1356.

Freedman, L. S., C. Clifford, and M. Messina (1990). Analysis of dietary fat, calories, body weight, and the development of mammary tumors in rats and mice: A review. *Cancer Res 50*, 5710–5719.

Freedman, L. S., R. L. Prentice, and C. Clifford, et al. (1993). Dietary fat and breast cancer: Where we are. *JNCI 85*, 764–765.

Friedenreich, C. M., G. R. Howe, and A. B. Miller (1991). An investigation of recall bias in the reporting of past food intake among breast cancer cases and controls. *Ann Epidemiol 1*, 439–453.

Friedenreich, C. M., G. R. Howe, and A. B. Miller (1994). Re: A comparison of prospective and retrospective assessments of diet in the study of breast cancer (letter). *Am J Epidemiol* 140, 579–580.

Frisch, R. E., G. Wyshak, N. L. Albright, T. E. Albright, I. Schiff, K. P. Jones, J. Witschi, E. Shiang, E. Kof, and M. Marguglio (1985). Lower prevalence of breast cancer and cancers of the reproductive system among former college athletes compared to nonathletes. *Br J Cancer* 52, 885–891.

Gaard, M., S. Tretli, and E. B. Loken (1995). Dietary fat and the risk of breast cancer: A prospective study of 25,892 Norwegian women. *Int J Cancer* 63, 13–17.

Giovannucci, E. (1995). Insulin and colon cancer. *Cancer Causes Control* 6, 164–179.

Giovannucci, E., M. J. Stampfer, G. A. Colditz, J. Manson, B. Rosner, M. Longnecker, F. Speizer, and W. C. Willett (1993). A comparison of prospective and retrospective assessments of diet in the study of breast cancer. *Am J Epidemiol* 137, 502–511.

Giovannucci, E., and W. C. Willett (1994). Re: A comparison of prospective and retrospective assessments of diet in the study of breast cancer (reply). *Am J Epidemiol* 140, 580–581.

Goldin, B. R., H. Adlercreutz, J. T. Dwyer, L. Swenson, J. H. Warram, and S. L. Gorbach (1981). Effect of diet on excretion of estrogens in pre-and postmenopausal women. *Cancer Res* 41, 3771–3773.

Graham, S., R. Hellmann, J. Marshall, J. Freudenheim, J. Vena, M. Swanson, M. Zielezny, T. Nemoto, N. Stubbe, and T. Raimondo (1991). Nutritional epidemiology of postmenopausal breast cancer in western New York. *Am J Epidemiol* 134, 552–566.

Graham, S., J. Marshall, C. Mettlin, T. Rzepka, T. Nemoto, and T. Byers (1982). Diet in the epidemiology of breast cancer. *Am J Epidemiol* 116, 68–75.

Gray, G. E., M. C. Pike, and B. E. Henderson (1979). Breast cancer incidence and mortality rates in different countries in relation to known risk factors and dietary practices. *Br J Cancer* 39, 1–7.

Gray, G. E., M. C. Pike, T. Hirayama, J. Tellez, V. Gerkins, J. B. Brown, J. T. Casagrande, and B. E. Henderson (1982a). Diet and hormone profiles in teenage girls in four countries at different risk for breast cancer. *Prev Med* 11, 108–113.

Gray, G. E., P. Williams, V. Gerkins, J. B. Brown, B. Armstrong, R. Phillips, J. T. Casagrande, M. C. Pike, and B. E. Henderson (1982b). Diet and hormone levels in Seventh-day Adventist teenage girls. *Prev Med* 11, 103–107.

Grodin, J. M., P. K. Siiteri, and P. C. MacDon-

ald (1973). Source of estrogen production in postmenopausal women. *J Clin Edocrinol Metab* 36, 207–214.

Hagerty, M. A., B. J. Howie, S. Tan, and T. D. Shultz (1988). Effect of low-and high-fat intakes on the hormonal milieu of premenopausal women. *Am J Clin Nutr* 47, 653–659.

Hankinson, S. E., J. E. Manson, S. J. London, W. C. Willett, and F. E. Speizer (1994). Laboratory reproducibility of endogenous hormone levels in postmenopausal women. *Cancer Epidemiol Biol Prev* 3, 51–56.

Hankinson, S. E., W. C. Willett, J. E. Manson, D. J. Hunter, G. A. Colditz, M. J. Stampfer, C. Longcope, and F. E. Speizer (1995). Alcohol, height, and adiposity in relation to estrogen and prolactin levels in postmenopausal women. *JNCI* 87, 1297–1302.

Helzlsouer, K. J., A. J. Alberg, T. L. Bush, C. Longcope, G. B. Gordon, and G. W. Comstock (1994). A prospective study of endogenous hormones and breast cancer. *Cancer Detect Prev* 18, 79–85.

Hems, G. (1978). The contributions of diet and childbearing to breast cancer rates. *Br J Cancer* 37, 974–982.

Hill, P., L. Garbaczewski, P. Helman, J. Huskisson, E. Sporangisa, and E. L. Wynder (1980). Diet, lifestyle, and menstrual activity. *Am J Clin Nutr* 33, 1192–1198.

Hirayama, T. (1978). Epidemiology of breast cancer with special reference to the role of diet. *Prev Med* 7, 173–195.

Hirohata, T., T. Shigematsu, A. M. Nomura, Y. Nomura, A. Horie, and I. Hirohata (1985). Occurrence of breast cancer in relation to diet and reproductive history: A case–control study in Fukuoka, Japan. *NCI Monogr* 69, 187–190.

Holmberg, L., E. M. Ohlander, T. Byers, M. Zack, A. Wolk, R. Bergstrom, L. Bergkvist, E. Thurfjell, A. Bruce, and H. O. Adami (1994). Diet and breast cancer risk—Results from a population-based, case–control study in Sweden. *Arch Intern Med* 154, 1805–1811.

Hopkins, G. J., and K. K. Carroll (1979). Relationship between amount and type of dietary fat in promotion of mammary carcinogenesis induced by 7,l2-dimethylbenz (α) anthracene. *JNCI* 62, 1009–1012.

Horn-Ross, P. L. (1995). Phytoestrogens, body composition, and breast cancer. *Cancer Causes Control* 6, 567–573.

Howe, G. R. (1985). The use of polytomous dual response data to increase power in case-control studies: An application to the association between dietary fat and breast cancer. *J Chronic Dis* 38, 663–670.

Howe, G. R., C. M. Friedenreich, M. Jain, and A. B. Miller (1991). A cohort study of fat intake and risk of breast cancer. *JNCI 83*, 336–340.

Howe, G. R., T. Hirohata, T. G. Hislop, J. M. Iscovich, J. M. Yuan, K. Katsouyanni, F. Lubin, E. Marubini, B. Modan, T. Rohan, P. Toniolo, and Y. Shunzhang (1990). Dietary factors and risk of breast cancer: Combined analysis of 12 case–control studies. *JNCI 82, 561–569.*

Huang, Z., S. E. Hankinson, G. A. Colditz, M. J. Stampfer, D. J. Hunter, J. E. Manson, C. H. Hennekens, B. Rosner, F. E. Speizer, W. C. Willett (1997). Dual effects of weight and weight gain on breast cancer risk. *JAMA 278*, 1407–1411.

Hunter, D. J., D. Spiegelman, H. O. Adami, L. Beeson, P. A. van den Brandt, A. R. Folsom, G. E. Fraser, R. A. Goldbohm, S. Graham, G. R. Howe, L. H. Kushi, J. R. Marshall, A. McDermott, A. B. Miller, F. E. Speizer, A. Wolk, S.-S. Yaun, and W. C. Willett (1996). Cohort studies of fat intake and the risk of breast cancer: A pooled analysis. *N Engl J Med 334*, 356–361.

Hunter, D. J., and W. C. Willett (1989). Human epidemiologic evidence on the nutritional prevention of cancer. In Moon, T., and Micozzi, M., (eds.): *Nutrition and Cancer Prevention.* New York: Marcel Dekker, pp. 83–100.

Hunter, D. J., and W. Willett (1993). Diet, body size, and breast cancer. *Epidemiol Rev 15*, 110–132.

Hunter, D. J., D. Spiegelman, and W. C. Willett (in press) Letter to the editor. *JNCI.*

Ingram, D. M. (1981). Trends in diet and breast cancer mortality in England and Wales 1928-1977. *Nutr Cancer 3*, 75–80.

Insull, W. J., T. Oiso, and K. Tsuchiya (1968). Diet and nutritional status of Japanese. *Am J Clin Nutr 21*, 753–777.

Ip, C. (1987). Fat and essential fatty acid in mammary carcinogensis. *Am J Clin Nutr 45(suppl)*, 218–224.

Ip, C. (1990). Quantitative assessment of fat and calorie as risk factors in mammary carcinogenesis in an experimental model. In Mettlin, C. J., and Aoki, K., (ed.): *Recent Progress in Research on Nutrition and Cancer.* Proceedings of a Workshop Sponsored by the International Union Against Cancer, held in Nagoya, Japan, November 1–3, 1989. New York: Wiley-Liss, Inc., pp 107–117.

Jenkins, D. J. A., T. M. S. Wolever, A. M. Ocana, V. Vuksan, S. C. Cunnane, M. Jenkins, G. S. Wong, W. Singer, S. R. Bloom, L. M. Blendis, and R. G. Josse (1990). Metabolic effects of reducing rate of glucose ingestion by single bolus versus continuous sipping. *Diabetes 39*, 775–781.

Jones, D. Y., A. Schatzkin, S. B. Green, G. Block, L. A. Brinton, R. G. Ziegler, R. Hoover, and P. R. Taylor (1987). Dietary fat and breast cancer in the National Health and Nutrition Examination Survey I Epidemiologic follow-up study. *JNCI 79*, 465–471.

Kamiyama, S., and O. Michioka (1982). Mutagenic components of diets in high and low-risk areas for stomach cancer. In Stich, H. F., (ed.): *Carcinogens and Mutagens in the Environment.* Boca Raton, FL: CRC Press, pp 29–42.

Karmali, R. A. (1987). Fatty acids: Inhibition. *Am J Clin Nutr 45(suppl)*, 225–229.

Kato, I., S. Miura, F. Kasumi, T. Iwase, H. Tashiro, Y. Fujita, H. Koyama, T. Ikeda, K. Fujiwara, and K. Saotome, et al. (1992). A case–control study of breast cancer among Japanese women: With special reference to family history and reproductive and dietary factors. *Breast Cancer Res Treat 24*, 51–59.

Katsouyanni, K., A. Trichopoulou, S. Stuver, Y. Garas, A. Kritselis, G. Kyriakou, M. Stoikidou, P. Boyle, and D. Trichopoulos (1994). The association of fat and other macronutrients with breast cancer: A case–control study from Greece. *Br J Cancer 70*, 537–541.

Key, T. J., S. C. Darby, and M. C. Pike (1987). Trends in breast cancer mortality and diet in England and Wales from 1911 to 1980. *Nutr Cancer 10*, 1–9.

Kinlen, L. J. (1982). Meat and fat consumption and cancer mortality: A study of strict religious orders in Britain. *Lancet 1*, 946–949.

Knekt, P., D. Albanes, R. Seppanen, A. Aromaa, R. Jarvinen, L. Hyvonen, L. Teppo, and E. Pukkala (1990). Dietary fat and risk of breast cancer. *Am J Clin Nutr 52*, 903–908.

Knox, E. G. (1977). Foods and diseases. *Br J Prev Soc Med 31*, 71–80.

Kolonel, L. N., J. H. Hankin, A. M. Nomura, and S. Y. Chu (1981). Dietary fat intake and cancer incidence among five ethnic groups in Hawaii. *Cancer Res 41*, 3727–3728.

Kushi, L. H., T. A. Sellers, J. D. Potter, C. L. Nelson, R. G. Munger, S. A. Kaye, and A. R. Folsom (1992). Dietary fat and postmenopausal breast cancer. *JNCI 84*, 1092–1099.

Landa, M. C., N. Frago, and A. Tres (1994).

Diet and the risk of breast cancer in Spain. *Eur J Cancer Prev 3*, 313–320.

La Vecchia, C., E. Negri, S. Franceschi, A. Decarli, A. Giacosa, and L. Lipworth (1995). Olive oil, other dietary fats, and the risk of breast cancer (Italy). *Cancer Causes Control 6*, 545–550.

Le, M. G., L. H. Moulton, C. Hill, and A. Kramar (1986). Consumption of dairy produce and alcohol in a case–control study of breast cancer. *JNCI 77*, 633–636.

Le Marchand, L., L. N. Kolonel, M. E. Earle, and M. P. Mi (1988). Body size at different periods of life and breast cancer risk. *Am J Epidemiol 128*, 137–152.

London, S. J., F. M. Sacks, M. J. Stampfer, I. C. Henderson, M. Maclure, A. Tomita, W. C. Wood, S. Remine, N. J. Robert, and J. R. Dmochowski, et al. (1993). Fatty acid composition of the subcutaneous adipose tissue and risk of proliferative benign breast disease and breast cancer. *JNCI 85*, 785–793.

Longnecker, M. P. (1994). Alcoholic beverage consumption in relation to risk of breast cancer: Meta-analysis and review. *Cancer Causes Control 5*, 73–82.

Lubin, J. H., P. E. Burns, W. J. Blot, R. G. Ziegler, A. W. Lees, and J. F. Fraumeni, Jr. (1981). Dietary factors and breast cancer risk. *Int J Cancer 28*, 685–689.

Maclure, M., L. B. Travis, W. C. Willett, and B. MacMahon (1991). A prospective cohort study of nutrient intake and age at menarche. *Am J Clin Nutr 54*, 649–656.

Malik, I. A., S. Sharif, F. Malik, A. Hakimali, W. A. Khan, and S. H. Badruddin (1993). Nutritional aspects of mammary carcinogenesis: A case–control study. *J Pak Med Assoc 43*, 118–120.

Manson, J. E., W. C. Willett, M. J. Stampfer, G. A. Colditz, D. J. Hunter, S. E. Hankinson, C. H. Hennekens, and F. E. Speizer (1995). Body weight and mortality among women. *N Engl J Med 333*, 677–685.

Marshall, J. R., and S. Graham (1993). Letter to the editor. *Am J Epidemiol 137*, 249–252.

Marshall, J. R., Y. Qu, J. Chen, B. Parpia, and T. C. Campbell (1992). Additional ecological evidence: Lipids and breast cancer mortality among women aged 55 and over in China. *Eur J Cancer 28A*, 1720–1727.

Martin-Moreno, J. M., W. C. Willett, L. Gorgojo, J. R. Banegas, F. Rodriguez-Artalejo, J. C. Fernandez-Rodriguez, P. Maisonneuve, and P. Boyle (1994). Dietary fat, olive oil intake and breast cancer risk. *Int J Cancer 58*, 774–780.

McMichael, A. J., and G. G. Giles (1988). Cancer in migrants to Australia: Extending descriptive epidemiological data. *Cancer Res 48*, 751–756.

Meyer, F., J. Moisan, D. Marcoux, and C. Bouchard (1990). Dietary and physical determinants of menarche. *Epidemiology 1*, 377–381.

Michels, K. B., and W. C. Willett (1992). The Women's Health Initiative: Daughter of Politics or Science? *Principles Practices Oncol 6*, 1–11.

Micozzi, M. S. (1985). Nutrition, body size, and breast cancer. *Yearbook Phys Anthropol 28*, 175–206.

Miller, A. B., A. Kelly, N. W. Choi, V. Matthews, R. W. Morgan, L. Munan, J. D. Burch, J. Feather, G. R. Howe, and M. Jain (1978). A study of diet and breast cancer. *Am J Epidemiol 107*, 499–509.

Mills, P. K., J. F. Annegers, and R. L. Phillips (1988). Animal product consumption and subsequent fatal breast cancer among Seventh-day Adventists. *Am J Epidemiol 127*, 440–453.

Mills, P. K., W. L. Beeson, R. L. Phillips, and G. E. Fraser (1989). Dietary habits and breast cancer incidence among Seventh-day Adventists. *Cancer 64*, 582–590.

Morgan, R. W., M. Jain, A. B. Miller, N. W. Choi, V. Matthews, L. Munan, J. D. Burch, J. Feather, G. R. Howe, and A. Kelly (1978). A comparison of dietary methods in epidemiologic studies. *Am J Epidemiol 107*, 488–498.

National Cancer Institute (1984). *Cancer Prevention: Good News; Better News; Best News.* DHHS Publication No. (NIH) 84-2671. Washington, DC: Department of Health and Human Services.

National Research Council Committee on Diet and Health (1989). *Diet and Health: Implications for Reducing Chronic Disease Risk.* Washington, DC. National Academy Press.

Nukada, A. (1975). Industrialization as a factor for secular increase in physiques of school children in Japan. In: Asahina, K., and Shigiya, R., (eds.): *Physiological Adaptability and Nutritional Status of the Japanese.* Tokyo: University of Tokyo Press, p 108.

Paffenbarger, R. S., Jr., J. B. Kampert, and H. G. Chang (1980). Characteristics that predict risk of breast cancer before and after the menopause. *Am J Epidemiol 112*, 258–268.

Pariza, M. W., and R. K. Boutwell (1987). Historical perspective: calories and energy expenditure in carcinogenesis. *Am J Clin Nutr 45(suppl)*, 151–156.

Pathak, D. R., and A. S. Whittemore (1992). Combined effects of body size, parity, and menstrual events on breast cancer incidence in seven countries. *Am J Epidemiol 135,* 153–168.

Phillips, R. L. (1975). Role of life-style and dietary habits in risk of cancer among Seventh-day Adventists. *Cancer Res 35,* 3513–3522.

Phillips, R. L., L. Garfinkel, J. W. Kuzma, W. L. Beeson, T. Lotz, and B. Brin (1980). Mortality among California Seventh-day Adventists for selected cancer sites. *JNCI 65,* 1097–1107.

Phillips, R. L., and D. A. Snowdon (1983). Association of meat and coffee use with cancers of the large bowel, breast, and prostate among Seventh-day Adventists: Preliminary results. *Cancer Res 43(suppl),* 2403S–2408S.

Pike, M. C., M. D. Krailo, B. E. Henderson, J. T. Casagrande, and D. G. Hoel (1983). "Hormonal" risk factors, "breast tissue age" and the age-incidence of breast cancer. *Nature 303,* 767–770.

Potter, J. D. (1987). Dietary fat and the risk of breast cancer (letter). *N Engl J Med 317,* 166.

Prentice, R., D. Thompson, C. Clifford, S. Gorbach, B. Goldin, and D. Byar (1990). Dietary fat reduction and plasma estradiol concentration in healthy postmenopausal women. The Women's Health Trial Study Group. *JNCI 82,* 129–134.

Prentice, R. L. (1996). Measurement error and results from analytic epidemiology: Dietary fat and breast cancer. *JNCI 88,* 1738–1747.

Prentice, R. L., F. Kakar, S. Hursting, L. Sheppard, R. Klein, and L. H. Kushi (1988). Aspects of the rationale for the Women's Health Trial. *JNCI 80,* 802–814.

Prentice, R. L., and L. Sheppard (1990). Dietary fat and cancer. Consistency of the epidemiologic data, and disease prevention that may follow from a practical reduction in fat consumption. *Cancer Causes Control 1,* 81–97.

Rich-Edwards, J. W., M. B. Goldman, W. C. Willett, D. J. Hunter, M. J. Stampfer, G. A. Colditz, and J. E. Manson (1994). Adolescent body mass index and infertility caused by ovulatory disorder. *Am J Obstet Gynecol 171,* 171–177.

Rich-Edwards, J. W., J. E. Manson, M. J. Stampfer, G. A. Colditz, W. C. Willett, B. Rosner, F. E. Speizer, and C. H. Hennekens (1995). Height and the risk of cardiovascular disease in women. *Am J Epidemiol 142,* 909–917.

Rose, D. P., A. P. Boyar, C. Cohen, and L. E. Strong (1987a). Effect of a low-fat diet on hormone levels in women with cystic breast disease. I. Serum steroids and gonadotrophins. *JNCI 78,* 623–626.

Rose, D. P., L. A. Cohen, B. Berke and A. P. Boyar (1987b). Effect of a low-fat diet on hormone levels in women with cystic breast disease. II. Serum radioimmunoassayable prolactin and growth hormone and bioactive lactogenic hormones. *JNCI 78,* 627–631.

Rose, D. P., J. M. Connolly, R. T. Chlebowski, I. M. Buzzard, and E. L. Wynder (1993). The effects of a low-fat dietary intervention and tamoxifen adjuvant therapy on the serum estrogen and sex hormone-binding globulin concentrations of postmenopausal breast cancer patients. *Breast Cancer Res Treat 27,* 253–262.

Rosner, B., W. C. Willett, and D. Spiegelman (1989). Correction of logistic regression relative risk estimates and confidence intervals for systematic within-person measurement error. *Statist Med 8,* 1051–1069.

Schatzkin, A., D. Y. Jones, R. N. Hoover, P. R. Taylor, L. A. Brinton, R. G. Ziegler, E. B. Harvey, C. L. Carter, L. M. Licitra, and M. C. Dufour, et al. (1987). Alcohol consumption and breast cancer in the epidemiologic follow-up study of the first National Health and Nutrition Examination Survey. *N Engl J Med 316,* 1169–1173.

Schrauzer, G. N., D. A. White, and C. J. Schneider (1977). Cancer mortality correlation studies—III: Statistical associations with dietary selenium intakes. *Bioinorg Chem 7,* 23–31.

Sonnenschein, E., L. Glickman, M. Goldschmidt, and L. McKee (1991). Body conformation, diet, and risk of breast cancer in pet dogs: A case–control study. *Am J Epidemiol 133,* 694–703.

Spicer, D. V., E. A. Krecker, and M. C. Pike (1995). The endocrine prevention of breast cancer. *Cancer Invest 13,* 495–504.

Stampfer, M. J., W. C. Willett, G. A. Colditz, and F. E. Speizer (1987). Intake of cholesterol, fish and specific types of fat in relation to risk of breast cancer. In Lands, W. E. (ed.): *Proceedings of the AOCS Short Course on Polyunsaturated Fatty Acids and Eicosanoids.* Mississippi, May 13–16, 1987. Champaign, IL: American Oil Chemists' Society, pp. 248–252.

Staszewski, J., and W. Haenszel (1965). Cancer mortality among the Polish-born in the United States. *JNCI 35,* 291–297.

Steinmetz, K. A., and J. D. Potter (1991). Vegetables, fruit and cancer. I. Epidemiology. *Cancer Causes Control 2,* 325–357.

Stephen, A. M., and N. J. Wald (1990). Trends in individual consumption of dietary fat in the United States, 1920–1984. *Am J Clin Nutr 52*, 457–469.

Stocks, P. (1970). Breast cancer anomalies. *Br J Cancer 24*, 633–643.

Swanson, C. A., D. Y. Jones, A. Schatzkin, L. A. Brinton, and R. G. Ziegler (1988). Breast cancer risk assessed by anthropometry in the NHANES I epidemiological follow-up study. *Cancer Res 48*, 5363–5367.

Talamini, R., C. La Vecchia, A. Decarli, S. Franceschi, E. Grattoni, E. Grigoletto, A. Liberati, and G. Togoni (1984). Social factors, diet and breast cancer in a Northern Italian population. *Br J Cancer 49*, 723–729.

Tannenbaum, A., and H. Silverstone (1953). Nutrition in relation to cancer. *Adv Cancer Res 1*, 451–501.

Toniolo, P., E. Riboli, R. E. Shore, and B. S. Pasternack (1994). Consumption of meat, animal products, protein, and fat and risk of breast cancer: A prospective cohort study in New York. *Epidemiology 5*, 391–397.

Toniolo, P. G., M. Levitz, A. Zeleniuch-Jacquotte, S. Banerjee, K. L. Koenig, R. E. Shore, P. Strax, and B. S. Pasternack (1995). A prospective study of endogenous estrogens and breast cancer in postmenopausal women. *JNCI 87*, 190–197.

Tretli, S. (1989). Height and weight in relation to breast cancer morbidity and mortality. A prospective study of 570,000 women in Norway. *Int J Cancer 44*, 23–30.

Tretli, S., and M. Gaard (1996). Lifestyle changes during adolescence and risk of breast cancer: An ecologic study of the effect of World War II in Norway. *Cancer Causes Control 7*, 507–512.

Trichopoulos, D. (1990). Is breast cancer initiated in utero? *Epidemiology 1*, 95–96.

Ursin, G., L. Bernstein, and M. C. Pike (1994). Breast Cancer. *Cancer Surv 19–20*, 241–264.

Valaoras, V. G., B. MacMahon, D. Trichopoulos, and A. Polychronopoulou (1969). Lactation and reproductive histories of breast cancer patients in greater Athens, 1965–67. *Int J Cancer 4*, 350–363.

Van den Brandt, P. A., P. Van't Veer, and R. A. Goldbohm, et al. (1993). A prospective cohort study on dietary fat and the risk of postmenopausal breast cancer. *Cancer Res 53*, 75–82.

Vatten, L. J., K. S. Bjerve, A. Andersen, and E. Jellum (1993). Polyunsaturated fatty acids in serum phospholipids and risk of breast cancer: A case–control study from the Janus serum bank in Norway. *Eur J Cancer 29A*, 532–538.

Vatten, L. J., and S. Kvinnsland (1990). Body height and risk of breast cancer. A prospective study of 23,831 Norwegian women. *Br J Cancer 61*, 881–885.

Vatten, L. J., K. Solvoll, and E. B. Loken (1990). Frequency of meat and fish intake and risk of breast cancer in a prospective study of 14,500 Norwegian women. *Int J Cancer 46*, 12–15.

Willett, W. C. (1987). Implications of total energy intake for epidemiologic studies of breast and large-bowel cancer. *Am J Clin Nutr 45(suppl)*, 354S–360S.

Willett, W. C. (1994). Diet and health: What should we eat? *Science 264*, 532–537.

Willett, W. C. (1998). Is dietary fat a major determinant of body fat? *Am J Clin Nutr*, (in press).

Willett, W. C. (1997b). Specific fatty acids and risks of breast and prostate cancer: Dietary intake. *Am J Clin Nutr* (in press).

Willett, W. C., M. L. Browne, C. Bain, R. J. Lipnick, M. J. Stampfer, B. Rosner, G. A. Colditz, C. H. Hennekens, and F. E. Speizer (1985a). Relative weight and risk of breast cancer among premenopausal women. *Am J Epidemiol 122*, 731–740.

Willett, W. C., D. J. Hunter, M. J. Stampfer, G. A. Colditz, J. E. Manson, D. Spiegelman, B. Rosner, C. H. Hennekens, and F. E. Speizer (1992). Dietary fat and fiber in relation to risk of breast cancer: An 8-year follow-up. *JAMA 268*, 2037–2044.

Willett, W. C., L. Sampson, M. J. Stampfer, B. Rosner, C. Bain, J. Witschi, C. H. Hennekens, and F. E. Speizer (1985b). Reproducibility and validity of a semiquantitative food frequency questionnaire. *Am J Epidemiol 122*, 51–65.

Willett, W. C., and M. J. Stampfer (1990). Dietary fat and cancer: Another view. *Cancer Causes Control 1*, 103–109.

Willett, W. C., M. J. Stampfer, G. A. Colditz, B. A. Rosner, C. H. Hennekens, and F. E. Speizer (1987a). Dietary fat and the risk of breast cancer. *N Engl J Med 316*, 22–28.

Willett, W. C., M. J. Stampfer, G. A. Colditz, B. A. Rosner, C. H. Hennekens, and F. E. Speizer (1987b). Moderate alcohol consumption and the risk of breast cancer. *N Engl J Med 316*, 1174–1180.

Willett, W. C., M. J. Stampfer, G. A. Colditz, B. A. Rosner, and F. E. Speizer (1990). Relation of meat, fat, and fiber intake to the risk of colon cancer in a prospective study among women. *N Engl J Med 323*, 1664–1672.

Wolk, A., R. Bergstrom, D. Hunter, W. C. Willett, H. Ljung, L. Holmberg, L. Bergkvist, A. Bruce, and H. O. Adami, H. (1998). A prospective study of association of monounsaturated and other types of fat with risk of breast cancer. *Arch Intern Med* 158, 41–45.

Wynder, E. L., F. MacCornack, P. Hill, L. A. Cohen, P. C. Chan, and J. H. Weisburger (1976). Nutrition and the etiology and prevention of breast cancer. *Cancer Detect Prev 1*, 293–310.

Wyshak, G., and R. E. Frisch (1982). Evidence for a secular trend in age of menarche. *N Engl J Med 306*, 1033–1035.

Yuan, J. M., Q. S. Wang, R. K. Ross, B. E. Henderson, and M. C. Yu (1995). Diet and breast cancer in Shanghai and Tianjin, China. *Br J Cancer 71*, 1353–1358.

Zaridze, D., Y. Lifanova, D. Maximovitch, N. E. Day, and S. W. Duffy (1991). Diet, alcohol consumption and reproductive factors in a case–control study of breast cancer in Moscow. *Int J Cancer 48*, 493–501.

Ziegler, R. G., R. N. Hoover, M. C. Pike, A. Hildesheim, A. M. Nomura, D. W. West, A. H. Wu-Williams, L. N. Kolonel, P. L. Horn-Ross, and J. F. Rosenthal (1993). Migration patterns and breast cancer risk in Asian-American women. *JNCI 85*, 1819–1827.

17

Diet and Coronary Heart Disease

According to the classic "diet–heart" hypothesis (Fig. 17–1), high intake of saturated fats and cholesterol and low intake of polyunsaturated fats increase the level of serum cholesterol, which leads to development of atheromatous plaques. Accumulation of these plaques narrows the coronary arteries, reduces blood flow to the heart muscle, and finally leads to myocardial infarction. The focus of this chapter is to examine the epidemiologic evidence addressing this hypothesis and to consider additional hypotheses relating diet to heart disease. Several relevant areas, including vast literatures on animal studies and metabolic experiments relating diet with blood lipid levels, are mentioned only briefly; these are reviewed in detail elsewhere (Wissler and Vesselinovitch, 1975; American Heart Association, 1984; Anonymous, 1985; National Research Council, Committee on Diet and Health, 1989; Grundy, 1991).

The inception of the diet–heart hypothesis has been recounted by Gordon (1988);

much of the early stimulus derived from the demonstration during the 1930s that dietary cholesterol can cause arterial lesions in animals and that this effect is mediated largely through elevation in plasma cholesterol (Katz and Stamler, 1953; Anitschkow, 1967; Wissler and Vesselinovitch, 1975; Grundy et al., 1982). The further development of the diet–heart hypothesis appears to have been influenced heavily by two lines of epidemiologic evidence, the first being ecologic correlations relating diet to rates of heart disease. These data, along with findings from migrant studies and special populations, are discussed in the next section. The other primary line of evidence derives from studies of serum cholesterol. These studies have related dietary factors to serum cholesterol and, in separate investigations, serum cholesterol to the risk of coronary heart disease. These are discussed briefly in a following section as such studies do not directly address the relation of diet to heart disease.

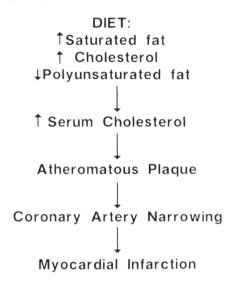

DIET:
↑Saturated fat
↑ Cholesterol
↓Polyunsaturated fat

↓

↑ Serum Cholesterol

↓

Atheromatous Plaque

↓

Coronary Artery Narrowing

↓

Myocardial Infarction

Figure 17–1. Classic diet–heart hypothesis.

DESCRIPTIVE STUDIES OF DIET AND CORONARY HEART DISEASE

Ecologic Studies

The most influential descriptive study on diet and coronary heart disease (CHD) was the work of Keys (1980) relating the mean intake of dietary factors of 16 defined populations in seven countries to the incidence of heart disease in those same groups. As shown in Figure 17–2, intake of saturated fat as a percentage of calories was strongly correlated with coronary death rates ($r = 0.84$). In Keys' sample, the countries with low saturated fat intake and low incidence of CHD were less industrialized and were likely to have differed in many ways from the wealthier countries, in particular in physical activity, obesity, and, at that time, smoking habits. Indeed, the slope of the line relating saturated fat to risk of CHD death is nearly 2.5 times greater than would be expected if saturated fat operated only by raising serum cholesterol level. In the same study, the percentage of energy from total fat had little relationship with CHD incidence or mortality. Indeed, populations with the highest fat intake (about 40% of energy) included the region with the highest CHD rate (Finland), as well as

that with the lowest rate (Crete). In an extended follow-up of these populations, CHD rates were found to vary four to fivefold among countries with similar mean serum cholesterol levels, indicating the importance of factors other than those related to cholesterol (Verschuren et al., 1995).

In another ecologic study, a strong association ($r = 0.67$) was observed between the percentage of calories from total fat in 12 countries and prevalence of raised atherosclerotic lesions in autopsy cases from the same geographic area (Scrimshaw and Guzman, 1968). As with any correlational study, this result may reflect confounding by other risk factors. The clearest message from these data and other comparisons (McGill, 1968) is that rates of CHD differ dramatically among countries and that those in the highly developed countries are highest. Other correlational studies are cited in the review by Grundy and coworkers (1982).

Migrant Studies

CHD incidence rates among three defined Japanese populations living in Japan, Hawaii, and San Francisco have been compared (Kato et al., 1973; Robertson et al., 1977). Saturated fat intake as a percentage

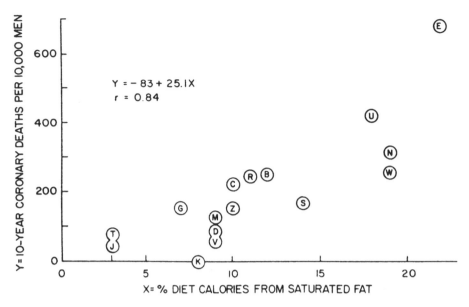

Figure 17–2. Ten-year coronary death rates of the cohorts plotted against the percentage of dietary calories supplied by saturated fatty acids.

(From Keys, 1980; reproduced with permission.)

of calories in the three populations was said to be 7%, 23%, and 26%, respectively (see Table 17–1).* With transition to the United States, mean relative weight (but not height) and serum cholesterol level increased in parallel with the saturated fat intake, mean alcohol intake markedly decreased, and dietary cholesterol was unchanged. Age-adjusted CHD incidence rates were 1.6 per 1,000 person-years in Japan, 3.0 in Hawaii, and 3.7 in San Francisco. These data indicate that the substantial differences in rates of CHD among the three areas cannot be explained by genetic factors and are consistent with the hypothesis that dietary saturated fat may contribute to the difference. However, because other strong dietary and nondietary risk factors, such as alcohol intake and obesity, vary dramatically among the groups, specific causal factors cannot

be firmly identified on the basis of this type of data.

Secular Trends

Data on secular trends in CHD mortality rates are of interest, but do not provide clear support for the classic diet–heart hypothesis. During World War II, major reductions in total and animal fat consumption occurred in Finland, Norway, and other areas in Europe. Decreases in deaths ascribed to arteriosclerosis occurred during this period, similar to decreases observed during World War I (Katz and Stamler, 1953). Within North America, CHD mortality rates rose dramatically over the first half of this century (Anderson, 1979), although the increase in total and saturated fat consumption was slight, and polyunsaturated fat intake rose two- to threefold (Friend, 1967; Page and Marston, 1979). Kahn (1970) has estimated that these changes in dietary fats would account for only a 10 mg/dl increase in serum cholesterol and an 8% rise in incidence of CHD. Since the late 1960s, age-specific mortality

---

* These saturated fat values must be seriously in error as intakes for the U.S. population as a whole at that time were close to 16% to 17% of energy. Nevertheless, there is little doubt that intake was substantially higher in the United States than in Japan.

Table 17–1. Mean levels of potential coronary heart disease risk factors in the Ni-Ho-San Study

	Japan	Hawaii	California
Saturated fat (% energy)	7	23	26
Cholesterol (mg/day)	464	545	533
Alcohol (% energy)	8.9	3.7	2.5
Serum cholesterol (mg/dl)	181	218	228
>120% Relative weight	22%	56%	63%

From Kato et al., 1973.

rates have decreased steadily by a total of over 40% in the United States (Anonymous, 1993; U.S. Department of Health and Human Services, 1994). During this period, dairy fat and lard continued to be replaced by vegetable fat, with the overall effect of increasing polyunsaturated fat intake and slightly decreasing saturated fat intake (Page and Marston, 1979; Stamler, 1985). Whether CHD *incidence* has also decreased is less well documented, and it is likely to have declined to a lesser degree than has mortality (Sytkowski et al., 1996). Because of uncertainty about recent time trends in incidence as well as the changes over time in many factors, including smoking habits, exercise, body weights, vitamin supplements, and multiple dietary factors, attribution of secular changes to any particular factor is treacherous.

In summary, the studies of diet and coronary heart disease that use population groups as units of observation provide convincing evidence that rates of disease differ dramatically among populations and that these differences are primarily due to environmental rather than genetic factors. Although these studies tend to be consistent with the classic diet–heart hypothesis, confounding factors cannot be excluded with confidence.

STUDIES OF BLOOD CHOLESTEROL LEVEL AS AN INTERMEDIARY FACTOR

Studies of blood cholesterol level as an intermediary factor between diet and CHD are considered in two parts: those relating diet to blood cholesterol level and those relating blood cholesterol level to CHD.

Studies of Diet and Blood Cholesterol Level

Relationships between dietary factors and blood lipid levels are best studied by randomized controlled, and preferably blinded, feeding trials in human subjects. The number of subjects required is usually small (typically 10 to 50), and hundreds of such studies have been conducted. Although there continues to be some debate about details of the shape of the dose–response relationships (Keys, 1984; Hegsted, 1986), there is no question that a higher intake of dietary cholesterol and saturated fats and a lower intake of polyunsaturated fats increase blood total cholesterol levels. Data from many metabolic studies have been summarized by Hegsted and colleagues (1993) and by Grande and colleagues (1965) as equations that predict serum total cholesterol level from intake of saturated fat, polyunsaturated fat, and cholesterol (see Chapter 9 for these equations). Most commonly, such studies have manipulated the proportions in the diet of saturated fat (high in palm oil and most animal fats), polyunsaturated fat (usually as corn oil, but also high in soybean oil and safflower oil), monounsaturated fat (usually as olive oil), and dietary cholesterol. Monounsaturated fat was not found to influence total serum cholesterol level appreciably relative to carbohydrate intake and thus was not included in the prediction equations.

The relationship of dietary lipids to blood cholesterol level has also been studied cross-sectionally in human populations. For example, intake of fat-containing foods assessed using a simple frequency questionnaire was not associated with serum cholesterol level among men participating in the Tecumseh Heart Study (Nichols et al., 1976); this has sometimes been cited as evidence against the diet–heart hypothesis

(Mann, 1977). Except for exploratory types of analyses, however, a cross-sectional study design is not optimal to define the effects of dietary factors on blood lipids levels. As noted in Chapter 1 and by Jacobs and colleagues (1979), the true correlation between saturated fat or dietary cholesterol and a single blood measurement of total cholesterol within a general U.S. population is expected to be very low because controlled metabolic studies show that most of the between-person variation in cholesterol level is unrelated to dietary fats. Hence, a very large sample size would be needed to detect any positive correlation between diet and blood cholesterol level. An association has been seen between dietary fat intake, expressed as the Keys score, and serum total cholesterol level among the nearly 2,000 men participating in the Western Electric Study (Shekelle et al., 1981), but, as expected, this correlation was low ($r = 0.08$). The Keys equation indicates that the relationship between cholesterol intake and blood level is nonlinear, being related to the square root of cholesterol intake; thus, perhaps a stronger correlation would be seen among populations with a lower cholesterol distribution. A strong correlation was observed between cholesterol intake and blood level among vegetarians (Kushi et al., 1988) and an Indian population living in Mexico (Connor et al., 1978); both groups consumed little cholesterol.

Frequent underlying assumptions in the use of the Keys and Hegsted equations have been that serum cholesterol level represents a surrogate endpoint and that a dietary factor that changes serum cholesterol will also change risk of CHD in a similar manner. However, this logic weakened as it became apparent that total serum cholesterol level represents several subcomponents, including the deleterious low-density lipoprotein (LDL) and very-low-density lipoprotein (VLDL) fractions, as well as the beneficial high-density lipoprotein (HDL) component. Thus, the effect of a specific dietary change on total serum cholesterol level might increase, decrease, or not influ-

ence risk of CHD, depending on which cholesterol components were changed. More recent metabolic feeding studies have measured a variety of lipid fractions and have consistently observed the effect demonstrated in Figure 17–3. As expected, substitution of carbohydrate for saturated fat reduces total cholesterol levels (and LDL cholesterol), but also reduces HDL-cholesterol (HDL-C) and increases triglyceride levels. Substitution of monounsaturated fat for saturated fat similarly reduces LDL cholesterol (LDL-C) but does not reduce HDL or increase triglycerides. Studies of specific cholesterol fractions have been summarized in new prediction equations by Mensink and Katan (1992) (Table 17–2). Although the prior observations by Keys and Hegsted for total cholesterol were confirmed, saturated fat when compared with carbohydrate was shown to raise serum HDL-C in proportion to the increase in LDL or total cholesterol. Thus, the ratio of total cholesterol to HDL-C, which appears to summarize best the relationship between serum lipid levels and CHD (see below), is not appreciably influenced by saturated fat intake. However, when monounsaturated fat replaces carbohydrate, HDL-C increases and LDL changes little. Thus, the lipid pattern on a high monounsaturated fat diet is favorable compared with a diet in which a similar amount of energy is provided by either saturated fat or carbohydrate. Mensink and Katan (1992) also noted that the effect of polyunsaturated fat on serum cholesterol levels appeared to be relatively weak in recent studies; the reason is unclear but could relate to the higher baseline polyunsaturated fat in contemporary diets (about 6% of energy) than in diets in the 1950s when polyunsaturated fat intake was about 3% of energy.

Blood Cholesterol Levels and Risk of CHD

Few relationships are as well established as that between blood total cholesterol levels and risk of CHD. The number of studies in which this has been observed are too nu-

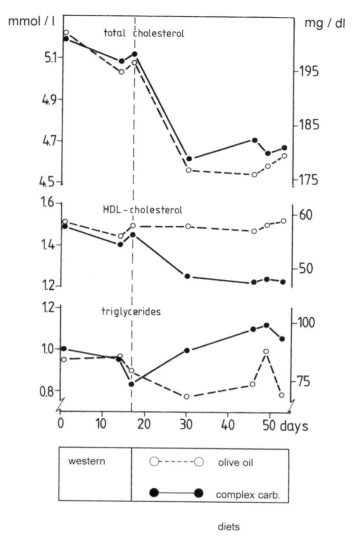

Figure 17–3. Mean serum total and HDL-C and serum triglyceride concentrations throughout the experiment. All 48 subjects first received a western-type diet high in saturated fat for 17 days. For the next 36 days half of the subjects received an olive-oil-rich diet (○) and the other half a diet low in fat and high in complex carbohydrates and fiber (●). From Mensink and Katan, 1987; reproduced with permission.)

merous to review or enumerate here. The findings from the largest of these studies, based on 356,222 men screened for participation in the Multiple Risk Factor Intervention Trial (MRFIT) (1982) study, are displayed in Table 17–3 (Stamler et al., 1986). As can be seen, the relationship is monotonic and without a threshold over a wide range of cholesterol values.

Because the relationship between serum cholesterol level and the incidence of CHD found in MRFIT and most other studies was based on a single cholesterol determination, an appreciable degree of measurement error will have occurred. The effect of this misclassification is to attenuate or reduce the relationship between true long-term average serum cholesterol level for an individual and risk of disease. The magnitude of this attenuation can be estimated from the intraclass correlation for repeated serum cholesterol measurements, which is

Table 17–2. Equations predicting effects of dietary fats on serum lipid fractions[a]

Total cholesterol = 1.51 (carb → sat) − 0.12 (carb → mono) − 0.60 (carb → poly)

LDL-C = 1.28 (carb → sat) − 0.24 (carb → mono) − 0.55 (carb → poly)

HDL-C = 0.47 (carb → sat) + 0.34 (carb → mono) + 0.28 (carb → poly)

Triglycerides = −2.22 (carb → sat) − 1.99 (carb → mono) − 2.47 (carb → poly)

[a] All equations predict change expected as a result of 1% daily dietary energy intake as carbohydrate replaced by a particular fatty acid. Changes in lipids are in mg/dl.

From Mensink and Katan, 1992.

equivalent to the regression coefficient for a single measurement (independent variable) predicting the true long-term average level (dependent variable). In the study of Shekelle and coworkers (1981), this coefficient (γ) for repeated measures at a 2-year interval was 0.65. As described in Chapter 12, γ can be used to approximate the true relative risk unattenuated by measurement error, specifically, true relative risk = $\exp(\beta/\gamma)$, where β is the observed logistic regression coefficient. From the study of Stamler and coworkers (1986), the observed relative risk for a 20 mg/dl (0.5 mmol/L) difference in serum cholesterol level was 1.17. Thus, the true relative risk for a long-term difference of 20 mg/dl in serum cholesterol level would be approximately $\exp(\ln 1.17/0.65) = 1.27$. One implication of the attenuation observed in typical studies is that the predicted effects of a dietary change on CHD rates will be somewhat underestimated unless correction is made for attenuation, because the assumed relationship between serum cholesterol level and CHD is erroneously weak.

The prediction of CHD risk using serum total cholesterol level is less direct, and thus less powerful, than by using the component lipid fractions, especially since they are related to risk in opposite directions. The relation of LDL-C, the major component of total cholesterol, to CHD risk has been re-

viewed in detail by Law and colleagues (1994), who have provided the intraclass correlation data needed to de-attenuated associations with this lipid fraction. Others have investigated the various lipid fractions to evaluate which combinations maximally predict risk of CHD (Castelli et al., 1983; Stampfer et al., 1991). As indicated in Figure 17–4, risk of CHD increases with higher total cholesterol levels, but even more strongly with low HDL levels. The ratio of total cholesterol divided by HDL-C provided the strongest prediction in risk. Further follow up of this cohort has suggested that nonfasting triglyceride levels provide additional independent prediction of CHD risk (Stampfer et al., 1996).

The consistent and clear dose–response relationship from many studies combined with a plausible mechanism leaves little doubt that the association between blood cholesterol level and LDL-C in particular and risk of CHD is causal. This conclusion was strengthened by the findings of randomized trials in which lowering LDL-C by drugs has reduced the risk of CHD (Lipid Research Clinics Program, 1984; Shepherd et al., 1995; Sacks et al., 1996). In addition to substantiating the causal association between blood LDL-C levels and CHD, these studies documented that the excess risk can be reversed, at least in part, within 5 years.

The ratio of serum total cholesterol level to HDL-C level predicts CHD risk better than does total serum cholesterol level, and substitution of carbohydrate for saturated fat does not influence this ratio; this raises serious questions about the validity of the hypothesis that replacing saturated fat with carbohydrate reduces CHD risk and the use of total cholesterol level as a surrogate endpoint to predict the effect of diet on CHD risk. Relative risks for 14% versus 8% of energy from saturated fat can be predicted by international correlations (as in Fig. 17–1) or by a two-step process using the effects of saturated fat on various blood lipid fractions in controlled metabolic studies and the relationship between blood lipid

Table 17–3. Relation between serum cholesterol and 6-year coronary heart disease mortality among 356,222 screenees in MRFIT[a]

Decile	Serum cholesterol, mg/dl (mmol/L)	Mean serum cholesterol, mg/dl (mmol/L)	CHD mortality		
			No. of deaths	Rate per 1,000	Relative risk
1	≤167 (≤4.32)	153.2 (3.962)	95	3.16	1.00
2	168–181 (4.34–4.68)	175.0 (4.526)	101	3.32	1.05
3	182–192 (4.71–4.97)	187.1 (4.838)	139	4.15	1.31
4	193–202 (4.99–5.22)	197.6 (5.110)	149	4.21	1.33
5	203–212 (5.25–5.48)	207.5 (5.366)	203	5.43	1.72
6	213–220 (5.51–5.69)	216.1 (5.588)	192	5.81	1.84
7	221–231 (5.72–5.97)	225.9 (5.842)	261	6.94	2.20
8	232–244 (6.00–6.31)	237.7 (6.147)	272	7.35	2.33
9	245–263 (6.34–6.80)	253.4 (6.553)	352	9.10	2.88
10	≥264 (≥6.83)	289.5 (7.486)	494	13.05	4.13

[a] CHD, coronary heart disease; MRFIT, Multiple Risk Factor Intervention Trial. Analysis is age standardized.
From Stamler et al., 1986.

fraction and CHD risk in epidemiologic studies (see Table 17–4). Depending on the assumptions, the effects range from strong to nonexistent if the effect of saturated fat operates by its influence on the total cholesterol to HDL ratio. (Note: The contrast of 14% versus 8% of energy from saturated fat intake represents the difference between the U.S. average and the Step II American Heart Association Diet and is thus a large increment.)

Some have argued that the reductions in HDL resulting from a high carbohydrate diet do not have the same adverse effect as similar reductions caused by other factors (Brinton et al., 1991). Although this argument is difficult to address directly, other factors that influence HDL levels, including alcohol, estrogens, obesity, smoking, exercise, and medications, affect CHD risk in the predicted direction (Manttari et al., 1990; Sacks and Willett, 1991). Some have

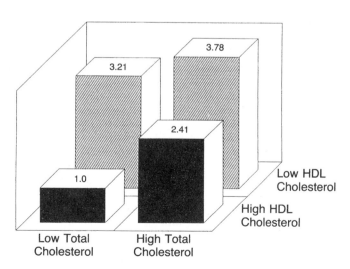

Figure 17–4. Relative risks of myocardial infarction for subjects with values above and below the median for total and HDL cholesterol levels. (From Stampler et al., 1991; reproduced with permission. Copyright 1991 Massachusetts Medical Society. All rights reserved.)

Table 17–4. Predicted relative risks of coronary heart disease from international comparisons and metabolic studies for 14% vs. 8% of energy from saturated fat

	Relative risk
International comparisons[a]	
Total coronary heart disease	1.6
Fatal coronary heart disease	2.2
Keys equation	
Coronary heart disease predicted from effect of saturated fat on total serum cholesterol[b]	1.2
Mensink and Katan equations	
Coronary heart disease predicted from effect of saturated fat on serum LDL-C	1.1
Coronary heart disease predicted by effect of saturated fat on serum total/HDL-C	1.0

[a] Data from Keys (1980).

[b] Calculated assuming a change in serum total cholestrol (mg/dl) $= 1.35 \ (2\Delta S - \Delta P) + 1.5\Delta Z$, where ΔS and ΔP are changes in % of energy contributed by saturated and polyunsaturated fat, respectively, and ΔZ is the change of square root of dietary cholesterol in mg/4 MJ (Keys et al., 1965), and assuming that reduction in total serum cholesterol of 0.6 mmol/L will cause a 24% decrease in risk of coronary heart disease (Lipid Research Clinics Program, 1984).

Adapted from Ascherio et al. (1996)

pointed to the international correlations as indicating that reductions in HDL-C by diet are not relevant to risk. However, the total cholesterol-to-HDL ratio is generally low in poor countries with low CHD rates and thus provides no evidence against the importance of HDL, because LDL levels tend to be very low (Castelli et al., 1983; Chen et al., 1990). It is troublesome that the crudest and clearly confounded epidemiologic evidence continues to be used as the ultimate basis for dietary recommendations. Ideally, uncertainties regarding the relevance of dietary effects on various lipid fractions should be resolved by evaluating the effects of diet on risk of myocardial infarction itself either in carefully conducted case–control and cohort studies or in randomized trials.

CASE–CONTROL AND COHORT STUDIES OF DIET AND CHD

The well-documented relationships between specific dietary lipids and blood cholesterol level and between blood cholesterol level and CHD strongly suggest that dietary lipids influence the risk of CHD. Nevertheless, this conclusion cannot be drawn with certainty from such data due to the complex and incompletely understood pathophysiology of CHD. For example, the manipulation of a dietary factor may decrease blood total cholesterol level and thus may appear to be beneficial, but have a counterbalancing deleterious effect on another physiologic parameter such as HDL-C or a nonlipid parameter such as coagulation factors. Even if a change in dietary lipids influences the incidence of CHD in the direction predicted by its effect on total blood cholesterol level, the quantitative relationship between this dietary change and risk of disease is uncertain because of the possibility of many other potential physiologic effects of this dietary manipulation. The classic diet–heart hypothesis would thus be strengthened by demonstrating that individuals who consume more saturated fat and cholesterol and less polyunsaturated fat actually have a higher risk of CHD.

The strongest evidence for this hypothesis would be derived from randomized, ideally double-blinded, trials of dietary manipulation in a human population initially free of CHD. In the customary development of a hypothesis, however, such a trial would be preceded by case–control or cohort studies that, if an association with diet were seen, would provide further justification for the expense of a long-term trial. For the classic diet–heart disease hypothesis, however, trials were pilot tested or initiated without evidence from case–control or cohort studies. This leap to trials may reflect the strength of the belief in the hypothesis and the failure to find an association between dietary lipids and serum cholesterol level in many cross-sectional studies. This lack of association, as noted earlier, has been attributed to homogeneity of diet among the general population and to an inability to measure the diets of free-living subjects with sufficient accuracy rather than to the relative unresponsiveness of serum cholesterol level to moderate changes in diet. Whatever the reasons, relatively few case–control or cohort studies of diet and CHD have been published, and most of these are quite recent.

Case–Control Studies of Diet and CHD

Only two case–control studies of diet and CHD seem to have been published until recently, both during the 1960s, and are noted primarily for historical interest. Meredith and colleagues (1960) interviewed 162 North Dakota men with incident or recurring CHD and compared their pre-hospitalization diets with those of 324 age-matched population controls. Using a 135-item food-frequency questionnaire, dietary intake was collected. Finegan and colleagues (1968) interviewed 100 Irish men hospitalized for CHD using a dietary history interview focused on a hypothetical "average week" and compared responses with those from 50 men admitted for minor surgical problems. In neither study were any appreciable associations between dietary lipids and CHD risk observed. However, these studies are far from definitively null as they were small and confidence limits would have been wide had they been calculated. No information was provided on the true variation in dietary intake within the study populations, and the possibility of distortions due to biased recall of diet are almost impossible to exclude in the context of a case–control study, especially among a recently hospitalized group.

More recently, additional aspects of diet have been evaluated in several case–control studies of myocardial infarction. In an Italian study among women (Gramenzi et al., 1990), increased risk of myocardial infarc-

tion was associated with higher consumption of meat, butter, and total fat and with lower intakes of fish, carrots, green vegetables, and fresh fruit. Ascherio and colleagues (1994a) reported higher risks of CHD among men and women with higher intake of *trans*-fatty acids. In a Greek case–control study, no clear associations were seen with saturated fat, but those who reported cooking with margarine had a relative risk of 1.87 (0.82 to 4.28) for first myocardial infarction, first positive coronary arteriogram, or both (Tzonou et al., 1993).

Prospective Cohort Studies of Diet and CHD

Because biases related to selection of control subjects and the recall of past diet are eliminated in prospective cohort studies, these investigations should provide more consistent findings on diet and CHD. Most of the available studies, however, were not primarily designed as investigations of diet and heart disease and thus have many limitations. These studies are summarized in Table 17–5 and are briefly discussed here.

Between 1956 and 1966, Morris and colleagues (1977) collected information on food intake using 1-week weighed dietary records from 337 men as part of an effort to develop a simple questionnaire that could be used in epidemiologic studies. Although the effort was abandoned, they nevertheless continued to follow the participants for up to 20 years and later analyzed the incidence of fatal or nonfatal myocardial infarction, based on 45 cases, in relation to their earlier diet. A strong inverse association was found between total energy intake and risk of CHD; the relative risk was 0.3 for those in the highest third compared with those in the lowest third (the interpretation of total energy intake is discussed in Chapter 11). This relationship was particularly strong during the first 5 years of follow up, for which the relative risk was 0.1. An inverse association was also seen with intake of dietary fiber; when

Table 17–5. Prospective cohort studies of dietary factors in relation to risk of coronary heart disease[a]

Study	Population	Dietary method	CHD cases	Energy	Sat fat	Poly fat	Diet chol	Lipid score[b]	Fiber	Fish	Alcohol	Comments
Morris et al. (1977)	337 U.K. bank clerks	7-day record, weighed	45	↓	0	—	0	—	↓	—	—	Trend of ↓ risk with high P/S[d] ratio
Shekelle et al. (1981, 1985)	1,900 U.S. men	Diet history interview	~200 CHD deaths	—	0	→	↑	↑	—	→	—	
Garcia-Palmieri et al. (1980)	8,218 Puerto Rican men	24-hour recall	163	↓	0	0	0	—	—	—	→	Inverse relation with starch intake
Gordon et al. (1981), Dawber et al. (1982)	895 Framingham men	24-hour recall	51	↓	0	0	0	—	—	—	→	No association with egg intake
McGee et al. (1984)	7,088 Honolulu men	24-hour recall	309	↓	↑[c]	0	↑	—	—	—	→	Dietary fat values were divided by calories
Kromhout et al. (1982, 1984, 1985)	857 Zutphen men (Dutch)	Diet history interview	30 CHD deaths	↓	0	0	0	—	↓	→	0	Inverse relation with fiber not significant when divided by calories
Kushi et al. (1985)	1,001 Irish and Boston men	Diet history interview	110 CHD deaths	0	↑[c]	0	0	↑	↓	—	—	Dietary fat values were divided by calories
Snowdon et al. (1984)	25,153 U.S. Seventh day Adventists	28-item frequency questionnaire	1599	—	—	—	—	—	—	—	—	Positive association with meat intake (RR=1.5)
Khaw and Barrett (1987)	California men and women	24-hour recall	65 CHD deaths	0	—	—	0	0	↓	—	0	
Burr et al. (1982)	10,943 Welsh vegetarians	Short food-frequency questionnaire	585	—	—	—	—	—	0	—	—	Vegetarians had lower CHD mortality
Lapidus et al. (1986)	1,462 Swedish women	24-hour recall	28 infarctions	→	—	—	—	—	—	—	—	
Norell et al. (1986)	10,966 Swedish men and women	?	800 CHD deaths	—	—	—	—	—	—	→	—	

Reference	Population	Dietary assessment	No. of CHD events								Comments
Fraser et al. (1992)	31,208 Seventh Day Adventists	65-item food frequency questionnaire	463 incident CHD deaths	—	—	—	—	↓	—	—	Nuts significantly related to lower risk of fatal and nonfatal CHD; inverse relationship for fiber is whole-wheat bread vs. white bread consumption
Fehily, et al. (1993)	2,512 Men from South Wales	50-item food frequency questionnaire	148	↓	0	—	0	—	—	→	Total fiber intake lower in those having an incident IHD event, but not independent of total calories
Goldbourt et al. (1993)	10,059 Israeli civil service Men	Short dietary questionnaire	1,098 CHD deaths	—	↑c	↓c	—	—	—	—	Independent dietary influence on CHD rates not strong
Dolecek (1992)	6,250 Men from usual care group from MRFIT	24 hour dietary recall	175 CHD deaths	—	—	↓c	—	↓c	—	—	Inverse association between polyunsaturated fat intake and CHD marginally significant
Posner et al. (1991)	420 younger and 343 older Framingham men	24-hour recall	99 / 114	→ / 0	↑ / 0	0 / 0	0 / 0	0 / 0	— / —	— / —	Positive association with total and monounsaturated fat (mainly from meat) in younger men only
Ascherio et al. (1996), Rimm et al. (1996a)	43,757 male health professionals	13-item food-frequency questionnaire	734 (229 CHD deaths)	0	0	0	0	→	0	—	Positive associations with saturated fat in age-adjusted analyses were attenuated by adjustment for other risk factors and fiber
Pietinen et al. (1997)	21,930 smoking men	276-item questionnaire	1,399 (635 CHD deaths)	0	0	0	0	→	0	—	Trans-fatty acid and ω-3 fatty acids from fish both associated with higher risk of CHD and CHD death.
Hu et al. (1997), Rimm et al. (1998)	80,082 female nurses	116-item questionnaire	939 (281 CHD deaths)	0	0	0	→	0	↑	→	Trans-fatty acid intake was strongly associated with risk of CHO

↓, inverse association; ↑, positive association; 0, no statistically significant association; —, no information.

[a] Sat, saturated; Poly, polyunsaturated; Chol, cholesterol; IHD, ischemic heart disease; MRFIT, Multiple Risk Factor Intervention Trial.

[b] Lipid score refers to Keys or Hegsted scores for predicting serum cholesterol.

[c] Expressed as percent of total calories, which may create an artifactual positive association.

[d] Polyunsaturated/saturated fat ratio.

fiber intake was further subdivided according to its food source, the inverse relationship was found to be entirely attributable to cereals rather than to fiber from fruits, vegetables, legumes, or nuts. No association was observed with percentage of calories from saturated fat or with cholesterol intake divided by calories; however, a nonsignificant inverse trend was noted with the ratio of polyunsaturated to saturated fatty acids, which was particularly strong during the first 5 years of follow up.

Shekelle and colleagues (1981) used the average of two detailed diet history interviews, each of which included information on the use of 195 foods consumed during the previous 28 days, as baseline information for the follow up of 1,900 men employed by the Western Electric Company. During the next 20 years approximately 200 men (the exact number is not given) died of CHD. Dietary intakes of saturated fat, polyunsaturated fat, and cholesterol were combined as scores for predicting serum cholesterol level as described by Keys and by Hegsted (see Chapter 9); a highly significant positive but small association was observed with these scores. Notably, this effect was seen even with serum cholesterol level included in a multivariate model, indicating an influence that was not mediated by serum cholesterol level. From the data provided, it can be estimated that the relative risk was 1.25 for a one standard deviation change in the Keys score. Although this finding provides general support for the specific hypothesis, practical decisions regarding diet must be based on information about the individual components of the predictor scores. In this study, specific nutrients were evaluated as nutrient densities. The overall positive association with the predictor score was primarily the result of an inverse relationship with polyunsaturated fat intake and a positive association with dietary cholesterol (Shekelle and Stamler, 1989); saturated fat intake was not significantly related with CHD risk. Because of the detailed dietary data collected in this investigation and the rela-

tively large population, this has been one of the most informative single studies of diet and CHD.

In 1965, a single 24-hour recall was incorporated in three populations (Framingham, MA; Puerto Rico; and Honolulu, HI) being followed prospectively to identify determinants of CHD. Follow-up analyses have been presented for each center individually (Garcia-Palmieri et al., 1980; Dawber et al., 1982; McGee et al., 1984) and also analyzed jointly by Gordon and coworkers (1981). An inverse relationship between total energy intake and incidence of CHD was found in all three studies. An inverse association with starch intake was also found in the Puerto Rican study, and positive associations were seen in the Hawaiian data with saturated fat and cholesterol intakes when presented as nutrient densities. These associations, however, are likely to have been in part the result of confounding because total energy intake was not included in the models (see example in Chapter 11). In a further analysis of the Framingham data, Dawber and colleagues (1982) found no association between egg consumption and incidence of CHD despite a 10-fold difference in average consumption between the first and third tertiles.

In 1960, detailed information on usual diet during the previous 6 to 12 months was collected by interview of both participants and their spouses for 857 men free of CHD living in Zutphen, the Netherlands, one of the centers of the Seven-Countries study organized by Keys (Kromhout et al., 1985). During the next 10 years, 30 participants died of CHD. For men in the highest quintile of total energy intake the relative risk of CHD was only about 0.2 compared with the those in the lowest quintile. Within the same study population, an inverse relationship was also seen with fiber intake (Kromhout and de Lezenne Coulander, 1984), although this did not remain significant when expressed as a ratio with calories. In addition, men consuming greater quantities of fish experienced a lower rate of death due to CHD (Kromhout et al., 1985), and those with higher intakes of isoflavonoids had reduced risk of CHD (Hertog et al., 1995).

Kushi and colleagues (1985) traced the mortality experience of 1,001 men living in Ireland and Boston who had completed a dietary history interview approximately 20 years earlier. During this period 110 men died of CHD. An inverse association between total energy intake and risk of CHD was observed; however, this did not attain statistical significance. Significant positive associations were seen with the predictor scores of Keys or Hegsted, which appeared to be largely attributable to a positive association with saturated fat intake. A marginally significant inverse association between fiber intake and risk of CHD death was also seen when expressed as a nutrient density.

In small studies by Lapidus and coworkers (1986), Khaw and Barrett-Connor (1987), and Fehily and colleagues (1993), dietary lipids were not associated with CHD risk (see Table 17–5). Goldbourt et al. (1993) collected dietary data from 10,059 Israeli civil servants in 1963 using a short food-frequency questionnaire, and 1,098 CHD deaths were ascertained during follow up. When expressed as nutrient densities, saturated fat was positively and polyunsaturated fat was inversely associated with risk of CHD; however, total energy was not accounted for in the analysis. Using dietary data collected by multiple 24-hour recalls from men in the control group of the MRFIT study, Dolecek (1992) found a marginally significant lower risk of fatal CHD among those with higher intake of total polyunsaturated fat intake and a stronger inverse association with intake of omega-3 fatty acids.

Among 44,895 men in the Health Professionals Follow-up Study who were followed for 6 years, a positive association between intake of saturated fat and CHD was seen, similar in magnitude to that predicted by the international correlations, when adjusted only for age and total energy intake

(Ascherio et al., 1996). However, this association weakened appreciably when adjusted for cigarette smoking and standard risk factors and vanished entirely when also adjusted for dietary fiber, which was inversely related to risk (Rimm et al., 1996a). The 95% confidence interval for saturated fat excluded the magnitude of association predicted by the international correlations (see Table 17–4), even after correction for measurement error. Some suggestion of a positive association remained for fatal CHD alone, although this was not significant. There was little evidence for any association between linoleic acid intake and risk of CHD.

Farchi and colleagues (1994) followed a cohort of 1,536 rural Italian men who completed a diet history questionnaire in 1965 for 20 years. Total energy intake and the percentage of energy from carbohydrate were associated with decreased CHD mortality, but saturated fat was unrelated to risk. An empirically derived dietary score was strongly associated with CHD rate. As the authors noted, however, predictive scores derived from the same data will tend to overestimate the prediction in that data. This is particularly problematic in dietary studies because a number of associations will arise even by chance if a large number of variables are examined. If these chance associations are then combined into a score, the prediction can be deceptively strong (see Chapter 13).

An alternate way of creating a total dietary score was used by Trichopoulou and colleagues (1995) to examine total dietary patterns in relation to total mortality in a small cohort of elderly Greeks. One point was given each of the eight characteristics of the diet determined a priori to be consistent with the traditional Mediterranean diet; this score was found to be inversely related to risk of death.

The most detailed prospective analysis of diet and CHD has been that conducted by Hu and colleagues (1997) using 14-year follow-up data from the Nurses' Health Study. The study was particularly powerful because over 80,000 women were included who developed over 900 cases of first myocardial infarction or fatal CHD and because four cycles of dietary data were collected over the follow-up period. A multivariate nutrient density analysis was used that allowed each type of fat to be compared not only with carbohydrate, but also with other types of fat. In comparison with carbohydrate providing the same percentage of energy, polyunsaturated fat was strongly inversely related to risk of CHD, as was monounsaturated fat, although less strongly. Saturated fat was weakly and nonsignificantly associated with higher risk, and *trans* fat was strongly positively associated with CHD.

In addition to the studies described previously in which an assessment of diet was obtained that allowed the calculation of nutrients, several other studies have been reported in which only a limited number of foods were examined. Snowdon and colleagues (1984) examined the association between meat intake, assessed using a short food-frequency questionnaire, and 1,599 subsequent deaths due to CHD among a population of 25,153 California Seventh-day Adventists. The risk of CHD death was 1.5 times greater for nonvegetarians than vegetarians, and within the nonvegetarian group a dose–response relationship was seen with frequency of meat intake among men but not among women. Also in a population of Seventh-day Adventists, Fraser and colleagues (1992) found a reduced risk of coronary heart disease among those who consumed higher amounts of nuts. Burr and Sweetnam (1982) followed a cohort of nearly 11,000 men and women who were identified by their interest in "health foods" and who completed a short but incompletely described dietary questionnaire. Although vegetarians had a lower CHD mortality rate than nonvegetarians, neither fish intake nor use of whole-meal bread was related to this outcome. Norell and colleagues (1986) collected information regarding fish intake by an unspecified method among 10,966 Swedish men and women. During 14 years of follow up an inverse relationship with myocardial infarction was found; for those consuming "high" amounts of fish, the relative risk was 0.70 compared with those consuming "low" amounts.

Summary of Prospective Cohort Studies of Diet and CHD

Viewed together, the most consistent finding in the prospective studies of diet and CHD is that men or women with higher total energy intake experience lower rates of disease. The interpretation of this finding, as discussed in Chapter 11, is not that an overall increase in food consumption will lead to a reduced risk of CHD, particularly as obesity is positively related to rates of this disease. As pointed out by Morris and colleagues (1977), this inverse relationship almost surely represents a protective effect of physical activity; increased physical activity leads to a higher energy intake and reduced risk of CHD. Thus, it is ironic that the existing studies of diet and CHD provide better support for the influence of exercise than they do for any primary effect of diet. Although the reported studies do provide some general support for the classic diet–heart hypothesis, data for specific dietary lipids are weak and inconsistent; a positive association with saturated fat intake was seen in only a few studies and not in the detailed study of Shekelle and colleagues (1981). Also, a positive association with cholesterol intake was found in only two studies, and an inverse relationship with polyunsaturated fat intake in only four.

In addition to these inconsistencies, the interpretation of the published findings is made difficult by the strong inverse association of total energy intake with risk of CHD observed in most of the studies. As pointed out in Chapter 11, this relationship causes specific nutrients to be inversely associated with risk of disease even if the composition of the diet has no effect. Several authors have recognized this problem and attempted to address it by presenting their findings as nutrient densities, that is, nutrient intake divided by total energy. Dividing by a confounding variable, such as caloric intake, however, does not control confounding; instead, this tends to make variables positively associated with risk of CHD (see Table 11–4). Until recently, none of the original publications used a theoretically more appropriate analysis, such as adjustment for total energy using residuals or by adding total energy to a model including the nutrient density, although Shekelle and colleagues (1987) noted that the results of their study (Shekelle et al., 1981) were essentially unaltered when using regression analysis.

Although existing studies do not provide consistent findings for any specific dietary lipid, they should not be interpreted as providing strong negative evidence. Many of these studies had major limitations, largely stemming from the fact that most were opportunistic analyses of data not originally intended to be used for that purpose. The most obvious limitation of the published studies is their small size; many of these had fewer than 100 endpoints. A second limitation of many studies relates to the method of dietary assessment. In several studies, a single 24-hour recall was used to represent exposure for a period of up to 12 years. Although this does provide some information on diet, as indicated by the consistent finding of an inverse relationship with total energy intake, the degree of misclassification can be substantial and varies among nutrients (see Chapter 3). A third limitation of many studies is the prolonged follow-up period. Although a long follow-up period is frequently viewed as an advantage, this would not be true if dietary exposure tended to change over time and recent exposure is relevant to risk of disease; this shorter time frame was suggested by an effect of blood cholesterol reduction within several years in trials using pharmacologic lipid lowering (Lipid Research Clinics Program, 1984; Shepherd et al., 1995; Sacks et al., 1996). With prolonged follow up, misclassification of dietary ex-

posures increases over time. Furthermore, this problem is exacerbated by the tendency for most of the disease in a cohort to occur toward the later part of the follow-up period as the effects of selecting a healthy population at entry will have waned and the participants will have aged. The most desirable solution is to assess diet repeatedly during the follow up period; alternate analyses can then be conducted with variable lag periods between measurement of dietary intake and occurrence of CHD and between degrees of change in diet and CHD. Unfortunately, of the studies reported to date, only Hu et al. (1997) has included reassessments of dietary intake. Another approach if one measurement is available is to subdivide the follow up period in the analysis of the data; however, this exacerbates the problem of small study size. Such an analytic approach was used in the study by Morris and coworkers (1977), who found that associations with diet generally tended to be stronger for disease occurring during the first 5 years than for disease occurring later.

A fifth limitation of most published studies is that they did not address potential confounding by other dietary factors. As discussed below, an inverse association with dietary fiber or other factors in plant foods has been seen in many studies, and it is likely that persons consuming higher amounts of saturated fat will tend to consume fewer of these foods. In one of the few examples where the intercorrelation of dietary factors was addressed, Ascherio et al. (1996) found that adjustment for dietary fiber reduced the association between saturated fat and CHD risk.

The possibility of detecting an association between dietary factors and risk of CHD in a cohort study depends strongly on the degree of variation in dietary intake among study participants; a perceived lack of heterogeneity of diets within the U.S. population has led some to believe that associations with saturated fat or cholesterol intake cannot be found. Many lines of evidence, however, indicate that dietary heterogeneity does exist within U.S. populations, including the findings of reasonable correlations between nutrient intake assessed by independent methods (see Chapter 6) and the associations, even if not consistent for some nutrients, between specific dietary factors and risk of CHD in the prospective studies cited earlier. The degree of variation, however, is modest for many nutrients, with the result that associations with disease rates are also likely to be modest. Potential magnitudes of association for saturated fat intake can be estimated from the data in Table 17–4, based on a comparison of 14% versus 8% of energy, which was similar to the medians for extreme quintiles observed in the study of Ascherio and colleagues (1996) after taking measurement error into account. If the international correlations represent the true relationship between saturated fat intake and CHD risk, the expected relative risk of 1.6 to 2.2 should be detectable with several hundred endpoints. However, if the effect of saturated fat is mediated only by its effect on total cholesterol level, the expected relative risk of 1.2 is small and is not detectable in an observational study or a randomized trial unless extremely large. These estimates assume that the effect of diet is mediated only by lipids and that diet during the preceding few years is considered the relevant exposure. Interestingly, the relative risk observed in the study by Shekelle and colleagues (1981) was 1.4 for the highest tertile of Keys score compared with the lowest, a finding somewhat larger than that predicted. Most of the other prospective studies that failed to find an association between dietary lipids and risk of CHD were too small to have excluded a relative risk of this magnitude. Clearly, studies to quantify the relationships of diet with CHD realistically will need to be large, and some issues may be difficult to resolve directly.

The strong associations seen in the 14-year analysis of the Nurses' Health Study are likely the result of addressing many of the shortcomings noted above. Controlling for *trans* fat was critical to appreciating the relationships with polyunsaturated and monounsaturated fat because all standard databases for poly and monounsaturates include the *trans* isomers and because they have common sources, such as margarines. Also, even with the large study size, the inverse association with polyunsaturated fat was much less clear when only the baseline questionnaire was used rather than a cumulative average based on all questionnaires. Because almost all of the previous studies have been much smaller, used only a single baseline questionnaire, and did not account for *trans* isomers, the lack of clear and consistent associations is not surprising. Available evidence from larger cohort studies suggests that the magnitude of association between saturated fat intake and risk of CHD predicted by the international correlation is likely to be seriously overstated, which is consistent with metabolic studies indicating little effect on the total cholesterol/HDL-C ratio when compared to carbohydrates. However, the larger cohort studies do suggest an important beneficial role for polyunsaturated fat.

STUDIES USING BIOCHEMICAL MARKERS OF FATTY ACIDS INTAKE AND RISK OF CHD

As an alternative to measuring dietary intake, some investigators have used biochemical analyses of plasma lipid fractions, platelet or red cell membranes, or subcutaneous fat as markers of fatty acid intake (see Chapter 9) to study relationships with risk of CHD. Although intakes of the major saturated and monounsaturated fatty acids are of great interest, these are poorly reflected in tissue levels as these fatty acids are also synthesized endogenously from carbohydrates. For this reason, levels of fatty acids that are not synthesized by humans generally provide better markers of diet.

In an ecologic study comparing regional mortality rates from CHD and mean levels of fatty acids in adipose of persons from these areas, Riemersma and colleagues

(1986) found the lowest levels of adipose linoleic acid in North Karelia, Finland, where CHD mortality was highest, and the highest levels in Italy, where CHD mortality was lowest. Lower levels of adipose linoleic acid were found in 75 men with myocardial infarction compared with 25 controls (Kirkeby et al., 1972b), but levels were similar in British men dying of CHD and those dying of other causes (Thomas and Scott, 1981). In a cross-sectional study of Scottish men, Wood and colleagues (1984) found significantly lower levels of linoleic acid in the 28 men with previously unidentified CHD than in the healthy men who provided dietary records. In a case–control study including 80 incident cases of myocardial infarction, the same group found that the risk of infarction decreased with higher levels of adipose linoleic acid (Wood et al., 1987); however, cigarette smokers had lower levels of linoleic acid than nonsmokers, and adjustment for smoking in a multivariate analysis eliminated the association between linoleic acid and myocardial infarction. In a group of healthy men who provided dietary records, the authors found that smokers consumed a substantially lower percentage of their fat as linoleic acid compared with nonsmokers, thus indicating that lower adipose levels in smokers were not simply a metabolic effect of smoking. In the same study, patients with angina pectoris had lower adipose linoleic acid levels than healthy controls; this inverse relationship was reduced, but remained statistically significant after adjusting for smoking. Inconsistent relationships between linoleic acid levels in platelet membranes, plasma or serum cholesteryl esters, or red cell membranes and risk of CHD have been noted in other small case–control studies (Lewis, 1958; Schrade et al., 1961; Renaud et al., 1970; Kirkeby et al., 1972a; Lea et al., 1982; Simpson et al., 1982).

In the context of a case–control study, the validity of plasma and platelet fatty acid measurements will always be open to some question as it is possible that they may be affected by acute events, such as those due to infarction, or be the result of dietary or other behaviors that change after the diagnosis of the disease. This problem is avoided by using blood specimens that were collected before the occurrence of CHD. Thus, Miettinen and coworkers (1982) used serum that had been collected and stored for a cohort of 1,222 men to measure fatty acid levels of 33 men who died of CHD and compared these levels with those from 64 men matched on the basis of hyperlipidemia and other risk factors and who remained free of CHD. A low content of linoleic and linolenic acids and high levels of palmitic and stearic acids (both saturated fats) in the serum phospholipids were found to be predictive of fatal CHD; however, these associations were not present for fatty acids measured in the cholesteryl ester or triglyceride fraction.

Biochemical analyses of blood or tissue fatty acids have the potential for providing information about diet that may be difficult to obtain from questionnaires as the type of fat used in prepared foods and the degree to which it has been modified by processing may be difficult for an individual to know. The studies noted previously, however, do not provide a clear or consistent picture of the relationship between fatty acid intake and risk of CHD. Although lower levels of linoleic acid have been seen in several tissues of patients with CHD in some studies, no independent association was found in others. As noted by Wood and colleagues (1987), many of these studies were small, the cases and sources of controls were often inadequately described, and the effects of potential confounders, such as cigarette smoking, were frequently not reported. Notably, no independent association of adipose linoleic acid level with myocardial infarction was noted in the study of Wood and coworkers (1987), which was one of the larger and better conducted investigations. Although improvements in the size and design of future studies should provide valuable and more consistent results, the interpretation of tissue fatty acid analyses is still subject to several limitations (see Chapter 9). First, these data provide an indication of the *proportion* of fatty acids in the specific tissues; thus the percentage of one fatty acid will be affected by changes in other fatty acids. For this reason, controlling for a measure of total fat intake, necessarily assessed by questionnaire, could enhance the interpretation of findings; however, this has never been done to date. In addition, tissue levels of fatty acids are affected by factors other than dietary intake, such as individual differences in absorption and metabolism as well as selective incorporation into tissues or blood lipid fractions. Even for fatty acids not produced endogenously, the relationship between intake and tissue level will vary by fatty acid and tissue. For example, although the levels of linoleic acid in the diet (as a percentage of total fatty acids) are reflected nearly proportionally in adipose tissue, levels in serum lipid fractions and red cell membranes are only slightly sensitive to intake (see Chapter 9).

TRIALS OF DIETARY FAT MODIFICATION FOR PREVENTION OF CHD

The most direct test of the classic diet–heart hypothesis is to conduct a randomized trial to determine whether changes in dietary lipids can reduce the risk of CHD. Two general strategies have been used: replacement of saturated fat by polyunsaturated fat (which would be expected to reduce risk on the basis of blood lipid changes) or replacement of saturated fat by carbohydrate (which might not alter risk due to adverse effects on HDL and triglycerides).

Early trials of primary prevention of CHD were conducted among institutionalized men, specifically residents of the Los Angeles Veterans Administration Hospital (Dayton et al., 1969) and two Finnish mental hospitals (Turpeinen et al., 1979). In both studies, patients passively received modified diets; cholesterol intake was reduced largely by a decrease in egg consumption, and polyunsaturated fats were increased to approximately 20% of calories by substitution for saturated fats in many foods. In the U.S. Veterans study, 846 men were randomized to either of the above diets and followed for up to 8 years. Seventy-one control men and 54 men on the special diets developed definite myocardial infarction or sudden death; this difference was not statistically significant. When cerebral infarction and other secondary endpoints were included, however, 47.7% of the control group and 31.3 % of the experimental group developed an event ($p = 0.02$). In the Finnish study, approximately 250 men in one hospital received the modified diet, and a similar number in the other served as a control; after 6 years the diets were reversed for the two institutions. CHD rates were reduced on the modified diet: 51% lower for CHD deaths alone ($p = 0.10$) and 67% lower for CHD deaths or major electrocardiogram change ($p = 0.001$). Although the hospitals were crossed over after 6 years, the interpretation of this study is limited by the fact that the unit of randomization was the institution rather than the individual, thus providing an effective randomized sample size of two. In a more recent U.S. study of similar design among institutionalized patients, little evidence was seen for a reduction in CHD among the group with modified fat intake (Frantz et al., 1989); however, the duration of follow up in this study (mean duration on diet was 1 year) may have been too limited to observe an association.

Although promising results were provided by the two studies of institutionalized patients, greater interest existed in demonstrating that the diets of free-living individuals could be modified to lower serum cholesterol level sufficiently to reduce CHD rates. Therefore, the National Diet Heart Study was initiated to serve as a pilot study for a large-scale national trial (National Diet Heart Study Research Group, 1968). Foods were modified and provided to participants in a double-blind manner. Over a 1-year period, serum cholesterol levels dropped about 11 % in the modified diet group compared with the control group. Despite this successful reduction of serum cholesterol level, a full-scale trial was never mounted because of the large number of subjects and accompanying costs required to detect a reduction in CHD.

To reduce the number of study subjects required, two large trials were mounted to evaluate the effect on CHD rates of dietary modification with simultaneous reduction of other risk factors. Such a study design can provide information that is applicable in practice, but may be difficult to interpret because the interventions are completely confounded, and reduced incidence could be due to only one, or any combination, of the interventions. In the MRFIT, over 12,000 U.S. men at high risk of CHD were randomly assigned to either an intensive program of dietary modification, smoking cessation, and blood pressure control (special intervention [SI] group) or to annual check-up (usual care group) (Multiple Risk Factor Intervention Trial Research Group, 1982). Interventions for both smoking (45% quit rate) and blood pressure control (approximately 11 mmHg reduction in diastolic blood pressure) were both highly successful. The dietary intervention was not only less successful (serum cholesterol level was reduced by 7.2% in the SI group), but a similar reduction also occurred in the control group. Thus, the difference between groups in serum cholesterol level during the intervention period was only about 2%, clearly an insufficient contrast to test the diet–heart hypothesis. No significant reduction in CHD mortality was found between the groups during the 10-year follow-up period, and the difficulty of distinguishing between the effects of simultaneous interventions was not encountered. In an extended follow-up of the MRFIT cohort, a marginally significant reduction in deaths due to acute myocardial infarction, but not all CHD deaths, was seen at 16 years (Multiple Risk Factor Intervention

Trial Research Group, 1996), but again, no inference regarding diet is possible for reasons noted (Multiple Risk Factor Intervention Trial Research Group, 1996).

More convincing support for the diet–heart hypothesis was obtained from the Oslo Heart Study (Hjermann et al., 1981; 1986). In this trial, 1,232 normotensive men with high serum cholesterol levels, 80% of whom also smoked, were randomly assigned to either a program of dietary intervention and smoking cessation or to a control group. Men who were already following a lipid-lowering diet, based on responses to a simple eight-item questionnaire, were excluded before randomization. Dietary intervention involved primarily a reduction in saturated fat and cholesterol; polyunsaturated fat intake increased only slightly. These changes were accompanied by an increase in total carbohydrates and fiber intake. During the intervention period, serum cholesterol level fell by 17% compared with the control group after 1 year, and after 5 years it was 13% lower in the intervention group. The smoking intervention was less successful; only 25% of the smokers in the intervention group stopped compared with 17% in the control group. After 5 years, the incidence of nonfatal myocardial infarction and fatal CHD was 47% lower in the intervention group compared with controls ($p = 0.03$). The authors conducted a series of multivariate analyses to assess the relative effects of dietary intervention (assessed by change in serum cholesterol level) and smoking cessation, thus treating the data as an observational study rather than a randomized trial. As is apparent by the relatively ineffective impact on smoking cessation, they concluded that most of the reduction in CHD incidence in this trial could be attributable to reduction in serum cholesterol level. Although active intervention stopped in this population after 5 years, a similar reduction (approximately 45%) was observed after 102 months, and the difference in total mortality had become marginally significant (19 deaths in the intervention group compared with 31 in the control group).

The contrast between the unimpressive findings of the MRFIT and the clear results of the Oslo study, in both serum cholesterol reduction and effect on incidence of CHD, may be in part related to the selection of subjects. It has been pointed out by Caggiula and colleagues (1983) that the initial serum cholesterol levels of the Oslo participants (325 mg/dl) were substantially higher than those of the MRFIT participants (254 mg/dl) and that for MRFIT participants with levels over 300 mg/dl the decrease in the intervention group was 14%. Among the MRFIT men with high baseline serum cholesterol levels, however, the control group also decreased 11%. The overall differences in serum cholesterol levels between the two studies is notable, and the overall decline in serum cholesterol levels of the MRFIT control group clearly contributed to difficulty in creating a contrast between the groups. The reductions in serum cholesterol level for both the MRFIT intervention and control participants with high levels on the first screening test, however, are suggestive of regression toward the mean and are not directly comparable with the Oslo data, which used the mean of three baseline cholesterol determinations for their initial values. Perhaps more importantly, men who were already following a cholesterol-lowering diet were excluded from the Oslo trial, whereas this was not true for the MRFIT study. As shown in Table 17–6, control participants in the Oslo study at 4 years after randomization (who, if anything, should have altered their diets in a favorable direction) had appreciably higher intakes of total and saturated fat and cholesterol than did MRFIT participants at baseline. The intervention groups for the two studies, however, achieved very similar intakes of saturated and polyunsaturated fat and cholesterol during the trial.

Given the recruitment methods for the MRFIT, participants were likely to be volunteers with above-average health consciousness and "better" diets. Indeed, the nutrient data obtained at baseline in the MRFIT study indicated that participants consumed less saturated fat and dietary cholesterol and more polyunsaturated fat than had been anticipated, so the potential for lowering serum cholesterol level was reduced (Caggiula et al., 1983). Thus, the MRFIT study tended to enroll men with high serum cholesterol levels who were less likely to be responsive to diet, and the Oslo study tended to exclude men whose high serum cholesterol levels would be unresponsive to diet. The finding that dietary intervention appeared to be more effective in the Oslo study should thus not be surprising.

This point illustrates an often overlooked principle in designing dietary intervention trials; subjects are frequently selected on the basis of an intermediary factor (e.g., serum cholesterol level) or on the basis of high overall risk of a clinical outcome (such as CHD or cancer). It is generally better, however, to select a population susceptible to the intervention on the basis of the dietary factors that will be directly altered by the intervention, such as high saturated fat and cholesterol intake. Although the number of endpoints can be increased by selecting a high-risk population on the basis of other factors, such as genetic predisposition, the statistical power of a study can actually be reduced by including persons whose increased risk is not influenced by the intervention (Stampfer et al., 1988c). In the case of CHD, for which serum cholesterol level is an intermediary factor that is partly determined by diet, a maximally susceptible population can be identified on the basis of both diet and serum cholesterol level. For other diseases, such as many cancers for which an intermediary factor has not been identified, baseline intake would appropriately assume greater weight in the selection criteria for a dietary intervention study.

In addition to trials of dietary change among persons without CHD at entry, several studies have examined the influence of dietary change among persons with exist-

Table 17–6. Dietary intake among a sample of control and intervention subjects in the Oslo Diet and Antismoking Trial and among the special intervention participants in the MRFIT study at baseline and during the intervention period

| | Oslo study, 4-year data | | MRFIT, special intervention group | |
	Control (n = 23)	Intervention (n = 23)	Baseline (n = 12,847)	Intervention[a] (n = 5,308)
Total calories/day	2,331	2,248	2,488	—
Total fat (% cal)	44.1	27.9	38.3	—
Saturated fat (% cal)	18.3	8.2	14.0	10
Polyunsaturated fat (% cal)	7.1	8.3	6.4	8.7
Cholesterol (mg/day)	527	289	451	265

[a]Mean values for years 1–3.

From Hjermann et al., 1981, and Caggiula et al., 1981.

ing CHD (Morrison, 1960; Koranyi, 1963; Ball et al., 1965; Rose et al., 1965; Morris et al., 1968; Leren, 1970; Woodhill et al., 1978; Burr et al., 1989; Singh et al., 1992; Watts et al., 1992; de Lorgeril et al., 1994). These are described elsewhere (Willett and Lenart, 1996) and discussed by Sacks (1994), who noted that the trials emphasizing overall fat reduction had minimal effect on serum total cholesterol levels or CHD incidence. However, in trials focusing on the substitution of unsaturated for saturated fats, both serum cholesterol level and CHD incidence was reduced (Fig. 17–5). Law et al. (1994) have summarized data from the largest primary and secondary dietary prevention studies by follow-up interval. They estimated that, for a 10% reduction in serum cholesterol level (0.6 mmol/L), the risk of nonfatal myocardial infarction was reduced by 9% in the first 2 years of follow up, 14% from years 2 to 5, and by 37% with more than 5 years of follow up. However, the results for 5 or more years of experience include a total of only 30 events and are based almost entirely on the Los Angeles Veterans Study, which used a high fat diet with 20% of energy from polyunsaturated fat.

In two recent randomized trials among patients with CHD, the interventions were comprehensive dietary changes that resulted in only slight differences in total fat intake, but major decreases in CHD inci-

dence with minimal changes in blood lipid levels. Singh and colleagues (1992) advised 505 Indian men and women with a recent myocardial infarction to replace animal and hydrogenated fats with liquid vegetable oil and then randomized half to special advice on increasing fruits, vegetables, lentils, nuts, and fish. Both CHD mortality and total cardiac events were reduced by about 40% in the special intervention group. A large (70%) reduction was seen among French patients assigned to a "Mediterranean diet" compared with those receiving an American Heart Association diet (de Lorgeril et al., 1994). As the special diet included a high intake of monosaturated fat, high intake of omega-3 fatty acids, and relatively low intake of omega-6 fatty acids, as well as abundant consumption of fruits and vegetables, it is not possible to attribute the findings to a single dietary component.

Several other dietary intervention studies, not reviewed here, have used changes in coronary occlusion assessed by angiography as the endpoint. One such study has been used by Ornish (1990) to promote an extremely low fat diet, less than 10% of energy. However, the intervention included a complete modification of lifestyle, including exercise, weight and stress reduction, and increased intake of vegetables and fruits; thus, attributing any benefit to a single aspect of this package is impossible.

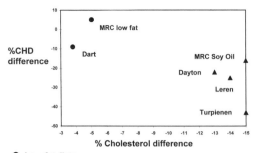

Figure 17–5. Controlled trials of diet therapy and coronary heart disease. Adapted (from Sacks, 1994; reproduced with permission.)

Also, the same diet that might be beneficial for patients with coronary artery disease may not necessarily be desirable as a lifelong diet for a population, particularly as rates of hemorrhagic stroke are seen in populations with diets extremely low in fat and animal protein (Jacobs et al., 1992; Willett, 1994).

Due to the practical difficulties in conducting primary prevention trials of diet and heart disease among free-living humans, studies in animals play an important role. Although the relevance of many animal models to human CHD can be questioned, studies among nonhuman primates are likely to be particularly germane and do contribute support to the diet–heart hypothesis. For example, Wissler and Vesselinovitch (1975) compared the development of atherosclerotic lesions in rhesus monkeys fed an average American diet with lesions among monkeys fed a "prudent diet" that was lower in calories, saturated fat, and cholesterol. Although monkeys fed the usual American diet developed four times as many coronary atherosclerotic lesions as the prudently fed animals, it is difficult to determine whether this was related to the composition of the diet as the prudent diets were nearly 40% lower in total energy availability, and the animals fed this diet must have been substantially leaner. More recently, Eggen and coworkers (1987) have demonstrated that diet-induced atherosclerotic lesions in rhesus monkeys can regress if cholesterol is removed from the diet.

In summary, intervention trials have contributed important support to the diet–heart hypotheses, even though the ideal randomized trial of primary prevention among a free-living population has not been and may never be conducted. Although most studies have had important limitations, in particular small sample sizes and limited durations of follow up, a reduction in CHD incidence has generally been observed in trials that replaced saturated fat with polyunsaturated fat. Evidence regarding the replacement of saturated fat by carbohydrate is more limited, but is generally unsupportive of benefit.

CRITIQUE OF THE CLASSIC DIET–HEART HYPOTHESIS

Despite decades of intensive scientific interest and scrutiny, the classic diet–heart hypothesis relating dietary saturated and polyunsaturated fat and cholesterol intake to risk of CHD remains unproven by the most rigorous scientific standards, specifically, replicated randomized experiments (Ahrens, 1985). Nevertheless, a large body of indirect evidence provides general support for the hypothesis. Serum LDL-C level is clearly causally related to risk of CHD, and a reduction of serum LDL-C level, which can be achieved by alterations in dietary lipids, all else being equal, reduces the incidence of CHD. Like most maturing hypotheses, however, the original formulation of the classic diet–heart hypothesis requires refinements. The next sections discuss the inadequacies of the classic diet–heart hypothesis, indicates further questions that merit investigation, and suggests additional dietary hypotheses that are not mutually exclusive.

Inadequacies of the Classic Diet–Heart Hypothesis

One obvious oversimplification of the diet–heart hypothesis is that total serum cholesterol level does not represent the complete effect of blood lipids on risk of CHD. Partly as a result of improved analytic methods, blood lipids have been fractionated into successively finer components. Total serum cholesterol has been subdivided by several methods, including ultracentrifugation, electrophoresis, and precipitation techniques. One of the most useful and well-established distinctions has been between HDL-C, LDL-C, and VLDL-C; as described earlier, HDL-C is strongly protective for CHD. HDL-C has been further fractionated into HDL-2 and HDL-3, and LDL subtypes have been further defined on the basis of particle size; the epidemiologic importance of these additional subdivisions is less well established, and thus far they have not been shown to predict CHD independently.

Another hypothesis, distinct from the LDL theory, suggests that transient postprandial elevations in blood lipids, including triglycerides and chylomicrons, increase atherogenesis and CHD incidence (Zilversmit, 1979). CHD patients have had higher peak postprandial concentrations of triglycerides or delays in chylomicron clearance than controls (Karpe et al., 1994; Nikkila et al., 1994), independent of other blood lipid fractions. In the prospective Physicians' Health Study, postprandial triglycerides significantly predicted CHD independently of other lipid risk factors, particularly HDL and LDL diameter (Stampfer et al., 1996). A greater percentage of energy from carbohydrate in the diet increases postprandial lipid responses in normal persons and those with noninsulin-dependent diabetes mellitus (Jeppesen et al., 1995), whether as mixed carbohydrate, sucrose, or fructose. The adverse metabolic effects of high carbohydrate intake on blood HDL-C and triglyceride levels are related to the degree of insulin resistance (Jeppesen et al., 1997), which is directly related to excess body fat and sedentary lifestyle. The dietary fat composition also affects the postprandial response with saturated fatty acids producing the largest rise and longest duration, monounsaturated and omega-6 polyunsaturated fatty acids less, and the highly polyunsaturated fish oil the least (Harris et al., 1988; Ginsberg et al., 1994).

Evidence that LDL-C is not actively taken up by tissue macrophage in the arterial wall (unless it is oxidatively modified) has added another dimension of complexity to the relation between blood lipid levels and CHD risk (Steinberg et al., 1989; Jialal and Devaraj, 1996; Shireman, 1996). This concept implies that the degree to which LDL particles are atherogenic will depend not only on their plasma level but also on their susceptibility to oxidative modification (in part determined by their polyunsaturated fatty acid content), factors that increase oxidative stress (such as cigarette smoking) (Morrow et al., 1995), and availability of antioxidants (discussed in more detail below). The concept of LDL oxidizability is closely entwined with the relationship between type of dietary fat and CHD because the source of dietary fat not only influences the level of LDL and susceptibility to oxidative modification (related to the degree of polyunsaturation) but also is a primary determinant of vitamin E intake, the most important lipid-soluble dietary antioxidant. For example, most sources of animal fat will tend to raise LDL levels and also contain little antioxidants. Polyunsaturated vegetable oils reduce LDL levels and generally contain higher amounts of vitamin E in rough proportion to the number of double bonds (the vitamin E is presumably present in seeds to protect them from oxidation and ensure their viability through additional seasons). Soybean oil, the primary vegetable fat in the United States, is a special case because its main form of vitamin E, gammatocopherol, is an effective antioxidant for protecting the seed or the extracted oil from oxidation, but is rapidly excreted by humans (Tran and Chan, 1992; Traber et al., 1993). Thus, consumption of soybean oil provides a high intake of double bonds that creates susceptibility to oxidation but a low level of effective antioxidant protection (Gey, 1994). Olive oil reduces LDL to an almost similar degree as high polyunsaturated vegetable oils, but is relatively resistant to oxidation because it is primarily monounsaturated fat and also contains an unusually high amount of vitamin E (and other non-nutrient antioxidants) in relation to its polyunsaturated fat content (Kushi et al., 1995). Berry et al. (1995) fed various diets to subjects to study directly their influence on the susceptibility of LDL-C to oxidation. Oxidizability was lowest when the dietary fat was olive oil and was higher with both saturated and polyunsaturated fat. When carbohydrate was substituted for fat, LDL oxidizability was also elevated, possibly in part by reduced antioxidant intake. These findings indicate the need to study the sources of dietary fats, not just the fatty acid content, of diets. They also suggest that the low rates of CHD disease in Mediterranean countries may be in part the result of using olive oil as the principal source of fat, but not simply due to beneficial effects on blood lipid levels.

A second oversimplification of the classic diet–heart hypothesis is that serum cholesterol does not represent the full effect of diet on blood lipids. Although dietary lipids clearly influence total serum cholesterol and LDL-C (the major component of total cholesterol), some aspects of diet, such as alcohol intake, have major effects on HDL-C but relatively small effects on total cholesterol. In addition, total energy balance, reflected in degree of adiposity, is more strongly related to HDL-C (inversely) and VLDL-C (positively) than to total serum cholesterol (Rhoads et al., 1976).

Accumulating evidence also indicates that the blood cholesterol responses of individuals differ substantially in response to changes in dietary lipids (Jacobs et al., 1983; Katan et al., 1986). For the same increase in dietary cholesterol or saturated fat, the cholesterol levels of most persons will increase, but some will remain essentially unchanged, and a few will increase dramatically. These differences in response are reproducible within individuals, indicating that this variation in response is not simply random statistical variability. Similarly, it has long been noted that the mean

cholesterol levels are frequently distinctly different for populations with markedly different rates of CHD, but that within each of these populations there exists a substantial degree of variability among persons. Factors that predict response to dietary changes are incompletely defined at present, but are likely to be largely genetic (Dreon and Krauss, 1992). It is thus likely that a fully developed diet–heart hypothesis must include a strong interaction with genetic predisposition to hypercholesterolemia and CHD.

A third limitation of the classic diet–heart hypothesis is that atherosclerosis and progressive coronary narrowing do not fully represent the pathophysiology of acute myocardial infarction. Indeed, the common clinical presentation of sudden, unheralded, catastrophic chest pain is not adequately accounted for by a slowly progressive process that develops over decades. With the advent of routine angiography performed at the time of infarction, it has become clear that acute thrombosis (to which atherosclerotic lesions may predispose) plays a central role in the development of myocardial infarction (DeWood et al., 1980; Rentrop et al., 1984). It is thus important to consider the possible effects of diet on factors that influence thrombosis (Ulbricht and Southgate, 1991). Higher fibrinogen levels and factor VII increase the risk of CHD (Meade et al., 1986), and dietary fiber intake has been associated with lower fibrinogen levels (Fehily et al., 1982). In a controlled metabolic study, a low fat, high fiber diet reduced levels of factor VII and increased fibrinolytic activity, but did not change fibrinogen levels (Marckmann et al., 1993). However, in two other controlled metabolic studies, reduction in total fat intake did not influence levels of fibrinogen, factor VII, or other factors thought to influence thrombosis (Marckmann et al., 1992; Wierik et al., 1996). Thus, foods containing fiber appear to influence propensity for thrombosis, but the details need further study. Platelet aggregability, which also alters the likelihood of thrombosis, clearly has a major influence on risk of CHD (Steering Committee of the Physicians' Health Study Research Group, 1988), and dietary factors may well act by this mechanism. For example, substituting unsaturated for saturated fats tends to reduce platelet aggregation in vitro (MacIntyre et al., 1984), although very high intake of omega-6 polyunsaturated fatty acids may increase platelet aggregation (Renaud et al., 1986). In addition, polyunsaturated fats may reduce the propensity for serious cardiac arrhythmias so that mild ischemia does not lead to a fatal cardiac event (Hetzel et al., 1989; Charnock et al., 1992). The possibility that the effects of diet on risk of CHD are not entirely mediated by total serum cholesterol was supported by the findings of Shekelle and coworkers (1981), who found an association between lipid intake and CHD mortality after controlling for serum cholesterol level in a multivariate analysis. Thus, additional diet–heart hypotheses must be considered whereby multiple aspects of the diet act through one or more pathways to influence the probability of thrombosis formation in the coronary arteries or the development of fatal arrhythmias.

Further Questions Regarding the Diet–Heart Hypothesis

Independent Effects of Dietary Saturated Fat, Cholesterol, and Polyunsaturated Fat

Even if it is accepted that diets high in saturated fat and cholesterol and low in polyunsaturated fat increase the risk of CHD, knowledge of the independent effects of these three components is of great practical importance as they can be manipulated separately in diets. For example, cholesterol intake is greatly influenced by changes in egg consumption without major changes in saturated or polyunsaturated fat intake. Substantial increases in polyunsaturated fat intake can be made by the substitution of vegetable oils for either other fats or carbohydrates, which may or may not change intake of saturated fat or cholesterol.

Available data do not provide a clear indication of the independent quantitative effects of these three lipid components. The optimal level of polyunsaturated fat intake is particularly unclear. Based simply on the relationship with total serum cholesterol, one would conclude that maximizing the intake would be desirable, and it has been suggested that current intake be increased to 10% of energy (compared with U.S. averages of about 3% in the 1950s and 6% at present, while simultaneously decreasing saturated fat, to attain a ratio of polyunsaturated to saturated fats of 1.0 (Anonymous, 1985). Using platelet aggregability rather than serum cholesterol level to evaluate the effect of diet, Renaud and colleagues (1986) have suggested that a dietary polyunsaturated-to-saturated fat ratio of 0.6 to 0.8 may be superior to a ratio of 1.0. Furthermore, some evidence suggests that higher intake of polyunsaturated fat may reduce sudden death by raising the threshold for ventricular arrhythmias (Charnock et al., 1992). Because the dose–response relationship between polyunsaturated fat intake and risk of CHD has not been determined directly, the optimal intake remains uncertain.

Fatty Acid Structure: Double-Bond Position and Chain Length

Saturated and polyunsaturated fats have frequently been treated as specific entities; however, the importance of their heterogeneity is becoming increasingly recognized. For example, the physiologic effects of omega-6 (primarily represented in the diet by linoleic acid) and omega-3 fatty acids (represented largely by linolenic acid and longer chain fatty acids derived from marine sources) are sometimes opposing (Leaf and Weber, 1988). The possibility that these types of polyunsaturated fats may compete with each other at enzymatic sites suggests that their interaction needs to be considered in epidemiologic studies. In addition, not all saturated fats have a similar effect on serum cholesterol. Butter and other dairy fats (high in 14:0, myristic acid) most strongly increase LDL, beef fat (containing palmitic acid, 16:0, and stearic acid, 18:00) raise LDL to a lesser degree, and cocoa butter (containing largely stearic acid) raises LDL only slightly (Denke and Grundy, 1991; Mensink and Katan, 1992). Medium chain saturated fats, such as those found in coconut fat, appear to be more atherogenic in animals than predicted solely on the basis of their relationship with serum cholesterol (Wissler and Vesselinovitch, 1975).

Trans-fatty acids are produced when liquid vegetable oils, which normally have all double bonds in the *cis* position, are heated in the presence of metal catalysts to form vegetable shortening and margarine. This process, called *partial hydrogenation,* was discovered around the turn of the twentieth century, and production increased steadily until about the 1960s as processed vegetable fats displaced animal fats in the U.S. diet, first because of costs and then because of purported health benefits. A similar increase has occurred worldwide; for example, in parts of India, a partially hydrogenated fat containing approximately 60% of fat as *trans* isomers is being widely used as a replacement for ghee (butter fat) (Achaya, 1987). Per capita consumption of *trans*-fatty acids has decreased slightly in the United States because of the increased use of softer margarine, which typically contain less than the 40% content of these isomers often found in the older stick margarines.

Concern that *trans*-fatty acids might have adverse effects on CHD risk (Senti, 1988) was greatly heightened by a careful metabolic study conducted by Mensink and Katan (1992). In this study, which used monounsaturated fat as a comparison, a diet with 10% of energy as *trans*-fatty acids raised LDL-C to a similar degree as did saturated fat. However, HDL-C was reduced by *trans* isomers but unaffected by saturated fat. Thus, the increase in the ratio of total cholesterol to HDL-C due to *trans* isomers was about twice that seen with sat-

urated fat. These findings have been reproduced in other metabolic studies (Nestel et al., 1992; Zock and Katan, 1992; Judd et al., 1994), including adverse effects on blood lipids when *trans*-fatty acids constituted 3% and 6% of energy (see Fig. 17–6 for a summary of metabolic studies). Also, *trans*-fatty acids have been found to increase blood levels of Lp(a), another potential risk factor for CHD, in several metabolic studies (Mensink et al., 1992; Nestel et al., 1992) and to adversely affect platelet activity (MacIntyre et al., 1984), which could increase thrombosis.

Although the uniquely adverse effects of *trans* isomers on blood lipids are alone sufficient to raise serious concern about consumption of these synthetic fats, positive associations between intake of these fats and risk of CHD have also been observed. In the Nurses' Health Study, women with the highest intake of *trans*-fatty acids from processed vegetable fats assessed in 1980 experienced the highest risk of myocardial infarction during the next 8 years (Willett et al., 1993). When those women whose intake of margarine had greatly increased or decreased over the previous 10 years were excluded, the risk was nearly 80% higher for those in the highest 20% of intake compared with those in the lowest 20%. Margarine, cookies, and white bread contributed most to intake and the excess risk of CHD. A further analysis in the Nurses' Health Study used food-frequency questionnaires collected four times during 14 years of follow up to update information on intake of *trans* fatty acids and other types of fat (Hu et al., 1997). The positive association with *trans* isomers was confirmed and inverse associations with consumption of polyunsaturated and monounsaturated fat were seen. Women with the highest intake of *trans* fat and lowest intake of polyunsaturated fat had a threefold higher risk of myocardial infarction than those with low consumption of *trans* fat and high intake of polyunsaturated fat. Positive associations with myocardial in-

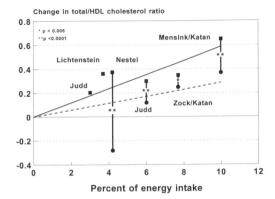

Figure 17–6. Change in the ratio of total cholesterol to HDL-C by percent of energy from *trans*-fatty acids (■) and saturated fat (●) compared with natural unsaturated fat (for *trans*-fat, $\beta = 0.059$, $p < 0.001$; for saturated fat, $\beta = 0.029$, $p = 0.10$; test for differences in slopes, $p = 0.03$). (From Willett and Ascherio, 1995; reproduced with permission.)

farction were also seen in a case–control study primarily among men (Ascherio et al., 1994a), and with the degree of atherosclerosis in a cross-sectional angiographic study (Siguel and Lerman, 1993). In one study of 22,000 Finnish smokers, intake of *trans*-fatty acids was significantly related to coronary deaths (relative risk, 1.39; 95% confidence interval, 1.04 to 1.78; p for trend 0.004) (Pietinen et al., 1997). In the Health Professionals Follow-up Study, higher intakes of *trans*-fatty acids were associated with both myocardial infarction and fatal CHD, although this was slightly attenuated by fiber intakes (Ascherio et al., 1996).

In a small case–control study of sudden cardiac death (66 cases), no association was seen with levels of *trans*-fatty acids in adipose tissue (Roberts et al., 1995). In a considerably larger multicenter case–control study of nonfatal myocardial infarction conducted in Europe, levels of *trans*-fatty acids varied greatly among countries (Aro et al., 1995). Levels of *trans*-fatty acids were by far the lowest in the two centers in Spain (which was the region with lowest CHD rates), so that nearly all participants in those centers were in the lowest quartile of the overall distribution of *trans*-fatty acids. When the outlying Spanish centers were excluded, the risk of CHD was approximately 40% greater among persons with the highest adipose *trans*-fatty acid levels, although the test for trend was not quite statistically significant. Thus, metabolic studies clearly indicate an adverse effect of *trans*-fatty acids fat on blood lipid fractions, and epidemiologic studies provide quite consistent support for an adverse effect on CHD risk.

Recent rapid changes in the food supply raise doubt as to whether additional studies of *trans*-fatty acids and CHD can be conducted at present in the United States and Europe. Although margarines were the major dietary source in the early 1980s, both decreases in the degree of hydrogenation (in part aimed at increasing the polyunsaturated fat content) and the trend to low fat margarines have reduced the contribution from this source substantially and has created great heterogeneity among margarines. However, in about 1990 the fast food industry converted from using beef fat to heavily hydrogenated vegetable fats for deep frying (Dupont et al., 1991), greatly increasing this as a source of *trans*-fatty acids. If the effect of *trans*-fatty acids is cumulative over a period of years, these changes seriously violate the basic assumption in nutritional epidemiology that the nutrient content of a food is reasonably constant among various samples of the same food and over time. The most extreme limitation in the epidemiologic investigation of *trans*-fatty acids has occurred in Europe: Because of the evidence regarding CHD, the food industry in a number of countries has committed itself to near zero levels, and even by the end of 1995 this had been achieved for margarines (Katan, 1995).

The sustained heating of fats, as used in

the deep frying processes of the fast food industry, can lead to the oxidation of polyunsaturated fatty acids. These oxidized fats can be absorbed and incorporated into plasma lipoproteins (Staprans et al., 1994). As described later, oxidized LDL particles are thought to be particularly atherogenic; thus this aspect of food preparation deserves further consideration.

Nutrients and Foods

Investigations and discussions of diet and CHD have largely focused on nutrients rather than on foods. Although this has scientific justification, practicality dictates that intake of foods should also be examined because nutrients are not usually consumed in pure chemical form (see Chapter 2). For example, high consumption of eggs might increase the risk of CHD due to their high cholesterol content. This cannot, however, be concluded with certainty as eggs contain a wide variety of other substances that could conceivably counterbalance an adverse effect of the cholesterol. Few studies have examined the relationship of egg intake with CHD incidence, and none has provided clear evidence of an association. Conversely, Shekelle and colleagues (1981) reported a positive association between cholesterol intake and risk of CHD, but did not report whether this was attributable to any particular food(s). Had this been attributable largely to meat rather than eggs, this would have suggested that other factors in meat, such as the protein or heme iron, were responsible for the association with dietary cholesterol. Furthermore, findings of an association between intake of foods or groups of foods and risk of CHD may provide guidance for selecting diets, even when the responsible nutrient or substance is not yet identified. As is discussed later, fiber intake has been inversely related to risk of CHD in several studies. Although interesting, further information on the fiber-containing foods that contributed to this protective effect would be extremely helpful, because not all forms or sources of

fiber have the same physiologic effects. This type of information was provided by Morris and colleagues (1977), who found that only fiber from grain sources contributed to a reduced risk of CHD. In the Health Professionals Follow-up Study (Rimm et al., 1996a), fiber from grain, vegetable, and fruit sources each contributed to reduced risk of CHD, suggesting that fiber per se may be beneficial. In addition, perhaps factors other than fiber in these foods, such as magnesium, are responsible for the reduced incidence of disease; the identification of foods that appear protective may provide the basis of alternate hypotheses that can be tested in other data. Thus, the investigation of foods in relation to occurrence of CHD is likely to further our basic understanding of this disease as well as provide practical guidance for eating.

Additional Diet–Heart Hypotheses

Although substantial indirect evidence supports the classic diet–heart hypothesis, the magnitude of any association is likely to be modest for ranges of diet found within western culture or attainable by realistic dietary changes if the effects predicted by metabolic studies are correct. Indeed, it is quite possible that intakes of saturated and polyunsaturated fats and cholesterol are considerably less important than other dietary factors in determining risk of CHD within the United States or similar populations. In addition to acting through total serum cholesterol, effects of other dietary factors could be mediated by other lipid fractions, platelet aggregability, fibrinogen levels, blood pressure, glucose levels, insulin resistance, endothelial damage, obesity, and other mechanisms that have yet to be discovered. In this section some additional hypotheses relating dietary factors to CHD are briefly discussed. The objective is not to list exhaustively all possible hypotheses or to explore them in depth, but rather to provide a sense of the scope of other factors that deserve consideration.

Obesity

Energy balance, as reflected by degree of adiposity, represents an important influence of diet on risk of CHD that is beyond the scope of this chapter but that may well be much more important than the composition of the diet (Manson et al., 1987; Grundy, 1992; Willett et al., 1995). The effect of obesity is mediated through numerous mechanisms, including hypertension, hyperglycemia, reduced HDL-C, increased LDL-C, and only to a slight extent through total serum cholesterol (Rhoads et al., 1976; Rosner et al., 1992).

Alcoholic Beverages

Among the various dietary factors that have been examined in epidemiologic studies of CHD, the most consistent association has been an inverse relationship with moderate alcohol intake. This relationship has been reviewed elsewhere (Moore and Pearson, 1986; Stampfer et al., 1988b; Rimm, 1996; Rimm et al., 1996b); in the summary by Moore and Pearson (1986), a protective relationship was observed in 7 of 8 case–control and in 12 of 14 cohort studies. In general, consumption of one or two drinks of beer, wine, or liquor per day has corresponded to a reduction in risk of approximately 30% to 70%. Alcohol from each of these beverages is associated with a similar reduction in risk of CHD, implicating alcohol per se as the primary protective factor (Rimm et al., 1996b). Alcohol increases blood levels of HDL-C, which is likely to be the most important mechanism underlying its protective effect (Gaziano et al., 1993), although an increase in plasminogen activator, which increases fibrinolysis, may also contribute (Ridker et al., 1994). An inverse relationship with CHD existed even after controlling for level of HDL-C, supporting the contribution of additional causal pathways (Criqui et al., 1987). At higher consumption levels, the risk of death attributed to CHD has been found to be similar to or even higher than the risk among nondrinkers (Moore and Pearson, 1986), which may be due to direct myocardial toxicity or the tendency for alcohol to induce arrhythmias, resulting in the assignment of myocardial infarction as a cause of death.

Despite the large body of evidence indicating that moderate alcohol intake is associated with a reduced risk of CHD, some have been reluctant to accept this as a causal relationship. One argument has been that nondrinkers include a substantial number of former alcoholics who continue to be at excess risk of CHD, thus creating the perception of elevated risk among this group relative to moderate drinkers. This hypothesis, however, was not supported by the findings of Rosenberg and colleagues (1981), who found a reduction in risk among moderate drinkers relative to lifetime nondrinkers or by Rimm and colleagues (1991) who found an inverse relationship even after excluding nondrinkers.

A second argument against the hypothesis of reduced risk has been that alcohol intake primarily causes an elevation in levels of HDL-3 fraction, whereas it is HDL-2 rather than HDL-3 that is related to reduced risk of CHD. In general, the use of a hypothetical mechanism as evidence against a large body of empirical data provides a very weak argument. In this instance, the data indicating that alcohol exclusively affects HDL-3 are based on a very small study (Haskell et al., 1984) contradicted by other findings (Camargo et al., 1985; Valimaki et al., 1986; Gaziano et al., 1993). Furthermore, a protective relationship has been observed between HDL-3 and risk of CHD in several studies (Miller, 1987; Stampfer et al., 1988a). Even if HDL-3 was not a primary intervening variable, it would not mean that alcohol could not be reducing CHD by other mechanisms.

Fiber

A growing literature suggests that certain types of fiber in the diet can reduce hyperglycemia (Rivellese et al., 1980; Potter et al., 1981) and exert a beneficial effect on blood lipids (Anderson et al., 1984; Behall et al., 1984). The relationship between fiber intake and risk of CHD has been reported in at least seven epidemiologic studies, and an inverse relationship has been noted in all but one (Table 17–5). Morris and colleagues (1977) found that men in the highest third of dietary fiber consumption experienced about one-third the risk of CHD during the next 20 years. These authors recognized that this relationship was partly explained by the tendency for men with low total energy intake to have an elevated risk of CHD (as a result of reduced physical activity); however, even when expressed as a nutrient density (g/1,000 kcal), the inverse relationship with fiber intake remained statistically significant. The protective effect was entirely attributable to fiber from grains; fiber from fruits, vegetables, and other sources was not associated with CHD incidence. Kushi and coworkers (1985), in a follow-up study of Irish siblings, found that those in the highest third of fiber consumption had about only about half the risk of CHD death compared with those in the lowest third. This finding persisted after adjustment for other risk factors, including total serum cholesterol level and blood pressure. When adjusted for total energy intake, however, this relationship was no longer statistically significant (Kushi, 1987). A similar inverse relationship was seen in the follow-up study of Dutch men conducted by Kromhout and colleagues (1982). Khaw and Barrett-Connor (1987), in a study based on a 12-year follow-up after obtaining a single 24-hour recall, found an inverse relationship between dietary fiber intake and CHD mortality among both men and women. Overall, the relative risk for a 6-g increase in dietary fiber, corresponding to about 1 standard deviation, was 0.74 (95% confidence interval, 0.58 to 0.94).

Among Seventh-day Adventists, the use of whole wheat, as opposed to white bread, was associated with reduced risk of CHD (Fraser et al., 1992), but in a small study in Wales only a nonsignificant inverse association was seen (Fehily et al., 1993). In the most detailed study of this relationship, Rimm and colleagues (1996a) evaluated fiber intake among 43,757 men who completed a food-frequency questionnaire in 1986 and were followed for 6 years. Dietary fiber intake was inversely associated with risk of CHD (relative risk, 0.64; 95% confidence interval, 0.47 to 0.87) for the highest versus the lowest quintile, even after controlling for a variety of other nutrients primarily obtained from plant sources. Both soluble and insoluble fiber appeared to contribute to reduced risk, but the association was strongest with insoluble fiber. In the only randomized trial, conducted among patients with a recent infarction, no reduction in risk was seen among those assigned to higher intake of fiber (Burr et al., 1989).

Although many of these studies of dietary fiber have been quite small, the consistency of the findings is remarkable. Nevertheless, a cautious interpretation of the data would suggest that some aspect of plant products, not necessarily a specific type of fiber, may reduce the risk of CHD. This relationship certainly deserves further examination, with focus on types and sources of fiber as well as a full consideration of other factors in fruits and vegetables.

Fish and Omega-3 Fatty Acids

Low rates of CHD in Japan and Greenland have led to speculation that the high consumption of fish in these areas might be protective (Bang et al., 1980; Kagawa et al., 1982). This hypothesis was supported by the finding of Kromhout and coworkers (1985) that Dutch men consuming more than 30 g of fish per day had only about half the risk of fatal CHD compared with men who consumed none. Lower rates of CHD mortality among persons who consumed higher amounts of fish were also observed in prospective studies reported by

Shekelle and colleagues (1985), Norell and colleagues (1986), Dolecek (1992), Kromhout and colleagues (1995) and Daviglus and colleagues (1997), but not in large prospective studies of CHD incidence or mortality conducted among Norwegian men (Vollset et al., 1985), Japanese men living in Hawaii (Curb and Reed, 1985), men in the Health Professionals Follow-up Study (Ascherio et al., 1995), male physicians (Morris et al., 1995), or a cohort of Finnish men (Pietinen, et al., 1997). In the Physicians' Health Study, fish consumption was inversely related to sudden death but not overall incidence of coronary disease (Albert et al., 1998).

Measurements of long chain (20- and 22-carbon) omega-3 fatty acids in blood and tissue can provide markers of past fish intake, providing another method to examine the relationship between fish intake and risk of CHD. In two small case–control studies, each including fewer than 30 patients with CHD, no significant associations were reported between risk of CHD and long chain omega-3 fatty acid levels in adipose tissue or platelets (Wood et al., 1984) or in specific serum lipid fractions (Schrade et al., 1961). Wood and colleagues (1987) measured adipose tissue and platelet fatty acid levels in 80 men with acute myocardial infarction, 108 men with angina pectoris, and 391 men without CHD. In both adipose and platelets, the long chain omega-3 fatty acid levels were consistently lower for patients with CHD, and for several comparisons these differences were statistically significant. Using frozen sera from a prospective study, Miettinen and colleagues (1982) found that phospholipid omega-3 fatty acid levels tended to be lower among the 33 men who subsequently developed myocardial infarctions than among a series of 64 men who remained free of CHD. The reverse was true, however, for omega-3 fatty acid levels in the triglyceride fraction. However, in a much larger study among 14,916 male physicians, no relationship was seen between levels of long chain omega-3 fatty acids in plasma fractions and risk of CHD (Guallar et al., 1995). In a case–control study of sudden cardiac arrest, higher fish consumption (ascertained from spouses) and blood levels of long chain omega-3 fatty acids were associated with reduced risk (Siscovick et al., 1995). The interpretation of findings based on tissue measurements of long chain omega-3 fatty acids must be tempered by the findings that some endogenous conversion may occur from alpha-linolenic acid (the 18-carbon omega-3 fatty acid obtained primarily from vegetables and vegetable oils) and that omega-6 fatty acids, such as linoleic acid, may competitively inhibit this synthesis.

In the one intervention study of fish consumption and risk of CHD, persons with a previous myocardial infarction were randomized to advice to eat fish regularly or to no such advice (Burr et al., 1989). Although there was no difference in total reinfarction rate, those advised to eat fish experienced a 32% reduction in cardiac death.

The hypothesis that fish intake may reduce the occurrence of CHD receives support from evidence that omega-3 fatty acids, which are predominantly provided by fish and other marine animals, have a wide variety of presumably favorable physiologic effects. These effects include a potent reduction in VLDL, inhibition of thromboxane production, and increase in prostacyclin synthesis with a resulting reduction in thrombotic tendency, reduction in blood viscosity, increase in fibrinolytic activity, slight reduction in blood pressure, and possibly a reduced tendency for ventricular fibrillation (Leaf and Weber, 1988; Morris et al., 1993; Leaf, 1995). However, high intake of omega-3 fatty acids may slightly increase LDL-C (Kestin et al., 1990).

The likelihood that higher intake of fish or supplements of omega-3 fatty acids may substantially reduce the incidence of CHD appears somewhat diminished by recent prospective studies that have been much larger and more statistically powerful than earlier studies, yet have found no relationship. These recent studies have been based on both blood levels of long chain omega-3 fatty acids (Guallar et al., 1995) and on fish consumption (Ascherio et al., 1995; Morris et al., 1995). However, the inconsistency of findings among studies is troublesome and begs explanation. One proposed explanation has been that the dose–response relationship is highly nonlinear: Only a low level of long chain omega-3 fatty acid in the diet is necessary to achieve the full benefit. This appeared to be true in the earlier study from Holland (Kromhout et al., 1985), but such a relationship has not been seen in other studies. If a low threshold effect of omega-3 fatty acids exists, it is conceivable that background increases in the alpha-linolenic acid content of the diet now provide sufficient precursors for conversion to the long chain omega-3 fatty acids so that a dose–response relationship between intake of fish consumption or long chain omega-3 fatty acids and risk of CHD no longer exists. While difficult to document, it is likely that consumption of alpha-linolenic acid has increased substantially in the United States and Europe over the last 15 years due to reduced hydrogenation of soybean oil (which comprises 80% of the vegetable fat in the United States) and increased intake of canola oil. One reason for partial hydrogenation is specifically to destroy alpha-linolenic acid because, by having three double bonds, it is prone to oxidation and thus rancidity if left "on the shelf" for weeks. However, in the mid 1980s liquid soybean oil sold for home use was no longer partially hydrogenated, and, as noted earlier, the degree of the hydrogenation of margarines was reduced (Dupont et al., 1991). Another possibility is that the original hypothesis, that omega-3 fatty acids reduce risk of CHD by decreasing the propensity for thrombosis, was incorrect, but that other mechanisms are operative.

More recently, it has been suggested that omega-3 fatty acids may act primarily by increasing the threshold for ventricular fibrillation (Leaf, 1995); if so, there may be little relationship with nonfatal CHD, and the benefit may be only for fatal CHD and sudden death. Such a hypothesis is consistent with evidence that the apparent protective effects were seen most clearly in studies restricted to fatal CHD (Kromhout et al., 1985; Shekelle et al., 1985; Norell et al., 1986; Dolecek, 1992; Albert et al., 1998), and the protective effect was limited to fatal CHD in the trial Burr et al. (1989). Also, the dramatic reduction of CHD mortality in the secondary prevention trial of de Lorgeril et al. (1994), which included a greatly increased intake of alpha-linolenic acid, is compatible with this hypothesis. This area clearly deserves further investigation; in doing so it will be important to account for intakes of both long chain omega-3 fatty acids from fish and alpha-linolenic acid and to examine both fatal and nonfatal CHD events. This topic also illustrates the potential for changes in the food supply and processing, which may be almost invisible to nutritionists and epidemiologists, to greatly impact national disease rates both adversely and beneficially.

Animal Protein

In numerous laboratory experiments, animal protein (usually beef protein or casein) has induced hypercholesterolemia and accelerated atherogenesis (Munro et al., 1965; Vahouny et al., 1984). In a recent meta-analysis, the substitution of soy for animal protein reduced serum LDL-C in humans without reducing HDL levels (Anderson et al., 1995). Potter and colleagues (1980, 1981) have suggested that saponins contained in some soybean protein preparations, and which sequester bile acids in the colon, may be responsible for the hypocholesterolemic effects seen in some experiments that attributed this effect to the amino acid composition of the vegetable product. The relationship of type of protein with risk of CHD has received little attention in epidemiologic studies. In the 14-year follow-up of the Nurses' Health Study, total and animal protein were inversely related to risk of CHD when compared with the same percentage of energy from carbohydrate, which is consistent with metabolic studies demonstrating an improvement in the blood lipid pattern associated with insulin resistance (Hu et al., 1998).

Complex and Simple Carbohydrates

As described earlier in this chapter, high intakes of complex carbohydrate or sugar increase blood triglyceride levels and reduce HDL-C levels, and thus could increase the risk of CHD. In two early studies, total carbohydrate intake was inversely related to risk of CHD (Gordon et al., 1981; McGee et al., 1984), although in the Puerto Rican data it is not clear that this effect was independent of total caloric intake. Also, because carbohydrate is the major source of energy in almost all diets, any substantial change in intake will need to be accompanied by a compensatory change in the other sources of energy, mainly fat, if weight is to be stable (see chapter 11). Thus, the effect of changes in carbohydrate intake should depend on the type of fat for which it is exchanged. In a detailed analysis in the Nurses' Health Study comparing total carbohydrate with specific types of fat, Hu et al. (1997) observed an apparent beneficial effect of higher carbohydrate intake if exchanged for *trans* fat, a slight beneficial effect if exchanged for saturated fat, and adverse effects if exchanged for polyunsaturated or monounsaturated fat.

The type of carbohydrate may also be important for risk of CHD. Jenkins and coworkers (1981, 1988) have suggested that carbohydrate quality may be characterized by the glycemic index, which is the area under the curve for blood glucose levels after ingesting a standard weight of carbohydrate. The glycemic index depends largely on the rapidity of absorption of carbohydrate; for example, whole grain products (typically high in fiber) and legumes have a lower index than do white bread and potatoes. Foods with a low glycemic index, also referred to as *lente carbohydrates*, generate a reduced insulin demand and, possibly, a reduced growth hormone response compared with foods with a high glycemic index (Jenkins et al., 1995). Thus, foods with a low glycemic index may have less tendency than rapidly absorbed carbohydrates to reduce HDL-C levels and to elevate triglyceride levels, blood pressure, and catecholamine excretion (Rowe et al., 1981; Young and Landsberg,1981).

Yudkin (1963) has proposed that sucrose is a major determinant of CHD, largely based on international comparisons. Although this hypothesis has been questioned (McGandy et al., 1967), it has not been securely confirmed or refuted. Whether sucrose has a somewhat greater adverse effect on HDL-C levels than other forms of carbohydrate is not clear (Albrink and Ullrich, 1986). In monkeys, a fructose-rich diet appeared to be atherogenic (Kritchevsky et al., 1974).

The influence of carbohydrate type and quality on risk of CHD has received little attention in epidemiologic studies. Salmeron and colleagues have examined the dietary glycemic load (the sum for all foods of the glycemic index for each food multiplied by its total carbohydrate content, adjusted for total energy intake) in relation to incidence of noninsulin-dependent diabetes in both men (Salmeron et al., 1997) and women (Salmeron et al., 1995). In both populations, risk increased with higher glycemic load, especially in combination with low intake of cereal fiber. As the overrefining of carbohydrate-containing foods may increase risk of CHD by increasing the glycemic index of the diet, as well as by reducing the original content of fiber and micronutrients (including folic acid and vitamin E), this aspect of the diet deserves additional attention in etiologic studies of CHD.

Vitamins A, C, and E

An antioxidant hypothesis, analogous to that suggested for cancer, has been proposed for CHD in which multiple nutrients that function as antioxidants, such as vitamin E, beta-carotene, and vitamin C, or components of antioxidative enzymes, such as selenium or copper, act jointly to protect the arterial intima from degradation or "aging" (Harmon, 1982; Gey, 1986). Subsequently, Steinberg and colleagues (1989) have suggested a specific mechanism whereby vitamin E and other antioxidants can block the oxidative modification of LDL-C, which appears to be an important step in the uptake of cholesterol into the arterial wall (Parthasarathy et al., 1990). Epidemiologic studies of these relationships are difficult because oxidative modification is thought to occur primarily in the arterial wall and is thus beyond the reach of routinely available biologic samples. Thus, it will probably be necessary to investigate these relationships indirectly; for example, by measuring the susceptibility of LDL to oxidation (Parthasarathy et al., 1990), markers of oxidative stress (Morrow et al., 1995), and intake of levels of antioxidants.

Vitamin E has long attracted popular attention as a potential agent to reduce CHD symptoms. Gey and colleagues (1991, 1993) have reported ecologic data based on blood samples and national CHD rates in Europe suggesting that the combination of low plasma alpha-tocopherol and ascorbate levels are associated with high CHD rates. In short-term intervention studies, vitamin E has not clearly reduced symptoms due to angina pectoris (Rinzler et al., 1950; Anderson and Reid, 1974). In a poorly controlled trial, patients with intermittent claudication treated with vitamin E were said to improve (Haeger, 1973).

The relationship of antioxidant intake from food and supplements, a major source in the United States, has been examined in several large cohort studies (Rimm et al., 1993; Stampfer et al., 1993; Kushi et al., 1996; Losonczy et al., 1996). In three of these cohorts, use of vitamin E supplements was associated with substantially reduced risks of CHD; risk was reduced by approximately 40% among those who had used vitamin E supplements containing more than 100 IU daily for more than 2 years. Among male health professionals, carotenoid intake was associated with reduced risk only among those who smoked, and vitamin C intake was not associated with incidence of CHD (Rimm et al., 1993). In a large prospective study among women (Kushi et al., 1996), vitamin E intake from dietary sources also appeared to be inversely associated with lower risk of CHD; overall, vitamin E supplement use was not associated with CHD risk, but few women used levels that had been associated with lower risk in other studies, and data on duration of use were not collected. Use of vitamin E supplements containing at least 100 IU per day has been associated with a reduced progression of coronary artery atherosclerosis assessed by serial angiography (Hodis et al., 1995).

Levels of antioxidants in blood and other tissues have also been examined in relation to risk of CHD. In a study among patients being evaluated by angiography, the degree of coronary occlusion was inversely related to blood leukocyte ascorbate levels among both smokers and nonsmokers (Ramirez and Flowers, 1980). Levels of blood carotenoids have been inversely associated with future risk of risk of CHD in several prospective studies (Gey et al., 1993; Morris et al., 1994; Street et al., 1994). In a multicenter case–control study in Europe, levels of beta-carotene in adipose tissue were inversely associated with risk of CHD (Kardinaal et al., 1993); in this and the prospective study by Morris and colleagues (1994), the inverse association was limited to smokers. In contrast with findings for blood carotenoids levels, in prospective studies using serum levels (Salonen et al., 1985; Kok et al., 1987; Gey et al., 1993; Street et al., 1994) and in a case–control study using adipose measurements (Kardinaal et al., 1993), vitamin E (alpha-tocopherol) has not been associated with risk of CHD.

The discordance between the studies of vitamin E intake and biochemical markers seems puzzling, but several possible explanations exist. First, in the studies of intake, the clearest evidence for protection was for high doses of supplements used for at least several years, and supplement use may have been low in the populations studied with biochemical indicators. Also, the biochemical studies used a single measurement and thus could not identify persons who would have had high levels for an extended time, as can be done by asking questions about duration of supplement use. In addition, vitamin E levels are much less sensitive to intake compared with, say, carotenoids (see Chapter 9). Vitamin E levels are strongly correlated with serum cholesterol levels and thus seriously confounded by this important risk factor (see Chapter 9). Some studies have addressed this by dividing vitamin E levels by cholesterol level, but this, analogous to the use of nutrient density to control for total energy intake, creates a variable confounded by the inverse of cholesterol; regression analysis is required to adjust appropriately for serum cholesterol. Finally, all the studies using biomarkers were much smaller than the prospective studies of vitamin E intake, and a protective effect could have been missed due to lack of statistical power.

The effect of beta-carotene supplement use on risk of CHD has been evaluated in three large randomized trials (The Alpha-Tocopherol Beta-Carotene Cancer Prevention Study Group, 1994; Hennekens et al., 1996; Omenn et al., 1996); in one no relation with risk of CHD was seen, and in two others, which included either smoking Finnish men or men and women exposed to asbestos or smoking, a modest but statistically significant increase was found (The Alpha-Tocopherol Beta-Carotene Cancer Prevention Study Group, 1994; Omenn et al., 1996). Although the prior evidence that beta-carotene supplements

specifically might reduce the risk of CHD was not strong, the increase in risk seen in Finnish men was unexpected. Potential reasons for the related increase in risk of lung cancer in the same trial are discussed in Chapter 15; one possibility is that beta-carotene is itself inactive, but that a pharmacologic dose interferes with the bioavailability of other factors, including other carotenoids, that are protective. In the Finnish trial, men assigned to a vitamin E supplement experienced only a small and nonsignificant risk of CHD mortality; however, the dose (50 IU daily) was substantially less than that observed to be protective in the large prospective cohort studies (Rimm et al., 1993; Stampfer et al., 1993). In the same trial, a small but statistically significant reduction (9%) in risk of angina pectoris was seen in men randomized to vitamin E supplementation (Rapola et al., 1996). Although this effect was small, a larger effect would not be expected on the basis of epidemiologic studies. This study does provide important evidence of biologic activity of vitamin E in prevention of CHD. In a randomized trial among patients with known CHD, those assigned to 400 or 800 IU daily of vitamin E experienced a 47% reduction in risk of CHD compared with the placebo group (Stephens et al., 1996).

At present, neither vitamin C nor beta-carotene intakes above those generally recommended to avoid deficiency appear to play a role in prevention of CHD. However, the evidence that vitamin E intake well above the usually recommended levels reduces the risk of CHD is strong, based on the epidemiologic findings, laboratory studies indicating effectiveness in blocking the oxidation of LDL-C, and evidence of benefit in two randomized trials. Ongoing randomized trials will provide further evidence about the causal relationship of vitamin E intake to risk of CHD, and additional data from large epidemiologic studies can provide further details on the dose–response and temporal relationships.

Folic Acid, Vitamin B₆, and Blood
Homocysteine Levels

More than 40 years ago, Rinehart and
Greenberg (1951) demonstrated that low
vitamin B_6 intake produced arterial intimal
damage in monkeys. Olszewski and Mc-
Cully (1993), noting the clinical syndrome
of homocysteinuria, which is characterized
by the homozygous deficiency of cystathionine synthase and fulminant atherosclerosis by age 20, hypothesized that less
extreme levels of homocysteinemia might
also increase CHD risk (Olszewski and
McCully, 1993). These observations are
linked by the roles of vitamin B_6 as a co-
factor for cystathionine synthase, the enzyme that metabolizes homocysteine, and
of folate and vitamin B_{12}, which are cofac-
tors in another metabolic pathway that
converts homocysteine back to methionine
(Fig. 17–7). Inadequate levels of any of
these vitamins can increase blood homocysteine levels. Diet can also influence levels of homocysteine through higher intakes
of its precursor methionine, which is particularly abundant in meat and high-
protein dairy products.

A substantial body of evidence supports
the role of blood homocysteine level as an
independent risk factor for CHD (Malinow,
1996; Rosenberg, 1996). Positive associations with risk of peripheral and coronary
arterial disease have been seen in a number
of case–control studies (Kang et al., 1986;
Clarke et al., 1991). Also, positive associations were observed between plasma homocysteine level measured in blood samples
collected at baseline and subsequent risk of
CHD in the Physicians' Health Study and a
Norwegian cohort (Stampfer et al., 1992;
Arnesen et al., 1995).

In a recent analysis in the Framingham
Heart Study population, Selhub and colleagues (1995) assessed the cross-sectional
relationships between intake of folic acid
and vitamins B_6 and B_{12}, blood levels of
these nutrients, blood levels of homocysteine, and degree of carotid stenosis. Intakes and blood levels of both folic acid

and vitamin B_6 were inversely related to
level of homocysteine, but for vitamin B_{12}
only blood levels, not intake, were associated with lower homocysteine, presumably
because variation in absorption rather than
dietary intake is the main determinant of
vitamin B_{12} levels in older persons. Intakes
of folic acid and vitamin B_6 and blood levels of all three nutrients were inversely associated with lower risk of stenosis. Having
all pieces of the pathway from diet to stenosis is particularly valuable, because this
documents that diet, not just genetic factors (although genetics play a role), is a primary determinant of the outcome and
indicates which aspects of diet are metabolically limiting in the population being
studied. In a similar approach, Verhoef and
colleagues (1996) examined these factors in
a case–control study of acute myocardial
infarction. This analysis included blood
levels of additional amino acids related to
the pathway described in Figure 17–7 and
provided evidence that folic acid was the
primary limiting nutrient in this population. Rimm and colleagues (1998) found
that intakes of both folic acid and vitamin
B_6 were associated with reduced risk of
CHD in the Nurses' Health Study cohort;
both supplements and dietary sources of
these vitamins contributed to lower risk.

From the standpoint of minimizing
blood homocysteine levels, a large proportion of the U.S. population, indeed a substantial majority, appears to have suboptimal intake of folic acid and probably
vitamin B_6 (Selhub et al., 1993; Stampfer
and Willett, 1993). Furthermore, supplementation with these vitamins, even in the
amounts contained in standard multiple vitamins, appears to normalize levels of homocysteine in most persons (Malinow, 1990;
Naurath et al., 1995). Thus, ensuring
optimal intakes of folic acid and vitamin B_6
may be an important means of preventing
CHD; Boushey et al. (1995) have estimated
that up to 10% of CHD deaths might be
avoided by adequate folic acid intake. Defining optimal intakes is an important chal-

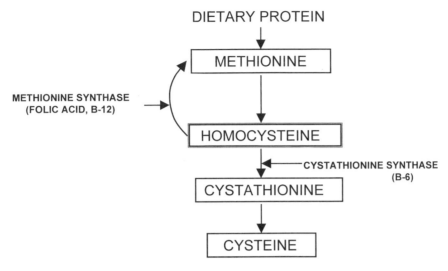

Figure 17–7. Pathway relating dietary factors to blood homocysteine levels. (From Willett and Lenart, 1996; reproduced with permission.)

lenge to nutritional epidemiologists. For folic acid, this will be complicated by the recent decision in the United States and some other countries to fortify flour with folic acid (see Chapter 18).

Selenium
Salonen and colleagues (1982) reported an inverse association between selenium levels in prospectively collected blood samples and subsequent risk of CHD in Finland, where selenium intake has historically been quite low due to relatively deficient levels in soil. This finding has been confirmed and extended to stroke in a larger study from the same country (Virtamo et al., 1985). In a small study from southern Finland, it was suggested that this inverse association may result from confounding by intake of fish, which, in Finland, is major source of both long chain omega-3 fatty acids and selenium (Miettinen et al., 1983). Although fish is a relatively less important source of selenium in the United States, this study underlines the need for simultaneous measurements of multiple nutritional factors in epidemiologic studies. In a Dutch case–control study, selenium levels in toenail

clippings, but not in serum, were inversely associated with risk of CHD (Kok et al., 1989). In one U.S. study, an inverse association between blood selenium levels and degree of atherosclerosis has been found among patients undergoing coronary artery angiography (Moore et al., 1984). In a large prospective U.S. study no relation was seen between plasma selenium levels and CHD risk (Salvini et al., 1995). At present, the relation between selenium levels in blood or tissue and risk of CHD remains unsolved and will require additional large prospective studies.

Iron
Iron might possibly increase risk of CHD by catalyzing the production of free radicals (Halliwell, 1989; Sullivan, 1989; Lauffer, 1991; McCord, 1991). Interest in this relationship was heightened by a report from a prospective Finnish study in which serum ferritin levels and iron intake were positively associated with subsequent incidence of CHD (Salonen et al., 1992). A relationship with iron status was not confirmed in a report using serum iron and iron-binding capacity in the NHANES fol-

low-up study; however, serum iron is not a good indicator of iron stores (Sempos et al., 1994). In a prospective study, nonheme iron, the primary form of this mineral in our diet, was not associated with risk of CHD (Ascherio et al., 1994b). However, intake of heme iron, primarily from red meat, was related to an increased risk of myocardial infarction. If tissue iron levels are important with regard to CHD, it is likely that heme iron would play a special role because the absorption of nonheme is greatly downregulated in subjects with adequate iron stores, whereas heme iron is not (Cook, 1990).

Calcium and Magnesium
A large and inconclusive literature has examined the relationship between water hardness, primarily although not uniquely characterized by high calcium and magnesium levels, and CHD (Marx and Neutra, unpublished data). However, this is a weak way of evaluating this issue because, in addition to the usual limitations of ecologic studies, most individuals obtain these minerals primarily through food rather than water. An inverse relationship between drinking water magnesium and risk of CHD was seen in a small case–control study that used direct measurements of water samples (Luoma et al., 1983) and in a larger study of similar design in Sweden (Rubenowitz et al., 1996). Magnesium intake from dietary sources has not been reported in other epidemiologic studies of CHD. Adequate magnesium intake is necessary to prevent CHD in animals (Seelig and Heggtveit, 1974; Seelig, 1980) and to maintain electrical stability in animals and humans (Karppanen, 1981). The strength of association between magnesium in drinking water and CHD incidence seen in some ecologic studies and the two case–control studies is difficult to reconcile with the very modest intake from this source. This suggests the likelihood of confounding by unmeasured variables; however, the relationship deserves further examination in studies that measure a full range of dietary

and other risk factors because a specific explanation has not been provided.

Although a role of calcium in reducing blood pressure has been suggested, in a meta-analysis of intervention studies, little effect was seen (Cutler and Brittain, 1990). The relationship of calcium intake to risk of CHD has not been evaluated in any detail in prospective cohort studies.

Other Minerals
Internationally, countries with higher chromium intake have lower rates of CHD (Anderson, 1981), and, in a small case–control study, hair levels of chromium were inversely associated with risk of CHD; the relative risk for extreme quartiles was 6.4 (Cote et al., 1979). Chromium may reduce CHD risk by improving glucose tolerance, reducing total serum cholesterol level, and increasing HDL-C (Levine et al., 1968; Schroeder et al., 1970; Riales and Albrink, 1981; Anderson et al., 1983), although the latter effect did not always attain statistical significance (Anderson et al., 1983). One problem in addressing relationships of chromium with disease is that blood levels are extremely low and easily contaminated. Keratinous tissues, however, concentrate this element, and supplements have been shown to raise levels in hair (Anderson et al., 1983).

Klevay (1975, 1983) has hypothesized that low intake of copper, particularly when coupled with high zinc intake, increases the risk of CHD. Although speculation has existed for some time that these minerals may influence CHD risk, there are few prospective data relating either their intake or tissue levels to CHD risk in humans. Based on prospectively collected sera, Kok and colleagues (1988) reported that higher levels of copper were associated with a 3.5-fold increased risk of fatal coronary heart disease and that zinc levels had no clear relationship with disease. It remains unclear, however, whether these associations represent differences in intake or in metabolism or even chance, as the study included only 62 cases.

SUMMARY

Abundant indirect evidence supports the hypothesis that specific dietary fatty acids play a role in both the cause and prevention of CHD. Nevertheless, the dose–response relationships between specific fatty acids and cholesterol intake and rates of CHD are not clearly defined. Modest reductions in CHD rates by further reductions in saturated fat and cholesterol intake are possible if saturated fat is replaced by unsaturated fat, but little or no benefit is likely if saturated fat is replaced by carbohydrate. Furthermore, aspects of diet other than fat and type of fat appear likely to influence risks of CHD substantially, and these may act by a variety of mechanisms, many unrelated to their effects on blood lipids. Strong evidence indicates that moderate alcohol intake reduces risk, and other data suggest that some aspects of plants, probably including dietary fiber and folic acid, are also associated with lower rates. Excess body fat is a powerful risk factor for CHD and may be quantitatively more important than any specific aspect of dietary composition. A number of other hypotheses based on animal studies and theoretical mechanisms remain to be investigated fully in human populations. Finally, data relating intake of specific foods to risk of CHD are extremely limited. Further epidemiologic data are needed to provide sound dietary guidance for persons wishing to reduce their risk of CHD.

REFERENCES

Achaya, K. T. (1987). Fat status of Indians—A review. *J Sci Indust Res 46*, 112–126.

Ahrens, E. H., Jr. (1985). The diet–heart question in 1985: Has it really been settled? *Lancet 1*, 1085–1087.

Albert, C. M., C. H. Hennekens, C. J. O'Donnell, U. A. Ajani, V. J. Carey, W. C. Willett, J. N. Ruskin, and J. E. Manson (1998). Fish consumption and risk of sudden cardiac death. *JAMA 279*, 23–28.

Albrink, M. J., and I. H. Ullrich (1986). Interaction of dietary sucrose and fiber on serum lipids in healthy young men fed high carbohydrate diets. *Am J Clin Nutr 43*, 419–428.

American Heart Association (1984). Recommendations for treatment of hyperlipidemia in adults: A joint statement of the Nutrition Committee and the Council on Atherosclerosis. *Circulation 69*, 1067A–1090A.

Anderson, J. W., B. M. Johnstone, and M. E. Cook-Newell (1995). Meta-analysis of the effects of soy protein intake on serum lipids. *N Engl J Med 333*, 276–282.

Anderson, J. W., L. Story, B. Sieling, W. J. Chen, M. S. Petro, and J. Story (1984). Hypocholesterolemic effects of oat-bran or bean intake for hypercholesterolemic men. *Am J Clin Nutr 40*, 1146–1155.

Anderson, R. A. (1981). Nutritional role of chromium. *Sci Total Environ 17*, 13–29.

Anderson, R. A., M. M. Polansky, N. A. Bryden, K. Y. Patterson, C. Veillon, and W. H. Glinsmann (1983). Effects of chromium supplementation on urinary Cr excretion of human subjects and correlation of Cr excretion with selected clinical parameters. *J Nutr 113*, 276–281.

Anderson, T. W. (1979). The male epidemic. In Havlik, R. J., and Feinleib, M., (eds.): *Proceedings of the Conference on the Decline in Coronary Heart Disease Mortality*. NIH Publication No. 79-1610. Washington, DC: U.S. Dept Health, Education, and Welfare, Public Heath Service, pp 42–47.

Anderson, T. W., and D. B. Reid (1974). A double-blind trial of vitamin E in angina pectoris. *Am J Clin Nutr 27*, 1174–1178.

Anitschkow, N. (1967). A history of experimentation on arterio atheroschlerosis in animals. In Blumenthal, H. T. (ed.): *Cowdry's Arterioschlerosis* (2nd ed. Springfield: Macmillan, pp. 21–44.

Anonymous (1985). Consensus Conference. Lowering blood cholesterol to prevent heart disease. *JAMA 253*, 2080–2086.

Anonymous (1993). Heart disease mortality: International comparisons. *Statist Bull Metropolitan Insurance Companies 74*, 19–26.

Arnesen, E., H. Refsum, and K. H. Bonaa, et al. (1995). Serum total homocysteine and coronary heart disease. *Int J Epidemiol 24*, 704–709.

Aro, A., A. F. Kardinaal, I. Salminen, J. D. Kark, R. A. Riemersma, M. Delgado-Rodriguez, J. Gomez-Aracena, J. K. Huttunen, L. Kohlmeier, B. C. Martin, J. M. Martin-Moreno, V. P. Mazaev, J. Ringstad, M. Thamm, P. van't Veer, and F. J. Kok (1995). Adipose tissue isomeric *trans* fatty acids and risk of myocardial infarction in nine countries: the EURAMIC study. *Lancet 345,* 273–278.

Ascherio, A., C. H. Hennekens, J. E. Buring, C. Master, M. J. Stampfer, and W. C. Willett (1994a). *Trans* fatty acids intake and risk of myocardial infarction. *Circulation 89,* 94–101.

Ascherio, A., E. B. Rimm, E. L. Giovannucci, D. Spiegelman, M. J. Stampfer, and W. C. Willett (1996). Dietary fat and risk of coronary heart disease in men: Cohort follow up study in the United States. *BMJ 313,* 84–90.

Ascherio, A., E. B. Rimm, M. J. Stampfer, E. Giovannucci, and W. C. Willett (1995). Dietary intake of marine n-3 fatty acids, fish intake and the risk of coronary disease among men. *N Engl J Med 332,* 977–982.

Ascherio, A., W. C. Willett, E. B. Rimm, E. L. Giovannucci, and M. J. Stampfer (1994b). Dietary iron intake and risk of coronary disease among men. *Circulation 89,* 969–974.

Ball, K. P., E. Hanington, P. M. McAllen, T. R. E. Pilkington, J. M. Richards, D. E. Sharland, G. S. C. Sowry, P. Wilkinson, J. A. C. Clarke, C. Murland, J. Wood, and Medical Research Council Committee (1965). Low-fat diet in myocardial infarction—A controlled trial. *Lancet 2,* 501–504.

Bang, H. O., J. Dyerberg, and H. M. Sinclair (1980). The composition of the Eskimo food in North Western Greenland. *Am J Clin Nutr 33,* 2657–2661.

Behall, K. M., K. H. Lee, and P. B. Moser (1984). Blood lipids and lipoproteins in adult men fed four refined fibers. *Am J Clin Nutr 39,* 209–214.

Berry, E. M., S. Eisenberg, Y. Friedlander, D. Harats, N. A. Kaufmann, Y. Norman and Y. Stein (1995). Effects of diets rich in monounsaturated fatty acids on plasma lipoproteins—the Jerusalem Nutrition Study: Monounsaturated vs saturated fatty acids. *Nutr Metab Cardiol Dis 5,* 55–62.

Boushey, C. J., S. A. A. Beresford, G. S. Omenn, and A. G. Motulsky (1995). A quantitative assessment of plasma homocysteine as a risk factor for vascular disease: Probable benefits of increasing folic acid intakes. *JAMA 274,* 1049–1057.

Brinton, E. A., S. Eisenberg, and J. L. Breslow (1991). Increased apo A-I and apo A-II fractional catabolic rate in patients with low high density lipoprotein-cholesterol levels with or without hypertriglyceridemia. *J Clin Invest 87,* 536–544.

Burr, M. L., A. M. Fehily, J. F. Gilbert, S. Rogers, R. M. Holliday, P. M. Sweetnam, P. C. Elwood, and N. M. Deadman (1989). Effects of changes in fat, fish, and fibre intakes on death and myocardial reinfarction: Diet and reinfarction trial (DART). *Lancet 2,* 757–761.

Burr, M. L., and P. M. Sweetnam (1982). Vegetarianism, dietary fiber, and mortality. *Am J Clin Nutr 36,* 873–877.

Caggiula, A. W., G. Christakis, M. Farrand, S. B. Hulley, R. Johnson, N. L. Lasser, J. Stamler, and G. Widdowson (1981). The Multiple Risk Factor Intervention Trial (MRFIT)—IV. Intervention on blood lipids. *Prev Med 10,* 443–475.

Caggiula, A. W., T. J. Orchard, and L. H. Kuller (1983). Epidemiologic studies of nutrition and heart disease. In Feldman, E. B. (ed.): *Nutrition and Heart Disease.* New York: Churchill Livingstone, pp 1–27.

Camargo, C. A., Jr., P. T. Williams, K. M. Vranizan, J. J. Albers, and P. D. Wood (1985). The effect of moderate alcohol intake on serum apolipoproteins A-I and A-II: A controlled study. *JAMA 253,* 2854–2857.

Castelli, W. P., R. D. Abbott, and P. M. McNamara (1983). Summary estimates of cholesterol used to predict coronary heart disease. *Circulation 67,* 730–734.

Charnock, J. S., P. L. McLennan, and M. Y. Abeywardena (1992). Dietary modulation of lipid metabolism and mechanical performance of the heart. *Mol Cell Biochem 116,* 19–25.

Chen, J., T. C. Campbell, L. Junyao, and R. Peto (1990). *Diet, Life-style and Mortality in China: A Study of the Characteristics of 65 Chinese Counties.* Oxford. Oxford University Press.

Clarke, R., L. Daly, K. Robinson, E. Naughten, S. Cahalane, B. Fowler, and I. Graham (1991). Hyperhomocysteinemia: An independent risk factor for vascular disease. *N Engl J Med 324,* 1149–1155.

Connor, W. E., M. T. Cerqueira, R. W. Connor, R. B. Wallace, M. R. Malinow, and H. R. Casdorph (1978). The plasma lipids, lipoproteins, and diet of the Tarahumara Indians of Mexico. *Am J Clin Nutr 31,* 1131–1142.

Cook, J. D. (1990). Adaptation in iron metabolism. *Am J Clin Nutr 51,* 301–308.

Cote, M., L. Munan, and M. Gagne-Billon, et al. (1979). Hair chromium concentration and arteriosclerotic heart disease. In Shapcott, D., and Hubert, J. (eds.): *Chromium in Nutrition and Metabolism.* New York: Elsevier/North Holland Biomedical Press, pp. 223–228.

Criqui, M. H., L. D. Cowan, H. A. Tyroler, S. Bangdiwala, G. Heiss, R. B. Wallace, and

R. Cohn (1987). Lipoproteins as mediators for the effects of alcohol consumption and cigarette smoking on cardiovascular mortality: Results from the Lipid Research Clinics Follow-Up Study. *Am J Epidemiol 126*, 629–637.

Curb, J. D., and D. M. Reed (1985). Fish consumption and mortality from coronary heart disease (letter). *N Engl J Med 313*, 820–824.

Cutler, J. A., and E. Brittain (1990). Calcium and blood pressure. An epidemiologic perspective. *Am J Hypertens 3*, 137S–146S.

Daviglus M. L., J. Stamler, A. J. Orencia, A. R. Dyer, K. Liu, P. Greenland, M. K. Walsh, D. Morris, and R. B. Shekelle (1997). Fish consumption and the 30-year risk of fatal myocardial infarction. *New Engl J Med., 336*(15), 1046–1053.

Dawber, T. R., R. J. Nickerson, F. N. Brand, and J. Pool (1982). Eggs, serum cholesterol, and coronary heart disease. *Am J Clin Nutr 36*, 617–625.

Dayton, S., M. L. Pearce, S. Hashimoto, W. J. Dixon, and U. Tomiyasu (1969). A controlled clinical trial of a diet high in unsaturated fat in preventing complications of atherosclerosis. *Circulation 40(suppl II)*, 1–63.

de Lorgeril, M., S. Renaud, N. Mamelle, P. Salen, J. L. Martin, I. Monjaud, J. Guidollet, P. Touboul, and J. Delaye (1994). Mediterranean alpha-linolenic acid–rich diet in secondary prevention of coronary heart disease. *Lancet 343*, 1454–1459.

Denke, M. A., and S. M. Grundy (1991). Effects of fats high in stearic acid on lipid and lipoprotein concentrations in men. *Am J Clin Nutr 54*, 1036–1040.

DeWood, M. A., J. Spores, R. Notske, L. T. Mouser, R. Burroughs, M. S. Golden, and H. T. Lang (1980). Prevalence of total coronary occlusion during the early hours of transmural myocardial infarction. *N Engl J Med 303*, 897–902.

Dolecek, T. A. (1992). Epidemiological evidence of relationships between dietary polyunsaturated fatty acids and mortality in the multiple risk factor intervention trial. *Proc Soc Exp Biol Med 200*, 177–182.

Dreon, D. M., and R. M. Krauss (1992). Gene–diet interactions in lipoprotein metabolism. In Lusis, A. J., Rotter, J. I., and Sparkes, R. S., (eds.): *Molecular Genetics of Coronary Artery Disease. Candidate Genes and Processes in Atherosclerosis.* Basel: Karger, pp. 325–349.

Dupont, J., P. J. White, and E. B. Feldman (1991). Saturated and hydrogenated fats in food in relation to health. *J Am Coll Nutr 10*, 577–592.

Eggen, D. A., J. P. Strong, W. P. Newman, G. T. Malcom, and C. Restrepo (1987). Regression of experimental atherosclerotic lesions in rhesus monkeys consuming a high saturated fat diet. *Arteriosclerosis 7*, 125–134.

Farchi, G., F. Fidanza, S. Mariotti, and A. Menotti (1994). Is diet an independent risk factor for mortality? 20 year mortality in the Italian rural cohorts of the Seven Countries Study. *Eur J Clin Nutr 48*, 19–29.

Fehily, A. M., J. E. Milbank, J. W. Yarnell, T. M. Hayes, A. J. Kubiki, and R. D. Eastham (1982). Dietary determinants of lipoproteins, total cholesterol, viscosity, fibrinogen, and blood pressure. *Am J Clin Nutr 36*, 890–896.

Fehily, A. M., J. W. G. Yarnell, P. M. Sweetnam, and P. C. Elwood (1993). Diet and incident ischaemic heart disease: The Caerphilly Study. *Br J Nutr 69*, 303–314.

Finegan, A., N. Hickey, B. Maurer, and R. Mulcahy (1968). Diet and coronary heart disease: Dietary analysis on 100 male patients. *Am J Clin Nutr 21*, 143–148.

Frantz, I. D. J., E. A. Dawson, P. L. Ashman, L. C. Gatewood, G. E. Bartsch, K. Kuba, and E. R. Brewer (1989). Test of effect of lipid lowering by diet on cardiovascular risk: The Minnesota Coronary Survey. *Arteriosclerosis 9*, 129–135.

Fraser, G. E., J. Sabate, W. L. Beeson, and T. M. Strahan (1992). A possible protective effect of nut consumption on risk of coronary heart disease. The Adventist Health Study. *Arch Intern Med 152*, 1416–1424.

Friend, B. (1967). Nutrients in the United States Food Supply: A review of trends, 1909–1913 to 1965. *Am J Clin Nutr 20*, 907–914.

Garcia-Palmieri, M. R., P. Sorlie, J. Tillotson, R. Costas Jr., E. Cordero, and M. Rodriguez (1980). Relationship of dietary intake to subsequent coronary heart disease incidence: The Puerto Rico Heart Health Program. *Am J Clin Nutr 33*, 1818–1827.

Gaziano, J. M., J. E. Buring, J. L. Breslow, S. Z. Goldhaber, B. Rosner, M. VanDenburgh, W. Willett, and C. H. Hennekens (1993). Moderate alcohol intake, increased levels of high-density lipoprotein and its subfractions and decreased risk of myocardial infarction. *N Engl J Med 329*, 1829–1834.

Gey, K. F. (1986). On the antioxidant hypothesis with regard to arteriosclerosis. *Bibl Nutr Diet 37*, 53–91.

Gey, K. F. (1994). Optimum plasma levels of antioxidant micronutrients. Ten years of antioxidant hypothesis on arteriosclerosis. *Bibl Nutr Diet 51*, 84–99.

Gey, K. F., U. K. Moser, P. Jordan, H. B. Stahelin, M. Eichholzer, and E. Ludin (1993). Increased risk of cardiovascular disease at suboptimal plasma concentrations of essential antioxidants: An epidemiological update with special attention to carotene and vitamin C. *Am J Clin Nutr 57(suppl)*, 787S–797S.

Gey, K. F., P. Puska, P. Jordan, and U. K. Moser (1991). Inverse correlation between plasma vitamin E and mortality from ischemic heart disease in cross-cultural epidemiology. *Am J Clin Nutr 53(suppl)*, 326S–334S.

Ginsberg, H. N., W. Karmally, S. L. Barr, C. Johnson, S. Holleran, and R. Ramakrishnan (1994). Effects of increasing dietary polyunsaturated fatty acids within the guidelines of the AHA step 1 diet on plasma lipid and lipoprotein levels in normal males. *Arterioscler Thromb 14*, 892–901.

Goldbourt, U., S. Yaari, and J. H. Medalie (1993). Factors predictive of long-term coronary heart disease mortality among 10,059 male Israeli civil servants and municipal employees: A 23-year mortality follow-up in the Israeli ischemic heart disease study. *Cardiology 82*, 100–121.

Gordon, T. (1988). The diet–heart idea. Outline of a history. *Am J Epidemiol 127*, 220–225.

Gordon, T., A. Kagan, M. Garcia-Palmieri, W. B. Kannel, W. J. Zukel, J. Tillotson, P. Sorlie, and M. Hjortland (1981). Diet and its relation to coronary heart disease and death in three populations. *Circulation 63*, 500–515.

Gramenzi, A., A. Gentile, M. Fasoli, E. Negri, F. Parazzini, and C. La Vecchia (1990). Association between certain foods and risk of acute myocardial infarction in women. *BMJ 300*, 771–773.

Grande, F., J. T. Anderson, C. Chlouverakis, M. Proja, and A. Keys (1965). Effect of dietary cholesterol on man's serum lipids. *J Nutr 87*, 52–62.

Grundy, S. M. (1991). Evaluation of publicly available scientific evidence regarding certain nutrient–disease relationships. In Office, L. S. R. (ed.): Task order no. 9 *Lipids and Cardiovascular Disease*, vol 9. Bethesda, MD: Federation of American Societies for Experimental Biology, pp. 1–38.

Grundy, S. M. (1992). How much does diet contribute to premature coronary heart disease? In Stein et al. (eds.): *Atherosclerosis IX. Proceedings of the 9th International Symposium on Atherosclerosis*. Tel Aviv, Israel. Creative Communications Ltd., pp. 471–478.

Grundy, S. M., D. Bilheimer, H. Blackburn, W. V. Brown, P. O. Kwiterovich Jr., F. Mattson, G. Schonfeld, and W. H. Weidman (1982). Rationale of the diet–heart statement of the American Heart Association. Report of Nutrition Committee. *Circulation 65*, 839A–854A.

Guallar, E., C. H. Hennekens, F. M. Sacks, W. C. Willett, and M. J. Stampfer (1995). A prospective study of plasma fish oil levels and incidence of myocardial infarction in U.S. male physicians. *J Am Coll Cardiol 25*, 387–394.

Haeger, K. (1973). Walking distance and arterial flow during long term treatment of intermittent claudication with d-α-tocopherol. *Vasa 2*, 280–287.

Halliwell, B. (1989). Free radicals, reactive oxygen species and human disease: A critical evaluation with special reference to atherosclerosis. *Br J Exp Pathol 70*, 737–757.

Harmon, D. (1982). The free radical theory of aging. In Pryor, W. A. (ed.): Free radicals in biology, volume 5. San Diego. Academic Press, pp. 255–275.

Harris, W. S., W. E. Connor, N. Alam, and D. R. Illingworth (1988). Reduction of postprandial triglyceridemia in humans by dietary n-3 fatty acids. *J Lipid Res 29*, 1451–1460.

Haskell, W. L., C. Camargo, Jr., P. T. Williams, K. M. Vranizan, R. M. Krauss, F. T. Lindgren, and P. D. Wood (1984). The effect of cessation and resumption of moderate alcohol intake on serum high-density-lipoprotein subfractions. A controlled study. *N Engl J Med 310*, 805–810.

Hegsted, D. M. (1986). Serum-cholesterol response to dietary cholesterol: A re-evaluation. *Am J Clin Nutr 44*, 299–305.

Hegsted, D. M., L. M. Ausman, J. A. Johnson, and G. E. Dallal (1993). Dietary fat and serum lipids: An evaluation of the experimental data. *Am J Clin Nutr 57*, 875–883.

Hennekens, C. H., J. E. Buring, J. E. Manson, M. J. Stampfer, B. Rosner, N. R. Cook, C. Belanger, F. LaMotte, J. M. Gaziano, P. M. Ridker, W. C. Willett, and R. Peto (1996). Lack of effect of long-term supplementation with beta carotene on the incidence of malignant neoplasms and cardiovascular disease. *N Engl J Med 334*, 1145–1149.

Hertog, M. G. L., D. Kromhout, C. Aravanis, H. Blackburn, R. Buzina, F. Fidanza, S. Giampaoli, A. Jansen, A. Menotti, S. Nedelijkovic, M. Pekkarinen, B. Simic, H. Toshima, E. J. M. Feskens, P. C. H. Hollman, and M. B. Katan (1995). Flavonoid intake and long-term risk of coronary heart disease and cancer in the Seven Countries Study. *Arch Intern Med 155*, 381–386.

Hetzel, B. S., J. S. Charnock, T. Dwyer, and P. L. McLennan (1989). Fall in coronary heart disease mortality in U.S.A. and Australia due to sudden death: Evidence for the role of polyunsaturated fat. *J Clin Epidemiol 42*, 885–893.

Hjermann, I., I. Holme, and P. Leren (1986). Oslo Study Diet and Antismoking Trial; results after 102 months. *Am J Med 80*, 7–11.

Hjermann, I., K. Velve Byre, I. Holme, and P. Leren (1981). Effect of diet and smoking intervention on the incidence of coronary heart disease. Report from the Oslo Study Group of a randomised trial in healthy men. *Lancet 2*, 1303–1310.

Hodis, H. N., W. J. Mack, L. LaBree, L. Cashin-Hemphill, A. Sevanian, R. Johnson, P. Azen (1995). Serial coronary angiographic evidence that antioxidant vitamin intake reduces progression of coronary artery atherosclerosis. *JAMA 273*, 1849–1854.

Hu, F. B., M. J. Stampfer, J. E., Manson, E. Rimm, G. A. Colditz, B. A. Rosner, C. H. Hennekens, W. C. Willett (1997). Dietary fat intake and the risk of coronary heart disease in women. *N Engl J Med, 337*, 1491–1499.

Hu, F. B., M. J. Stampfer, J. E. Manson, E. B. Rimm, G. A. Colditz, F. E. Speizer, C. H. Hennekens, and W. C. Willett (1998). Dietary protein and risk of coronary heart disease in women. (Submitted).

Jacobs, D., G. Blackburn, M. Higgins, D. Reed, H. Iso, G. McMillan, J. Neaton, J. Nelson, J. Potter, B. Rifkind, J. Rossouw, R. Shekeller, S. Usuf, and DPHIL (1992). Report of the Conference on Low Blood Cholesterol: Mortality Associations. *Circulation 86*, 1046–1060.

Jacobs, D. R., Jr., J. T. Anderson, and H. Blackburn (1979). Diet and serum cholesterol: Do zero correlations negate the relationship? *Am J Epidemiol 110*, 77–87.

Jacobs, D. R., Jr., J. T. Anderson, P. Hannan, A. Keys, and H. Blackburn (1983). Variability in individual serum cholesterol response to change in diet. *Arteriosclerosis 3*, 349–356.

Jenkins, D. J., R. G. Josse, A. L. Jenkins, T. M. Wolever, and V. Vuksan (1995). Implications of altering the rate of carbohydrate absorption from the gastrointestinal tract. *Clin Investi Med 18*, 296–302.

Jenkins, D. J., T. M. Wolever, G. Buckley, K. Y. Lam, S. Giudici, J. Kalmusky, A. L. Jenkins, R. L. Patten, J. Bird, and G. S. Wong, et al. (1988). Low-glycemic-index starchy foods in the diabetic diet. *Am J Clin Nutr 48*, 248–254.

Jenkins, D. J., T. M. Wolever, R. H. Taylor, H. Barker, H. Fielden, J. M. Baldwin, A. C. Bowling, H. C. Newman, A. L. Jenkins, and D. V. Goff (1981). Glycemic index of foods: a physiological basis for carbohydrate exchange. *Am J Clin Nutr 34*, 362–366.

Jeppesen, J., Y. D. Chen, M. Y. Zhou, T. Wang, and G. M. Reaven (1995). Effect of variations in oral fat and carbohydrate load on postprandial lipemia. *Am J Clin Nutr 62*, 1201–1205.

Jeppesen, J., P. Schaaf, G. Jones, M. Y. Zhou, Y. D. I. Chen, G. M. Reaven (1997). Effects of low-fat, high-carbohydrate diets on risk factors for ischemic heart disease in postmenopausal women. *Am J Clin Nutr, 65(4)*, 1027–1033.

Jialal, I., and S. Devaraj (1996). The role of oxidized low density lipoprotein in atherogenesis. *J Nutr 126(suppl)*, 1053S–1057S.

Judd, J. T., B. A. Clevidence, R. A. Muesing, J. Wittes, M. E. Sunkin, and J. J. Podczasy (1994). Dietary *trans* fatty acids: Effects of plasma lipids and lipoproteins on healthy men and women. *Am J Clin Nutr 59*, 861–868.

Kagawa, Y., M. Nishizawa, M. Suzuki, T. Miyatake, T. Hamamoto, K. Goto, E. Motonaga, H. Izumikawa, H. Hirata, and A. Ebihara (1982). Eicosapolyenoic acids of serum lipids of Japanese islanders with low incidence of cardiovascular diseases. *J Nutr Sci Vitaminol 28*, 441–453.

Kahn, H. A. (1970). Change in serum cholesterol associated with changes in the United States civilian diet, 1909–1965. *Am J Clin Nutr 23*, 879–882.

Kang, S. S., P. W. K. Wong, H. Y. Cook, M. Norusis, and J. V. Messer (1986). Protein bound homocyst(e)ine—A possible risk factor for coronary artery disease. *J Clin Invest 77*, 1482–1486.

Kardinaal, A. F., F. J. Kok, J. Ringstad, J. Gomez-Aracena, V. P. Mazaev, L. Kohlmeier, B. C. Martin, A. Aro, J. D. Kark, and M. Delgado-Rodriguez, et al. (1993). Antioxidants in adipose tissue and risk of myocardial infarction: The EURAMIC Study. *Lancet 342*, 1379–1384.

Karpe, F., G. Steiner, K. Uffelman, T. Olivecrona, and A. Hamsten (1994). Postprandial lipoproteins and progression of coronary atherosclerosis. *Atherosclerosis 106*, 83–97.

Karppanen, H. (1981). Epidemiological studies on the relationship between magnesium intake and cardiovascular diseases. *Artery 9*, 190–199.

Katan, M. B. (1995). Exit *trans* fatty acids. *Lancet 346*, 1245–1246.

Katan, M. B., A. C. Beynen, J. H. de Vries, and A. Nobels (1986). Existence of consistent hypo-and hyperresponders to dietary cholesterol in man. *Am J Epidemiol 123*, 221–234.

Kato, H., J. Tillotson, M. Z. Nichaman, G. G. Rhoads, and H. B. Hamilton (1973). Epidemiologic studies of coronary heart disease and stroke in Japanese men living in Japan, Hawaii and California. *Am J Epidemiol 97*, 372–385.

Katz, L. N., and J. S. Stamler (1953). *Experimental Atheroschlerosis*. Springfield, IL: Charles C. Thomas.

Kestin, M., P. Clifton, G. B. Belling, and P. J. Nestel (1990). N-3 fatty acids of marine origin lower systolic blood pressure and triglycerides but raise LDL cholesterol compared with N-3 and N-6 fatty acids from plants. *Am J Clin Nutr 51*, 1028–1034.

Keys, A. (1980). *Seven Countries: A Multivariate Analysis of Death and Coronary Heart Disease*. Cambridge, MA: Harvard University Press.

Keys, A. (1984). Serum-cholesterol response to dietary cholesterol. *Am J Clin Nutr 40*, 351–359.

Keys, A., J. T. Anderson, and F. Grande (1965). Serum cholesterol response to changes in the diet. II. The effect of cholesterol in the diet. *Metabolism 14*, 759–765.

Khaw, K. T., and E. Barrett-Connor (1987). Dietary fiber and reduced ischemic heart disease mortality rates in men and women: A 12-year prospective study. *Am J Epidemiol 126*, 1093–1102.

Kirkeby, K., P. Ingvaldsen, and I. Bjerkedal (1972a). Fatty acid composition of serum lipids in men with myocardial infarction. *Acta Med Scand 192*, 513–519.

Kirkeby, K., S. Nitter-Hauge, and I. Bjerkedal (1972b). Fatty acid composition of adipose tissue in male Norwegians with myocardial infarction. *Acta Med Scand 191*, 321–324.

Klevay, L. M. (1975). Coronary heart disease: the zinc/copper hypothesis. *Am J Clin Nutr 28*, 764–774.

Klevay, L. M. (1983). Copper and ischemic heart disease. *Biol Trace Element Res 5*, 245–255.

Kok, F. J., A. M. de Bruijn, R. Vermeeren, A. Hofman, A. van Laar, M. de Bruin, R. J. J. Hermus, and H. A. Valkenburg (1987). Serum selenium, vitamin antioxidants, and cardiovascular mortality: A 9-year follow-up study in the Netherlands. *Am J Clin Nutr 45*, 462–468.

Kok, F. J., A. Hofman, and J. C. Witteman, et al. (1989). Decreased selenium levels in acute myocardial infarction. *JAMA 261*, 1161–1164.

Kok, F. J., C. M. Van Duijn, A. Hofman, G. B. Van der Voet, F. A. De Wolff, C. H. Paays, and H. A. Valkenburg (1988). Serum copper and zinc and the risk of death from cancer and cardiovascular disease. *Am J Epidemiol 128*, 352–359.

Koranyi, A. (1963). Prophylaxis and treatment of the coronary syndrome. *Ther Hung 12*, 17–20.

Kritchevsky, D., L. M. Davidson, J. J. van der Watt, P. A. Winter, and B. I. (1974). Hypercholesterolemia and atherosclerosis induced in vervet monkeys by cholesterol-free, semisynthetic diets. *S Afr Med J 48*, 2413–2414.

Kromhout, D., E. B. Bosschieter, and C. de Lezenne Coulander (1982). Dietary fiber and 10-year mortality from coronary heart disease, cancer and all causes: The Zutphen Study. *Lancet 2*, 518–522.

Kromhout, D., E. B. Bosschieter, and C. de Lezenne Coulander (1985). The inverse relation between fish consumption and 20-year mortality from coronary heart disease. *N Engl J Med 312*, 1205–1209.

Kromhout, D., and C. de Lezenne Coulander (1984). Diet, prevalence and 10-year mortality from coronary heart disease in 871 middle-aged men: The Zutphen Study. *Am J Epidemiol 119*, 733–741.

Kromhout, D., E. J. M. Feskens, and C. H. Bowles (1995). The protective effect of a small amount of fish on coronary heart disease mortality in an elderly population. *Int J Epidemiol 24*, 340–345.

Kushi, L. H. (1987). Total energy intake: Implication for epidemiologic analyses (letter). *Am J Epidemiol 126*, 981–982.

Kushi, L. H., A. R. Folsom, R. J. Prineas, P. J. Mink, Y. Wu, and R. M. Bostick (1996). Dietary antioxidant vitamins and death from coronary heart disease in postmenopausal women. *N Engl J Med 334*, 1156–1162.

Kushi, L. H., E. B. Lenart, and W. C. Willett (1995). Health implications of Mediterranean diets in light of contemporary knowledge. 2. Meat, wine, fats and oils. *Am J Clin Nutr 61 (suppl)*, 1416S–1427S.

Kushi, L. H., R. A. Lew, F. J. Stare, C. R. Ellison, M. el Lozy, G. Bourke, L. Daly, I. Graham, N. Hickey, R. Mulcahy, and J. Kevancy (1985). Diet and 20-year mortality from coronary heart disease: The Ireland–Boston Diet–Heart study. *N Engl J Med 312*, 811–818.

Kushi, L. H., K. W. Samonds, J. M. Lacey, P. T. Brown, J. G. Bergan, and F. M. Sacks (1988). The association of dietary fat with serum cholesterol in vegetarians: The effect of dietary assessment on the correlation coefficient. *Am J Epidemiol 128*, 1054–1064.

Lapidus, L., H. Andersson, C. Bengtsson, and I. Bosaeus (1986). Dietary habits in relation to incidence of cardiovascular disease and death in women: A 12-year follow-up of participants in the population study of women in Gothenburg, Sweden. *Am J Clin Nutr 44*, 444–448.

Lauffer, R. B. (1991). Iron stores and the international variation in mortality from coronary artery disease. *Med Hypoth 35*, 96–102.

Law, M. R., N. J. Wald, and S. G. Thompson (1994). By how much and how quickly does reduction in serum cholesterol concentration lower risk of ischaemic heart disease? *BMJ 308*, 367–372.

Lea, E. J., S. P. Jones, and D. V. Hamilton (1982). The fatty acids of erythrocytes of myocardial infarction patients. *Atherosclerosis 41*, 363–369.

Leaf, A. (1995). Omega-3 fatty acids and prevention of ventricular fibrillation. *Prostaglandins Leukotrienes Essential Fatty Acids 52*, 197–198.

Leaf, A., and P. C. Weber (1988). Cardiovascular effects of n-3 fatty acids. *N Engl J Med 318*, 549–557.

Leren, P. (1970). The Oslo diet–heart study. Eleven-year report. *Circulation 42*, 935–942.

Levine, R. A., D. H. Streeten, and R. J. Doisy (1968). Effects of oral chromium supplementation on the glucose tolerance of elderly human subjects. *Metabolism 17*, 114–125.

Lewis, B. (1958). Composition of plasma cholesterol ester in relation to coronary-artery disease and dietary fat. *Lancet 2*, 71–73.

Lipid Research Clinics Program (1984). The lipid research clinics coronary primary prevention trial results. Reduction in incidence of coronary heart disease. *JAMA 251*, 351–364.

Losonczy, K. G., T. B. Harris, and R. J. Havlik (1996). Vitamin E and vitamin C supplement use and risk of all-cause and coronary heart disease mortality in older persons: The established populations for epidemiologic studies of the elderly. *Am J Clin Nutr 64*, 190–196.

Luoma, H., A. Aromaa, S. Helminen, H. Murtomaa, L. Kiviluoto, S. Punsar, and P. Knekt (1983). Risk of myocardial infarction in Finnish men in relation to fluoride, magnesium and calcium concentration in drinking water. *Acta Med Scand 213*, 171–176.

Ma, J., M. J. Stampfer, C. H. Hennekens, P. Frosst, J. Selhub, J. Horsford, M. R. Malinow, W. C. Willett, and R. Rozen (1996). Methylenetetrahydrofolate reductase polymorphism, plasma folate, homocysteine, and risk of myocardial infarction in U.S. physicians. *Circulation 94*, 2410–2416.

MacIntyre, D. E., R. L. Hoover, M. Smith, M. Steer, C. Lynch, M. J. Karnovsky, and E. W. Salzman (1984). Inhibition of platelet function by *cis*-unsaturated fatty acids. *Blood 63*, 848–857.

Malinow, M. R. (1990). Hyperhomocyst(e)inemia: A common and easily reversible risk factor for occlusive atherosclerosis. *Circulation 81*, 2004–2006.

Malinow, M. R. (1996). Plasma homocyst(e)ine—A risk factor for arterial occlusive diseases. *J Nutr 126(suppl)*, S1238–S1243.

Mann, G. V. (1977). Diet–heart: End of an era. *N Engl J Med 297*, 644–650.

Manson, J. E., M. J. Stampfer, C. H. Hennekens, and W. C. Willett (1987). Body weight and longevity. A reassessment. *JAMA 257*, 353–358.

Manttari, M., J. K. Huttunen, P. Koskinen, V. Manninen, L. Tenkanen, O. P. Heinonen, and M. H. Frick (1990). Lipoproteins and coronary heart disease in the Helsinki Heart Study. *Eur Heart J 11*, 26h–31h.

Marckmann, P., B. Sandstrom, and J. Jespersen (1992). Fasting blood coagulation and fibrinolysis of young adults unchanged by reduction in dietary fat content. *Arterioscler Thromb 12*, 201–205.

Marckmann, P., B. Sandstrom, and J. Jespersen (1993). Favorable long-term effect of a low-fat/high-fiber diet on human blood coagulation and fibrinolysis. *Arterioscler Thromb 13*, 505–511.

McCord, J. M. (1991). Is iron sufficiency a risk factor in ischemic heart disease? *Circulation 83*, 1112–1114.

McGandy, R. B., D. M. Hegsted, and F. J. Stare (1967). Dietary fats, carbohydrates, and atherosclerotic vascular disease. *N Engl J Med 277*, 245–247.

McGee, D. L., D. M. Reed, K. Yano, A. Kagan, and J. Tillotson (1984). Ten-year incidence of coronary heart disease in the Honolulu Heart Program: Relationship to nutrient intake. *Am J Epidemiol 119*, 667–676.

McGill, H. C. J. (ed.) (1968). *The Geographic Pathway of Atherosclerosis*. Baltimore: Williams & Wilkins.

Meade, T. W., S. Mellows, M. Brozovic, G. J. Miller, R. R. Chakrabarti, W. R. North, A. P. Haines, Y. Stirling, J. D. Imeson, and S. G. Thompson (1986). Haemostatic function and ischaemic heart disease: Principal results of the Northwick Park Heart Study. *Lancet 2*, 533–537.

Mensink, R. P., and M. B. Katan (1987). Effect of monounsaturated fatty acids versus complex carbohydrates on high-density lipoprotein in healthy men and women. *Lancet 1*, 122–125.

Mensink, R. P., and M. B. Katan (1992). Effect of dietary fatty acids on serum lipids and lipoproteins: A meta-analysis of 27 trials. *Arterioscler Thromb 12*, 911–919.

Mensink, R. P., P. L. Zock, M. B. Katan, and G. Hornstra (1992). Effect of dietary *cis* and *trans* fatty acids on serum lipoprotein [a] levels in humans. *J Lipid Res 33*, 1493–1501.

Meredith, A. P., P. E. Enterline, B. Peterson, and J. G. Pekover (1960). An epidemiologic diet study in North Dakota. *J Am Diet Assoc 37*, 339–343.

Miettinen, T. A., G. Alfthan, J. K. Huttunen, J. Pikkarainen, V. Naukkarinen, S. Mattila, and T. Kumlin (1983). Serum selenium concentration related to myocardial infarction and fatty acid content of serum lipids. *BMJ 287*, 517–519.

Miettinen, T. A., V. Naukkarinen, J. K. Huttunen, S. Mattila, and T. Kumlin (1982). Fatty-acid composition of serum lipids predicts myocardial infarction. *BMJ 285*, 993–996.

Miller, N. E. (1987). Associations of high-density lipoprotein subclasses and apolipoproteins with ischemic heart disease and coronary atherosclerosis. *Am Heart J 113*, 589–597.

Moore, J. A., R. Noiva, and I. C. Wells (1984). Selenium concentrations in plasma of patients with arteriographically defined coronary atherosclerosis. *Clin Chem 30*, 1171–1173.

Moore, R. D., and T. A. Pearson (1986). Moderate alcohol consumption and coronary artery disease: A review. *Medicine 65*, 242–267.

Morris, D. L., S. B. Kritchevsky, and C. E. Davis (1994). Serum carotenoids and coronary heart disease: The Lipid Research Clinics Coronary Primary Prevention Trial and Follow-Up Study. *JAMA 272*, 1439–1441.

Morris, J. N., K. P. Ball, and A. Antonis, et al. (1968). Controlled trial of soya-bean oil in myocardial infarction. *Lancet 2*, 693–699.

Morris, J. N., J. W. Marr, and D. G. Clayton (1977). Diet and heart: A postscript. *BMJ 2*, 1307–1314.

Morris, M. C., J. E. Manson, B. Rosner, J. E. Buring, W. C. Willett, and C. H. Hennekens (1995). Fish consumption and cardiovascular disease in the Physicians' Health Study: A prospective study. *Am J Epidemiol 142*, 166–175.

Morris, M. C., F. Sacks, and B. Rosner (1993). Does fish oil lower blood pressure? A meta-analysis of controlled trials. *Circulation 88*, 523–533.

Morrison, L. M. (1960). Diet in coronary atherosclerosis. *JAMA 173*, 884–888.

Morrow, J. D., B. Frei, A. W. Longmire, J. M. Gaziano, S. M. Lynch, Y. Shyr, W. E. Strauss, J. A. Oates, and L. J. 2. Roberts (1995). Increase in circulating products of lipid peroxidation (F2-isoprostanes) in smokers. Smoking as a cause of oxidative damage. *N Engl J Med 332*, 1198–1203.

Multiple Risk Factor Intervention Trial Research Group (1982). Multiple Risk Factor Intervention Trial: Risk factor changes and mortality results. *JAMA 248*, 1465–1477.

Multiple Risk Factor Intervention Trial Research Group (1996). Mortality after 16 years for participants randomized to the Multiple Risk Factor Intervention Trial. *Circulation 94*, 946–951.

Munro, H. N., M. H. Steele, and W. Forbes (1965). Effect of dietary protein level on deposition of cholesterol in the tissues of the cholesterol-fed rabbit. *Br J Exp Pathol 46*, 489–496.

National Diet Heart Study Research Group (1968). National Diet Heart Study Final Report. *Circulation 37(s1)*, 1–428.

National Research Council, Committee on Diet and Health (1989). *Diet and Health: Implications for Reducing Chronic Disease Risk*. Washington, DC: National Academy Press.

Naurath, H. J., E. Joosten, R. Riezler, S. P. Stabler, R. H. Allen, and J. Lindenbaum (1995). Effects of vitamin B-12, folate, and vitamin B-6 supplements in elderly people with normal serum vitamin concentrations. *Lancet 346*, 85–89.

Nestel, P., M. Noakes, and B. E. A. Belling (1992). Plasma lipoprotein and Lp [a] changes with substitution of elaidic acid for oleic acid in the diet. *J Lipid Res 33*, 1029–1036.

Nichols, A. B., C. Ravenscroft, D. E. Lamphiear, and L. D. Ostrander Jr. (1976). Independence of serum lipid levels and dietary habits. The Tecumseh Study. *JAMA 236*, 1948–1953.

Nikkila, M., T. Solakivi, T. Lehtimaki, T. Koivula, P. Laippala, and B. Astrom (1994). Postprandial plasma lipoprotein changes in relation to apolipoprotein E phenotypes and low density lipoprotein size in men with and without coronary artery disease. *Atherosclerosis 106*, 149–157.

Norell, S. E., A. Ahlbom, M. Feychting, and N. L. Pedersen (1986). Fish consumption and mortality from coronary heart disease. *BMJ 293*, 426.

Olszewski, A. J., and K. S. McCully (1993). Homocysteine metabolism and the oxidative modification of proteins and lipids. *Free Rad Biol Med 14*, 683–693.

Omenn, G. S., G. E. Goodman, M. D. Thornquist, J. Balmes, M. R. Cullen, A. Glass, J. P. Keogh, F. L. Meyskens, B. Valanis, J. H. Williams, S. Barnhart, and S. Hammar (1996). Effects of a combination of beta carotene and vitamin A on lung cancer and cardiovascular disease. *N Engl J Med 334*, 1150–1155.

Ornish, D. (1990). *Dr. Dean Ornish's Program for Reversing Heart Disease*. New York: Balantine Books.

Page, L., and R. M. Marston (1979). Food consumption pattern—US diet. In Havlik, R. J., and Feinleib, M. (eds.): *Proceedings of the Conference on the Decline in Coronary Heart Disease Mortality*. NIH Publication No. 79-1610. Washington, DC: U.S. Department of Health, Education and Welfare, Public Health Service, pp. 236–243.

Parthasarathy, S., J. C. Khoo, E. Miller, J. Barnett, J. L. Witztum, and D. Steinberg (1990). Low density lipoprotein rich in oleic acid is protected against oxidative modification: Implications for dietary prevention of atherosclerosis. *Proc Natl Acad Sci USA 87*, 3894–3898.

Pietinen, P., A. Ascherio, P. Korhonen, A. M. Hartman, W. C. Willett, D. Albanes, and J. Virtamo (1997). Intake of fatty acids and risk of coronary heart disease in a cohort of Finnish men: The ATBC Study. *Am J Epidemiol 145*, 876–887.

Posner, B. M., J. L. Cobb, A. J. Belanger, L. A. Cupples, R. B. D'Agostino, and J. Stokes III (1991). Dietary lipid predictors of coronary heart disease in men. The Framingham Study. *Arch Intern Med 151*, 1181–1187.

Potter, J. G., K. P. Coffman, R. L. Reid, J. M. Krall, and M. J. Albrink (1981). Effect of test meals of varying dietary fiber content on plasma insulin and glucose response. *Am J Clin Nutr 34*, 328–334.

Potter, J. G., R. J. Illman, G. D. Calvert, D. G.

Oakenfull, and D. L. Topping (1980). Soya, saponins, plasma lipids, lipoproteins, and fecal bile acids: A double-blind crossover study. *Nutr Rep Int 22*, 521–528.

Ramirez, J., and N. C. Flowers (1980). Leukocyte ascorbic acid and its relationship to coronary artery disease in man. *Am J Clin Nutr 33*, 2079–2087.

Rapola, J. M., J. Virtamo, J. K. Haukka, O. P. Heinonen, D. Albanes, P. R. Taylor, and J. K. Huttunen (1996). Effect of vitamin E and beta carotene on the incidence of angina pectoris—A randomized, double-blind, controlled trial. *JAMA 275*, 693–698.

Renaud, S., F. Godsey, E. Dumont, C. Thevenon, E. Ortchanian, and J. L. (1986). Influence of long-term diet modification on platelet function and composition in Moselle farmers. *Am J Clin Nutr 43*, 136–150.

Renaud, S., K. Kuba, C. Goulet, Y. Lemire, and C. Allard (1970). Relationship between fatty-acid composition of platelets and platelet aggregation in rat and man. Relation to thrombosis. *Circ Res 26*, 553–564.

Rentrop, K. P., F. Feit, H. Blanke, P. Stecy, R. Schneider, M. Rey, S. Horowitz, M. Goldman, K. Karsch, H. Meilman, et al. (1984). Effects of intracoronary streptokinase and intracoronary nitroglycerin infusion on coronary angiographic patterns and mortality in patients with acute myocardial infarction. *N Engl J Med 311*, 1457–1463.

Rhoads, G. G., C. L. Gulbrandsen, and A. Kagan (1976). Serum lipoproteins and coronary heart disease in a population of Hawaiian Japanese men. *N Engl J Med 294*, 293–298.

Riales, R., and M. J. Albrink (1981). Effect of chromium chloride supplementation on glucose tolerance and serum lipids including high-density lipoprotein of adult men. *Am J Clin Nutr 34*, 2670–2678.

Ridker, P. M., D. E. Vaughan, M. J. Stampfer, R. J. Glynn, and C. H. Hennekens (1994). Association of moderate alcohol consumption and plasma concentration of endogenous tissue-type plasminogen activator. *JAMA 272*, 929–933.

Riemersma, R. A., D. A. Wood, S. Butler, R. A. Elton, M. Oliver, M. Salo, T. Nikkari, E. Vartiainen, P. Puska, and F. Gey, et al. (1986). Linoleic acid content in adipose tissue and coronary heart disease. *BMJ 292*, 1423–1427.

Rimm, E. B. (1996). Invited commentary—Alcohol consumption and coronary heart disease: Good habits may be more important than just good wine. *Am J Epidemiol 143*, 1094–1098.

Rimm, E. B., A. Ascherio, E. Giovannucci, D. Spiegelman, M. J. Stampfer, and W. C. Willett (1996a). Vegetable, fruit, and cereal fiber intake and risk of coronary heart disease among men. *JAMA 275*, 447–451.

Rimm, E. B., E. L. Giovannucci, W. C. Willett, G. A. Colditz, A. Ascherio, B. Rosner, and M. J. Stampfer (1991). A prospective study of alcohol consumption and the risk of coronary disease in men. *Lancet 338*, 464–468.

Rimm, E. B., A. Klatsky, D. Grobbee, and M. J. Stampfer (1996b). Review of moderate alcohol consumption and reduced risk of coronary heart disease: Is the effect due to beer, wine, or spirits? *BMJ 312*, 731–736.

Rimm, E. B., M. J. Stampfer, A. Ascherio, E. Giovannucci, G. A. Colditz, and W. C. Willett (1993). Vitamin E consumption and the risk of coronary heart disease in men. *N Engl J Med 328*, 1450–1456.

Rimm, E. B., W. C. Willett, F. B. Hu, L. Sampson, G. A. Colditz, J. E. Manson, C. Hennekens, and M. J. Stampfer (1998). Folate and vitamin B_6 from diet and supplements in relation to risk of coronary heart disease among women. *JAMA 279*, 359–364.

Rinehart, J. F., and L. D. Greenberg (1951). Pathogenesis of experimental arteriosclerosis in pyridoxine deficiency. *Arch Pathol 51*, 12–18.

Rinzler, S. H., H. Bakst, Z. H. Benjamin, A. L. Bobb, and J. Travell (1950). Failure of alpha tocopherol to influence chest pain in patients with heart disease. *Circulation 1*, 288–293.

Rivellese, A., G. Riccardi, A. Giacco, D. Pacioni, S. Genovese, P. L. Mattioli, and M. Mancini (1980). Effect of dietary fibre on glucose control and serum lipoproteins in diabetic patients. *Lancet 2*, 447–450.

Roberts, T. L., D. A. Wood, R. A. Riemersma, P. J. Gallagher, and F. C. Lampe (1995). *Trans* isomers of oleic and linoleic acids in adipose tissue and sudden cardiac death. *Lancet 345*, 278–282.

Robertson, T. L., H. Kato, G. G. Rhoads, A. Kagan, M. Marmot, S. L. Syme, T. Gordon, R. M. Worth, J. L. Belsky, D. S. Dock, M. Miyanishi, and S. Kawamoto (1977). Epidemiologic studies of coronary heart disease and stroke in Japanese men living in Japan, Hawaii and California: Incidence of myocardial infarction and death from coronary heart disease. *Am J Cardiol 39*, 239–243.

Rose, G. A., W. B. Thomson, and R. T. Williams (1965). Corn oil in treatment of ischaemic heart disease. *BMJ i*, 1531–1533.

Rosenberg, I. H. (1996). Homocysteine, vitamins and arterial occlusive disease—an overview. *J Nutr 126(suppl)*, S1235–S1237.

Rosenberg, L., D. Slone, S. Shapiro, D. W. Kaufman, O. S. Miettinen, and P. D. Stolley (1981). Alcoholic beverages and myocardial infarction in young women. *Am J Public Health 71*, 82–85.

Rosner, B., D. Spiegelman, and W. C. Willett (1992). Correction of logistic regression relative risk estimates and confidence intervals for random within-person measurement error. *Am J Epidemiol 136*, 1400–1413.

Rowe, J. W., J. B. Young, K. L. Minaker, A. L. Stevens, J. Pallotta, and L. Landsberg (1981). Effect of insulin and glucose infusions on sympathetic nervous system activity in normal man. *Diabetes 30*, 219–225.

Rubenowitz, E., G. Axelsson, and R. Rylander (1996). Magnesium in drinking water and death from acute myocardial infarction. *Am J Epidemiol 143*, 456–462.

Sacks, F. (1994). Dietary fats and coronary heart disease. Overview. *J. Cardiovasc Risk 1*, 3–8.

Sacks, F. M., M. A. Pfeffer, L. A. Moye, J. L. Rouleau, J. D. Rutherford, C. T. G., L. Brown, J. W. Warnica, J. M. Arnold, C. C. Wun, B. R. Davis, and E. Braunwald (1996). The effect of pravastatin on coronary events after myocardial infarction in patients with average cholesterol levels—Cholesterol and Recurrent Events Trial investigators. *N Engl J Med 335*, 1001–1009.

Sacks, F. M., and W. C. Willett (1991). More on chewing the fat—The good fat and the good cholesterol. *N Engl J Med 325*, 1740–1742.

Salmeron, J., A. Ascherio, E. Rimm, G. Colditz, D. Spiegelman, and M. Stampfer (1995). Carbohydrate quality and risk of non-insulin-dependent diabetes in women (abstract). *Am J Epidemiol 141*, S67.

Salmeron, J., A. Ascherio, E. B. Rimm, G. A. Colditz, D. Spiegelman, D. J. Jenkins, M. J. Stampfer, A. L. Wing, and W. C. Willett (1997). Dietary fiber, glycemic load, and risk of NIDDM in men. *Diabetes Care 20*, 545–550.

Salonen, J. T., G. Alfthan, J. K. Huttunen, J. Pikkarainen, and P. Puska (1982). Association between cardiovascular death and myocardial infarction and serum selenium in a matched-pair longitudinal study. *Lancet 2*, 175–179.

Salonen, J. T., K. Nyyssonen, H. Korpela, J. Tuomilehto, R. Seppanen, and R. Salonen

(1992). High stored iron levels are associated with excess risk of myocardial infarction in Eastern Finnish men. *Circulation* 86, 803–811.

Salonen, J. T., R. Salonen, I. Pnettila, J. Herranen, M. Jauhiainen, M. Kantola, R. Lappetelainen, P. H. Maenpaa, G. Alfthan, and P. Puska (1985). Serum fatty acids, apolipoproteins, selenium and vitamin antioxidants, and the risk of death from coronary artery disease. *Am J Cardiol 56*, 226–231.

Salvini, S., C. H. Hennekens, J. S. Morris, W. C. Willett, and M. J. Stampfer (1995). Plasma levels of the antioxidant selenium and risk of myocardial infarction among US physicians. *Am J Cardiol 76*, 1218–1221.

Schrade, W., R. Biegler, and E. Bohle (1961). Fatty-acid distribution in the lipid fractions of healthy persons of different age, patients with atherosclerosis and patients with idiopathic hyperlipidaemia. *J Atheroscler Res 1*, 47–61.

Schroeder, H. A., A. P. Nason, and I. H. Tipton (1970). Chromium deficiency as a factor in atherosclerosis. *J Chronic Dis 23*, 123–142.

Scrimshaw, N. S. and M. A. Guzman (1968). Diet and atherosclerosis. *Lab Invest 18*, 623–628.

Seelig, M. (1980). *Magnesium Deficiency in the Pathogenesis of Disease.* New York: Plenum Press.

Seelig, M. S., and H. A. Heggtveit (1974). Magnesium interrelationships in ischemic heart disease: A review. *Am J Clin Nutr 27*, 59–79.

Selhub, J., P. F. Jacques, A. G. Bostom, R. B. D'Agostino, P. W. F. Wilson, A. J. Belanger, D. H. O'Leary, P. A. Wolf, E. J. Schaefer, and I. H. Rosenberg (1995). Association between plasma homocysteine concentrations and extracranial carotid-artery stenosis. *N Engl J Med 332*, 286–291.

Selhub, J., P. F. Jacques, P. W. F. Wilson, D. Rush, and I. H. Rosenberg (1993). Vitamin status and intake as primary determinants of homocysteinemia in an elderly population. *JAMA 270*, 2693–2698.

Sempos, C. T., A. C. Looker, R. F. Gillum, and D. M. Makuc (1994). Body iron stores and the risk of coronary heart disease. *N Engl J Med 330*, 1119–1124.

Senti, F. R. (1988). *Health Aspects of Dietary Trans Fatty Acids: August 1985.* Bethesda, MD: Federation of American Societies for Experimental Biology.

Shekelle, R. B., L. Missell, O. Paul, A. M. Shryock, and J. Stamler (1985). Fish consumption and mortality from coronary heart disease (letter). *N Engl J Med 313*, 820–824.

Shekelle, R. B., M. Z. Nichaman, and W. J. Raynor Jr. (1987). Re: total energy intake: implication for epidemiolgic analyses (letter). *Am J Epidemiol 126*, 980–983.

Shekelle, R. B., A. M. Shryock, O. Paul, M. Lepper, J. Stamler, S. Liu, and W. J. Raynor, Jr. (1981). Diet, serum cholesterol, and death from coronary heart disease: The Western Electric Study. *N Engl J Med 304*, 65–70.

Shekelle, R. B., and J. Stamler (1989). Dietary cholesterol and ischemic heart disease. *Lancet 1*, 1177–1179.

Shepherd, J., S. M. Cobbe, I. Ford, C. G. Isles, A. R. Lorimer, P. W. MacFarlane, J. H. McKillop, and C. J. Packard (1995). Prevention of coronary heart disease with pravastatin in men with hypercholesterolemia—West of Scotland Coronary Prevention Study Group. *N Engl J Med 333*, 1301–1307.

Shireman, R. (1996). Formation, metabolism and physiologic effects of oxidatively modified low density lipoprotein. Overview. *J Nutr 126 (suppl)*, 1049S–1052S.

Siguel, E. N., and R. H. Lerman (1993). Trans fatty acid patterns in patients with angiographically documented coronary artery disease. *Am J Cardiol 71*, 916–920.

Simpson, H. C., K. Barker, R. D. Carter, E. Cassels, and J. I. Mann (1982). Low dietary intake of linoleic acid predisposes to myocardial infarction. *BMJ 285*, 683–684.

Singh, R. B., S. S. Rastogi, R. Verman, B. Laxmi, R. Singh, S. Ghosh, and M. A. Niaz (1992). Randomised controlled trial of cardioprotective diet in patients with recent acute myocardial infarction: Results of one year follow up. *BMJ 304*, 1015–1019.

Siscovick, D. S., T. E. Raghunathan, I. King, S. Weinman, K. G. Wicklund, J. Albright, V. Bovbjerg, P. Arbogast, H. Smith, L. H. Kushi, L. A. Cobb, M. K. Copass, B. M. Psaty, R. Lemaitre, B. Retzlaff, M. Childs, and R. H. Knopp (1995). Dietary intake and cell membrane levels of long-chain N-3 polyunsaturated fatty acids and the risk of primary cardiac arrest. *JAMA 274*, 1363–1367.

Snowdon, D. A., R. L. Phillips, and G. E. Fraser (1984). Meat consumption and fatal ischemic heart disease. *Prev Med 13*, 490–500.

Stamler, J. (1985). The marked decline in coronary heart disease mortality rates in the United States, 1968–1981: Summary of findings and possible explanations. *Cardiology 72*, 11–22.

Stamler, J., D. Wentworth, and J. D. Neaton (1986). Is the relationship between serum cholesterol and risk of premature death from coronary heart disease continuous and graded? Findings in 356,222 primary screenees of the Multiple Risk Factor Intervention Trial (MRFIT). *JAMA 256*, 2823–2828.

Stampfer, M. J., G. A. Colditz, W. C. Willett, J. E. Manson, R. A. Arky, C. H. Hennekens, and F. E. Speizer (1988a). A prospective study of moderate alcohol drinking and risk of diabetes in women. *Am J Epidemiol 128*, 549–558.

Stampfer, M. J., G. A. Colditz, W. C. Willett, F. E. Speizer, and C. H. Hennekens (1988b). A prospective study of moderate alcohol consumption and the risk of coronary disease and stroke in women. *N Engl J Med 319*, 267–273.

Stampfer, M. J., C. H. Hennekens, J. E. Manson, G. A. Colditz, B. Rosner, and W. C. Willett (1993). Vitamin E consumption and the risk of coronary disease in women. *N Engl J Med 328*, 1444–1449.

Stampfer, M. J., R. M. Krauss, J. Ma, P. J. Blance, L. G. Holl, F. M. Sacks, and C. H. Hennekens (1996). A prospective study of triglyceride level, low-density lipoprotein particle diameter, and risk of myocardial infarction. *JAMA 276*, 882–888.

Stampfer, M. J., M. R. Malinow, W. C. Willett, L. M. Newcomer, B. Upson, D. Ullmann, P. V. Tishler, and C. H. Hennekens (1992). A prospective study of plasma homocyste(e)ine and risk of myocardial infarction in US physicians. *JAMA 268*, 877–881.

Stampfer, M. J., F. M. Sacks, S. Salvini, W. C. Willett, and C. H. Hennekens (1991). A prospective study of cholesterol, apolipoproteins, and the risk of myocardial infarction. *N Engl J Med 325*, 373–381.

Stampfer, M. J., and W. C. Willett (1993). Homocysteine and marginal vitamin deficiency—The importance of adequate vitamin intake. *JAMA 270*, 2726–2727.

Stampfer, M. J., W. C. Willett, and C. H. Hennekens (1988c). Selection of population. In Moon, T., and Micozzi, M. (eds.): *Nutrition in Cancer Prevention*. New York: Plenum Press, pp. 473–482.

Staprans, I., J. H. Rapp, X. M. Pan, K. Y. Kim, and K. R. Feingold (1994). Oxidized lipids in the diet are a source of oxidized lipid in chylomicrons of human serum. *Arterioscler Thromb 14*, 1900–1905.

Steering Committee of the Physicians' Health Study Research Group (1988). Preliminary report: Findings from the aspirin component of the ongoing Physicians' Health Study. *N Engl J Med 318*, 262–264.

Steinberg, D., S. Pathasarathy, T. E. Carew, J. C. Khoo, and J. L. Witztum (1989). Beyond cholesterol. Modifications of low-density lipoprotein that increase its atherogenicity. *N Engl J Med 320*, 915–924.

Stephens, N. G., A. Parsons, P. M. Schofield, F. Kelly, K. Cheeseman, M. J. Mitchinson, and M. J. Brown (1996). Randomised controlled trial of vitamin E in patients with coronary disease: Cambridge Heart Antioxidant Study (CHAOS). *Lancet 347*, 781–786.

Street, D. A., G. W. Comstock, R. M. Salkeld, W. Schuep, and M. J. Klag (1994). Serum antioxidants and myocardial infarction. Are low levels of carotenoids and alpha-tocopherol risk factors for myocardial infarction? *Circulation 90*, 1154–1161.

Sullivan, J. L. (1989). The iron paradigm of ischemic heart disease. *Am Heart J 117*, 1177–1188.

Sytkowski, P. A., R. B. D'Agostino, A. Belanger, and W. B. Kannel (1996). Sex and time trends in cardiovascular disease incidence and mortality: The Framingham Heart Study, 1950–1989. *Am J Epidemiol 143*, 338–350.

The Alpha-Tocopherol Beta-Carotene Cancer Prevention Study Group (1994). The effect of vitamin E and beta carotene on the incidence of lung cancer and other cancers in male smokers. *N Engl J Med 330*, 1029–1035.

Thomas, L. H., and R. G. Scott (1981). Ischaemic heart disease and the proportions of hydrogenated fat and ruminant-animal fat in adipose tissue at post-mortem examination: A case–control study. *J Epidemiol Commun Health 35*, 251–255.

Traber, M. G., Y. A. Carpentier, H. J. Kayden, M. Richelle, N. F. Galeano, and R. J. Deckelbaum (1993). Alterations in plasma alpha–and gamma-tocopherol concentrations in response to intravenous infusion of lipid emulsions in humans. *Metab Clin Exp 42*, 701–709.

Tran, K., and A. C. Chan (1992). Comparative uptake of alpha- and gamma-tocopherol by human endothelial cells. *Lipids 27*, 38–41.

Trichopoulou, A., A. Kouris-Blazos, M. L. Wahlqvist, C. Gnardellis, P. Lagiou, E. Polychronopoulos, T. Vassilakou, L. Lipworth, and D. Trichopoulos (1995). Diet and overall survival in elderly people. *BMJ 311*, 1457–1460.

Turpeinen, O., M. J. Karvonen, M. Pekkarinen, M. Miettinen, R. Elosuo, and E. Paavilainen (1979). Dietary prevention of coronary heart disease: The Finnish Mental Hospital Study. *Int J Epidemiol 8*, 99–118.

Tzonou, A., A. Kalandidi, A. Trichopoulou, C. C. Hsieh, N. Toupadaki, W. Willett, and D. Trichopoulos (1993). Diet and coronary heart disease: A case–control study in Athens, Greece. *Epidemiology 4*, 511–516.

Ulbricht, T. L. V., and D. A. T. Southgate (1991). Coronary heart disease: Seven dietary factors. *Lancet 338*, 985–992.

U.S. Department of Health and Human Services (1994). *National Heart, Lung, and Blood Institute Report of the Task Force on Research in Epidemiology and Prevention of Cardiovascular Disease.* Washington, DC: U.S. Department of Health and Human Services.

Vahouny, G. V., W. Chalcarz, S. Satchithanandam, I. Adamson, D. M. Klurfeld, and D. Kritchevsky (1984). Effect of soy protein and casein intake on intestinal absorption and lymphatic transport of cholesterol and oleic acid. *Am J Clin Nutr 40*, 1156–1164.

Valimaki, M., E. A. Nikkila, M. R. Taskinen, and R. Ylikahri (1986). Rapid decrease in high density lipoprotein subfractions and postheparin plasma lipase activities after cessation of chronic alcohol intake. *Atherosclerosis 59*, 147–153.

Verhoef, P., M. J. Stampfer, J. E. Buring, J. M. Gaziano, R. H. Allen, S. P. Stabler, R. D. Reynolds, F. J. Kok, C. H. Hennekens, and W. C. Willett (1996). Homocysteine metabolism and risk of myocardial infarction: Relation with vitamins B_6, B_{12}, and folate. *Am J Epidemiol 143*, 845–859.

Verschuren, W. M., D. R. Jacobs, B. P. Bloemberg, D. Kromhout, A. Menotti, C. Aravanis, H. Blackburn, B. R., A. S. Dontas, and F. Fidanza, et al. (1995). Serum total cholesterol and long-term coronary heart disease mortality in different cultures. Twenty-five-year follow-up of the Seven Countries Study. *JAMA 274*, 131–136.

Virtamo, J., E. Valkeila, G. Alfthan, S. Punsar, J. K. Huttunen, and M. J. Karvonen (1985). Serum selenium and the risk of coronary heart disease and stroke. *Am J Epidemiol 122*, 276–282.

Vollset, S. E., I. Heuch, and E. Bjelke (1985). Fish consumption and mortality from coronary heart disease (letter). *N Engl J Med 313*, 820–821.

Watts, G. F., B. Lewis, J. N. H. Brunt, E. S. Lewis, D. J. Coltart, L. D. Smith, J. I. Mann, and A. V. Swan (1992). Effects of coronary artery disease of lipid-lowering diet, or diet plus cholestyramine, in the St. Thomas' Atherosclerosis Regression Study (STARS). *Lancet 339*, 563–569.

Wierik, E. J. M. V. T., C. Kluft, H. Vandenberg, and J. A. Weststrate (1996). Consumption of reduced-fat products, haemostatic parameters and oral glucose tolerance test. *Fibrinolysis 10*, 159–166.

Willett, W. C. (1994). Diet and health: What should we eat? *Science 264*, 532–537.

Willett, W. C., and A. Ascherio (1995). Response to the International Life Sciences Institute report on *trans* fatty acids. *Am J Clin Nutr 62*, 524–526.

Willett, W. C., and E. B. Lenart (1996). Dietary factors. In Manson, J. E., Ridker, P. M., Gaziano, J. M., and Hennekens, C. H. (eds.). *Prevention of Myocardial Infarction.* New York: Oxford University Press, pp. 351–383.

Willett, W. C., J. E. Manson, M. J. Stampfer, G. A. Colditz, B. Rosner, F. E. Speizer, and C. H. Hennekens (1995). Weight, weight change, and coronary heart disease in women: Risk within the "normal" weight range. *JAMA 273*, 461–465.

Willett, W. C., M. J. Stampfer, J. E. Manson, G. A. Colditz, F. E. Speizer, B. A. Rosner L. A. Sampson, and C. H. Hennekens (1993). Intake of trans fatty acids and risk of coronary heart disease among women. *Lancet 341*, 581–585.

Wissler, R. W. and D. Vesselinovitch (1975). The effects of feeding various dietary fats on the development and regression of hypercholesterolemia and atherosclerosis. *Adv Exp Med Biol 60*, 65–76.

Wood, D. A., S. Butler, R. A. Riemersma, M. Thomson, M. F. Oliver, A. Fulton, A. Birtwhistle, and R. Elton (1984). Adipose tissue and platelet fatty acids and coronary heart disease in Scottish men. *Lancet 2*, 117–121.

Wood, D. A., R. A. Riemersma, S. Butler, M. Thomson, C. Macintyre, R. A. Elton, and M. F. Oliver (1987). Linoleic and eicosapentaenoic acids in adipose tissue and platelets and risk of coronary heart disease. *Lancet 1*, 177–183.

Woodhill, J. M., A. J. Palmer, B. Leelarthaepin, C. McGilchrist, and R. B. Blacket (1978). Low fat, low cholesterol diet in secondary prevention of coronary heart disease. *Adv Exp Med Biol 109*, 317–330.

Young, J. B., and L. Landsberg (1981). Effect of oral sucrose on blood pressure in the spontaneously hypertensive rat. *Metab Clin Exp 30*, 421–424.

Yudkin, J. (1963). Nutrition and palatability with special reference to obesity, myocardial infarction, and other diseases of civilisation. *Lancet 1,* 1335–1338.

Zilversmit, D. B. (1979). Atherogenesis: A postprandial phenomenon. *Circulation 60,* 473–485.

Zock, P. L., and M. B. Katan (1992). Hydrogenation alternatives: Effects of trans fatty acids and stearic acid versus linoleic acid on serum lipids and lipoproteins in humans. *J Lipid Res 33,* 399–410.

18

Folic Acid and Neural Tube Defects

Neural tube defects (NTDs) are the most common major congenital abnormalities in the United States and in many other countries. They result from failure of the embryonic neural tube to close completely at about the 28th day of pregnancy and are manifested as two main clinical abnormalities, anencephaly and spina bifida. The topic of folic acid and NTDs illustrates how astute clinical observations, basic nutritional biochemistry, nutritional epidemiology, randomized trials, and molecular genetics have each contributed to our understanding of a definitive and important causal relationship. This relationship also has wider implications because it establishes a major beneficial effect of a nutrient intake at intakes well above those that prevent classic deficiency, thus calling into question the basic paradigm of nutritional deficiency. This case also illustrates that knowledge of a causal relationship may not be sufficient to guide preventive measures and that further contributions from nutri-

tional epidemiology are needed to establish and evaluate effective public health policy.

DESCRIPTIVE EPIDEMIOLOGY

A genetic component in the etiology of NTDs has been long suspected because a previously affected pregnancy and a family history of an affected pregnancy are risk factors. However, other epidemiologic features clearly indicate major nongenetic contributions to risk (Elwood and Elwood, 1980). Rates have varied greatly by geographic area, including a striking increasing gradient from south to north in the United Kingdom and Ireland. Groups who have migrated from these high-risk areas to the south of Britain or to the United States have much lower risks of a pregnancy with an NTD. Rates of NTDs have also changed markedly over time within areas. For example, an epidemic of NTDs, recognized only in retrospect, appears to have occurred in Boston during the Great Depression, and rates have steadily declined afterward (Fig. 18–1). Although war and other social disruptions have been associated with increases in rates, in most areas rates have been declining, even before regular screening during pregnancy further reduced their occurrence. For example, in Dublin the prevalence at birth declined from 4.7/1,000 in 1980 to 1.3/1,000 over a 12-year period, during which time breakfast cereals were fortified with folic acid and vitamin B_{12} (Kirke et al., 1993).

CLINICAL OBSERVATIONS AND EARLY INTERVENTION STUDIES

Because of observations that rates of NTDs were high in economically disadvantaged populations that appeared to have poor diets, Smithells and colleagues in the United Kingdom assessed the diets and blood levels of mothers of children with NTDs; values were low for several micronutrients, including folic acid (Smithells et al., 1976). Further observations that some drugs that interfere with folate metabolism increase the risk of NTDs suggested that low intake of this nutrient was likely to be etiologically important (Rhoads and Mills, 1984; Milunsky, 1986). Because of a suggested benefit of folic acid and ethical concerns about the use of a placebo, Smithells et al. were constrained from conducting a randomized prevention trial. Thus, he and others undertook a nonrandomized intervention trial in the United Kingdom using a multivitamin, multimineral supplement among women who had already experienced an NTD pregnancy (Smithells et al., 1980, 1981). Women who were otherwise eligible and presented for antenatal care after the 6th week from their last menstrual period (at which time the neural tube normally closes) served as controls. A large reduction in risk was seen among supplemented women (1/200 pregnancies, 0.5%) compared with unsupplemented women (13/300, 4%; $p < 0.01$). Smithells and coworkers (1983) repeated this protocol and

again found a large reduction in NTD pregnancies among supplemented women (2/234 supplemented and 11/215 unsupplemented women, $p < 0.01$). Reductions in NTDs were also seen in other small, nonrandomized intervention studies and in one very small randomized trial (Laurence et al., 1981; Holmes-Siedle et al., 1982; Vergel et al., 1990), but the results were not statistically significant. Collectively, the reduction in risk was greater than fourfold.

CASE–CONTROL AND COHORT STUDIES OF FOLIC ACID INTAKE

In part concurrent with the early intervention studies, the relationship of folic acid intake to risk of NTDs was examined in several case–control studies (Table 18–1). Most of these studies examined the use of multiple vitamins, which typically contain 0.4 mg of folic acid (or 0.8 mg in prenatal preparations), which is substantially greater than the average daily dietary folate intake in the United States (about 0.2 mg/day); only four studies assessed folate from diet. (The contrast between folic acid from supplements and folate from foods is actually even greater because the food sources are only about half as bioavailable as the chemically pure folic acid in supplements [Gregory, 1995].) A major potential advantage of evaluating use of vitamin supplements is that they are started and stopped at distinct times, and thus their use during the critical first 4 weeks of gestation can be assessed. However, prenatal multiple vitamins containing folate are routinely prescribed during pregnancy; because they are often started after the time of neural tube closure, errors by only a few weeks in commencement of vitamin supplement use can result in misclassification.

The first two large case–control studies generated enormous controversy because they came to opposite conclusions. The Atlanta study conducted by Mulinare et al. (1988) identified cases ascertained by a birth defect registry; both a general popu-

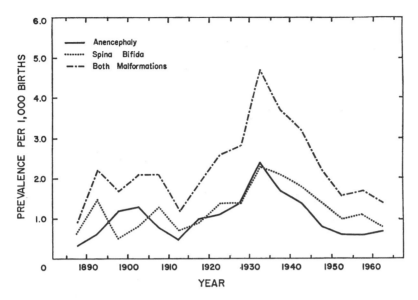

Figure 18–1. Frequency of anencephaly and Spina bifida in the two hospitals combined, 1885–1965. (From MacMahon and Yen, 1971; reproduced with permission.)

lation sample and children with other birth defects served as controls. Mothers of cases and controls were asked in retrospect about periconceptional use of multiple vitamins; for some women this referred to a pregnancy up to 14 years earlier. Risk of an NTD was about 60% lower for women who used supplements, and the association was similar using either control series. In contrast, no association was seen by Mills et al. (1989) in a large study conducted in California and Illinois. Strong apparent protective effects of periconceptional multiple vitamin use were also seen by Bower and Stanley (1989) and Werler et al. (1993). Shaw et al. (1995) also found an inverse association for use of folate-containing multiple vitamins before pregnancy and during the first 3 months of gestation. As this large case–control study was conducted in California, it was of particular interest because Mills et al. (1989) had speculated that the somewhat lower rates of NTDs in that state might have explained the lack of association between folic acid intake and NTDs. However, Shaw and colleagues (1995) also found a similar reduc-

tion in risk associated with use of multiple vitamins started after the first 3 months of pregnancy, which raises concern about the causal nature of their findings.

The relationship between periconceptional folic acid supplements and risk of NTDs was examined in only one prospective study, conducted by Milunsky et al. (1989). In this study, women who provided either blood or amniotic fluid samples at the end of the first trimester of pregnancy for purposes of birth defect screening were interviewed by telephone immediately after submitting the specimens and then before diagnosis. This proximity to the critical period for neural tube closure allowed a detailed assessment of timing and type of multiple vitamin preparation. A strong inverse association (relative risk [RR] 0.27; 95% confidence interval [CI], 0.12 to 0.59) was seen between use of a folic acid–containing multiple vitamin during the first 6 weeks of pregnancy and risk of NTD (Table 18–2). This was highly specific because use starting after this time was unrelated to risk.

In each of the four studies that examined

Table 18–1. Case–control studies of periconceptional multiple vitamin use and risk of NTDs

Study	Supplement use		RR (95% CI)
	Cases	Controls	
Mulinare et al. (1988)	24/178	404/1,470	0.4 (0.3–0.7)
Mills et al. (1989)	100/565	103/567	0.9 (0.8–1.1)
Bower and Stanley (1989)	12/77	16/77	0.7 (0.3–1.8)
Werler et al. (1993)	34/436	339/1,253	0.6 (0.4–0.8)
Shaw et al. (1995)	88/538	98/539	0.7 (0.5–0.9)

intake of folate from diet, inverse associations with risk of NTDs were seen among women who did not take supplements. Milunsky et al. (1989) found an increase in risk only among women with the lowest folic acid intake assessed by a limited food-frequency questionnaire (RR, 0.4; 95% CI, 0.16 to 1.15 for 0.1 mg/day vs. ≤ 0.1 mg /day), but the analysis was limited by the small number of cases among supplement nonusers. Werler et al. (1993) found a significant inverse dose–response relationship with dietary intake assessed by a food-frequency questionnaire; the relative risk for more than 0.3 mg/day was 0.6 compared with intakes less than 0.2 mg/day, p value for trend = 0.02. Inverse associations with dietary intake were also seen by Bower and Stanley (1989) and Shaw et al. (1995). Although these data on folate from food sources add further support for an effect within the range of existing diets, because of the limited number of cases the confidence intervals were too wide to convey precision regarding the dose–response relationship.

With one exception, the case–control and cohort studies have supported a protective effect of periconceptional use of multiple vitamins and are consistent with the randomized trials as discussed below. It may be of value to consider, in retrospect, possible methodologic reasons for the lack of association found in the study by Mills et al. (1989). At face value, this study appeared superior to the study by Mulinare et al. (1988) because it was designed specifically to address this issue and mothers were interviewed as soon as possible after identification of the birth defect. However, the percentage of case mothers who were contacted and interviewed may have been as low as 43%, and those who were lost are likely to have been less health conscious and less likely to use vitamin supplements (Shaw et al., 1995). Also, women were specifically told not to report vitamin use that was started because of the pregnancy, which is likely to have excluded a substantial proportion of vitamin use before neural tube closure; even this definition was apparently not systematically applied because spontaneous reports of such use by the participants were included (Mills et al., 1990; Milunsky et al., 1990). The wording of the question regarding multiple vitamin use was not included in the original report so that this potential for misclassification was not apparent. Although some role of chance, and possibly other factors, cannot be excluded, this experience suggests that shortcomings in the implementation of epidemiologic studies can lead to serious biases and also suggests the value of including in published reports the exact wording of questions used to define exposure, perhaps as an appendix.

Viewed collectively, the inverse relationship between periconceptional multiple vitamin use and risk of NTDs observed in all but one of the previously noted studies is highly unlikely to be the result of chance. Because of the variety of study designs and sources for controls, recall bias or other methodologic artifacts are also unlikely explanations of these collective results. The main concern, given this evidence, is the possibility of confounding at two levels; first, that women who used multiple vitamins were at decreased risk of NTDs for

Table 18–2. Prevalence of neural tube defects according to intake of folic acid–containing multivitamins and their time of use[a]

	None	Weeks 1–6		Weeks 7+ only	
		Folic acid +	Folic acid −	Folic acid +	Folic acid −
No. of cases	11	10	3	25	0
Total	3,157	10,713	926	7,795	66
Prevalence per 1,000	3.5	0.9	3.2	3.2	—
Prevalence ratio estimate	1.00	0.27	0.93	0.92	—
95% confidence interval	—	0.12–0.59	0.26–3.3	0.45–1.87	—

[a] As reported in response to the question, "Did you take a multivitamin in the first 3 months of pregnancy?" If yes, "What week of pregnancy did you start the multivitamin?" (in practice based on date of last menstrual period).

(From Milunsky et al., 1989; reproduced with permission.).

reasons unrelated to folate intake (perhaps socioeconomic or behavioral differences) and, second, that vitamins other than folic acid in the multiple vitamin preparations were responsible for the reduction in NTDs. Although confounding by unmeasured socioeconomic or behavioral risk factors is, in principle, a possible explanation for the observed inverse associations, this is unlikely for several reasons. First, to account for the magnitude of association in most of the studies—overall approximately fourfold in the nonrandomized intervention studies and approximately threefold in the case–control and cohort studies apart from that of Mills et al. (1989)—would require an even stronger unknown risk factor that was also highly correlated with multiple vitamin use. Although multiple vitamin use has usually been found to be associated with indicators of higher education and income, these associations have been too weak to account for confounding by even a very strong unmeasured variable. Also, all of the case–control and cohort studies, including the null study of Mills et al. (1989), measured and controlled for a variety of socioeconomic variables; doing so did not appreciably alter the associations in any of these studies. Had there been some change in the magnitude of associations when these

potential confounders were controlled, the possibility of residual confounding by imperfectly measured lifestyle factors would have been more plausible; the robustness of the associations diminishes the likelihood of this source of confounding. The second level of potential confounding, due to other components in the multiple vitamins, could not be refuted by the case–control and cohort studies because most multiple vitamins contained folic acid, precluding the ability to study separately preparations with and without folic acid.

CASE–CONTROL AND COHORT STUDIES OF FOLIC ACID BLOOD LEVELS

Studies of blood levels of folic acid and NTDs are difficult to conduct because the specimen collection should occur just before conception or within a few weeks thereafter. If obtained later, serious misclassification will result because many women will have started supplements, and their blood levels will not represent levels during the critical period of exposure. Also, plasma folate is labile and should be stored at an ultra-low temperature to avoid degradation. Because of these strict requirements, few studies using blood folic acid levels have been published; these are relatively recent and small.

The most detailed evaluation of blood folate levels and risk of NTDs has been conducted by Daly and colleagues (1995), who enrolled 56,049 Irish women in a prospective study. Blood samples were collected at the time of the first antenatal visit, separated into plasma and whole blood, and frozen. In this cohort, 84 women who had provided blood had pregnancies affected by NTDs; using a nested case–control design, these cases were matched 1:3 with unaffected control pregnancies. Both plasma and red cell folic acid levels were lower for cases than for controls. A continuous linear dose–response relationship with red cell folate was seen without indication of any plateau (Fig. 18–2). Importantly, increased risks were seen at red cell folic acid levels even well above those thought to represent deficiency (140 mg/ml).

Wald and colleagues (1996) have provided a meta-analysis of studies of blood folic acid levels and risk of NTDs; as observed by Daly and colleagues (1995), inverse relationships were seen with both serum or plasma and red cell folic acid levels for bloods collected at the time of first antenatal visit or the first trimester. Not surprisingly, in studies that used blood collected after delivery there was little overall association.

RANDOMIZED TRIALS

The clearest evidence on the relationship of folic acid and NTDs has come from the Medical Research Council's randomized trial in five European countries, Israel, and Canada (MRC Vitamin Study Research Group, 1991). In a 2 × 2 factorial design, women with a previous neural tube pregnancy were randomized to 4 mg of folic acid daily or to a placebo and to other vitamins usually contained in multivitamins or their placebo. The high dose of folic acid was chosen to minimize the chance of a negative result, not because the investigators had any biologic basis for believing this dose was necessary. The trial was stopped early because a statistically significant 72% protective effect of folic acid was observed; no significant effect of the other vitamins was seen (Table 18–3).

Another large randomized trial was conducted in Hungary by Czeizel and Dudas (1992) among women without a previous history of NTDs. The supplement was a multivitamin/multimineral tablet taken daily that included 0.8 mg of folic acid. The trial was stopped prematurely because six pregnancies with NTDs had occurred among women taking placebo and none among those taking the active supplement, and to continue was deemed unethical. Interestingly, congenital abnormalities other than NTDs were also reduced among pregnancies of women receiving the supplement (Czeizel, 1993).

STUDIES OF GENETIC MARKERS AND METABOLIC INDICATORS

The demonstration that folic acid has a major role in the prevention of NTDs has fueled further research into its mechanism and the possibility of nutrient–gene interactions, in particular that some individuals are more susceptible to low folate intakes. This research has also been stimulated by the discovery of a functionally important variant of a gene coding an enzyme that metabolizes folic acid.

The implicated metabolic pathway is the same as that linking homocysteine to coronary heart disease (and is extended in Fig. 18–3). Although higher levels of homocysteine resulting from low activity of methionine synthase are hypothesized to increase risk of cardiovascular disease, low activity of this enzyme would also lead to lower availability of methionine. Methionine availability, by providing methyl groups for methylation of DNA, influences gene expression, and thus perhaps embryogenesis. Other mechanisms are also possible because the availability of methyl groups is essential for many reactions; it remains

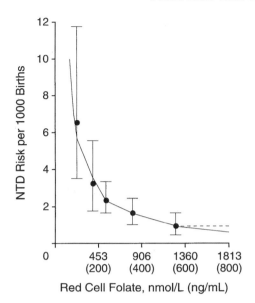

Figure 18–2. Relationship of red cell folate levels to neural tube defect (NTD) risk. The solid line gives the predicted risk using logistic regression. (From Daly et al., 1995; reproduced with permission.)

possible that homocysteine is itself toxic to the developing embryo. The findings that higher maternal homocysteine levels both after (Steegers-Theunissen et al., 1994) and during (Mills et al., 1995) pregnancy are associated with risk of NTDs has supported a role for this metabolic pathway.

In 1995, Frosst and colleagues reported a common polymorphism (677C→T) in the 5,10-methylenetetrahydrofolate reductase (MTHFR) gene that is associated with reduced activity of this enzyme. Persons who are homozygous for this polymorphism (about 5% of Whites) have higher plasma levels of homocysteine, presumably because inadequate amounts of 5-methyltetrahydrofolate are available for maximal activity of the methionine synthase enzyme. These elevations in homocysteine can be corrected with higher intake of folic acid (Ma et al., 1996). In a Dutch case–control study (van der Put et al., 1995), an increased prevalence of the homozygous MTHFR polymorphism was seen in both infants with NTDs (13%) and

their parents (16% of mothers and 10% of fathers) compared with unaffected controls (5%) (odds ratio [OR], 2.9; 95% CI, 1.0 to 7.9 for affected infants vs. controls). This genotype by itself thus accounted for 9% of NTD pregnancies. This finding has been confirmed by Whitehead et al. (1995), who observed a relative risk of 3.5 (95% CI, 1.3 to 9.4) for affected cases and of 3.5 (95% CI, 1.2 to 10.2) for parents of cases; the population attributable risk was 13%. Ou et al. (1996) also found a positive association (RR, 7.2; 95% CI, 1.8 to 30.3) for affected cases. The gene–environment interaction (i.e., between intake of folic acid and MTHFR genotype) was not examined directly in these studies. However, the relationship between this genotype and NTDs is likely to explain, in part, the role of folic acid because higher intake is needed in the presence of reduced activity of MTHFR to provide the same level of methionine synthase function. Because the attributable risk due to this genotype is small compared with that for low folate intake, which has been estimated to be 50% to 70% (Centers for Disease Control and Prevention, 1992), either other genetic susceptibilities exist or folic acid also reduces risk in persons without a specific susceptibility.

In the search for other genetic susceptibilities, a variant in the gene coding methionine synthase is an obvious suspect. Support for a critical role of this enzyme in the causation of NTDs was provided by Kirke et al. (1993), who found that lower plasma vitamin B_{12} levels in blood samples collected at the first antenatal clinic visit predicted risk of defects independently of folic acid level. This finding implicates methionine synthase because it is the only enzyme that requires both folate and vitamin B_{12}. Further evidence was provided by Adams and colleagues (1995), who found that maternal midtrimester levels of a metabolic indicator of low vitamin B_{12} availability, serum methylmalonic acid, were strongly associated with risk of NTDs. However, in the meta-analysis of Wald and colleagues

Table 18–3. Prevalence of neural tube defects (NTDs) according to randomization group in the MRC study

Folic acid	Other vitamins	NTD/alt		Relative risk: folic acid *vs.* nonfolic acid (95% CI)
+	−	2/298	} 6/593 (1.0%) }	
+	+	4/295		
−	−	13/300	}21/602 (3.5%) }	0.28 (0.12–0.71)
−	+	8/302		

(From the MRC Vitamin Study Research Group, 1991; reproduced with permission.)

(1996), which included the data of Kirke and colleagues (1993), a crude association between blood vitamin B_{12} levels and risk of defect was no longer apparent after controlling for levels of folic acid. It is also notable that in women in the MRC trial assigned to multiple vitamins without folic acid, but did include vitamin B_{12}, no reduction in risk was seen. The relationship of vitamin B_{12} to risk of NTDs is presently unresolved; however, lack of an association would not exclude a role of genetic variation in the function of methionine synthase. Although functionally important polymorphisms have not been identified at this time, they are being actively sought in multiple laboratories.

A SYNTHESIS OF DATA

The possibility of a relationship between folic acid intake and risk of NTDs raised a

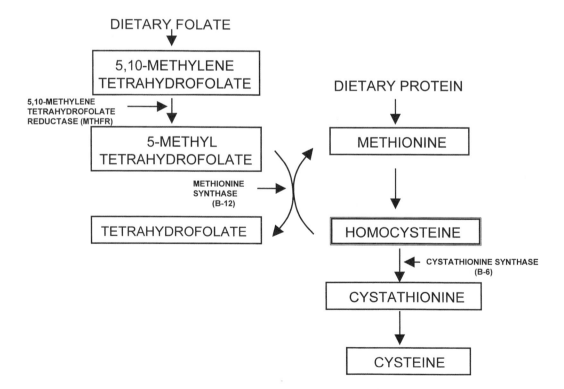

Figure 18–3. Pathways of folate metabolism.

series of important practical questions, including

1. Is low intake of folic acid causally related to risk of defects?
2. Will higher intake prevent defects in pregnancies that have not been preceded by an affected pregnancy or recurrent defects?
3. What is the dose–response relationship? In particular, what is the minimal intake that will produce maximal reduction in incidence?
4. What percentage of cases could be prevented by additional folic acid?
5. Can women be identified who are particularly susceptible to affected pregnancies and who would benefit from higher folate intake?

No single study has been able to provide answers to more than one or two of these questions, and a maximal understanding requires the synthesis of data from a variety of sources. Although other evidence that folic acid prevented NTDs was strong, the MRC trial (MRC Vitamin Study Research Group, 1991) provided the clearest documentation of a causal effect and that folic acid itself was the active component of multiple vitamins. Although prevention programs might have been based on the provision of multiple vitamins without this knowledge, this degree of specificity is needed to embark on fortification programs.

Largely for reasons of statistical power, the MRC study was conducted among women who had already experienced an NTD pregnancy. Because of this, there was reluctance to generalize the findings to the prevention of first occurrences (Willett, 1992); indeed, the initial guidelines issued by the Centers for Disease Control only included women with a previous affected pregnancy (Centers for Disease Control and Prevention, 1991). The large majority of NTDs occur without a history of a previously affected pregnancy; thus, recommendations limited to high-risk women would have limited impact. The body of

evidence available provides an excellent example of how data from observational epidemiologic and randomized trials can be most informative when viewed as being complementary. In the case–control and cohort studies indicating a benefit of multiple vitamins, the large majority of cases were first occurrences, thus providing a strong empirical basis for generalizing the findings to the population as a whole. Subsequently, the randomized trial by Czeizel and Dudas (1992) conducted among women without a previously affected pregnancy, although based on small numbers because of the ethical imperative to stop, provided further direct support for generalizing to first occurrences.

The dose of folic acid used in the MRC trial was 4 mg daily, a level far above the average dietary intake (about 0.2 mg per day in the United States); this was chosen to ensure a large contrast and because this dose had been used in a small intervention study that appeared to show benefit (Laurence et al., 1981). However, in the observational studies, including the prospective study by Milunsky et al. (1989) in which the reduction in risk was identical to the MRC trial, the multiple vitamins used typically contained 0.4 mg of folic acid. Also, the doses were 0.36 mg/day in the intervention study by Smithells and colleagues (1983) and 0.8 in that by Czeizel and Dudas (1992). Collectively, these findings provide strong evidence that a supplement dose much lower than 4 mg/day, including 0.4 mg/day, would be similarly effective, at least for the prevention of first occurrences. Whether higher doses are needed for prevention of recurrences cannot be known for certain. Although the etiology of first occurrences and recurrences must overlap considerably (because the pattern of familial risk does not behave as a highly penetrant genetic defect), it is possible that families with a history of NTDs are enriched with individuals having a very high requirement for folic acid.

The level of folic acid intake needed for maximal prevention of NTDs might also be estimated using intermediate markers of risk if, in turn, good dose–response relationships were available relating these markers to risk. Plasma and red cell folate are obvious potential markers; as noted above, the data relating levels to risk are limited. In the most detailed data available, Daly et al. (1995) found no evidence for a threshold above which higher intake would not further reduce risk of NTDs. On the basis of data relating intake to blood levels, they estimated that consuming an extra 0.4 mg/day of folic acid in addition to existing diets would prevent 48% of NTDs and that higher levels of supplementation would have only a small additional benefit. Whether blood levels of homocysteine are directly related to the etiology of NTDs or are only an indicator of folic acid intake, they can provide another criterion for estimating optimal intake. Using this approach, a roughly similar conclusion was reached by Oakley et al. (1996).

The percentage of NTDs in a population that are potentially preventable by supplementation with folic acid can be estimated as the preventable fraction multiplied by the proportion of cases in a population that were not already exposed to supplements (population preventable fraction = $PF \times P_1$). The preventable fraction is $(1 - RR)$, where the relative risk is obtained from an observational study or a randomized trial (Rothman, 1986). For example, in the prospective study of Milunsky and colleagues (1989) (Table 18–2), the relative risk was 0.27 and the proportion of cases who were unexposed (i.e., their mothers did not take folic acid supplements during the critical period) was 0.82. Thus,

$$\text{Population preventable fraction} = (1 - 0.27) \times 0.82 = 0.60$$

The relative risk from the MRC trial of recurrent defects was similar (0.28), which, if applied to a population with the same existing rate of supplement usage, would yield virtually the same preventable fraction. Using this approach in combination

with the full literature, the Centers for Disease Control (1992) has estimated that 50% of cases of NTDs in the United States could be prevented by universal supplementation with folic acid among women in the reproductive ages. In absolute numbers, this corresponds to about 1,500 of the approximately 3,000 cases of spina bifida or anencephaly that occur annually in the United States. The population preventable fraction, of course, depends on the background dietary intake of folic acid and the percentage of women already using supplements. For example, the percentage reduction would probably have been considerably higher in Northern Ireland, where rates of NTDs were extremely high before fortification of breakfast cereals (Kirke et al., 1993). Even for the United States, however, the potential reduction of an important disease is large, particularly for a modest nutritional modification.

A genetic susceptibility has been long suspected because a family history of an NTD is a risk factor for this condition. Although this could have resulted from a familial behavior, such as avoidance of folate-rich foods, the documentation that the 677C→T polymorphism in the MTHFR gene is associated with NTD occurrence establishes a genetic risk. Whether polymorphisms in MTHFR account for the known familial risk is not clear. As shown in the MRC study, those with a family history of NTD benefit substantially from folic acid supplements; those with the homozygous MTHFR polymorphisms probably do, but this has not been directly documented. Whether other genetic susceptibilities will be found is presently unclear.

POLICY IMPLICATIONS

Although low folic acid intake conclusively increases risk of NTDs and many details of this relationship are known, the appropriate policy responses are not totally clear and have been the topic of great controversy (Willett, 1992; Beresford, 1994; Wald, 1994; Oakley et al., 1995, 1996;

Wald and Bower, 1995; Mills et al., 1996; Rayburn et al., 1996). Given the need to increase folic acid intake, three main strategies are possible: increase intake of foods rich in folic acid (particularly certain fruits and vegetables), use vitamin supplements, and fortify the food supply with folic acid.

A strong tradition appears to exist among nutritionists that goals for nutrient intakes should be achieved by changing food intake. There is some reason for this; increasing intake of fruits and vegetables would augment intake of many nutrients and phytochemicals believed to be beneficial for a variety of conditions, and toxicity would be extremely unlikely. A general increase in intake of fruits and vegetables is desirable for many reasons, and the associations between dietary folate intake and risk of NTDs consistently seen in case–control and cohort studies indicate that improvement in diets can have a beneficial impact. However, there is also evidence that pursuing this as a public health strategy will have limited effect on occurrence of NTDs. The first reason is that, as described above, large increases in intakes and blood levels appear to be needed to achieve maximal benefits. Despite intensive national programs to increase fruits and vegetables, only very modest changes have been seen. In addition, folate contained in foods has rather low and variable bioavailability compared with pure folic acid itself (Gregory, 1995). In the Framingham Heart Study population, only participants in the highest decile of dietary folate intakes (about 0.55 mg/day on average) had intakes sufficient to maximally reduce plasma homocysteine levels, and their plasma folate levels were still lower than those taking a folate supplement (Tucker et al., 1996). A small randomized trial of various strategies to increase folate levels has been conducted by Cuskelly and colleagues (1996), who compared supplementation (0.4 mg/day), food fortification, free provision of folate-rich foods, dietary advice to eat folate-rich foods, and a control group. Dietary advice increased plasma levels by about 60%, which was not statistically significant. In contrast, provision of folate-rich foods and fortification more than doubled plasma levels, and supplementation tripled levels. As many practical barriers exist to making major dietary changes, including price and availability to low income populations, the effectiveness of this approach will be limited.

The second general strategy for prevention would be to recommend folic acid supplements for women during their reproductive years. This strategy is most directly supported by epidemiologic intervention studies and has been recommended by the Centers for Disease Control (1992). Specifically, all women who could potentially become pregnant are advised to take 0.4 mg of folic acid daily, and those with a previously affected pregnancy or other special indications, as noted above, are advised to take 4 mg daily. The recommendation applies to all potentially pregnant women because the critical period for neural tube closure occurs before pregnancy is recognized by many women. The cost of this is modest as multiple vitamins containing folic acid can be purchased for as low as $10 to $20 per year, which is minor compared with the cost of doubling fruit and vegetable consumption. The primary limitation of this approach is that not all women will be compliant; this is most likely to be problematic among low income groups who could benefit the most. Nevertheless, this strategy will be effective among those who comply. It is now supported by the Preventive Medicine Task Force (U.S. Preventive Services Task Force, 1996), and failure of a physician to advise women appropriately might well be considered negligence if a child was affected with an NTD.

Strategies to increase folic acid intake by dietary advice or by supplementation could be targeted to the population at large or by screening individuals at high risk and focusing interventions on them. However, a basis for screening is not established. An obvious screening test might be blood folic acid level. However, this can fluctuate over time, requiring repeated monitoring, and would be costlier than providing supplements to everyone. Moreover, the data of Daly et al. (1995) suggest that the majority of the population is at some increased risk. A genetic marker of susceptibility might be more practical as this would be performed only once. However, as noted above, the one established marker, the homozygous polymorphism of MTHFR, accounts for only a small fraction of cases. Thus, at present there does not appear to be a basis for screening, beyond asking about family and personal history of NTDs, to identify a limited group for intervention.

The third main strategy for increasing a population's intake of folic acid is fortification of the food supply. This has strong precedent as flour in the United States and many countries is already fortified with iron and other B vitamins. As a public health strategy, this is potentially the most effective because it can reach almost the entire population and does not depend on constant education and motivation. Although attractive, the level of fortification has generated major controversy because of uncertainties regarding the amount needed to minimize risk of NTDs coupled with concern about the safety of high intakes. Concern about safety is related to the capacity of folic acid to correct anemia due to vitamin B_{12} deficiency, thus delaying the diagnosis and allowing the neurologic complications of B_{12} deficiency to progress (the so-called masking of vitamin B_{12} deficiency). There is considerable controversy about the level of folic acid needed for masking and the frequency with which it occurs; this is clearly a rare event as few, if any, cases have been noted in recent decades despite the use of multiple vitamin supplements containing 0.4 mg of folic acid by about 25% of U.S. adults. Given a mandate to avoid any appreciable risk, the Food and Drug Administration has considered intake above 1.0 mg/day from food plus supplements to be of concern, but others have argued that even somewhat higher

levels would entail minimal risks (Wald, 1994; Oakley et al., 1995).

Individuals consume different amounts of foods that might be fortified, for example, flour. Thus, fortification would shift the population distribution of folic acid intake to higher levels by adding the distribution due to fortification to the distribution from usual food sources and supplements. The combined effect has been evaluated by using food intake data from several populations based on multiple diet records per subject, assigning values for folic acid or total folate to products made from flour assuming different fortification policies and recalculating the population distribution of intake for each of these several scenarios (Fig. 18–4). Using this approach, it becomes apparent that to increase substantially intakes for most of the population, for example, to the 0.4 mg of folic acid recommended by the Centers for Disease Control, median intakes need to be considerably higher. In the simulations (Fig. 18–4), fortifying flour with 0.35 mg of folic acid per 100 g of flour (about five times the level of wheat before milling) would increase average intake by about 0.25 mg per day, still leaving about 30% of women with total folate intakes below 0.4 mg/day (Oakley et al., 1995). However, total folate consumption from foods, supplements, and fortification in this scenario would be more than 1.0 mg for 15% of the population, almost all of them multiple vitamin users. Fortification with 0.14 mg/100 g of flour would increase average intake by only about 0.1 mg per day; because intake for women would increase by considerably less than this amount because of lower total energy intake, this strategy is likely to have only a modest effect on rates of NTDs. However, the Food and Drug Administration (1996) elected to use the 0.14 mg/100 g of flour as the fortification strategy, to be implemented in 1998.

The decision about level of fortification involves balancing of clear benefits for some against unproven and probably rare

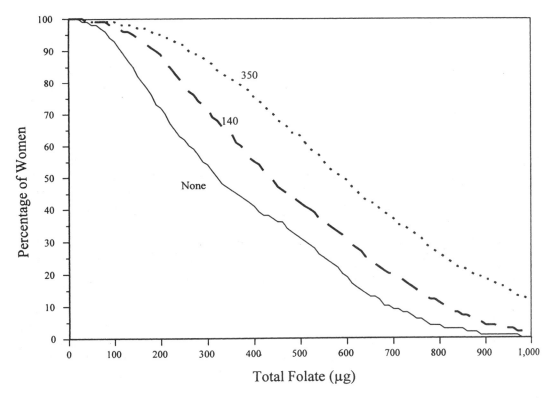

Figure 18–4. Percentage of women aged 19 to 50 years with mean daily intake of total folate greater than or equal to specified amount, by grain fortification level (ug/100g). (Courtesy of G. Oakley.)

hazards for others. Also part of a rational decision-making process is the unproven but likely reduction in coronary heart disease incidence that is probably numerically far greater than either NTDs or masking of vitamin B_{12} deficiency (Boushey et al., 1995; Tucker et al., 1996), as well as possible reduction in colon cancer incidence. The complexities of this decision-making process in the face of uncertainty is beyond the scope of this chapter. However, one solution that has been proposed is to require that folic acid supplements also contain 0.4 mg of vitamin B_{12}, which would ensure that almost all persons who would ingest more than 1.0 mg of folic acid would receive sufficient vitamin B_{12} to prevent deficiency (Oakley et al., 1996; Herbert and Bigaouette, 1997).

Uncertainties are best resolved by addi-

tional data, and it may be useful to consider the types of studies that are needed. To determine whether the level of fortification is adequate, in principle, rates of NTDs could be tracked to determine the degree to which the 50% to 70% reduction is achieved. This may be possible in several existing registries of birth defects, but the interpretation may be complicated because the rate has been steadily declining for many years and would be expected to decline further due to greater use of supplements by women who may conceive. An ancillary method could be to conduct an additional observational study of vitamin supplement use and occurrence of NTDs. If fortification is adequate, supplement use should no longer be protective. The development of a registry for masked pernicious anemia would be desirable to investigate incidence before and after fortification, but this may not be feasible. A case–control study of such events, perhaps imbedded in the registry, would be valuable to determine if they are associated with folic acid consumption. Finally, policies regarding folic acid fortification may ultimately be decided more by the relationship with coronary heart disease and colon cancer; thus more definitive data on these relationships are needed.

BROADER IMPLICATIONS FOR NUTRITIONAL EPIDEMIOLOGY

The definitive evidence that folic acid supplementation greatly decreases incidence of NTDs has major implications for our concepts of nutritional deficiency. The conventional wisdom in nutrition has been that, apart from secondary effects of other diseases, deficiencies do not exist in the United States and other affluent countries and that the use of vitamin supplements by apparently well persons has no benefit. The benefit of folic acid supplementation in prevention of NTDs is clear documentation that this paradigm is incorrect. Scott and colleagues (1994) have argued that NTDs may be the result of a metabolic defect rather than a deficiency of folic acid. However, this distinction becomes blurred when the susceptible genotype is common. For example, the homozygous MTHFR genotype associated with NTDs is 5% to 10% and still accounts for a minority of cases. A gene frequency this common is hard to define as a defect and suggests that it may even have some survival advantages. Indeed, we have observed that it is associated with a lower risk of colon cancer (Chen et al., 1996; Ma et al., 1996). Alternatively, these polymorphisms may be regarded as genetic determinants of the variations in nutrient requirements that are likely to exist for most dietary factors and that should be considered when setting Recommended Daily Allowances for populations.

The documented relationship between folic acid and NTDs provides an important additional reason to pursue other evidence that suboptimal intakes of many dietary factors may be important in the etiology of numerous chronic diseases. Progress has been remarkably rapid in the area of folic acid and NTDs, in part because of features that may be almost unique. First, the critical temporal window is very narrow and known a priori within a few days, in contrast to uncertainties measured by decades for most cancers. Second, the interval between the critical exposure and knowledge of the outcome is only several months, or even weeks if the defects are ascertained by screening during pregnancy. Third, the exposure can be assessed in multiple ways, including from diet, use of supplements, and with readily available biochemical indicators. Fourth, randomized trials can be conducted with relative ease as the intervention can be a safe and convenient supplement and the required duration of the intervention is short for reasons noted above. Fifth, the magnitude of effect of diet and supplementation is large and may be greater than most other diet–disease relationships. Although much can be learned from the experiences in elucidating the folic acid and NTD relationship, additional patience and perseverance will be needed to resolve other issues in nutritional epidemiology, and many may never be known with such certainty and precision.

The folic acid–NTD relationship represents one of the first areas in which modern molecular genetics has played a role in understanding a diet–disease relationship. Although the causal role of folic acid was established before the relationship between a polymorphism in the MTHFR gene and the occurrence of defects was discovered, it is interesting to consider the possibility that an earlier discovery of this relationship might have eliminated the need for a randomized trial. Prior to the randomized trial, the evidence from case–control and cohort studies was strong that some aspect of vitamin supplements reduced occurrence of NTDs, and there were multiple reasons to implicate folic acid. The main residual concern was that confounding by something else in the supplements or another lifestyle factor might explain the association. Because MTHFR has no other role than in folate metabolism, it would be hard to account for a clear and reproducible association between a functionally important polymorphism in this gene and risk of defect if folic acid were not causally related to risk. Although direct evidence from a supplementation trial may be more appealing, in circumstances when a randomized trial may be less feasible, a similar level of support for causal relationships may in the future be obtained from a combination of observational studies that include both measures of dietary or supplemental intake and genetic markers of nutrient metabolism.

SUMMARY

Evidence from a wide variety of sources, including case–control and cohort studies and randomized trials, has documented that use of multiple vitamins early in pregnancy can reduce the risk of NTDs by more than half, that the active factor in these supplements is primarily or entirely folic acid, and that the minimal dose for full benefit is approximately 0.4 mg per day. Although the basic relationship is established, additional work is needed to define possible gene–diet interactions, to determine the optimal level of food fortification, and to investigate whether suboptimal vitamin B_{12} status can contribute to the etiology of these defects.

REFERENCES

Adams, M. J., Jr., M. J. Khoury, K. S. Scanlon, R. E. Stevenson, G. J. Knight, J. E. Haddow, G. C. Sylvester, J. E. Cheek, J. P. Henry, S. P. Stabler, and R. H. Allen (1995). Elevated midtrimester serum methylmalonic acid levels as a risk factor for neural tube defects. *Teratology 51*, 311–317.

Beresford, S. A. A. (1994). Annotation: How do we get enough folic acid to prevent some neural tube defects? *Am J Public Health 84*, 348–350.

Boushey, C. J., S. A. A. Beresford, G. S. Omenn, and A. G. Motulsky (1995). A quantitative assessment of plasma homocysteine as a risk factor for vascular disease: Probable benefits of increasing folic acid intakes. *JAMA 274*, 1049–1057.

Bower, C., and F. J. Stanley (1989). Dietary folate as a risk factor for neural tube defects: Evidence from a case–control study in Western Australia. *Med J Aust 150*, 613–619.

Centers for Disease Control and Prevention (1991). Use of folic acid for prevention of spina bifida and other neural tube defects—1983–1991. *Morbid Mortal Weekly Rep 40*, 513–516.

Centers for Disease Control and Prevention (1992). Recommendations for the use of folic acid to reduce the number of cases of spina bifida and other neural tube defects. *Morbid Mortal Weekly Rep 41(No.RR-14)*, 1–7.

Chen, J., E. Giovannucci, K. Kelsey, E. B. Rimm, M. J. Stampfer, G. A. Colditz, D. Spiegelman, W. C. Willett, and D. J. Hunter (1996). A methylenetetrahydrofolate reductase polymorphism and the risk of colorectal cancer. *Cancer Res 56*, 4862–4864.

Cuskelly, G. J., H. McNulty, and J. M. Scott (1996). Effect of increasing dietary folate on red-cell folate: Implications for prevention of neural tube defects. *Lancet 347*, 657–659.

Czeizel, A. E. (1993). Prevention of congenital abnormalities by periconceptional multivitamin supplementation. *BMJ 306*, 1645–1648.

Czeizel, A. E., and I. Dudas (1992). Prevention of the first occurrence of neural tube defects by periconceptual vitamin supplementation. *N Engl J Med 327*, 1832–1835.

Daly, L. E., P. N. Kirke, A. Molloy, D. G. Weir, and J. M. Scott (1995). Folate levels and neural tube defects: Implications for prevention. *JAMA 274*, 1698–1702.

Elwood, J. M., and J. H. Elwood (1980). *Epidemiology of Anencephalus and Spina Bifida*. New York: Oxford University Press.

Food and Drug Administration (1996). Food standards: Amendment of standards of identity for enriched grain products to require addition of folic acid. *Fed Regr 61*, 8781–8797.

Frosst, P., H. J. Blom, R. Milos, P. Goyette, C. A. Sheppard, R. G. Matthews, G. J. H. Boers, M. den Heijer, L. A. J. Kluijtmans, L. P. van den Heuvel, and R. Rozen (1995).

A candidate genetic risk factor for vascular disease: A common mutation in methylenetetrahydrofolate reductase (letter). *Nat Genet 10*, 111–113.

Gregory, J. F. (1995). The bioavailability of folate. In Bailey, L. B. (ed.): *Folate in Health and Disease.* New York: Marcel Dekker, Inc., pp 195–235.

Herbert, V., and J. Bigaouette (1997). Call for endorsement of a petition to the Food and Drug Administration to always add vitamin B-12 to any folate fortification or supplement. *Am J Clin Nutr 65*, 572–573.

Holmes-Siedle, M., R. H. Lindenbaum, A. Galliard, and M. Borrow (1982). Vitamin supplementation and neural tube defects (letter). *Lancet 1*, 276.

Kirke, P. N., A. M. Molloy, L. E. Daly, H. Burke, D. G. Weir, and J. M. Scott (1993). Maternal plasma folate and vitamin B-12 are independent risk factors for neural tube defects. *Q J Med 86*, 703–708.

Laurence, K. M., N. James, M. H. Miller, G. B. Tennant, and H. Campbell (1981). Double-blind randomized, controlled trial of folate treatment before conception to prevent recurrence of neural-tube defects. *BMJ Clin Res Ed 282*, 1509–1511.

Ma, J., M. J. Stampfer, C. H. Hennekens, P. Frosst, J. Selhub, J. Horsford, M. R. Malinow, W. C. Willett, and R. Rozen (1996). Methylenetetrahydrofolate reductase polymorphism, plasma folate, homocysteine, and risk of myocardial infarction in U.S. physicians. *Circulation 94*, 2410–2416.

MacMahon, B., and S. Yen (1971). Unrecognized epidemic of anencephaly and spina bifida. *Lancet 1*, 31–33.

Mills, J. L., J. M. McPartlin, P. N. Kirke, Y. J. Lee, M. R. Conley, D. G. Weir, and J. M. Scott (1995). Homocysteine metabolism in pregnancies complicated by neural-tube defects. *Lancet 345*, 149–151.

Mills, J. L., G. G. Rhoads, H. T. Hoffman, J. L. Simpson, G. C. Cunningham, and M. R. Lassman (1990). Periconceptional use of multivitamins and the prevalence of neural-tube defects (reply). *N Engl J Med 322*, 1083–1084.

Mills, J. L., G. G. Rhoads, and J. L. Simpson, et al. (1989). The absence of a relation between the periconceptional use of vitamins and neural tube defects. *N Engl J Med 321*, 430–435.

Mills, J. L., J. M. Scott, P. N. Kirke, J. M. McPartlin, M. R. Conley, D. G. Weir, A. M. Molloy, and Y. J. Lee (1996). Homocysteine and neural tube defects. *J Nutr 126*, 756S–760S.

Milunsky, A. (1986). The prenatal diagnosis of neural tube and other congenital defects. In Milunsky, A. (ed.): *Genetic Disorders and the Fetus: Diagnosis, Prevention, and Treatment.* New York: Plenum Press, pp 453–519.

Milunsky, A., H. Jick, S. Jick, C. L. Bruell, D. S. MacLaughlin, K. J. Rothman, and W. C. Willett (1989). Multivitamin/folic acid supplementation in early pregnancy reduces the prevalence of neural tube defects. *JAMA 262*, 2847–2852.

Milunsky, A., H. Jick, S. S. Jick, and W. C. Willett (1990). Periconceptional use of multivitamins and the prevalence of neural-tube defects (letter). *N Engl J Med 322*, 1082–1083.

MRC Vitamin Study Research Group (1991). Prevention of neural tube defects: Results of the Medical Research Council Vitamin Study. *Lancet 338*, 131–37.

Mulinare, J., J. F. Cordero, J. D. Erickson, and R. J. Berry (1988). Periconceptional use of multivitamins and the occurrence of neural tube defects. *JAMA 260*, 3141–3145.

Oakley, G. P., Jr., M. J. Adams, and C. M. Dickinson (1996). More folic acid for everyone, now. *J Nutr 126*, 751S–755S.

Oakley, G. P., Jr., J. D. Erickson, and M. J. Adams Jr. (1995). Urgent need to increase folic acid consumption (editorial). *JAMA 274*, 1717–1718.

Ou, C. Y., R. E. Stevenson, V. K. Brown, C. E. Schwartz, W. P. Allen, M. J. Khoury, R. Rozen, G. P. Oakley Jr., and M. J. Adams Jr. (1996). 5,10-Methylenetetrahydrofolate reductase genetic polymorphism as a risk factor for neural tube defects. *Am J Med Genet 63*, 610–614.

Rayburn, W. F., J. R. Stanley, and E. Garrett (1996). Periconceptional folate intake and neural tube defects. *J Am Coll Nutr 15*, 121–125.

Rhoads, G. G., and J. L. Mills (1984). The role of the case–control study in evaluating health interventions. *Am J Epidemiol 120*, 803–808.

Rothman, K. J. (1986). *Modern Epidemiology.* Boston: Little, Brown and Company.

Scott, J. M., D. G. Weir, A. Molloy, J. McPartlin, L. Daly, and P. Kirke (1994). Folic acid metabolism and mechanisms of neural tube defects. *Ciba Found Symp 181*, 180–189.

Shaw, G. M., D. Schaffer, E. M. Velie, K. Morland, and J. A. Harris (1995). Periconceptual vitamin use, dietary folate and the ocurrence of neural tube defects in California. *Epidemiology 6*, 219–226.

Smithells, R. W., N. C. Nevin, M. J. Seller, S. Sheppard, R. Harris, A. P. Read, D. W. Fielding, S. Walker, C. J. Schorah, and J.

Wild (1983). Further experience of vitamin supplementation for prevention of neural tube defect recurrences. *Lancet 1*, 1027–1031.

Smithells, R. W., S. Sheppard, and C. J. Schorah (1976). Vitamin deficiences and neural tube defects. *Arch Dis Child 51*, 944–950.

Smithells, R. W., S. Sheppard, C. J. Schorah, M. J. Seller, N. C. Nevin, R. Harris, A. P. Read, and D. W. Fielding (1980). Possible prevention of neural-tube defects by periconceptional vitmain supplementation. *Lancet i*, 339–340.

Smithells, R. W., S. Sheppard, C. J. Schorah, M. J. Seller, N. C. Nevin, R. Harris, A. P. Read, and D. W. Fielding (1981). Apparent prevention of neural tube defects by periconceptional vitamin supplementation. *Arch Dis Child 56*, 911–918.

Steegers-Theunissen, R. P., G. H. Boers, F. J. Trijbels, J. D. Finkelstein, H. J. Blom, C. M. Thomas, G. F. Borm, G. A. Wouters, and T. K. Eskes (1994). Maternal hyperhomocysteinemia: A risk factor for neural-tube defects? *Metabolism 43*, 1475–1480.

Tucker, K. L., B. Mahnken, P. W. F. Wilson, P. Jacques, and J. Selhub (1996). Folic acid fortification of the food supply: Potential benefits and risks for the elderly population. *JAMA 276*, 1879–1885.

U.S. Preventive Services Task Force (1996). Screening for neural tube defects—including folic acid/folate prophylaxis. In *Guide to Clinical Preventive Services*, 2nd edition, Section One, Screening, Part G. Congenital Disorders. Washington, DC: U.S. Government Printing Office.

van der Put, N. M., R. P. Steegers-Theunissen, P. Frosst, F. J. Trijbels, T. K. Eskes, L. P. van den Heuvel, E. C. Mariman, M. den Heyer, R. Rosen, and H. J. Blom (1995). Mutated methylenetetrahydrofolate reductase as a risk factor for spina bifida. *Lancet 346*, 1070–1071.

Vergel, R. G., L. R. Sanchez, B. L. Heredero, P. L. Rodriguez, and A. J. Martinez (1990). Primary prevention of neural tube defects with folic acid supplementation: Cuban experience. *Prenat Diagn 10*, 149–152.

Wald, N. J. (1994). Folic acid and neural tube defects: The current evidence and implications for prevention. *Ciba Found Symp 181*, 192–211.

Wald, N. J., and C. Bower (1995). Folic acid and the prevention of neural tube defects. *BMJ 310*, 1019–1020.

Wald, N. J., A. K. Hackshaw, R. Stone, and N. A. Sourial (1996). Blood folic acid and vitamin $B_{1}2$ in relation to neural tube defects. *Br J Obstet Gynaecol 103*, 319–324.

Werler, M. M., S. Shapiro, and A. A. Mitchell (1993). Periconceptional folic acid exposure and risk of occurrent neural tube defects. *JAMA 269*, 1257–1261.

Whitehead, A. S., P. Gallagher, J. L. Mills, P. N. Kirke, H. Burke, A. M. Molloy, D. G. Weir, D. C. Shields, and J. M. Scott (1995). A genetic defect in 5,10 methylenetetrahydrofolate reductase in neural tube defects. *Q J Med 88*, 763–766.

Willett, W. C. (1992). Folic acid and neural tube defect: Can't we come to closure? *Am J Public Health 82*, 666–668.

19

Future Research Directions

Probably the most important accomplishment in nutritional epidemiology during the 1980s and early 1990s was the development and validation of methods for measuring dietary intake that are sufficiently inexpensive to be used in large populations and yet accurate enough to provide informative answers to numerous existing hypotheses. Of fundamental importance is the fact that relatively simple structured questionnaires can discriminate among persons in a general population with respect to intake of a wide variety of nutrients; this means that their diets are not so homogeneous as to preclude meaningful study. These developmental studies set the stage for a new generation of prospective investigations that are now producing a rapidly growing body of data that avoids some of the potential biases of case–control studies. These large studies were typically initiated to investigate cancer or cardiovascular disease incidence, but, with extended follow-up or pooling of results, the outcomes that can be examined have grown

rapidly to include most important human diseases, as well as functional impairment in aging populations.

DEVELOPMENT OF PROSPECTIVE COHORT DIETARY STUDIES

Prospective dietary studies are not a new phenomenon; valuable cohorts, such as thoseof Hirayama (1979) and Shekelle and colleagues (1981), were started as long as 30 years ago. The older studies, however, were limited by their narrow scope of questions (e.g., Hirayama's questionnaire included only five food items), the use of 24-hour recalls to assess dietary intake, study populations that were too small to assess any but the most common conditions, or lack of reassessment of diet during prolonged follow-up periods. A newer generation of prospective dietary studies is based on self-administered food-frequency questionnaires completed by groups sufficiently large to study important specific cancers and cardiovascular diseases (Table 19–1).

These studies now comprise nearly 3 million persons with diverse ethnic backgrounds. Because many of these cohorts were designed to study specific cancers of women, men in these studies are substantially outnumbered by women, in contrast to most of the older studies primarily designed to investigate coronary heart disease in men.

An obvious void is the relative lack of cohorts in nonwestern populations. Several cohorts have recently been started in Japan, which will provide unique insight into associations with aspects of diet impossible to assess in North American or European cohorts. Cohorts in developing countries are completely lacking, although some are being planned in Latin America. In many developing countries, mortality due to infectious diseases has been greatly reduced so that chronic diseases, which are likely to have important dietary etiologies, are already the major causes of death. The incidences of many infectious diseases that remain important problems are also likely to be influenced by dietary factors (Chandra and Kumari, 1994); this area has been relatively neglected by nutritional epidemiologists. Populations in developing countries are likely to have unique and different ranges of dietary factors, as well as possible genetic differences in susceptibility, that justify the establishment of well-designed cohort studies. Differences in dietary exposures may be the result of traditional diets or the modern food industry, which heavily influences the food supply of urban populations. For example, *trans*-fatty acids comprise over 50% of the partially hydrogenated "vegetable ghee" widely used in several Asian countries, which greatly exceeds levels in current western foods (Ascherio et al., 1996). Because education and infrastructure, such as mail services, may be less well developed in poorer countries, the use of interviewers and alternative methods for follow up may be required.

Another relatively neglected area is the effect of maternal diet during pregnancy on infant and maternal outcomes. As this is a nutritionally critical period in life, it is surprising that more has not been done. The critical need for adequate folate (see Chapter 18) and omega-3 fatty acid consumption in pregnancy (Nettleton, 1993) illustrates the importance of this area, but many other aspects of diet and infant outcomes have not been fully examined. Aspects of diet during childhood are hypothesized to have impacts on breast and other cancers, other diseases of later life, and possibly more immediate outcomes, such as asthma. An adolescent cohort comprised of offspring of Nurses' Health Study II participants (which should facilitate follow up) has been enrolled and should provide a resource for both current and future generations of epidemiologists.

As discussed in Chapter 13, the value of the prospective studies can be enhanced by a collaborative pooling of the primary data so that all datasets are analyzed in the same manner. This greatly enhances the precision of estimates of association, extends the range of dietary intakes that can be examined, and increases statistical power to evaluate interactions. In principle, the process can provide an opportunity to account for discrepancies in findings. However, the experience thus far in pooled analyses of fat and alcohol intake in relation to breast cancer (Hunter et al., 1996; Smith-Warner et al., 1997) has been that there was little or no statistical heterogeneity, which is itself reassuring (see Chapter 16). Because even weak or modest associations are potentially important when the disease and exposure are common, the power of pooled analyses is of great value for both establishing or excluding such relationships. For this reason, the process of pooling data to evaluate major issues is likely to become the norm in nutritional epidemiology.

An important future development in nutritional epidemiology will be to assess the impact of time, which has not been possible in most published studies because they have been based on a single measure of diet

Table 19–1. Large prospective studies of diet and disease using comprehensive food-frequency questionnaires

Study	Population	Started	Biologic specimens
Israeli IHD Study (Goldbourt et al., 1993)	10,000 M Israel	1963	No
Norwegian Cohort (Bjelke, 1974)	17,000 M+F Norway	1967	No
Adventist Health Study (Fraser et al., 1991)	40,000 M+F U.S.	1976	No
Nurses' Health Study (Willett et al., 1992)	90,000 F U.S.	1980	33,000 blood 68,000 nail
Canadian Breast Screening Study (Howe et al., 1991)	57,000 F Canada	1982	No
New York University Women's Health Study (Toniolo et al., 1994)	14,000 F U.S.	1985	14,000 blood, repeated samples
ATBC (The Alpha-Tocopherol Beta-Carotene Cancer Prevention Study Group, 1994a,b)[a]	29,000 M Finland	1985	29,000 blood
Northern Sweden Health and Diseases Study (G. Hallmans, personal communication)	55,000 M+F	1985	50,000 blood
Health Professionals Follow-up Study (Rimm et al., 1993)	52,000 M U.S.	1986	18,000 blood
Iowa Women's Health Study (Kushi et al., 1992)	42,000 F U.S.	1986	No
Netherlands Cohort Study (Van den Brandt et al., 1993)	121,000 M+F Holland	1986	No
Sweden Mammography Cohort (A. Wolk and H.-O. Adami, personal communication)	61,000 F Sweden	1987	No
ARIC (ARIC Investigators, 1989)	16,000 M+F U.S.	1987	16,000 blood
ORDET (Berrino et al., 1996)	11,000 F Italy	1987	11,000 blood, urine, and nails
Honolulu Heart Program (Kagan, 1996)	8,000 M U.S. (Japanese)	1988	Blood
Cardiovascular Health Study (Fried, L. P. et al., 1991)	5,880 M+F, 65+ yrs	1989	5,800 blood
Washington County, Maryland, U.S. (G. W. Comstock, personal communication)	30,000 M+F	1989	30,000 blood 20,000 nails
JPHC (S. Tsugane, personal communication)	140,000 M+F Japan	1990	49,000 blood

and relatively short follow-up period. Because many chronic diseases may develop over decades, studies with limited duration could potentially miss an important association. As discussed in Chapter 13, an optimal assessment of temporal relations will require both long follow-up period and repeated measures of diet. Thus far, only the Nurses' Health Study and the Health Professionals Follow-up Study include repeated dietary assessments, but this is being planned for other cohorts. The availability

Table 19-1. (continued)

Study	Population	Started	Biologic specimens
Melbourne Collaborative Cohort Study (Giles, 1990)	42,000 M+F Australian-born Italian and Greek migrants	1990	42,000 blood
Nurses' Health Study II (Rich-Edwards et al., 1994)	95,000 F U.S. young nurses	1991	~30,000 blood + urine[b]
American Cancer Society (M. Thun, personal communication)	184,000 M+F U.S.	1992	No
Canadian Study of Diet, Lifestyle, and Health (T. Rohan, personal communication)	100,000 M+F[b] Canada	1992	Hair + toenail for 97%
Women's Health Study (Buring and The Women's Health Study Research Group, 1992)[a]	40,000 F U.S.	1992	27,000 blood
EPIC (Riboli and Kaaks, 1997)	440,000 M+F 9 European countries	1993	350,000 blood
NCI (A. Schatzkin, personal communication)	540,000 M+F U.S.	1995	No
Multi-Ethnic Cohort (L. Kolonel, personal communication)	215,000 M+F U.S. (multiethnic)	1993	Blood and urine on subsets
Singapore Cohort Study (M.C. Yu, personal communication)	48,000 M+F Singapore (Chinese)[b]	1993	Blood and urine on subsets
Women's Health Initiative (Rossouw et al., 1994)[a]	165,000 F[b] U.S.	1993	164,500 blood, ~10,000 urine
Women's Antioxidant Cardiovascular Study (Manson et al., 1995)[a]	8,000 F	1994	5,800 blood
California Teachers' Study (W. Wright, personal communication)	132,000 F	1995	No
Black Women's Health Study (L. Rosenberg, personal communication)	65,000 F U.S. (black)	1995	No
Growing up in the '90s (G. Colditz, personal communication)	15,000 U.S. M+F adolescents	1996	No
Shanghai Women's Health Study (W. Zheng, personal communication)	75,000 F China	1996	20,000 blood and urine

[a] Dietary data collected within a randomized trial.

[b] Planned number, still enrolling.

of the repeated measures will also allow an assessment of change in diet, which is important in assessing the potential impact of interventions. The most effective analysis of repeated measures of diet will require further study.

VALIDATION STUDIES

Validation studies, in which a dietary questionnaire is compared with a detailed assessment method such as diet recording or with biochemical markers, have been conducted within most of the existing large prospective cohort investigations. These substudies, also called standardization or calibration studies, should be a component of any new major dietary study. In future reports from prospective studies, the validation substudy can provide a better estimate of the actual distributions of nutrient intakes within the study population. If only the data from a questionnaire are used, the true variation among subjects cannot be separated from variation due to measurement error.

If no diet–disease association is seen in a particular study, the validation study permits distinction between the possibilities that this is due to lack of variation in the dietary factor, that the questionnaire is insufficiently accurate, or that no association really exists within defined constraints of time and variation in diet. Although epidemiologic studies have only recently presented relative risks and confidence intervals corrected for measurement error, use of data from validation studies and relatively simple statistical methods for correcting measures of association should encourage the routine presentation of corrected results. Validation studies also allow the findings from multiple investigations to be combined in a manner that reflects the accuracy of the dietary data from each of the individual studies.

Many aspects of dietary questionnaire validity deserve further investigation. The performance of these questionnaires in other populations is of interest, particularly among less educated groups, children of various ages, and the populations of developing countries. An extension of validation studies to additional nutrients and nonnutritive aspects of diet, such as food additives and the chemical products of cooking and processing food, will also be useful. The use of biochemical markers as standards in validation studies is likely to be particularly helpful when the assumptions involved in calculating intakes are open to question (see Chapter 2). For example, a database has been created for calculation

of heterocyclic aromatic amines, which are potential human carcinogens, from information on the cooking of various meats (Sinha and Rothman, 1997; Sinha et al., 1997). Whether calculated intakes can provide a reasonable valid estimate of intake will remain uncertain until they can be compared with a biologic indicator of intake or response.

CASE–CONTROL STUDIES IN NUTRITIONAL EPIDEMIOLOGY

The future role of case–control studies in epidemiologic studies of diet and clinical disease is declining as results from large prospective studies become available. Many, or even most, of the case–control studies may have provided valid, unbiased estimates of dietary relationships, but the potential for biases in the selection of controls and in the recall of past diet makes it difficult to be confident in the results of any one study or even in the pooled results of many studies. As described later, case–control studies may play a larger role in the evaluation of preclinical endpoints.

Because uncommon diseases cannot be studied adequately even in the larger cohorts, case–control studies may provide the only opportunity to investigate some dietary relationships. Also, case–control studies may be appropriate when the primary exposure is a nondietary factor less subject to bias in measurement, such as a genotype or environmental electrical fields, and diet is a potential modifying or confounding factor. In conducting such a case–control study, special care must be taken to ensure high participation rates of cases and controls, as dietary relationships do appear to be sensitive to weakness in study design and conduct. Design features may include restrictions to populations or individuals who can be predicted a priori to have high participation rates, such as by avoiding large urban areas. In some instances the overall relationship of the dietary factors of interest to disease may already be known, which can provide a basis for judging, in retrospect, the validity of the dietary data. For rare diseases, a weak association with a dietary variable has little practical implication so that it may be appropriate to give credibility to only strong and robust associations, which are less likely to be the result of methodologic bias.

Expansion of Food Composition Databases

The range of dietary factors that can be examined by nutritional epidemiologic methods is constrained by food composition data. To be useful for calculating intakes, known or estimated values must be available for almost all foods on a questionnaire. Until recently, data have been available only for essential nutrients. However, because of the growing appreciation that many other biologically active constituents of plants may influence the occurrence of numerous diseases, efforts have begun to create databases for a wider range of natural chemicals in the food supply. For example, the creation of databases for carotenoids other than beta-carotene (Chug-Ahuja et al., 1993; Mangels et al., 1993) has allowed additional analyses of diet in relation to lung cancer (see Chapter 15); had these data been available earlier there might have been less enthusiasm for investing so heavily in intervention trials using beta-carotene. In addition to natural constituents in fruits and vegetables, databases are needed for chemicals created by food processors (such as *trans*-fatty acids and olestra), chemicals produced in food preparation (such as heterocyclic amines [Sinha and Rothman, 1997; Sinha et al., 1997] contaminants (such as mercury [MacIntosh et al., 1997]), and additives. Also, variables that reflect the physical characteristics and physiologic responses to foods (such as glycemic index [Wolever et al., 1991]) or the bioavailability of a constituent can be important to incorporate into databases. For many of these dietary constituents, numerous analyses have been conducted and published, but they are typically not useful for epidemiologists be-

cause one or more commonly consumed food sources were not included. For this reason, close collaboration between epidemiologists and analytic chemists will be required to maximize the value of food composition databases.

BIOCHEMICAL INDICATORS IN STUDIES OF DIET AND DISEASE

Studies of diet and disease could be substantially enhanced by new and better biochemical indicators of intake. The use and interpretation of many existing indicators can be improved by a better characterization of their relationship with dietary intake and their variation between persons and within persons over different periods of time. The search for new biochemical indicators of diet should concentrate on those that are likely to provide time-integrated measures, such as protein adducts and levels in fat stores or nails. Despite general enthusiasm for the use of biochemical indicators to assess the effects of diet, they are not likely to replace dietary questionnaires because practical indicators are not in sight for many nutrients of greatest interest, and dietary data can usually be collected for large populations at far less cost using self-administered questionnaires. For the latter reason, biochemical indicators may play a greater role in calibrating and improving questionnaires than in direct application in case–control or cohort studies.

ROLE OF NUTRITIONAL EPIDEMIOLOGY IN TRIALS

As dietary hypotheses become better defined and supported, an increasing number are likely to be evaluated by intervention trials. Nutritional epidemiology continues to play an important role in these trials. One important role will be to screen or identify persons for eligibility. As discussed in Chapter 1, the ability of a study to detect an effect of diet will be greatest among those who have not yet partially adopted the intervention, that is, those with high intake in a trial to reduce a dietary factor or those with low intake in a trial to increase a dietary factor. Therefore, simple assessment methods to identify those with diets most susceptible to intervention should be incorporated in such future trials.

Monitoring dietary compliance, at both the individual and treatment group levels, presents great challenges as persons who are being taught to modify their diet tend to report better compliance than is true (Forster et al., 1990). If dietary records are used, adherence to the diet may be better while keeping records than at other times (Buzzard et al., 1996). Because the possibility for biased information is especially great in this situation, objective markers of diet, such as biochemical measurements, will be especially important.

Although accurate measurements of individual compliance are useful for counseling and feedback, an accurate assessment of group compliance is most critical in an intervention trial. Thus, objective indicators that are responsive to change in the intervention variable can be valuable even if they are somewhat nonspecific. For example, by comparing the magnitude of decrease in plasma high-density lipoprotein cholesterol (HDL-C) due to a reduction in dietary fat with the change expected on the basis of controlled metabolic feeding studies, it was possible to substantiate the reported compliance in a fat reduction trial (Willett, 1998). Of course, when using nonspecific indicators such as HDL-C, it will be important to measure changes in other determinants and correct for them if they are important. Changes in variables such as plasma beta-carotene level can be used to assess changes in beta-carotene specifically or more general interventions, such as increases in fruit and vegetable consumption. In the latter case, several measures reflective of fruit and vegetable intake, such as vitamin C and folic acid, would also be useful. Even measures that classify individual intakes poorly, such as

random urine collections, can be valuable in estimating group compliance. If these are short-term indicators, it is essential that they be done on a "surprise" basis, because participants may increase compliance before clinic visits so that even objective measures would overstate compliance. It is indeed possible that the subjects in the alcohol reduction trial noted above did accurately report their alcohol intake during the week before clinic visits but that the HDL-C levels, which reflect alcohol consumption integrated over several weeks, reflected usual consumption. Because objective indicators of adherence are critically important in randomized dietary trials, further creativity in the development and application of such indicators is needed.

USE OF INTERMEDIATE AND PRECLINICAL ENDPOINTS

Future studies of dietary effects are likely to use premorbid endpoints with increasing frequency. Because individuals are frequently not aware of these conditions, problems of recall bias or changes in diet due to disease that can plague traditional case–control studies can often be avoided. Also, because these endpoints are often continuous variables or relatively common, such studies may be less costly. In the area of cardiovascular disease, epidemiologists have frequently studied determinants of risk factors for coronary heart disease, such as blood pressure or blood lipid levels. More recently, noninvasive methods are providing measurements of atherosclerosis at different sites in the body. Other examples of these endpoints could include dysplastic lesions, in situ neoplasms, or premalignant growths such as colon polyps. Although cancer epidemiologists have been hampered by lack of established intermediary markers of risk or accessible precursor lesions for many cancers, some of the large cohort studies will soon be providing data on hormonal and other biochemical determinants of cancer risk, which can then provide informative dependent variables for dietary studies.

The application of biochemical indicators of diet that are expensive or unstable during storage may be particularly well suited to case–control studies with preclinical endpoints as opposed to large cohort studies with clinical disease as an endpoint. In addition, intervention trials are making increased use of these endpoints because the number of subjects and follow-up time required are usually far less than for trials to prevent clinical outcomes. Nevertheless, studies of preclinical endpoints cannot completely substitute for investigations with the event of ultimate interest as the outcome because the effect on clinical disease may not always be predicted by the effect on a benign or premorbid lesion. For example, oral contraceptives have been shown to reduce the occurrence of benign breast lesions in many studies, but do not appear to reduce the risk of breast cancer. For some diseases, concordant findings from a combination of observational data with clinical disease as the outcome, as might be obtained from cohort studies, and intervention studies with premalignant lesions as an endpoint would be extremely compelling evidence of a causal relationship.

An examination of an association between a dietary factor and both a clinical disease and its precursor lesion can provide insight into the temporal relationship between dietary exposure and disease. For example, cigarette smoking has consistently been associated with colon adenomas, but little relation has been seen in most studies of colon cancer. As this suggested a possible effect of smoking on early events in colon carcinogenesis, Giovannucci and colleagues (1994a,b) examined various latency periods between smoking and colon cancer diagnoses. They observed a strong association with smoking 40 or more years in the past, but not with recent smoking. Because changes in diet are less well de-

marcated in time, this suggests that a follow-up period of at least several decades might be required to detect an association between diet and colon cancer if an association has been seen between diet and its precursor lesion. On the other hand, if no association is seen between a dietary factor and both clinical disease and its precursor lesion, this provides assurance that an important relationship has not been missed because of insufficient follow-up time. For these reasons, the evaluation of diet in relation to both clinical disease and its precursors within the same population can be extremely valuable.

Rapid advances in molecular and cell biology are providing new possibilities for future studies of dietary effects. A variety of measurements, such as excision products of DNA measured in the urine (Cathcart et al., 1984), sister chromatid exchange, and micronuclei counts, provide indicators of damage to DNA (Rosin et al., 1987; Hulka et al., 1990). These may be used as outcomes to evaluate the effect of dietary factors that are presumed either to reduce or to increase damage to macromolecules. Recognition that the sequence leading from normal tissue to invasion, clinical cancer, and metastasis is characterized by an accumulation of mutations in specific genes (Vogelstein et al., 1988) creates new opportunities for etiologic studies of diet. Although certain genes, for example p53, are commonly mutated in many cancers, cancers of the same site are almost always heterogenous in the specific genes that are mutated. For example, p53 mutations occur in only about 30% to 45% of breast cancers. Thus, subtypes of cancers may be classified according to which genes are mutated, and these subtypes could have specific relations with dietary factors. Furthermore, the mutated genes can often be further classified by the specific DNA mutations within the gene, which again may be related to specific etiologic factors, a relation that has been termed *fingerprinting*. For example, aflatoxin causes a specific mutation in codon

249 of the p53 gene (Vogelstein and Kinzler, 1992), and this relationship appears to be so specific that a liver cancer with this mutation can be presumed to be caused by aflatoxins. Also, ultraviolet light appears to cause CC to TT transitions in the p53 gene in actinic keratosis and squamous cell skin cancer (Brash et al., 1991).

Because most dietary factors are thought not to be directly genotoxic, but instead to influence risk indirectly such as by effects on hormonal or growth factors, it is unlikely that most dietary exposures will correspond to specific mutations on a one-to-one basis. However, even if a dietary factor is but one of several factors that increase risk of a specific mutation, linking a cancer subtype to the dietary factor could greatly increase the magnitude of a relative risk, and thus statistical power, because the association would otherwise be diluted by other subtypes unrelated to that exposure. Of course, a search for associations with subgroups of a disease creates the opportunity for multiple comparisons and a higher likelihood for associations to arise by chance. Thus, particularly when no significant overall association is seen and an association exists only with a subtype, repeated confirmation of this result is essential. Studies of dietary factors in relation to specific mutations will clearly be common in the coming years; the contribution that these will make to our knowledge of diet and disease is uncertain.

INTERACTION WITH INHERITED GENETIC FACTORS

Interactions between genetic and environmental factors, such as diet, have long been suspected to be important in the occurrence of many diseases. Until recently, a major limitation has been that genetic predisposition has not been directly measurable; usually only family history of disease has been available. However, rapid progress has been made in the last several years in the identification of inherited variants of genes, usually referred to as *polymor-*

phisms if they are common or *mutations* if their prevalence is less than 1% (Simopoulos and Nestel, 1997). Some of these polymorphisms result in functional differences that account, in full or in part, for familial increases in risk of disease. In some cases the genetic change may completely disrupt gene function so that the homozygous individual develops serious disease with a high probability; this is considered a highly penetrant polymorphism or mutation. Complete lack of function of the methylenetetrahydrofolate reductase gene, for example, results in the severe disease known as *homocysteinuria* (see Chapter 17). Other variants only modestly affect function and thus do not predictably result in disease, but still increase the risk of disease in some circumstances; these have been considered to be low penetrance polymorphisms. For example, a different polymorphism in methylenetetrahyrofolate reductase appears to increase by severalfold the occurrence of neural tube defects, even though the large majority of women with the genotype deliver normal infants (see Chapter 18). The identification of DNA polymorphisms can be done on small aliquots of white blood cells or whole blood and usually at relatively low cost using polymerase chain reaction and restriction fragment polymorphism methods (Austin et al., 1996). In some instances the DNA needs to be sequenced, which is more expensive, but technical advances will make this much more efficient in the near future.

The ability to identify persons at increased genetic risk for disease on the basis of DNA analyses can potentially add greatly to the statistical power of studies of diet and disease, particularly when evaluating diseases with multiple etiologies. If an effect of diet is limited to a subset of genetically susceptible persons, and other cases of disease occur that are unrelated to this dietary factor, the relative risk should be substantially higher in this subset than in the population as a whole. For example, if high intake of saturated fat increases risk of coronary heart disease (CHD) only in a subset of persons, the association between saturated fat and CHD will be much stronger and easier to detect in an analysis restricted to this subset than in the total population. This occurs because the association in the total population is diluted by the addition of other cases of CHD that are all unrelated to saturated fat intake. From a practical standpoint, being able to identify persons for whom dietary changes are particularly effective, or of no value, may be useful. The evaluation of interactions between diet and susceptibility factors is more complex than just testing for statistical heterogeneity because the effect of diet in a high-risk subgroup can be of great importance even when there is no formal statistical interaction.

In addition to providing greater statistical power and identifying persons who could most benefit by dietary change, the establishment of associations between specific polymorphisms and disease can sometimes provide powerful evidence for causality of diet and disease associations. As discussed in Chapter 18, repeatedly confirmed associations between higher folic acid intake and reduced risk of neural tube defects and between a functionally important polymorphism in an enzyme specifically involved in folic acid and risk of neural tube defects would constitute strong and perhaps sufficient evidence of a causal relationship between folic acid intake and neural tube defects. Because we are in essence randomized to various genotypes at conception, such a combination of evidence on nutrient and genotype association with disease might, in some cases, replace the need for randomized trials, in particular when the genotype is unknown to individuals. Even when the genetic polymorphism is not specifically related to the metabolism of the dietary factor in question, clear evidence of effect modification, or interaction, between a dietary factor and a genotype can provide important support for a causal relation between the dietary factor and disease. As another example, Roberts-Thomson et al. (1996) found an association between consumption of red meat and colon cancer only among persons with one of several polymorphisms of a gene potentially involved in the metabolism of heterocyclic amines produced by cooking meat. Because the existence of such an interaction would require that there be a biologic effect of cooked red meat, such evidence could add importantly to support for a causal relationship between cooked red meat and colon cancer and suggests that the carcinogens produced by cooking may be at least in part responsible. However, interactions may well occur by chance so that such an observation requires confirmation in carefully conducted and analyzed studies. Because randomized trials of dietary change are particularly difficult to conduct, particularly for diseases that develop over decades, the use of genetic polymorphisms as etiologic probes should be considered whenever possible.

Interactions between dietary factors and genotype will be widely studied during the coming years because the technology to do so is readily available and the potential for new and more solid knowledge is great. However, large well-designed studies will be needed to avoid the chaos in other areas of gene–disease relationships resulting from a plethora of small and haphazardly conducted case–control studies that have predictably been highly inconsistent. What will emerge from this exciting new dimension to nutritional epidemiology is impossible to know.

SUMMARY

The new generation of large prospective studies will provide an enormous increment of new data during the next decade on diet in relation to cancer, coronary heart disease, and other outcomes. These data are far less subject to the methodologic biases that can affect case–control studies and should provide a far more coherent and consistent picture of these relationships than is available today. Validation studies embedded in most of these new studies will allow quantitative estimates of associations unattenuated by measurement error.

As overall diet and disease relationships become well established, these studies should also provide relatively precise estimates of dose–response and temporal relationships and of interactions with other dietary and nondietary factors. The pooling of primary data from such studies will extend the range of dietary variables that can be examined and provide further precision in estimating associations. The use of premorbid endpoints and newer markers of tissue damage can enhance the plausibility of findings from studies with clinical disease as an endpoint and improve our understanding of the pathophysiology involved. The identification of individuals at high genetic risk of disease using DNA analysis has created new opportunities to study interactions between genetic factors and diet that can add greatly to the etiologic understanding of disease and its prevention.

REFERENCES

ARIC investigators, (1989). The Atherosclerosis Risk in Communities (ARIC) Study: Design and objectives. *Am J Epidemiol 129*, 687–702.

Ascherio, A., E. Cho, K. Walsh, F. M. Sacks, W. C. Willett, and A. Faruqui (1996). Premature coronary deaths in Asians (letter). *BMJ 312*, 508.

Austin, M. A., J. M. Ordovas, J. H. Eckfeldt, R. Tracy, E. Boerwinkle, M.-M. Lalouel, and M. Printz (1996). Guidelines of the National Heart, Lung, and Blood Institute Working Group on Blood Drawing, Processing, and Storage for genetic studies. *Am J Epidemiol 144*, 437–441.

Berrino, F., P. Muti, A. Micheli, G. Bolelli, V. Krogh, R. Sciajno, P. Pisani, S. Panico, and G. Secreto (1996). Serum sex hormone levels after menopause and subsequent breast cancer. *JNCI 88*, 291–296.

Bjelke, E. (1974). Epidemiologic studies of cancer of the stomach, colon and rectum; with special emphasis on the role of diet. *Scand J Gastroenterol (Suppl) 31*, 1–235.

Brash, D. E., J. A. Rudolph, J. A. Simon, A. Lin, G. J. McKenna, H. P. Baden, A. J. Halperin, and J. Ponten (1991). A role for sunlight in skin cancer: UV-induced p53 mutations in squamous cell carcinoma. *Proc Natl Acad Sci USA 88*, 10124–10128.

Buring, J. E., and The Women's Health Study Research Group (1992). The Women's Health Study: Summary of the study design. *J Myocardiol Ischemia 4*, 27–29.

Buzzard, I. M., C. L. Faucett, R. W. Jeffery, L. McBane, P. McGovern, J. S. Baxter, A. C. Shapiro, G. L. Blackburn, R. T. Chlebowski, R. M. Elashoff, and E. L. Wynder (1996). Monitoring dietary change in a low-fat diet intervention study: Advantages of using 24-hour dietary recalls vs food records. *J Am Diet Assoc 96*, 574–579.

Cathcart, R., E. Schwiers, R. L. Saul, and B. N. Ames (1984). Thymine glycol and thymidine glycol in human and rat urine; a possible assay for oxidative DNA damage. *Proc Natl Acad Sci USA 81*, 5633–5637.

Chandra, R. K., and S. Kumari (1994). Nutrition and immunity: An overview. *J Nutr 124(suppl)*, 1433S–1435S.

Chug-Ahuja, J. K., J. M. Holden, M. R. Forman, A. R. Mangels, G. R. Beecher, and E. Lanza (1993). The development and application of a carotenoid database for fruits, vegetables, and selected multicomponent foods. *J Am Diet Assoc 93*, 318–323.

Forster, J. L., R. W. Jeffery, M. VanNatta, and P. Pirie (1990). Hypertension prevention trial: Do 24-h food records capture usual eating behavior in a dietary change study? *Am J Clin Nutr 51*, 253–257.

Fraser, G. E., W. L. Beeson, and R. L. Phillips (1991). Diet and lung cancer risk in California Seventh-day Adventists. *Am J Epidemiol 133*, 683–693.

Fried, L. P. N. O. Borhani, P. Enright, C. D. Furberg, J. M. Gardin, R. A. Kronmal, L. H. Kuller, T. A. Manolio, M. B. Mittelmark, A. Newman, D. H. O'Leary, B. Psaty, P. Rautaharju, R. P. Tracy, and P. G. Weiler for the Cardiovascular Health Study Research Group (CHS) (1991). The Cardiovascular Health Study: Design and rationale. *Ann Epidemiology 1*, 263–276.

Giles, G. G. (1990). The Melbourne Study of Diet and Cancer. *Proc Nutr Soc Aust 15*, 61–68.

Giovannucci, E., G. A. Colditz, M. J. Stampfer, D. Hunter, B. A. Rosner, W. C. Willett, and F. E. Speizer (1994a). A prospective study of cigarette smoking and risk of colorectal adenoma and colorectal cancer in U.S. women. *JNCI 86*, 192–199.

Giovannucci, E., E. B. Rimm, M. J. Stampfer, G. A. Colditz, A. Ascherio, J. Kearney, and

W. C. Willett (1994b). A prospective study of cigarette smoking and risk of colorectal adenoma and colorectal cancer in U.S. men. *JNCI 86*, 183–191.

Goldbourt, U., S. Yaari, and J. H. Medalie (1993). Factors predictive of long-term coronary heart disease mortality among 10,059 male Israeli civil servants and municipal employees: A 23-year mortality follow-up in the Israeli ischemic heart disease study. *Cardiology 82*, 100–121.

Hirayama, T. (1979). Diet and cancer. *Nutr Cancer 1*, 67–81.

Howe, G. R., C. M. Friedenreich, M. Jain, and A. B. Miller (1991). A cohort study of fat intake and risk of breast cancer. *JNCI 83*, 336–340.

Hulka, B. S., T. C. Wilcosky, and J. D. Griffith (1990). *Biological Markers in Epidemiology*. New York: Oxford University Press.

Hunter, D. J., D. Spiegelman, H. O. Adami, L. Beeson, P. A. van den Brandt, A. R. Folsom, G. E. Fraser, R. A. Goldbohm, S. Graham, G. R. Howe, L. H. Kushi, J. R. Marshall, A. McDermott, A. B. Miller, F. E. Speizer, A. Wolk, S.-S. Yaun, and W. C. Willett (1996). Cohort studies of fat intake and the risk of breast cancer: A pooled analysis. *N Engl J Med 334*, 356–361.

Kagan, A. (ed.) (1996). *The Honolulu Heart Program: An Epidemiologic Study of Coronary Heart Disease and Stroke*. Amsterdam: Harwood Academic Press.

Kushi, L. H., T. A. Sellers, J. D. Potter, C. L. Nelson, R. G. Munger, S. A. Kaye, and A. R. Folsom (1992). Dietary fat and postmenopausal breast cancer. *JNCI 84*, 1092–1099.

MacIntosh, D. L., P. L. Williams, D. J. Hunter, L. A. Sampson, S. C. Morris, W. C. Willett, and E. B. Rimm (1997). Evaluation of a food frequency questionnaire–food composition approach for estimating dietary intake of inorganic arsenic and methylmercury. *Cancer Epidemiol Biomark Prev 6*, 1043–1050.

Mangels, A. R., J. M. Holden, G. R. Beecher, M. R. Forman, and E. Lanza (1993). Carotenoid content of fruits and vegetables: An evaluation of analytic data. *J Am Diet Assoc 93*, 284–296.

Manson, J. E., J. M. Gaziano, A. Spelsberg, P. M. Ridker, N. R. Cook, J. E. Buring, W. C. Willett, and C. H. Hennekens (1995). A secondary prevention trial of antioxidant vitamins and cardiovascular disease in women: Rationale, design, and methods. The WACS Research Group. *Ann Epidemiol 5*, 261–269.

Nettleton, J. A. (1993). Are n-3 fatty acids essential nutrients for fetal and infant development? *J Am Diet Assoc 93*, 58–64.

Riboli, E., and R. Kaaks (1997). The EPIC project: Rationale and study design. *Int J Epidemiol 26(suppl)*, S6–S14.

Rich-Edwards, J. W., M. B. Goldman, W. C. Willett, D. J. Hunter, M. J. Stampfer, G. A. Colditz, and J. E. Manson (1994). Adolescent body mass index and infertility caused by ovulatory disorder. *Am J Obstet Gynecol 171*, 171–177.

Rimm, E. B., M. J. Stampfer, A. Ascherio, E. Giovannucci, G. A. Colditz, and W. C. Willett (1993). Dietary antioxidant intake and risk of coronary heart disease among men. *N Engl J Med 328*, 1450–1456.

Roberts-Thomson, I. C., P. Ryan, K. K. Khoo, W. J. Hart, A. J. McMichael, and R. N. Butler (1996). Diet, acetylator phenotype, and risk of colorectal neoplasia. *Lancet 347*, 1372–1374.

Rosin, M. P., B. P. Dunn, and H. F. Stich (1987). Use of intermediate endpoints in quantitating the response of precancerous lesions to chemopreventive agents. *Can J Physiol Pharmacol 65*, 483–487.

Rossouw, J. E., L. P. Finnegan, W. R. Harlan, V. W. Pinn, C. Clifford, and J. A. McGowan (1994). The evolution of the Women's Health Initiative: Perspectives from the NIH. *JAMA 50*, 50–55.

Shekelle, R. B., A. M. Shryock, O. Paul, M. Lepper, J. Stamler, S. Liu, and W. J. Raynor, Jr. (1981). Diet, serum cholesterol, and death from coronary heart disease: The Western Electric Study. *N Engl J Med 304*, 65–70.

Simopoulos, A. P., and P. J. Nestel (eds.) (1997). Genetic variation and dietary response. *World Review of Nutrition and Dietetics*. Farmington, CT: S. Karger Publishers, Inc.

Sinha R., N. Rothman (1997). Exposure assessment of heterocyclic amines (hcas) in epidemiologic studies. *Mutation Res 376 (1–2)*, 195–202.

Sinha, R., N. Rothman, C. P. Salmon, M. G. Knize, E. D. Brown, C. A. Swanson, D. Rhodes, S. Rossi, J. S. Felton, and O. A. Levander (1997). Heterocyclic aromatic amine content of beef cooked by different methods and degrees of doneness and beef gravy made from roast. *Food Chem Toxicol* (submitted).

Smith-Warner, S. A., D. Spiegelman, S. S. Yaun, H. O. Adami, P. A. van den Brandt, A. R. Folsom, R. A. Goldbohm, S. Graham, G. R. Howe, J. R. Marshall, A. B. Miller, J. D. Potter, F. E. Speizer, W. C. Willett, A.

Wolk, and D. J. Hunter (1998). Alcohol and breast cancer in women: A pooled analysis of cohort studies. *JAMA 279*, 535–540.

The Alpha-Tocopherol Beta-Carotene Cancer Prevention Study Group (1994a). The Alpha-Tocopherol, Beta-Carotene Lung Cancer Prevention Study: Design, methods, participant characteristics, and compliance. *Ann Epidemiol 4*, 1–10.

The Alpha-Tocopherol Beta-Carotene Cancer Prevention Study Group (1994b). The effect of vitamin E and beta carotene on the incidence of lung cancer and other cancers in male smokers. *N Engl J Med 330*, 1029–1035.

Toniolo, P., E. Riboli, R. E. Shore, and B. S. Pasternack (1994). Consumption of meat, animal products, protein, and fat and risk of breast cancer—A prospective cohort study in New York. *Epidemiology 5*, 391–397.

Van den Brandt, P. A., P. Van't Veer, and R. A. Goldbohm, et al. (1993). A prospective cohort study on dietary fat and the risk of postmenopausal breast cancer. *Cancer Res 53*, 75–82.

Vogelstein, B., E. R. Fearon, S. R. Hamilton, S. E. Kern, A. C. Preisinger, M. Leppert, Y. Nakamura, R. White, A. M. Smits, and J. L. Bos (1988). Genetic alterations during colorectal-tumor development. *N Engl J Med 319*, 525–532.

Vogelstein, B., and K. Kinzler (1992). Carcinogens leave fingerprints. *Nature 355*, 209–210.

Willett, W. C. (1998). Is dietary fat a major determinant of body fat? *Am J Clin Nutr 67*(suppl), 556s–562s.

Willett, W. C., D. J. Hunter, M. J. Stampfer, G. A. Colditz, J. E. Manson, D. Spiegelman, B. Rosner, C. H. Hennekens, and F. E. Speizer (1992). Dietary fat and fiber in relation to risk of breast cancer: An 8-year follow-up. *JAMA 268*, 2037–2044.

Wolever, T. M. S., D. J. Jenkins, A. L. Jenkins, and R. G. Josse (1991). The glycemic index: methodology and clinical implications. *Am J Clin Nutr 54*, 846–854.

Index